Better Health Through Natural Healing

How to get well without drugs or surgery

Second Edition

Dr Ross Trattler N.D., D.O.

with the assistance of

Dr Adrian Jones N.D.

HB

HINKLER BOOKS

First published 1986 by McGraw-Hill

Second edition 2001
Hinkler Books Pty Ltd
17-23 Redwood Drive
Dingley Victoria, 3172 Australia

ISBN: 186515259 5

Printed and bound in Australia

DISCLAIMER
This book is not intended to replace the services of a physician. Any application
of the recommendations set forth in the following pages is at the reader's discretion and sole risk.

CONTENTS

Acknowledgments

I would like to give special thanks to Adrian Jones N.D. for his collaboration on this updated and revised edition, bringing *Better Health Through Natural Healing* into the 21st century. Doctors like Adrian are the best examples of why naturopathy is and will always be an evolving form of healing. Each generation of naturopaths adds to the ancient principles of the past, the foundation of naturopathy, new aspects, new techniques and new knowledge. It was my privilege to have Adrian as a student, later as a colleague and now as a co-author. Long life, Adrian!

I also want to thank my two sons, Kyle and Shea, who are an ever present source of entertainment and joy. What are a million smiles worth to your health? Much better than any elixir!

And finally I want to thank whatever wonderful *blessing* of luck or fate that has brought my wife Nancy into my life. She has taught me more about peace, love and happiness than any other of life's lessons. What a healing force is Love!

Introduction to Second Edition

This book has been written out of true need. As the years passed in my practice, I found that my memory was far from perfect. Treatments I once knew well and had used successfully would sometimes evade me at the very time they were needed most. In a busy practice, with patient following patient, a doctor is called upon to reach the essence of a problem and its cure with little time for pondering. Late in the afternoon and worn out by a hectic day, I often found myself unable to remember quickly a specifically useful prescription or other aspect of therapy, or which book it was in. The task was not easy, since, when this book was first written I used hundreds of reference books regularly. Unfortunately, at that time, there was no naturopathic equivalent to The Merck Manual where one could quickly look up essential details of a particular illness.

It has now been over 20 years since I first put pen to paper for the first volume. Now as I sit at my computer I wonder how such a reference book could have been written without the resources we now have. Information on and about naturopathy and naturopathic treatment is much more available today, especially with the use of computers and the Internet. With this in mind I have included a list of useful web sites to aid you in your search. I'm sure you will find these sites invaluable. I certainly have. Within these sites you can research any health topic you could think of, locate a qualified naturopath practicing near you and research a particular therapy, supplement or herb. Even with these new and accessible resources it often most useful to have one major text to refer to when the need arises. It is for this reason that I have decided to release a completely revised second edition of *Better Health Through Natural Healing*. I have revised and updated the book to include changes both in our approach to the treatment of a particular disorder and to incorporate changes made possible through the immense amount of nutritional research the has been going on over the last 20 years pertaining to natural therapies.

This book has been written with both the lay public and practitioner in mind. It is not always an easy marriage, and some sections do get a bit technical. It isn't a simple task to write a comprehensive text on naturopathic medicine, or even one approach to this field. In reality, naturopathic medicine, or the science and art of natural therapeutics, can never be written down completely. Each naturopath lives and breathes his or her own philosophy and therapies differ widely. Mine is no more correct than others, but it works well for me in my practice. It is my hope and desire to make these methods easier to understand and more accessible.

How to Use this Book

Naturopathic medicine is not a subject that easily lends itself to definition. After all is said and done, naturopathy is a way of life. When practicing as a naturopathic physician, one is forced to translate a philosophical conviction in the healing power of nature, breaking it down into fractions that can easily be understood. Too often the result of this dissection is that the listener begins to feel that naturopathy is diet, or fasting, or spinal manipulation, or botanical medicine—or any of its various parts.

As you read through each chapter, always bear in mind that disease as an entity does not exist. People are at *dis-ease*, each for his or her own unique set of causes. The role of the naturopath, whatever tools he or she may use, is to educate the patient and when necessary help direct and release the inner healing power of nature.

Part I of this book examines the philosophy behind natural therapeutics and presents a brief summary and description of its most frequently used tools. You will also find at the end of this section "Health Topics of Special Interest" Part II is the practical application of the philosophy and these therapeutic tools as they relate to the most common diseases. Most chapters begin with a brief definition and description of signs and symptoms. There then follows a list of factors possibly related to the cause of the disease. Here you will find most of the causes recognized by orthodox medicine, but, more importantly, factors as seen from a naturopathic perspective. In reviewing this list, consider how much each one may be a factor in your particular case. Obviously not all or even most of these contributing factors will be part of the cause in each individual case. They are included to act as mental triggers or signposts to help each person (or practitioner) recognize the obvious and also the sometimes more obscure conditions that set the stage for disease to be created. It is vitally important to recognize our role in disease creation so that we can learn how to undertake the responsibility for its cure. Next follows a general discussion drawing on the previous section, examining etiology, or causative factors, in more depth. Each discussion section should leave the reader with a clear understanding of what may cause the particular disorder.

Finally comes the treatment section, broken down into diet, physiotherapy, therapeutic agents, and botanicals. Here you will find many suggestions of therapy for each disorder. Obviously, not all of these should be employed in each case. Remember that people are unique in their requirements for cure. Therapies useful in an early stage of a health disorder may not apply later on. People vary widely in their response to therapy, and therefore individual dose prescriptions differ.

Disease is not a stagnant process. Dose prescriptions will vary as the condition changes. Also, the cause of a disease will vary from person to person, calling for different approaches to therapy.

I have tried to make the information as practical as possible for home use. Nothing, however, can replace the expertise and knowledge of an experienced and properly trained physician.

Dietary advice has been laid out in stages to represent progression of the disorder towards health; or, in some cases, as specific short-term regimens to be used as indicated. In the acute states of a disease it is generally best to begin with the most restricted regimen, such as a fast or mono diet (a diet containing only one substance). In some cases specific diets, such as the onion diet used for lung congestion, may be the best initial approach. As symptoms improve, one progresses to later stages until a full dietary range has been achieved, which coincides with the arrival of better health.

The choice of physiotherapy is usually very easy. In most conditions, you should do as much as possible. A proper regimen should keep you too busy getting well to stay sick. This, of course, does not apply to those with diseases causing extreme weakness or debilitation, in which case you should choose less vigorous techniques.

Special attention should be given to the sections on vitamins, minerals, and botanical medicines. Many remedial agents are mentioned here, but not all are to be taken with each disease. The choice of therapeutic agents is, by their sheer number, not easy. Individuals vary so widely in their needs during the disease process that only general guidelines are possible. I have given specific dose prescriptions as a general guide. I suggest that you obtain expert advice on your particular needs whenever possible.

Botanical medication is much more difficult to use wisely at home without some in-depth knowledge about individual properties of substances. To use herbs safely, however, I suggest researching each herb for its properties and general use prior to your use. Refer to Appendix III for botanical names appearing in the book.

You will probably notice the conspicuous absence of suggestions regarding homeopathy. I feel that homeopathy can only be prescribed individually, even more so than botanicals, to derive any therapeutic results. For serious or chronic ailments, it is always best to consult a trained physician.

Should you live in an area where professional help is simply not available, and by your own choice you decide to follow the suggestions made in this book, please use common sense. Do not allow the disease process to reach a critical stage without some medical supervision. Refer to Appendix II, Useful Web Sites to help in your search for a qualified naturopath in your area.

Most diseases are curable, but not all patients. The benefit you obtain from natural therapy will depend upon the amount of effort you expend. The process of cure does not end when your symptoms disappear, but continues each day as you live more and more according to the laws of nature. Let this book function as a trained guide, giving useful suggestions to help you along the path to self-cure. The rest is up to you.

REGARDING CORRESPONDENCE

When *Better Health Through Natural Healing* was first published I received frequent phone calls from around the world seeking personal health advice over the phone. As I hope you can appreciate, due to the complexity of most health problems it simply is not possible to give any meaningful advice in this manner.

Usually with a little research you will be able to find a competent naturopath or medical doctor with naturopathic leanings in your area. Try asking at your local health food store for recommendations. If you have other reason to contact either Dr Jones or myself you may send an e-mail to: RossTrattler@aol.com or ToHealth@fan.net.au to contact Adrian and we will respond to your enquiry. If you need to speak with me personally please call me on my home phone (+61 7) 5530-5962 between the hours of 7 p.m. to 9 p.m. weekdays or any time during the day on the weekends. Please remember the local time difference is 10 hours earlier the following day from New York time. Should you simply wish to make enormous philanthropic donations or invite us to gala events in exotic locations (all expenses paid) feel free to call me anytime.

Wishing you the best of health.
Ross Trattler N.D., D.O.

A Final Note

Advances in our understanding of clinical nutrition over the past 50 years have drastically altered the public conception of natural therapies and how these are applied by most naturopaths or naturopathic minded physicians. What originally was a science and philosophy of natural living and natural health maintenance and repair based on restoring proper equilibrium through diet, fasting, exercise, air and sun bathing, breathing and cultivation of inner peace, has now become based, sometimes almost solely, on the prescription of various vitamins, minerals and herbs. You will find in this book many such recommendations. Please bear in mind that even if every supplier of these specific supplements was to close their doors tomorrow, most health complaints could still be corrected and health restored through the time-honored techniques of what was once called "nature cure".

I truly hope I have not added to the impression that specific supplementation is essential to healing. While it is true that vitamins, minerals and herbs are extremely valuable aids to healing at specific stages of the disease or healing process, they are not irreplaceable

Certainly the application of pure nature cure has become more difficult in our modern world. Soil depletion and pesticides have rendered our fruit and vegetable supplies nutritionally deficient and even toxic to the human body, necessitating organically grown sources for health recovery. Water pollutants necessitate bottled sources or proper filtration. Air pollution may even require relocation in some chronic disorders like severe asthma. These are difficult changes, but they can be done if you are willing. For those unwilling or unable to make these basic changes, supplementation of specific condensed nutrients and herbs provides a useful and effective alternative.

Over the years of my practice I have headed away from excessive supplementation back to the roots of naturopathy. I encourage you to seek this path also as the best and final cure to your health problems.

PART I

What is Natural Medicine?

NATUROPATHIC MEDICINE

Natural therapies have been used to treat disease since our earliest beginnings. The first known written records mention herbs and their use in healing. Every known culture has attempted to harness the healing powers in plants. Both the Old and New Testaments speak of herbs and their uses. Hydrotherapy, or the use of water in healing disease, is also very ancient. Early written records describe various uses for water therapy well before either the Roman or Christian eras. These natural therapies were on a few occasions written down, but for the most part they were passed down as oral traditions, as was the case with the native Americans.

When naturopathy originated as a science distinct from these loosely gathered bits of natural therapy, no one can say. Hippocrates is considered the father of naturopathic medicine. The Hippocratic school treated disease with diet, fasting, herbs, hydrotherapy, exercise, and spinal manipulation, prescribed from a basis of principles of healing that are now used as the foundation of naturopathy. Their most basic tenet, *vis medicatrix naturae* (only nature heals), which emphasizes the body's ability to heal itself if given a chance, is still the central theme of naturopathic philosophy.

From these origins naturopathic medicine has grown and developed. Physicians throughout the world have worked within the context of natural therapies, often specializing in one particular aspect such as fasting, hydrotherapy, herbalism, or spinal manipulation, and so developing and perfecting each natural therapeutic tool.

A great surge of development in natural therapies occurred during the 19th century, when the orthodox medical profession drifted further and further towards the widespread use of drugs and surgery. It was not until the water cure was popularized by the work of Vincent Priessnitz, Sebastian Kneipp, and J. H. Kellogg that naturopathy once again emerged as a distinct discipline. Many schools of hydrotherapy, herbalism, and naturopathy sprang up and flourished in Europe and America. Great pioneers of naturopathy emerged at this time to help convince the skeptical public that nature, not drugs, was the path towards health. Many of these men attempted to prove their convictions by daredevil stunts, flaunting their health for all to witness. I remember reading with awe of early naturopaths swallowing vials of cholera-infected material, or fasting 40 or even 60 days, and then performing incredibly strenuous physical demonstrations to prove their unusual vigor obtained by natural means.

Many of these pioneers left written legacies of great value. Each book tells the story of powerful people of strength, conviction, and courage. Taking whatever assistance they could find from the past, they entered the labyrinth of disease only to discover not confusion, but simplicity. In an age when their colleagues of the orthodox school were finding more and more complexity in disease with the advent of the germ theory, these naturopathic physicians were discovering the very principles of health and disease.

Slowly but steadily orthodox medicine gained political power and united against the freely practicing naturopathic profession. Within a short time, most alternative medical schools were forced to close. Not only were naturopaths declared illegal and prosecuted, but so were midwives and many other health professionals who were seen as either a financial or philosophical threat.

The 1970s and 1980s were years of re-emergence for naturopathic physicians. With the 1960s came a rebirth of awareness and interest in all things "natural". A new generation arose that no longer accepted the status quo blindly. All aspects of modern society were scrutinized; among these the practice of modern medicine. Thalidomide in Europe, DES-induced cancer, and other recent drug-related tragedies have led the general public more and more to ask, not how effective a drug is, but how safe. With each new horror story of tragedies induced by drugs thought to be harmless for years, more people are seeking a safe alternative.

Now, as in the past, naturopathic physicians are offering that alternative. The naturopathic physicians' training today encompasses both traditional and modern techniques of diagnosis and therapy. They are trained in four-year accredited private naturopathic medical schools. The program includes all the basic science, diagnostic, and medical courses standard to any other medical training institution. In addition, the naturopath is trained in a wide variety of natural therapies to be used to help the body in its self-repairing efforts. The aim of naturopathy is to treat people, not disease; to remove the cause of disease, not merely its symptoms; and to cure disease, not just postpone it.

THE PHILOSOPHY OF NATUROPATHIC MEDICINE

The natural therapeutic approach maintains that the constant effort of the body's life force is always in the direction of self-cleansing, self-repairing and positive health. The philosophy maintains that even acute disease is a manifestation of the body's efforts in the direction of self cure. Disease, or downgraded health, may be eliminated only by removing from the system the real cause and by raising the body's general vitality so that its natural and inherent ability to sustain health is allowed to dominate. Natural therapeutic philosophy also maintains that chronic diseases are frequently the result of mistaken efforts to cure or attempted suppression of the physiological efforts of the body to cleanse itself.[1]

This short quote fully encompasses both the cause and treatment of nearly all disease. It begins by affirming the basic inner vitality that is life itself. The "great law of life" states that "Every living cell in an organized body is endowed with an instinct of self preservation which is sustained by an inherent force named The

4

Vital Force of Life."[2] The "great law of life" needs to be understood on many levels to be of real use. If all disease is a self-repairing effort aimed towards health, then why bother to treat disease at all, even with naturopathic therapy? Does this law not guarantee cure? Why not lie back and wait for our pneumonia, ulcer, heart disease, or diabetes to simply go away? The reason, of course, as common sense tells us, is that it probably won't.

This law means the general flow of life's energies is in the direction of positive health. If, however, this flow is hindered in any way, the final result may be less than perfect. To understand the many factors that may cause disease or hinder this life force, we must first understand what health is. Lindlahr's definition states that "Health is normal and harmonious vibration of the elements and forces composing the human entity on the physical, mental and moral (emotional) planes of being, in conformity with the constructive principle (great law of life) in nature."[3]

Disease is therefore an abnormal or inharmonious vibration of the elements and forces composing the human entity in one or more planes of being.[4] In the "perfectly normal" individual all aspects of life are kept in harmony. If this situation were possible to maintain, the body would live forever. The "ordinary" individual, however, is constantly being subjected to influences that upset his or her inner equilibrium. Normal changes in the physical environment, both internally and externally, are easily compensated for. The body is equipped with sophisticated defense mechanisms which have evolved over eons. It is designed to maintain a healthy internal environment, and can protect itself from any reasonable threat. If nothing catastrophic happens to the body other than ordinary changes, and if the life force is unhindered on all planes, the physical body would live significantly longer than the accepted three score and ten. This has been hinted at in various religious works and can be seen today in certain societies where the lifestyle is relatively harmonious.

Modern humanity, however, can no longer be considered either "normal" or "ordinary". Nearly every aspect of modern living causes disharmony in the physical, mental, and moral planes of our existence. Suddenly, in a minute fraction of our total existence on the evolutionary scale, we are being exposed to vast changes in both our internal and external environment. The physical body, designed for and requiring demanding physical exercise for its optimum functioning, now performs effortless tasks. Our diet, once composed of whole grains, nuts, raw fruits, fresh vegetables, simple proteins, and pure water, is now made up of refined, devitalized grains, highly salted nuts, frozen, canned, or poisoned fruits and vegetables, complex protein meals also poisoned by all manner of drugs and chemicals, and harmful liquids, such as coffee, tea, soda, and alcohol. Even the air is no longer pure.

As if this were not enough for the physical body to handle, many people take drugs and smoke cigarettes, pipes, cigars, and marijuana. We are exposed to toxic chemicals at work and at home. It is no wonder that the body reaches a point when it can no longer safely deal with these poisons.

Mental and emotional stresses have increased rapidly over the recent past. These are often of a nature that must be suppressed, such as in the employer–employee relationship, causing severe disruption of balance in the physical body.

We are equipped with various adaptive mechanisms which clear from the body a normal amount of unneeded, unwanted, or toxic substances. If, however, these safety channels are clogged, overburdened, or suppressed, the vital force can no longer slowly and safely maintain harmony, and disease results. This disease, however, is still the activity of the vital force to create balance. As such it is a positive action made to correct and remove hindrances to its proper function. Lindlahr states, "Every acute disease is the result of a healing effort of nature,"[5] expressing the truth that disease is an *action* made by the body as a result of a cause and effect relationship. To further understand the direction and purpose of the disease process, it is first necessary to better appreciate basic causes of disease.

Accumulation of toxic material within the body due to improper diet, poor circulation, poor eliminations, and lack of demanding exercise is a major factor in almost all disease. While it is acknowledged that other causes do exist, most factors that predispose to disease result in an accumulation of poisonous substances in the body which, when the channels of elimination cannot adequately remove them, will invariably initiate a disease process. These accumulations ultimately lead to changes within the cell and eventually within the whole body.

Incorrect or unbalanced diets lead to reduced vitality, nutritional deficiency, toxemia, poor eliminations, and local tissue degeneration. Modern food processing and refining leads to an unbalanced, low-fiber, unnatural diet which drastically decreases the nutrient value of food. High-yield fertilizer usage upsets the natural balance of the soil, producing nutritionally inferior and deficient food. Pesticides and additives place a further burden on the body to detoxify unwanted and poisonous substances. Improper diet is a major cause of nearly all forms of disease.

Improper posture and body mechanics due to habit, poor muscle tone, accident, or injury may interfere with normal nervous activity or the circulation of blood and lymph, leading to tissue degeneration and defective function. As the normal curves of the spine are altered by weak abdominal muscles, high heels, spinal trauma, or poor body mechanics in sitting or standing, the normal relationship of internal organs and their nervous, blood, and lymph supply (and consequently their nutrition) are severely affected. These changes may lead to poor local nutrition, reduced drainage, and reduced tissue vitality. The end result is congestion, toxic accumulation, and disease.

Destructive emotions such as fear, anxiety, hate, self-pity, and resentment can affect the body by upsetting digestion, blood flow, hormone balance, and the general biochemistry of the entire body. Psychological causes of disease are increasing as society itself places greater pressures on the individual.

The administration of suppressive drugs and vaccines, which inhibits the eliminative efforts of the body and places further demands on it for drug detoxification, is a growing cause of disease. Many drugs, and vaccines in particular, can cause allergic reactions, chronic allergies, and other long-term health problems. The incidence of drug-induced illness is on the increase, especially in older age groups where multiple prescriptions may cause toxic interactions.

Excessive use of alcohol, coffee, and tobacco are serious health threats. These social drugs, although widely accepted and used, are major factors in many disease processes. They can severely damage the liver, lungs, pancreas, thyroid, adrenal glands, and other parts of the body or mind.

Environmental causes of disease are becoming difficult to avoid. The air, water, and soil are all becoming more susceptible to pollution as population increases and we continue to treat the earth without proper respect.

Occupational hazards may also help cause disease. Chemical contact and poor air quality are common factors in downgraded health. Some substances that have been in use for years, such as asbestos, have been found to be toxic, and are a severe health risk. Work-related stress, however, may be the greatest cause of illness among workers.

Certain inherited factors or tendencies, congenital predisposition, or abnormalities may also leave an individual more susceptible to disease or unstable conditions. Often, however, these weaknesses only become manifest when the body comes under stress from one or more of the other causes of disease above.

Parasitic, virus, or germ infection is not a primary cause of disease but rather its result. Even Pasteur, the recognized father of the germ theory, began to understand the true relationship of germs to disease late in his life when he stated "The germ is nothing, the soil is everything," meaning that a germ can only thrive in a suitable environment. The body normally is host to millions of micro-organisms, some beneficial, others pathogenic. If "harmful" bacteria are allowed to multiply, then typical symptoms of disease result.

In a healthy body several factors can help keep harmful bacteria from gaining a strong foothold. The normal healthy bacterial flora in the digestive tract and vagina prevent others from proliferating, the way we would resist an intruder in our home. The body's secretions also act to prevent bacterial infection by their pH (their acidity or alkalinity) and their other qualities. Many mucous membranes are lined with tiny cilia, or hairs, that constantly move debris and bacteria towards the nearest exit. Glandular structures such as the tonsils are designed to screen foreign matter from the air, and internally from the circulation. Other glands perform a similar process throughout the entire lymphatic circulation, which filters the body's internal fluids. Foreign invaders that do manage to break through the body's first defenses are attacked by antibodies, consumed by white blood cells, and either digested or removed from the body.

The body is very well protected. Only when defenses are weakened can harmful bacteria gain a foothold. The factors that bring about reduced vitality are found above in the true causes of disease. When one or more of the causative factors predisposing to disease are present, the body is forced to act vigorously to re-establish proper equilibrium. The result is acute disease.

The body is equipped with various avenues of action to free itself of these burdens.

Fever increases the body's metabolic rate and circulation of blood and lymph, thereby speeding removal of toxins from the body, and nutrition to diseased areas. The increased circulation also acts as a carrier for the body's more complicated defenses such as white blood cells and antibodies. Fever also creates a less favorable environment for either bacteria or viruses, which generally have a very narrow temperature range for optimal growth. As fever increases, these organisms begin to die faster than they can reproduce. Hippocrates stated, "Give me fever and I will cure any disease."

Sweating carries toxins out of the system through the skin. It also helps keep the rising temperature within a range that will not endanger the long-term health of the body.

Mucous secretions also remove toxic material from the body. Cells of some mucous membranes protect against invasion by the action of the tiny cilia that move particles of foreign matter and debris towards the nearest outlet. These cilia are stimulated by external irritants, bacteria, viruses, or internal toxins.

Inflammation, swelling, and edema are actions by the body to localize a problem. Inflammation indicates a local increase in metabolic activity with increased blood and lymph supply, and an increased capillary supply to aid in transport of blood-borne defenses. Edema, or fluid accumulation, aids in diluting an undesirable, toxic, or irritating substance.

Local infection results from breakdown of vital tissues into waste matter, which then provides a suitable environment for bacterial spread until the body's forces can remove the waste material. The reduced vitality occurs first, the infection is secondary. Boils, acne, and other local infections may also be the result of an inner cleansing process.

Diarrhea and vomiting are obvious attempts by the body to rid itself of toxic substances. Local irritants may initiate this action, as will systemic toxins.

Pain is a natural mechanism by which the body draws attention to a problem area. Pain indicates that the malfunction can no longer be tolerated or compensated for, and that further derangement may become injurious.

Sneezing and coughing are vigorous attempts by the body to rid the respiratory system of irritants and toxins. The coughing up of mucus can reduce the spread of infection by preventing morbid material from stagnating, and also can help prevent blockage of smaller respiratory passageways. Sneezing effectively rids the upper respiratory passages of particles and irritants.

All these acute symptoms of "disease" are in fact the result of an intelligent action by the body to re-establish equilibrium and positive health. As such they are corrective and eliminative and should not be suppressed. What is commonly called *acute disease* is really the result of nature's efforts to eliminate waste matter or poisons from the body and to repair injured tissues. If this acute condition is not allowed to run its natural course, or is treated with suppressive methods and therefore not allowed to fulfil its intended function of elimination, then eventually *chronic disease* will result. Thus, Lindlahr defines chronic disease as:

"a condition of the organism in which lowered vibration (lowered vitality), due to the accumulation of waste materials and poisons with the consequent destruction of vital parts and organs, has progressed to such an extent that nature's constructive and healing forces are no longer able to act against the disease conditions by acute corrective efforts (healing crisis)."[6]

The chronic disease condition is therefore much more permanent and often involves radical changes in the body's structures and chemistry.

Although the body is composed of vastly different types of structural units, each cell requires the same three factors to maintain life. These are:
- Nutrition
- Drainage
- Coordination

These factors are also essential for the health of the total organism, which depends upon the health of its individual cells.

NUTRITION

The body is composed of a number of chemical elements which combine to form the basic units of protein, carbohydrates, and fats; as well as essential fatty acids, vitamins, and minerals.

Proteins are built up from building blocks called *amino acids*. Eight of these are considered *essential amino acids* since they cannot be synthesized within the body and therefore must be taken in with the normal diet.

Carbohydrates are essential units which must be supplied by the diet. Although complex by nature, the basic unit is glucose, which forms the major energy source for the body. Carbohydrates may be synthesized from proteins or fats within the body. In the case of proteins, this is an energy-expending pathway that yields less energy than required for the conversion and only functions when the body's dietary supply of carbohydrate is absent.

Fats are used partly as structural and functional material and partly as a storage form of food. Fats may be synthesized within the body; however, food acts as the major source.

Essential fatty acids (EFA): three polyunsaturated fatty acids (linolenic, linoleic, and arachidonic) have essential fatty acid activity. In humans only linoleic and arachidonic acids are considered essential. They play important roles in fat transport and metabolism and in maintaining the function and integrity of cellular membranes. They also act as precursors to prostaglandin formation. While the body can synthesize arachidonic and linolenic acids from linoleic acid, linoleic acid itself must be ingested and cannot be synthesized in the body.

Vitamins and minerals are essential to life and are used within the body's various structures as building material and are necessary for various biochemical functions. Normally these must be ingested; however, some may be synthesized within the body.

For normal maintenance of health all the above nutrients must constantly be ingested to provide the basic building blocks of life for the body's tissues to be repaired and remade, and to furnish an adequate energy supply for body action and maintenance.

DRAINAGE

Proper drainage of the cell is necessary to get rid of toxic end products of metabolism. If these wastes are not removed, the cell's function is reduced, which can downgrade the health of tissues, organs, and ultimately the entire body, if affecting many cells.

COORDINATION

Coordination within single cells and also within the total organism is essential for life. Intracellular regulation is controlled by chemical means while coordination throughout the entire system is controlled by both the nervous and hormonal systems. If either of these is not functioning properly, delicate balancing mechanisms can be upset, causing downgraded local or systemic health.

In health all three of these essentials, nutrition, drainage, and coordination, are functioning and in balance, while in disease there is either disharmony or lack of performance of one or more of these essentials of life. The body's constant effort is to establish this harmony. If harmony exists, inner vitality is then able to express itself fully. Such a person appears to have an unbounded source of life and energy.

In reality very few people have completely free-flowing vitality. The total vitality available to the ordinary person equals his or her life force, minus any obstructions to this energy being expressed. Just as the quality of television reception may depend on the television receiver or antenna, so it is with the human organism. These obstructions to the life force can be any one or any combination of the basic causes of disease. In order to relieve any diseased condition, it is necessary to remove from the body any obstructive factors which interfere with its life force, allowing the body to heal itself.

We truly are what we eat and drink, what we feel, and what we think. Health can only be attained and maintained by the coordination of our body, emotions, and mind. Cures cannot come from external measures, even if they are natural therapies. True healing can only come from within with the healing power of nature freely flowing.

THE TOOLS OF NATUROPATHY

Naturopathy is a method of curing disease by releasing inner vitality and allowing the body to heal itself. The methods that the naturopath uses should be looked on only as useful tools that help release this vital healing power. In and of themselves they are not intrinsically healing. Certainly this is evident when we consider that many of the herbs used routinely in practice are potent poisons if given in the wrong doses. The beneficial effect is not due to this poison, but in the direction it urges the body to take in its self-repairing process. With hydrotherapy, healing power is in the body's action, not due to any specific medicinal power of water. The use of "natural" therapy does not of its own constitute naturopathy. Naturopathy involves the use of natural therapies according to certain established principles. This is where naturopathy as a science must be distinguished from folk medicine or any other "natural" therapy. While these techniques or tools may be employed by the naturopath, they must be used according to the basic principles of naturopathy for the end result to be naturopathic medicine.

A herb may be used to stimulate the body to action, aid in elimination, help purge the body of toxic waste, or act as a nutrient. Used in these ways the herb works *with* the healing power of nature. It may, however, be used to *suppress* the body's healing efforts, just as a drug might be used, to rid the body of its distressing symptoms with little thought for real causes or cure. In such a case the herb is not used according to naturopathic principles. Hydrotherapy may be used to aid in circulation, nutrition, and generally to increase vitality so that the healing efforts of nature are allowed freer action. Hydrotherapy, however, can be used solely to suppress pain or discomfort without concern for the final cure. The tools of naturopathy can be used in proper or improper ways.

Not all naturopaths use the same therapeutic tools. Naturopathy in its essence is a philosophy of life, not a collection of rigid, learn-by-rote prescriptions. Once the philosophy is understood, the naturopath uses whichever agents or tools his or her temperament feels most comfortable with. Some naturopaths interpret the philosophy very narrowly and use only diet, fasting, exercise, sunlight, and hydrotherapy to guide the body's healing forces towards cure. These naturopaths shun the use of herbs unless used as nutrients, and even look distrustingly on vitamin or mineral supplements. These purist or "nature cure" naturopaths are just as right as others who have added spinal manipulation, massage, physiotherapy, vitamin and mineral therapy, homeopathy, botanical medicine, acupuncture, and many other non-toxic procedures. What is important is that the procedures be used according to the basic principles of naturopathy.

BOTANICAL MEDICINE

The earliest written records of nearly all civilizations mention the use of herbs for healing. Throughout human history there has been a close relationship between people and plants. Botany and medicine have always been closely associated. The *Pentsao*, or Great Herbal of China, which dates around 3000 B.C., discusses herbal treatments in detail. Another early herbal is the Ebers Papyrus of 1500 B.C., which lists over 800 botanical prescriptions used in various disorders. Early Greek literature also has many references to the medical use of plants. Hippocrates (460–355 B.C.) was the first to list plants by their use. Several lists of pharmaceutically active plants were made throughout Greek history. The first attempt at publication of a materia medica, however, was not made until the early 1500s A.D. by Paracelsus. The first official pharmacopoeia, mostly of botanical origin, appeared in 1564. The earliest one in English was the first United States pharmacopoeia, published in 1820. Currently, over 50 percent of all new prescriptions written in the United States contain at least one ingredient either produced directly from plants, or discovered from plant sources and later synthesized.

Modern medicine draws its origins from early herbal therapies. Until the advent of "synthetic" medicine within the past 50–100 years, all medical doctors prescribed herbs routinely. Later research into the chemistry of plants and plant products isolated what was considered the "active principle" from plants. The active principles were prescribed as drugs whose names often still reflect their botanical origins. A commonly known example of this is *Digitalis purpurea* (foxglove). This herb had been used as a heart stimulant in folk medicine for centuries prior to the isolation of its active principle, digitoxin. Another example is the isolation in 1947 of reserpine from *Rauwolfia serpentina* (Indian snakeroot), a plant native to India and clearly described for its pharmacological uses in the *Vedas*, India's earliest written records dating from 1500 B.C.

Within the decade 1940–1950, hundreds of new "wonder drugs" were discovered, nearly all of botanical origin. The amazing thing about the "discovery" of these potent and clearly therapeutic drugs was not their existence, since written history was literally pregnant with specific examples testifying to the medicinal use of plants, but rather how long modern researchers took to investigate them. This nearsighted attitude has been expressed by De Ropp in *Drugs and the Mind*:

The situation results, in part at least, from the rather contemptuous attitude which certain chemists and pharmacologists in the west have developed towards both folk remedies and drugs of plant origin.... They further fell into the error of supposing that because they had learned the trick of synthesizing certain substances, they were better chemists than Mother Nature who, besides creating compounds too numerous to mention, also synthesized the aforesaid chemist and pharmacologist.[7]

Unfortunately, this separation of herbs from their "drug actions" was the fall from grace of the medical profession. Not only was the active principle found to be much more potent than the herb from which it was obtained, it also was usually found to be much more dangerous, with more profound toxic effects. These toxic effects were termed "side effects", but in reality were merely the normal action of the active principle in the body acting in ways other than desired by the physician. With the development of drugs came an increase in diseases caused by medication. It is now estimated that at least one-third of all diseases today are iatrogenic or the result of medication given to treat disease.

The use of botanical medicine, or preparations derived from the entire complex of the botanical plant part used, is usually safer but slower in action than orthodox drug therapy. By utilizing not only the so-called "active principle" but also the "associated factors" which naturally occur in the plant, the practitioner of botanical medicine has been spared most of the problem of drug-related diseases. The beneficial use of a botanical preparation in fact does not rest solely with the active principle, of which there may be several for a single herb, but usually in the total interaction of all its constituents.

It is, however, a common misconception that botanical medications are completely safe and non-toxic. For the most part this is true if herbs are used in their proper doses; however, any medicine can cause toxic reactions when used improperly. The use of herbs such as thyme, sage, rosemary, dill, ginger, and garlic in cooking and seasoning is an example of how widespread the safe use of herbs really is in daily life. Herbal teas now abound in most food stores and are used as pleasant-tasting drinks or to obtain mild botanical effects such as the calmative effects of chamomile, or the digestive benefits of peppermint. Even commonly used herbal teas, however, should really be reserved for medicinal use and not taken routinely. Such commonly used herbs as comfrey, goldenseal, or lobelia can cause toxic reactions. A knowledge of botanical toxicology, therefore, is essential before one tries to treat disease with herbs. Even with this warning in mind it can be fairly said that botanical medicine is usually safer and more therapeutic than the use of drugs when prescribed and monitored properly.

Herbs may be used in many ways to treat disease. If a herb is used merely to suppress symptoms without regard for cause or cure, it is little better than a non-toxic drug. If used properly, herbs act as aids in stimulating or directing the body's own healing forces, thus promoting health from within.

Actions of Botanical Preparations

Botanical preparations, although often referred to as herbs, may be derived from any member of the plant kingdom, including leafy plants, weeds, trees, ferns, or lichens. The whole plant or a single part of the plant, such as its root, rhizome, bulb, stem, bark, flower, stylus, stigma, fruit, seed, or resin may be used. Each part has a known action or actions; each herb stimulates the body to act in one or more directions. These actions have names that are useful as aids in prescription. Some are summarized below.

ALTERATIVES
This herbal action elicits an alteration for the better in the course of an illness. Alteratives are often described as blood purifiers and are used to treat conditions arising from or causing toxicity. If given in proper doses over a prolonged period of time, these herbs improve the condition of the blood, accelerate elimination, improve digestion, and increase the appetite. Commonly used alteratives are:

Barberry (*Berberis vulgaris*)
Blue flag (*Iris versicolor*)
Burdock (*Arctium lappa*)
Chaparral (*Larrea tridentata*)
Echinacea (*Echinacea angustifolia*)
Figwort (*Scrophularia nodosa*)
Oregon grape root (*Berberis aquifolium*)
Plantain (*Plantago lanceolata*)
Poke root (*Phytolacca decandra*)
Prickly ash (*Xanthoxylum americanum*)
Queen's root (*Stillingia sylvatica*)
Red clover (*Trifolium pratense*)
Sarsaparilla (*Smilax ornata*)
Sassafras (*Sassafras officinale*)

Tree of life (*Thuja occidentalis*)
Wild indigo (*Baptisia tinctoria*)
Yellow dock (*Rumex crispus*)

ANODYNES/ANALGESICS

These herbs will relieve pain usually by reducing nerve excitability. These remedies are closely related to antispasmodics and sedatives. Commonly used herbs in this class are:

Catnip (*Nepeta cataria*)
Chamomile (*Matricaria recutita*)
Dong quai (*Angelica sinensis*)
Hops (*Humulus lupulus*)
Jamaica dogwood (*Piscidia erythrina*)
Mistletoe (*Viscum album*)
Skullcap (*Scutellaria lateriflora*)
Valerian (*Valeriana officinalis*)
White bryony (*Bryonia alba*)
Wild yam (*Dioscorea villosa*)
Wintergreen (*Gaultheria procumbens*)

ANTHELMINTICS

These include vermicides that kill intestinal worms, and vermifuges that aid in expelling worms. Most commonly used are:

Aloe
Bitterwood (*Picraena excelsa*)
Butternut (*Juglans cinerea*)
Elecampane (*Inula helenium*)
Garlic (*Allium sativum*)
Hyssop (*Hyssopus officinalis*)
Kousso (*Brayera anthelmintica*)
Male fern (*Dryopteris filixmas*)
Papaya (*Carica papaya*)
Pomegranate (*Puncia granatum*)
Pumpkin (*Curcurbita pepo*)
Santonica (*Artemisia santonica*)
Tansy (*Tanacetum vulgare*)
Worm grass (*Spigelia marilandica*)
Wormseed (*Chenopodium anthelminticum*)
Wormwood (*Artemisia absinthium*)

ANTIBIOTICS

These herbs inhibit the growth of or kill bacteria. They include:

Bearberry (*Arctostaphylos uva-ursi*)
Bitter orange (*Citrus aurantium*)

Cajuput (*Melaleuca cajuputi*)
Echinacea (*Echinacea angustifolia*)
Eucalyptus (*Eucalyptus globulus*)
Garlic (*Allium sativum*)
Goldenseal (*Hydrastis canadensis*)
Horseradish (*Cochlearia armoracia*)
Mullein (*Verbascum thapsus*)
Myrrh (*Commiphora myrrha*)
Nasturtium (*Tropaeolum majus*)
Onion (*Allium cepa*)
Peruvian bark (*Cinchona ledgeriana*)
Propolis (a resinous beeswax)
Watercress (*Nasturtium officinale*)

ANTISEPTICS

These herbs are used internally or externally to prevent breakdown of organic tissues or inhibit growth of microorganisms. Some are similar to alteratives, while others are astringents. Among these herbs are:

Barberry (*Berberis vulgaris*)
Calendula (*Calendula officinalis*)
Echinacea (*Echinacea angustifolia*)
Eucalyptus (*Eucalyptus globulus*)
Garlic (*Allium sativum*)
Goldenseal (*Hydrastis canadensis*)
Myrrh (*Commiphora myrrha*)
Pine (*Pinus* spp.)
St John's wort (*Hypericum perforatum*)
White pond lily (*Nymphaea odorata*)

ANTISPASMODICS

These herbs stop or prevent muscular spasm. They are used for muscle cramps, menstrual cramps, asthma, and other disorders with muscle irritability, spasm, or contraction. Commonly used herbs in this class are:

Black cohosh (*Cimicifuga racemosa*)
Blue cohosh (*Caulophyllum thalictroides*)
Chamomile (*Anthemis nobilis*)
Cramp bark or high-bush cranberry (*Viburnum opulus*)
Lady's slipper (*Cypripedium pubescens*)
Lobelia (*Lobelia inflata*)
Mistletoe (*Viscum album*)
Passion flower (*Passiflora incarnata*)
Skullcap (*Scutellaria lateriflora*)
Valerian (*Valeriana officinalis*)
Wild yam root (*Dioscorea villosa*)

ASTRINGENTS

These herbs act upon the albumin of the tissue to which they are applied, causing a hardening and contraction, leaving the area more dense and firm. They prevent bacterial infection, stop discharges, diarrhea, or hemorrhages. Most astringents contain tannin as a primary ingredient. Herbs used are:

Avens (*Geum urbanum*)
Bayberry (*Myrica cerifera*)
Bistort (*Polygonum bistorta*)
Blackberry (*Rubus* spp.)
Calendula (*Calendula officinalis*)
Cranesbill (*Geranium maculatum*)
Myrrh (*Commiphora myrrha*)
Pinus bark (*Tsuga canadensis*)
Tormentil (*Potentilla tormentilla*)
White oak bark (*Quercus alba*)
Witch hazel (*Hamamelis virginiana*)

CARMINATIVES (AROMATICS)

These herbs, usually having an agreeable taste or aromatic odor, relieve flatulence and flatulent pain (colic), and soothe the stomach. Many herbs fit into this category, such as:

Angelica (*Angelica archangelica*)
Anise (*Pimpinella anisum*)
Balm (*Melissa officinalis*)
Caraway (*Carum carvi*)
Cinnamon (*Cinnamomum zeylanicum*)
Cloves (*Eugenia carophyllus*)
Cumin (*Cuminum cyminum*)
Dill (*Anethum graveolens*)
Fennel (*Foeniculum dulce*)
Ginger (*Zingiber officinale*)
Peppermint (*Mentha piperita*)

CATHARTICS

These herbs cause copious bowel evacuation. They also usually stimulate bile secretion. Cathartics are used to expel worms after an anthelmintic herb has been used and whenever a complete bowel evacuation is desired. Their use in chronic constipation is not therapeutic and only causes further constipation as its secondary effect. Most often used are:

Black root (*Leptandra virginica*)
Butternut (*Juglans cinerea*)
Castor oil plant (*Ricinus communis*)
Jalapa (*Ipomoea jalapa*)
May-apple or American mandrake (*Podophyllum peltatum*)
Mountain flax (*Linum cartharticum*)

Rhubarb (*Rheum palmatum*)
Senna (*Cassia acutifolia*)

DEMULCENTS
These herbs soothe, soften, reduce irritation, and protect the mucous membranes. Their effect may be mechanical or medicinal, depending on the herb. Among this class we find:

Chickweed (*Stellaria media*)
Coltsfoot (*Tussilago farfara*)
Comfrey (*Symphytum officinale*)
Goldenseal (*Hydrastis canadensis*)
Irish moss (*Chrondrus crispus*)
Marshmallow (*Althaea officinalis*)
Slippery elm (*Ulmus fulva*)

DIAPHORETICS
These herbs increase perspiration and rid the body of waste material through the sweat glands. They are best given as hot infusions repeated frequently. Useful herbs in this class are:

Balm (*Melissa officinalis*)
Blue vervain (*Verbena hastata*)
Boneset (*Eupatorium perfoliatum*)
Catnip (*Nepeta cataria*)
Chamomile (*Matricaria recutita*)
Crawley root (*Corallorhiza odontorhiza*)
Ginger root (*Zingiber officinalis*)
Peppermint (*Mentha piperita*)
Pleurisy root (*Asclepias tuberosa*)
Spearmint (*Mentha viridis*)
Yarrow (*Achillea millefolium*)

DIURETICS
These herbs increase the flow of urine. Often used diuretics are:

Bearberry (*Arctostaphylos uva-ursi*)
Broom top (*Cytisus scoparius*)
Buchu (*Barosma betulina*)
Burdock (*Arctium lappa*)
Cleavers (*Calium aparine*)
Couch grass (*Agropyrum repens*)
Hydrangea (*Hydrangea arborescens*)
Juniper (*Juniperus communis*)
Parsley (*Petroselinum sativum*)
Parsley piert (*Alchemilla arvensis*)
Pellitory-of-the-wall (*Parietaria officinalis*)

Queen of the meadow (*Eupatorium purpureum*)
Stinging nettle (*Urtica urens*)
Stone root (*Collinsonia canadensis*)
Wild carrot (*Daucus carota*)
Yarrow (*Achillea millefolium*)

EMETICS

Herbs that induce vomiting include:

Ipecacuanha (*Psychotria ipecacuanha*)
Lobelia (*Lobelia inflata*)
Mustard seeds (*Brassica juncea*)

EMMENAGOGUES

These herbs promote menstrual flow. Useful among this class are:

Arrach (*Chenopodium olidum*)
Black cohosh (*Cimicifuga racemosa*)
Blazing star root (*Chamaelirium luteum*)
Blue cohosh (*Caulophyllum thalictroides*)
Cramp bark or high-bush cranberry (*Viburnum opulus*)
False unicorn root (*Helonias dioica*)
Life root (*Senecio aureus*)
Mugwort (*Artemisia vulgaris*)
Pennyroyal (*Hedeoma pulegioides*)
Pulsatilla (*Anemone pulsatilla*)
Rue (*Ruta graveolens*)
Southernwood (*Artemisia abrotanum*)
Squaw vine (*Mitchella repens*)
Tansy (*Tanacetum vulgare*)

LAXATIVES

Mild purgatives encouraging gentle bowel movements:

Cascara (*Cascara sagrada*)
Castor oil plant (*Ricinus communis*)
Chia seed (*Salvia columbariae*)
Flaxseed (*Linum usitatissimum*)
Licorice (*Glycyrrhiza glabra*)
Olive oil (*Olea europaea*)
Psyllium (*Plantago ovata*)
Rhubarb (*Rheum palmatum*)
Senna (*Cassia acutifolia*)

NERVINES/SEDATIVES

These herbs can calm nervous tension, nourish the nervous system, and favor
sleep. Many are also antispasmodics. Useful herbs in this class are:

Betony (*Betonica officinalis*)
Catnip (*Nepeta cataria*)
Chamomile (*Anthemis nobilis*)
European vervain (*Verbena officinalis*)
Hops (*Humulus lupulus*)
Lady's slipper (*Cypripedium pubescens*)
Mistletoe (*Viscum album*)
Passion flower (*Passiflora incarnata*)
Pulsatilla (*Anemone patens*)
Skullcap (*Scutellaria lateriflora*)
Valerian (*Valeriana officinalis*)

STIMULANTS
Herbs that excite and arouse nervous sensibility, and stimulate vital forces to action. They increase and strengthen the pulse and restore weakened circulation. Commonly used herbs in this class are:

Cayenne (*Capsicum frutescens*)
Ginger root (*Zingiber officinale*)
Horseradish (*Cochlearia armoracia*)
Poplar (*Populus tremuloides*)
Prickly ash (*Xanthoxylum americanum*)
Snake root (*Aristolochia reticulata*)
Wintergreen (*Gaultheria procumbens*)

STOMACHICS
Herbs that stimulate the secretion of gastric juices include:

Avens (*Geum urbanum*)
Bitterwood (*Picraena excelsa*)
Columbo (*Frasera carolinensis*)
Gentian (*Gentiana lutea*)
Meadowsweet (*Filipendula ulmaria*)
Sweet flag (*Acorus calamus*)

TONICS
Herbs that give vigor and strengthen the entire system or a particular set of organs or actions. Some improve general vitality while others strengthen the heart, nerves, stomach, liver, or circulation. Some examples are valerian (nerve tonic), hawthorn berries (heart tonic), and dandelion (liver tonic). Tonics must be chosen for the effect desired to obtain benefit.

These specific "properties" of botanical medication are useful in classifying herbs for easy reference, and help narrow the choice of herbs most useful with a particular condition. But these properties in themselves tell us little of the herb itself, its temperament or character. Many herbs have alterative (blood-purifying), diaphoretic (sweat-inducing), or laxative properties, but not all of these would be beneficial for everyone with a similar health complaint. Each of the herbs must slowly become known as one gets to know an old friend—each has its own personality. The relationship between botanical and practitioner is a distinctly personal one.

Since no two people with the same disease are alike and the causes of their imbalance are unique, no set herbal prescription can benefit all. Each person must be considered individually to determine the best course of botanical medicine required, if any. One must consider if the condition is acute or chronic, if the patient is weak or strong, the state of his or her internal organs, and the function of the avenues of elimination. Herbs must be chosen which aid and direct the healing powers within.

Methods of Preparation

Methods of preparing herbs depend on the part of the herb used and the manner in which it is to be taken or applied.

INFUSION

This preparation is one of the most common and is similar to that used for beverage teas, except in the amount of herb used. Infusions are made from leaves, flowers, or other soft parts of the plant, where botanical properties may be extracted by water. Place ½-1 oz (15-30 g) of dried or fresh herbs that have been thoroughly bruised in an enamel, porcelain, or glass container. Pour 1 pint (500 mL) of boiled hot water over the herbs and cover the container tightly. The herbs are allowed to steep for 10-20 minutes. Strain the liquid. The infusion may be taken hot, warm, or cool, depending on the herb and effect desired. The usual dose is ½-1 cup (125-250 mL) taken 3-4 times daily, or more frequently in acute disease. Occasionally honey as a sweetener is allowed although some remedies should not be sweetened. Since these herbal infusions decompose rapidly, they should be made freshly each day.

DECOCTION

A decoction is used to extract botanical principles that are not easily obtained by infusion, which is often the case with roots, coarse leaves, stems, or barks. Decoctions may be prepared by boiling 1 oz (30 g) of herb to 1 pint (500 mL) of water in a covered non-metallic container for 20-30 minutes. The liquid is then cooled and strained. Sometimes it is desirable to concentrate a decoction by simmering the mixture uncovered. This is not done if volatile principles are present that would be lost in steam. Softer leaves or flowers may be added in the last 2-3 minutes, or added after the pot has been removed from the heat and strained, as one would make an infusion, leaving the herbs to steep 10-20 minutes. Doses vary according to the herb—from 1 tsp (5 mL) to 1 cup (250 mL) taken three to six times daily. Decoctions, like infusions, rapidly deteriorate unless some preservative is used.

FLUID EXTRACT

These botanical preparations are the most concentrated form of the herb, and are prepared in a variety of ways to preserve the herb's maximum effectiveness.

The simplest preparation, a *green extract*, is made by thoroughly crushing the juicy parts of the herb and pressing out its juices. This is then strained. In medicinal effect, 1 fl oz (30 mL) of the fluid extract is equal to 1 oz (30 g) of the pure herb. Other methods requiring special machines are used commercially. Some herbs have properties that can only be obtained by the fluid extract process. However, this is rarely done at home, with commercial preparations being the main source. Fluid extracts also deteriorate rapidly.

TINCTURE
An herbal tincture is a solution of the herb's active botanical principles in alcohol. Many of the principles in herbs can only be extracted in this manner, as they are not soluble in water. Often, alcohol extractions are used to provide a stable, preservable extract for principles that easily deteriorate. Nearly any herb is obtainable in its tincture form from reliable botanical pharmaceutical houses. The difference between a standard drug and a botanical tincture is that a tincture is an extract of the entire herb portion used without isolating or concentrating one single active principle. Although they may be prepared at home, only by purchasing tinctures from reliable sources can the exact percent of alcohol and strength of preparation be assured, which is essential for accurate prescriptions. Tinctures take 2 weeks to prepare at home and within this time any herbal tincture you desire can be in your mailbox. As a physician I have no time to prepare tinctures and only rarely advise them to be prepared at home, except for local herbs unobtainable elsewhere.

To make a tincture at home add 4 oz (120 g) of coarsely powdered or cut herb to 1 pint (500 mL) of 90 proof vodka, gin, 80+ proof brandy, or, for more purity, grain alcohol. Let set for 2 weeks, shaking daily. Strain the brew and store in amber glass bottles. Tinctures may be diluted prior to storing to make a 50% alcohol dilution, depending on the percent of alcohol used. The usual dose is 25 drops in water 3-4 times daily. However, weaker herbs or weaker tinctures may require more. In some cases, the dose may reach 1-2 tsp (5-10 mL) three times daily.

SYRUP
Syrups are saturated solutions made with the herb and sugar, which is used as a preservative and to disguise the unpleasant taste of some medications. They are frequently employed as cough and sore throat medications. A syrup may be made in several ways. One is to add 1 oz (30 g) of herb to 2 cups (500 mL) of water and simmer down to 1½ cups (375 mL). Strain and add 1 fl oz (30 mL) honey or glycerine. Another method is to add 1 oz (30 g) herbs to a mixture of water and brown sugar. Simmer until the medicine is the correct consistency and then strain. Tinctures may be added after the syrup has thickened, and require no straining. Raw syrups may be made of onion or garlic merely by slicing the bulbs thinly and covering with a small amount of honey. Cover the container, let stand overnight, mash, and strain. Dose is 1 tsp (5 mL) three to six times daily.

POULTICE

This is a warm, moist application of crushed and bruised fresh herbs or moistened dry herbs made into a paste and applied externally directly on the surface of the body or between a thin layer of gauze. Crush and bruise the fresh herb and slightly moisten with hot water. If the dry herb is used, add a little hot water to wet it and pound the mixture to a pulp. The mixture should be just wet and not dripping. Apply directly to skin or place the mixture between gauze and strap on with tape or elastic bandage. Most poultices should be ¼-½ inch (1.25-2.5 cm) thick. These should be left on 3 hours or all night. An infusion or decoction may also be soaked into soft cotton and applied repeatedly or as a continuous application, like a compress. Moist heat may be applied over the poultice.

DOUCHE

Douches are usually made from herbal infusions or decoctions; however, dilutions of apple cider vinegar or yoghurt also are used, using a douche bag or enema bag with douche applicator. The bag is hung 1½-2 ft (45-60 cm) above the pelvis and the medicated fluid is allowed to enter the vagina slowly and gently, under low pressure. Some douches are done by continuously flushing the area, while others are retained for 10-20 minutes or even longer.

ENEMA

Herbal enemas are used in some cases to act locally or systemically by absorption through the mucous membranes. An infusion or decoction of the herb is made, and the enema instructions under Hydrotherapy are followed.

SUPPOSITORY

These are small cylinder-shaped preparations of herbs combined with cocoa butter, which are inserted vaginally or rectally. Often these may be purchased from reliable botanical supply houses. However, many useful suppositories have been withdrawn from production due to lack of demand. I often have the patient make the suppository by heating cocoa butter slowly and adding powdered herbs or tinctures as required. The cocoa butter is heated only until very soft and then is reshaped into large pencil shapes, cut into 1¼-inch (3 cm) segments, covered with wax paper, and refrigerated until used. The usual mixture is 1-3 oz (30-90 g) to 3 fl oz (90 mL) cocoa butter. Another method is to totally melt the cocoa butter, mix in herbs, and then pour the mixture into molds made of foil, 1¼ in. (3 cm) long and as deep and round as a large pencil. These are allowed to set, then covered with wax paper and refrigerated.

OINTMENT

Ointments are mixtures of herbs heated with cocoa butter, lanolin, and other oils or hardeners, such as beeswax. I rarely need to advise home production of ointments since they are readily available from botanical supply houses or health food stores. Details of their production at home may be found in *Herbal Medicine* by Dian Dincin Buchman. Basic ointments are made by heating dried or fresh herbs in fats or oils such as wheat germ oil, almond oil, and others desired, with lanolin, for several hours. This is strained and then reheated, adding beeswax as a hardener. The mixture is then poured into ointment jars to harden.

A good introductory book on herbalism which I suggest reading prior to using the botanical measures in this book is *The Way of Herbs* by Michael Tierra. It is simply written and will aid you in the proper choice of herbs found under each of the therapeutic sections.

DIET, FASTING, AND NUTRITIONAL THERAPY

One of the basic concepts of natural therapy has been expressed in the common phrase, "You are what you eat." It is becoming clearer now, that "You are what you digest and absorb". Our diet has, to a large extent, determined the diseases we suffer from. Over the past 100–150 years our basic diet has changed drastically. We have gone from fresh, wholesome, unrefined, unsprayed food to the opposite. Our foods now are picked unripened, frozen, canned, or refined, and treated with toxic pesticides, preservatives, colorings, and other chemicals. Mass food production techniques have given us more food but less nutrition as the soil becomes depleted of essential nutrients and its living balance upset by fertilizers and sprays. The refining of cereal grains strips them of their fiber and germ coatings, which contain the bulk of their protein, vitamins, and minerals, and leaves an unbalanced food composed primarily of starch. The consumption of refined sugar is also one of the most detrimental influences in the modern diet. Sugar consumption has increased phenomenally within the past 170 years. In 1815, the average intake of sugar was about 15 lb (6.75 kg) per year. By 1955 it had reached 120 lb. (54 kg) per year, and is even higher now.

Consider a typical teenager's diet: refined and sweetened cereal, two fried eggs (from chickens fed hormones and confined to a cage their whole lives), and white toast with butter for breakfast; a hamburger and french fries and a Coke for lunch; boiled frozen vegetables, meat, and white rice for supper, with two other soda beverages containing 7 tsp (35 g) of sugar and multiple other sweets each day. You can see how it is possible for people to eat more of less. We are literally starving ourselves nutritionally.

Not only is the *quality* of our diet extremely poor, but also its quantity is often as much of a problem. The old Chinese saying that nine-tenths of the food you eat is for your health while the last one-tenth is for your doctor is true. Whenever you eat more than the body can effectively deal with, disease is invited. This is true of the best, most nourishing foods as well as when the foods eaten are, of themselves, a health risk. A major cause of disease is accumulation of waste or toxins that cannot be silently dealt with, and overeating is one cause of this accumulation.

Another important factor in our foods' nutritional value is the manner in which it is prepared. Many foods have maximum value in their natural state, or as close to it as possible. For instance, when fruit is harvested green, unripened, many of the vitamins we traditionally associate with sun-ripened fruits are simply not present, and certainly not in adequate amounts. Certainly, for most fruit or vegetables heating destroys many of their enzymes and vitamins. In the case of water-soluble vitamins, these are lost if the food is boiled and the cooking water discarded. Long-term storage or canning also results in the loss of many of the less stable vitamins. Some foods, however, require heat to be made digestible, such as whole grains, some tuberous vegetables, a few fruits, and dried beans. Some nutritionists feel that a completely raw food diet is the only natural human diet and that cooked food is a major cause of suffering and disease. Raw foods are our most natural and nutritious foods and a person following such a diet with full knowledge of necessary nutritional requirements for health will experience profound physical vigor and resistance to disease.

Such a diet may be too extreme for the general population. The body is sufficiently adaptable to be able to handle a certain amount of cooked foods quite effectively. The type of diet I usually suggest is one containing a large amount of raw vegetables, fruits, seeds and nuts, with a smaller amount of lightly cooked vegetables, beans, and whole grains. For those who wish dairy products, free-range eggs and unpasteurized, unhomogenized, goat's milk products are advised. The question of the use of raw milk products is a subject of some dispute. Raw unpasteurized milk can carry brucellosis, as well as the more common salmonella organisms. To prevent these infections and still retain the benefit of raw milk, the milk source must be continually monitored for safety. Certainly, to prevent gastroenteritis, infants younger than 6 months must not be given raw milk from any source. All fluids given to infants must be boiled or pasteurized. Goat's milk, although a better source of general nutrition for infants than cow's milk, is commonly deficient in iron, vitamin D, and folic acid, increasing the incidence of megaloblastic anemia, unless care has been given to proper supplementation of these needs. Milk, even goat's milk, is rarely advisable for adults: fermented foods such as yoghurt and kefir are best. Raw goat's milk cheese is the best cheese product when available. Those desiring fleshy foods are directed first towards fish, then free-range chicken or turkey. Be aware that battery raised hens carry special health risks in the diet and should be avoided if at all possible.

The amount of red meat now consumed by the general public is a definite health risk. Many people eat meat or other animal products with each meal. If meat is to be included in the diet, it should be restricted to 2–3 times per week, or less. In general, it is wise to have at least two entirely lacto-vegetarian days each week.

For a proper diet to be of any use all food must be chewed slowly and thoroughly. Too many people rush their meals, putting an excess burden on their stomachs. In addition to this, the food must be eaten only when one is relaxed and under no tension. Stress completely stops the actions of the entire digestive system.

Many diseases can be directly related to improper dietary habits. The real proof, however, is seen when a disease process is reversed and cured by a simple change of diet. The prevention and cure of disease lies largely in proper diet.

Fasting and elimination diets

Aesculapius of ancient Greece advised, "Instead of using medicine, fast." Hippocrates routinely recommended prolonged fasting. Most religions advocate periods of abstinence from food to attain physical and spiritual purity. Christ fasted 40 days in meditation. Animals and babies retain their natural instincts and refuse food when ill. Most people remain uninformed of the beneficial effects of fasting when sick and continue to advise their loved ones to "Eat and keep up your strength." Nothing worse could be done to lower vitality in illness than eating.

During fasting there is an increase in the amount of energy available for the eliminative process due to absence of large amounts of food requiring digestion and assimilation, both of which require energy. The body is able to redirect this increased energy towards elimination of the obstructions to the vital force in the form of toxic waste. Since vitality equals the life force minus any obstructions, as these are removed higher levels of vital energy are available for more rapid elimination.

The initial elimination begins as soon as the first meal is missed. Sometime during the first 3 days of the fast, usually reaching its maximum on the third day, the elimination activity is manifested by the appearance of a coated tongue, bad breath, headaches, muscular aches, and general debility. These symptoms are due to the increase in toxins in the bloodstream and passing out of the channels of elimination. The sooner these unpleasant symptoms are present, the more toxic is the system. Often patients complain that if they miss a meal a severe headache results. These are the people who need to fast most urgently. By the morning of the fourth day, these eliminations are much less and a feeling of general well-being is often experienced, with great clarity of mind and abundant energy. This state lasts in degrees of varying intensity, interspersed with periods of lack of energy, fatigue, and difficulty in concentration as more toxins are eliminated. This period usually lasts until around the tenth day, when a *healing crisis* commonly occurs to a greater or lesser degree. During this process the body is able to eliminate a large amount of deep-seated toxins and waste matter. This manifests itself in a variety of ways from flu-like symptoms, skin eruptions, or other eliminative processes. Following this crisis, the patient once again will experience a further improvement in health and vigor.

The minimum period of fasting for cleansing purposes is 3 days, while a prolonged fast may safely last 3–4 weeks or even longer, *under supervision*. The length of the fast must be determined by monitoring the patient's reaction and general vitality during the fasting period. It is customary to continue a fast for 3, 7, 14, 21 (or other multiples of 7) days. *All fasts of 3 days or more are best supervised by a physician.*

It is essential that the fast be terminated with extreme care, especially in more prolonged regimens. In general, the longer the period of fasting, the longer the time needed before a full diet can be resumed. This must be a gentle process of adding easily digested foods first, to gradually recondition the digestive system. A common fast-breaker for prolonged fasts is stewed apples without their skin, while fresh fruit is acceptable after a 3-day fast. Fresh goat's yoghurt is also used in some cases, especially where enemas were used during the fast. This should be continued for 1 day if the fast has been less than 1 week, or 2–3 days for longer regimens. This is followed by the slow introduction of other fruits for 1 day and then at least 2 days of fresh fruit and salads or steamed vegetables. Gradually over the next 1–2 weeks a full diet is resumed. Food must be chewed until liquefied, especially when grains are reintroduced. The food to be eaten during this building-up period must be of the best quality since the body will be building tissue from these materials. As I tell most patients, it is easy to fast, but much more difficult to break a fast properly. All the beneficial effects of fasting may be undone in a very short time by adding too much food too soon, of the wrong type or quality.

The tongue is often considered the mirror of internal health and is used as a guide to the fasting length and progress. What usually occurs is that the tongue becomes heavily coated during the first 3 days of a fast and becomes progressively clearer until the healing crisis starts, or the fast is terminated. The clearing of the tongue after the healing crisis is a good indication that the fast may be ended. If the fast is allowed to continue until the tongue is clear, and it is broken gently with wholesome food, the result will be an increase in physical well-being, vitality, and mental clarity. The body will be at peace.

The type of fast performed determines to a large extent the rate of elimination achieved. In this way it is possible to control the elimination process required by the individual patient. Fasting by definition is the elimination of solid food. The strictest fast is the *water fast*, where the patient drinks only water whenever desired. *Fresh fruit juice or fresh vegetable juice* fasts are also used, depending on the case and desired result. The order of fast in degree of eliminative power is:

1. Water fast
2. Citrus juice fast
3. Subacid fruit juice fast
4. Vegetable juice fast

Although the water and citrus juice fasts are more eliminative than the subacid fruit juice or vegetable juice fasts, this does not necessarily mean that they are more desirable in every situation. Some disorders need a slower, less dramatic elimination than others, and not all patients can handle citrus in excess, or could go even 1 day on only water. The various fasts are, in reality, only members of the order of elimination diets. Many regimens are employed to effect an elimination of greater or lesser strength. The following is a list in order of eliminative effect:

Citrus fruit mono diet (a diet of only one type of fruit, plus its juice)
Subacid fruit mono diet (e.g. apple mono diet)
Mixed fruit diet (only one fruit type per meal; no bananas are allowed)
Raw fruit and vegetable diet
Raw vegetable mono diet (e.g. raw carrot and raw carrot juice)
Raw fruit, raw vegetables, and some cooked vegetables
Raw and cooked fruit and vegetables plus carbohydrates
Raw and cooked fruit and vegetables with carbohydrates and vegetarian
    proteins
Reasons for fasting are:
During any acute disease
In any case of lowered vitality or general debility

During any healing crisis
Repeatedly in most chronic diseases
To clear the mind

The following juice or mono diets are frequently used:

Apple juice or mono diet: this is a good alkaline diet for acid conditions such as gout or other inflammatory conditions.

Grape juice or mono diet: this is especially useful in heart conditions or where heavy activity has to be undertaken during the elimination. Black grapes are especially called for with heart complaints. Grapes are not as eliminative as most other fruit juices or mono diets.

Grapefruit juice or mono diet: this is especially useful in liver conditions, for general elimination, and with colds or mucous conditions. It is unsuitable for arthritis, ulcers, or hyperacidic states.

Orange fruit juice or mono diet: oranges are not frequently advised in too great a quantity since they tend to upset the liver. They are used primarily in mucous and lung complaints. Excess may cause inflammation and itching of the anus.

Lemon juice: in dilute form, lemon juice and water are highly eliminative. Most hydropathic health institutes fast their patients on cold or hot water with a slice of lemon.

Carrot juice or mono diet: especially useful in digestive problems such as colitis or ulcers. A very alkaline juice and therefore useful in all acid states.

Cabbage juice: this is most effective with ulcers. It is commonly mixed with carrot juice for this purpose.

Onion juice and mono diet: excellent for any condition with excess mucus, lung complaints, sinus congestion, colds, middle ear or Eustachian tube congestion, etc.

Nutritional therapy

Most naturopaths advise specific vitamin, mineral, or other food supplements, depending on the state of the patient. A great deal of research is now being done to further understand the physiological effects of these food factors. The use of these substances as food supplements or medication has been hotly contested by most medical doctors. The average conventional physician feels that all factors necessary for health can be obtained through a normal diet and that additional supplements are a waste of money. Naturopaths, however, feel strongly that the average diet no longer supplies these needed elements in sufficient quantities for several reasons. Our foods are now grown on soils depleted by years of intensive farming, without proper understanding of organic principles of land use and ecology. Essential minerals such as zinc are already deficient in the soil of many states. Even if the food eaten looks nutritious it no longer supplies the same proportion of minerals that food 100 years ago provided. The situation becomes even worse if these already-deficient foods are canned, stored for long periods, or cooked improperly. The average person has little or no awareness of how to prevent loss of water-soluble vitamins from food, or destruction of heat-labile vitamins in cooking. The refining of foods such as we see on nearly every super-market shelf is another obvious cause of reduced food value. The replacement of a few vitamins can in no way duplicate or make up for the wholesale destruction of our basic food groups.

Even if our food supply were the best available and we were careful to eat only organic and unprocessed foods, there still is the possibility that a certain per-centage of us would be nutritionally deficient. Dr Roger Williams first expressed the reason for this some years ago when he presented what is now termed the concept of "biochemical individuality". Briefly, this is the recognized fact that each person is unique in his or her biochemical makeup.[8] We, as members of the group *Homo sapiens*, are not exact replicas of a common ancestor, but rather evolving and genetically variable beings, with unique variations in our biochemical makeup and requirements.

Much evidence is now available to support this concept. Some 50 or more relatively rare conditions have been recognized where, due to a genetic bio-chemical alteration, an individual may need many times the recommended amount of a nutrient simply to maintain normal function and health. What is less well known and recognized, is that it is far more common for there to be a *partial* block in the ability of the body to utilize a nutrient. This metabolic fault may be genetic or acquired. An example of a genetic cause would be the production of abnormal enzymes that are either deficient in number or are unable to bind to their co-factors (vitamins are co-factors for enzyme functions). Without this bond many biochemical pathways arc unable to be completed, resulting in what may appear to be a nutritional deficiency of a single nutrient, when in fact an average, or even above average, amount of that nutrient is consumed in the diet. To correct this situation, a very large amount of the co-factor must be supplied to "force" the enzyme reaction to occur.

The exact manner in which this excess co-factor functions is not entirely clear, but it appears that in the case where the enzyme is normal in number, but slightly abnormal in structure, the saturation of co-factor bombarding the enzyme eventually finds a site of attachment, allowing the reaction to continue. In the situation where total enzyme production is low, but the enzyme is normal in structure, the increased supply of co-factors in some way stimulates the produc-tion of more enzymes.[9]

In addition to a reduced number of abnormal enzymes, other factors may result in a nutritional deficiency state, even with what should be an adequate diet. Impaired absorption from the gastrointestinal tract is a common problem. This may be due to gastric or pancreatic enzyme deficiency, which in turn may be partly genetic or acquired. There may also be impaired transport of nutrients into the cells, insensitivity of the tissues to a given nutrient, or increased excretion of a nutrient. Recent studies in animals have found that severe maternal deficiency of a single nutrient such as zinc can be passed on as an excess need for that nutrient, not only in the immediate progeny, but also as far as three generations later.[10, 11]

When we consider that even by the most orthodox estimates and techniques of estimating the biochemical need of a nutrient, as expressed by the recommended daily allowances of the known essential nutrients, 1-2 percent of the population will need more than the RDAs of an individual nutrient to maintain proper health. When we multiply this 1-2 percent by the 50 or so known essential nutrients, you can see how probable it is that a given individual might be nutritionally deficient in at least one if not more of these essential health factors, if the diet supplied only the RDA recommendations.

From these and similar observations emerged the concept of orthomolecular medicine. "Orthomolecular" literally means "right molecule" and describes a form of medicine that treats disease by supplying the right amount of individual nutrients, according to the individual needs of the patient.

Also, stress places a further burden on the body, rapidly depleting the stores of many vitamins. Cigarettes, alcohol, coffee, and air pollution do the same.

Obtain and retain as many vitamins, minerals, and other nutrients from food by using organically grown foods, increase the consumption of uncooked foods, and minimize cooking of foods that are cooked. If you take great care, you can obtain all the nutrients your body needs from a "normal diet". In this case, "normal" means a property balanced, organic, unrefined diet, and not the diet most people consume.

The aim of supplemental therapy is to supply essential elements deficient in the diet to aid in the healing process. On some occasions supplements are taken more for specific therapeutic effects. In such cases they are more like medicines and less like nutrients. An example is high doses of garlic taken to dissolve mucus or high doses of vitamins A and C to increase the effectiveness of the body's immune system.

Some naturopaths also employ glandular substances such as raw ovary concentrate, raw adrenal, raw pituitary, and others. These are used to nourish the body's glandular system and strengthen it, and not as a traditional doctor might use a hormone extract, which naturopaths feel weakens the gland.

Your body is continually undergoing a process of death and rebirth, with old cells being replaced by new. It is essential for this continual regeneration and repair that all of the necessary building blocks be made available. Diet is one of the most crucial factors in the production of health or disease.

Vitamins and vitamin-like substances

There are whole books written about the specific functions of particular vitamins, and it is not our purpose here to duplicate this information. This section is to provide some general guidance when it comes to selecting vitamins appropriate for your needs.

Vitamins are biologically active organic compounds, not able to be synthesized by the body, which are essential for normal health and growth, and without which disease will onset (sooner or later). Vitamins are available in the diet in small amounts, and once absorbed are carried in blood and lymph to act on target organs, tissues and cells.

FORMULATIONS AND SYNERGISTIC CO-FACTORS

There is a multitude of vitamin preparations through retail outlets such as health food shops, pharmacies and chemists, as well as increasingly through multi-level marketing organizations.

Take professional advice as to what particular requirements you may have for a specific vitamin. In other words, do not self-prescribe. This is one of the most common mistakes made by vitamin consumers today Without professional help there often is the tendency to choose natural health products to relieve a particular "symptom" and to fail to see the underlying cause.

This is not the proper application of naturopathy and involves the same thought process that medical doctors use to prescribe drugs to relieve the symptoms of disease. This is also one of the reasons that it is often difficult to get good nutritional advice from your medical doctor unless he or she has been schooled in naturopathic medical thought. Their basic philosophical view of disease termed allopathy is by definition "the curing of a diseased action by the inducing of a different kind" and the basic naturopathic philosophic understanding that allows the proper use of nutritional supplementation is often lacking. If you are supplement-shopping, patronize the health food shop before the chemist. They are generally more aware of health issues, their products of a higher standard and more likely to be organically sourced. It may be worthwhile discussing possible product purchases firstly with your naturopath.

Beware of the "multi-approach" to therapy. A multi-vitamin, multi-mineral regime will be useful for "maintenance" of vitality. That is why we recommend Celtic salt as a multi-mineral. But it may not be enough to achieve or recover vitality. You are more likely to need high doses of a specific vitamin or mineral in order to effect changes needed. For example, a multi-mineral tablet with some magnesium in it will not contain enough magnesium to assist with period cramps. For that, you need greater amounts than the multi-mineral tablet can provide.

This is why in this book we endeavor to give you some guide as to potential doses of specific nutrients in a particular situation. These are guides only. Each person's requirements will vary according to biochemical individuality, which reflects all sorts of parameters such as age, stress, health status (past and present), lifestyle factors, dietary factors, and perhaps genetic and family factors. The recommended dosages contained in this book are not intended to be prescriptive, but to act as a "ball park" guide.

Minerals

Minerals are supplied to the body via our food. Plants take up minerals (in the form of mineral salts) from the soils in which they grow, and we ingest these mineral salts as we eat the fruit, vegetables, herbs, that contain them, or eat animals that have ingested these minerals in their food.

Mineral salts are essential for our structural and functional well-being. This should not be surprising, considering that we came from a salty environment (our mother's womb filled with amniotic fluid) to start with. All our body fluids, blood, extracellular fluid, lymph, tears and sweat, are salty. Every cell in the body has to be constantly bathed in extracellular fluid ("the internal ocean"), a fluid with a salt composition very similar to that of the ocean. The skeletal system is composed of a complex matrix of different minerals, of which calcium is just one player. Proper levels of minerals are important also for nervous system function, all metabolic processes, and proper hydration of the lymphatic and vascular systems (electrolyte balance). Also, all nutrients such as vitamins, proteins, enzymes, amino acids, carbohydrates, fats, sugars, oils, etc. require mineral salts to be of any biological use at all. Mineral salts sometimes act as co-factors, as catalysts, or ionized energy conductors. All elements work together (synergistically) as a collective whole; if there is a shortage of one mineral, the balance of the body's chemistry can be upset, like the weak link in a chain. For example, lithium is a trace mineral that is an important player in the central nervous system when it comes to mood swings (either up, as in mania, or down as in anxiety and depression). Lithium is largely missing from soils used to grow foods these days, and what are we seeing? Epidemiologists tell us we are on the crest of a huge wave of anxiety/depression and mood swing disorders.

Given intensive farming practices which effectively alter soil biochemistry (irrigation leeches minerals, use of fertilizers creates unnatural mineral concentrations, etc.), and since many soils are often depleted in minerals to start with, we can no longer rely on food sources alone to ensure proper mineral intake. They are not usually deficient in calcium or magnesium, phosphorus or potassium (the base of most of the common fertilizers), but various soils in different places are found to be deficient in a whole range of trace minerals our body biochemistry needs to function properly. This is one reason why people are becoming much more interested in foods grown organically and in other more natural ways; studies demonstrate such organic foods contain better mineral values.

While in many disease processes a particular mineral may be required in more therapeutic doses, for every day requirements it is best to supplement with a broad spectrum mineral salt, such as unrefined sea salt. The minerals and trace elements found in sea water and harvested as natural, unrefined sea salt, work to maintain proper functioning of the body's systems and is preventative. Taking this unrefined salt on a daily basis is like taking a multi-mineral supplement, only it is cheaper, tastier, and probably better balanced than any multi-mineral tablet.

We need to take an enlightened look at salt, and understand the issues a little more clearly. There is "good" salt, and there is "bad" salt. Over the past 40 years, there has been a lot of good scientific advice suggesting that salt is a poison, like tobacco and alcohol. Since childhood, people have been taught that salt causes high blood pressure. This is still the general medical position, and this is certainly the case with *refined salt*. However, with *natural unrefined salt* it is definitely not so. All salt is not the same, and in the light of recent studies into salt, it is now timely to put the record straight.

Refined salt is basically just two mineral salts, sodium (Na^+) and chloride (Cl^-), together with other chemicals. Anti-caking agents (e.g. aluminosilicate of sodium), plus bleaches are used in refined salt; sometimes, inorganic iodine is also added (which incidentally causes obesity and sexual dysfunction), so then other chemicals are added to stabilize these iodine additives. Other chemicals to prevent water absorption and promote free-flow of the salt from the container are also added. None of these chemicals is compatible with human biochemistry, and simply contribute to the problems refined salt causes. Like anything which is isolated from its organic whole (i.e. refined), excessive concentrations of sodium and chloride can and will cause mineral and fluid imbalances in the body which can lead to any of the following problems: fluid retention, hypertension, excessive thirst, diarrhea, stiff gait, exhaustion (fatigue), tremors, seizures, hyperactivity, cognitive dysfunction, anemia, anorexia, and imbalances of other minerals.

Conversely, the current belief that our body can function on a no-salt or even on a low-salt intake causes more problems than it tries to solve. You cannot function without salt; you can't digest your food without salt; your heart cannot function; your adrenal glands can't function; neither can your liver nor kidneys, your lymphatic system will become sluggish and inefficient, as will the blood system, without proper intakes of mineral salts. Here are some problems a low- or no-salt diet can and will cause:

- Dehydration (salt helps the body retain the water needed for the fluid systems)
- Oedema (fluid retention—the other side of the dehydration coin)
- Massive adrenal exhaustion (fatigue)
- Kidney and liver problems
- High blood pressure
- Heart attack (heart valves can tire and lacerate)
- Accelerated aging, cellular degeneration, biochemical starvation
- Breathing difficulties

So don't be conned by the crusade against salt. It is certainly true that all salt is not the same. While we criticize refined salt which is indeed toxic and poisonous, causing as it does imbalance within human biochemistry, we also need to speak of the good salt, that which is totally unrefined and organic.

Celtic salt, (also called gray sea salt, or Brittany salt), if you can obtain it, is perhaps the very best available in the world today. This natural, unrefined salt is a multi-mineral, containing 84 minerals and trace elements, some of which are also referred to as electrolytes. These 84 minerals provide for all the needs of human biochemistry. In this unrefined state, sodium and chloride are therefore balanced and buffered by the other 82 elements, and the combined impact is very beneficial to our bodies.

There is available in shops (including health food shops) a wide range of salts, from the highly refined table salt, through to rock, macrobiotic, vegetable and various other salts. Each of these has negatives and positives, although there are no real positives the more refined anything is, including salt.

Celtic salt is totally unrefined, hand-harvested off the northwest coast of France, where there are cold, active, North Sea currents, 9 foot (3 metre) tides, and other suitable marine conditions such as pristine ponds and natural waterways edged with wild grasses and other green plants, the wind and sun evaporate the ocean water leaving a rich brine. The salt crystals are harvested in the age-old method by hand, with wooden rakes. The salt fields of northwest France (about 2,000 hectares) are lined with a natural layer of clay and sand. There is no intervention by modern chemistry, nothing is added, nothing removed, and it comes with organic certification.

Currently, there are plans to harvest a similar product from the coast of Tasmania in Australia, but until I see the finished product, we recommend Celtic salt on a daily basis for everyone, as a very low-cost way of ensuring proper intake of minerals.

HOMEOPATHY

Dr Samuel Hahnemann (1755–1843) is the father of homeopathy. Hahnemann, a medical doctor and researcher in pharmacology, gave up his busy practice after becoming disillusioned with the barbaric medical practices of his day. His daughter's severe illness sent him speculating whether safer techniques might be found to treat disease. Later, when translating a text on pharmacology, Hahnemann began to question the author's description of the action of Peruvian bark (cinchona). He decided that the only way to resolve the question was to take the drug himself and observe its actions. To his great surprise, he found that the action of the drug created exactly the same symptoms that it was commonly employed to cure! From this, he speculated that the first law of cure was in fact the law of similars: *Similia similibus curantur.* "Let likes be treated by likes."

This was an old concept dating back to the days of Hippocrates. It had, however, become bastardized into the simplistic concept that an herb, fruit, or food that "looked" like the disease was the best therapeutic agent. Thus, something red might be for blood building, a herb that looked like the heart was used for heart ailments, and so on.

Hahnemann set out to prove or disprove his initial findings by testing more drugs, both on himself and on others. The result was the rediscovery of the true law of similars, the foundation of homeopathy. According to Hahnemann, a medicine will cure a patient if his or her total set of symptoms corresponds almost exactly to the symptoms produced by the same medicine when given to a healthy person:

The curative power of medicines, therefore, depends on their symptoms, similar to the disease but superior to it in strength, so that each individual case of disease is most surely, radically, rapidly and permanently annihilated and removed only by a medicine capable of producing (in a healthy individual) in the most similar and complete manner the totality of its symptoms, which at the same time are stronger than the disease.[12]

This new or rediscovered science of homeopathy, or the treatment of disease with substances that produce symptoms *similar* to those of the disease, was diametrically opposed to the already established allopathic school, which by definition treated disease with agents that produce effects different from the symptoms of the disease.

From his early conclusions regarding the true law of similars Hahnemann further proposed that the only useful diagnosis could be made by compiling a detailed list of the patient's symptoms, both physical and mental, and then finding the "proven" medicine that matched those symptoms exactly. He felt that the tissue changes of a clinical case of disease were merely the results of disease but not the disease itself. Emphasizing a holistic concept, he often said, "There are no diseases, only sick people." This was entirely different from the typical allopathic approach, both then and now. Too often we naturopaths and homeopaths see patients who have been to every specialist in town and through almost every conceivable laboratory test, only to be told that they have nothing wrong with them, even though they may suffer from a multitude of symptoms. This physically undiagnosable condition, however, if left untreated, may eventually settle down into a clinical syndrome so that some time later, if no treatment has been introduced, the doctor will proclaim that you have kidney disease, liver disease, or heart disease, etc.

The problem, as Hahnemann explains, is that disease is a disorder of the vital life force first, which then is manifested in the physical (material) plane. Of this life force he says:

The material organism, without the vital force, is capable of no sensation, no function, no self-preservation; it derives all sensation and performs all functions of life solely by means of the immaterial being (the vital force) which animates the material organism in health and disease.[13]

The language of this vital force is first expressed as symptoms and only much later as tissue changes.

This concept of the vital force, or the inner person being the first cause of disease, led Hahnemann to the conclusion that tissue changes in no way indicated the remedy. As Dr James Tyler Kent explains, "Do not say the patient is sick because he has a white swelling, but that the white swelling is there because the patient is sick."[14]

Homeopathy specifically condemns the removal of external manifestations of disease by any external means whatsoever. If an external problem is thus removed (suppressed) the disease is driven inward, causing chronic disease. Early homeopaths warned that the final result of allopathic suppressive treatments would be a rapid increase in chronic disease in the future.

According to homeopathic philosophy, it is the inner person (vital force) that is ill, so the cure must take place from within, outwards. If properly treated in this manner disease follows a set path of elimination. Homeopathic physicians believe that disease elimination proceeds from more important to less important organs, from above downwards, from within outwards, and in reverse order of its origin. Thus, according to this philosophy, since all chronic disease has its origin on the surface and then progresses deeper, as proper cure is effected, first the inner manifestations of disease will be removed while the external manifestations will *resurface*, only later being removed as final cure results. This progression of symptoms tells the doctor that the disease is in fact once and for all being removed.

Not all conditions are treatable with homeopathic remedies. A condition such as appendicitis is better left to surgery.

The preparation of homeopathic remedies is unique. Hahnemann found that by diluting medicine to reduce its natural effect of aggravating the disease, which by definition was its therapeutic attribute, not only was the aggravation made less, but its beneficial effect was surprisingly enhanced. Later he came to realize that a vital disorder could only be corrected by a medicine similar in quality to the vital force. To attain this similarity in quality, medicines were "potentized" to be effective on the subtle forces of man. This "minimum dose" medicine is prepared by diluting one part of the original substance with nine parts of milk sugar, or in an 87% solution of alcohol, or diluted with water. This mixture is then treated in a specific way until it is uniformly dispersed. It is then known as the $1 \times$ dilution. The process is then repeated as many times as required, taking one part of the previous mixture and mixing it with nine parts as above, to create $2 \times$, $3 \times$ and so on up to $30 \times$, $200 \times$ and so on. The "higher" the dilution the more dilute the mixture.

This dilution process creates great difficulties for the physically minded scientist in understanding how a more dilute medicine may in fact be more therapeutic in a particular case than the more concentrated substance. The fact that these medicines are found by homeopathic physicians in practice to be even more effective in some cases than more concentrated doses supports Hahnemann's vital force concept of both the medicine and the disease itself.

According to Hahnemann,

The dose of the homeopathic remedy can never be sufficiently small as to be inferior to the power of the natural disease, which it can, at least, partially extinguish and cure, provided it be capable of producing only a small increase of symptoms immediately after it is administered."[15]

Actual diagnosis and treatment along homeopathic lines is extremely complex and not suited for self-administration. The patient must be interviewed in depth regarding symptoms, with each detail carefully noted. A remedy must be chosen with a complete understanding of its ability to be able to reproduce exactly the disease symptoms described. Homeopathic prescribing is not possible along "disease" categories. There is no set remedy useful for everyone with arthritis or migraines. It is in the subtle differences between each patient that the correct remedy is chosen, and its proper dilution prescribed. The treatment process is not stagnant, with the original dose being repeated until symptoms are removed. It is in fact by a change in symptoms that the homeopath judges the prescription and alters it as required.

In this book you will find few homeopathic remedies recommended. The treatment by homeopathy must be undertaken with the guidance of someone competent in homeopathy and is not easily applied with only a little knowledge at home. For homeopathic therapy, consult a qualified naturopathic or homeopathic physician.

HYDROTHERAPY

The history of hydrotherapy dates back well before Hippocrates. Water was worshipped by primitive peoples as far as recorded history, and probably before. Many great rivers such as the Nile in Egypt and the Ganges in India have long been considered to have sacred healing powers. Many cultures, such as those of the early Egyptians, Arabians, Mohammedans, Hebrews, Greeks, Hindus, Chinese, Japanese, and American Indians used mineral waters for healing purposes. Many centuries before Hippocrates, physician–priests established temples near thermal springs or mineral waters where the sick came to bathe, be massaged, and fast in communion with their gods. Hippocrates himself gave detailed prescriptions for the use of water in the treatment of many diseases. The Romans established extensive hydrotherapy spas for both social and health purposes. The Finnish, Turkish, and Russian sweat baths are other examples of water therapy with ancient origins.

In the early middle ages the Church set up opposition to the treatment of disease with water therapy, labeling it paganism. A dark cloud was then cast on the history of hydrotherapy in the western world until the late 1600s. Water therapy continued undaunted, however, in Japan and the eastern countries even during these dark times. In 1747 John Wesley, the founder of Methodism, wrote a text on hydrotherapy entitled *An Easy and Natural Method of Curing Disease*. Hydrotherapy as a science is commonly credited to Vincent Priessnitz, a Silesian peasant. In the early nineteenth century when Priessnitz was 17 years old, he suffered a severe accident that his doctors fully expected to be fatal. Having had some experience in treating his animals with water therapy, Priessnitz applied the same measures to himself, and in a short time was completely cured. Hearing of his remarkable cure peasants from near and later far came to Priessnitz for treatment. Soon his whole time was devoted to this new "hydrotherapy". He employed douches, wet sheet packs, cold purges, sweat baths, wet compresses, sitz baths, and other treatments commonly used today.

Unfortunately, Priessnitz did not record his therapies in book form. The first modern hydrotherapy text came out of Bavaria in 1886. Father Sebastian Kneipp was from youth a rather frail, sickly sort, until hearing of the use of cold water to harden and strengthen the body. He thereupon determined to give it a try and proceeded to take daily swims, first in summer and then in the heart of the icy Bavarian winters. Soon he developed extraordinarily good health and strength. Moved by the plight of the underprivileged poor, who he felt were too often neglected and forsaken, he expanded and developed hydrotherapy, and dedicated his life's work, *My Water-Cure*, to them. His hope was to send this newly rediscovered knowledge throughout the world and be relieved of his self-appointed task as healer of the tens of thousands who sought his aid. In this task he succeeded well. In less than 10 years his English translation had already undergone 50 printings, and made its way onto many orthodox physicians' bookshelves. Water-cure establishments or "hydros" sprang up all over Germany and Europe, later spreading to the United States.

Up until this time the use of water in the treatment of disease was based mostly on empirical results; in the late 1800s Dr J. Winternitz of Vienna developed the scientific theory that the action of water was upon the nervous system, and its effects were either direct or reflex. The extent of its influence depended upon the water's temperature, and the force with which it was applied. By 1906 Dr H. Kellogg of the United States had written *Rational Hydrotherapy*, the first scientific text on hydrotherapy, which still serves as the basic text on the subject.

Principles and physiology of hydrotherapy

Even though we now possess a better understanding of how the application of water at different temperatures affects the body, the science of hydrotherapy has advanced little since the days of Kellogg. To understand how something as simple as the application of water could profoundly affect the body, we must review the mechanisms of heat regulation since it is by these basic bodily responses that hydrotherapy is able to produce its reactions. The balance between heat gain and loss is controlled primarily by the nervous system. Numerous areas in the nervous system control changes in superficial and deep circulation of blood, sweating, shivering, and general metabolic rate in response to changes in the environment and body temperatures. In the central nervous system the most important area is the hypothalamus. This thermoregulatory center regulates general body temperature, responding to nerve impulses passing from the various parts of the body, or as a result of its direct sensitivity of the surrounding blood's temperature. Another part of the brain, the medulla oblongata, controls the vasoconstricting (narrowing) tone of the blood vessels and is modified by impulses coming from the cerebral cortex and hypothalamus. The parasympathetic and sympathetic branches of the nervous system control the constriction or dilation of blood vessels throughout the body, responding to nervous and hormonal stimulation.

The degree of threat to the body's temperature equilibrium determines the extent that the nervous system is brought into play. If the stimulus is local and at a temperature slightly higher than normal, only local nerves are excited. If the thermal threat is greater, more extensive spinal reflexes are stimulated. If the heating is more prolonged, of greater temperature, or over a larger area, the hypothalamus centers in the brain are brought into play and a general reaction throughout the system is initiated. In these general reactions the body responds with superficial dilation of the blood vessels, increased blood volume, increased cardiac output, and increased pulse rate. This rapidly increases the skin's circulation and permits heat loss by conduction, convection, and radiation. Sweating then results if further heat loss is needed. The secretion of adrenaline and thyroxin is inhibited.

When the application of heat is not sufficient to raise the general body temperature and therefore does not stimulate the heat loss center in the brain, spinal vasoconstrictor centers play an essential role in heat regulation. Nervous reflexes produced by heating the skin inhibit these centers and vasodilation results. This dilation of the blood vessels occurs not only in and about the heated area, but also in other areas reflexly related. It is in this distant reflex response that most of the beneficial results of the superficial application of heat occur for the treatment of internal disorders.

The effects of cold on the body are controlled primarily by the nervous system. Heat loss is reduced by superficial vasoconstriction of blood vessels. This reduces the amount of heat transferred from the central parts of the body to the surface. Heat production is then initiated by involuntary muscular activity which may be irregular and imperceptible as individual muscle units contract out of harmony with each other, often termed "thermal muscular tone"; or it may result in the regular in-phase contractions known to all as "shivering". Thus, the body can speed up its general metabolic rate 2–5 times and keep the body temperature at acceptable levels. Other mechanisms helping to control body temperature are the secretion of adrenaline and thyroid hormones, which increases the metabolic rate, a rise in blood pressure, an increase in heart rate, and the erection of the body's hairs ("goose flesh") to prevent heat loss.

The body responds to the application of water at different temperatures and pressure in a two-step process. The *initial* action of the body is the immediate response to a threatening external stimulus. It is strictly defensive in origin. For example, when ice-cold water is applied to the skin, the body acts to prevent heat loss by sudden vasoconstriction of the local blood supply. The opposite is true when hot water is applied to the skin, with vasodilation occurring to encourage heat loss.

If the application of either hot or cold stimuli is of short duration, a secondary reaction occurs in the body. This reaction begins just after the stimulus is removed and is usually complete within 20 minutes, and occurs due to reflex stimulation of the vasomotor and heat regulation centers. In general, the reaction is the opposite of the initial action made by the body.

The following tables summarize the body's initial actions and secondary reactions to both hot and cold stimuli if of short duration.

COLD

Action	Reaction
1. Contraction of small blood vessels of skin, with dilation of reflexly related with contraction of internal vessels	1. Dillation of small blood bessels of surface, internal vessels after a brief contraction
2. Pallor of skin	2. Redness of skin
3. Goose flesh and rough skin	3. Smooth, soft skin
4. Sense of chilliness	4. Sensation of warmth
5. Trembling, shivering, and some pain	5. Comfort and relaxation
6. Quickened pulse	6. Slowed pulse
7. Quick, gasping respiration	7. Free, slow, deep, and easy respiration
8. Cooking of skin	8. Warmth of skin
9. Perspiration halted	9. Perspiration increased

HEAT

Action	Reaction
1. Vasodilation of surface blood vessels	1. Surface congestion due to inactive dilated blood vessel
2. Redness	2. Pallor
3. Pulse slowed at first, then quickened	3. Pulse frequent
4. Perspiration increased	4. Perspiration decreased
5. General nervous excitation	5. Nervousness and mental tiredness, drowsiness, and depression
6. Increased muscular irritability	6. Muscular weakness, atonic,

The primary effect of cold is therefore excitant, while the secondary reaction is invigorating, restorative, and tonic. The primary effect of heat is also excitant, while its secondary reaction is depressant, sedative, and atonic. Neutral applications are calmative.

Hydropathic use of the primary effect of heat or cold

As a general rule the shorter the application and the more extreme the temperature, the more purely excitant will be the effect of heat or cold.

GENERAL PRIMARY EXCITANT EFFECTS

Any method of application may be used to initiate a *general primary excitant effect*. In practice, heat is usually employed for this purpose. The effect of alternate hot and cold applications of very short duration is to continually renew the excitant effect of heat. The cold source is applied only as long as is necessary to return the skin to its preheated temperature. These applications are usually 15 seconds for each temperature; however, heat may be prolonged slightly longer than cold with good effect. This technique allows an indefinite extension of the primary excitant qualities of heat without its depressant reaction. The general primary excitant effect of heat is useful in cases of severe exhaustion, collapse, fainting, shock, drowning, fright, or suffocation. *Extremes of temperature are not advised with heart conditions, advanced age, or in the very young.*

LOCAL PRIMARY EXCITANT EFFECTS

More extensive use is made of the *local primary excitant effect*. There is no more powerful method of increasing heart activity than short very cold applications over the chest or back. This is used only as a last resort to stimulate a failing heart into increased activity in emergency situations where no other help is available. Very short cold applications almost anywhere on the body, hands, checks, face, or trunk are useful to arouse one from a faint. Intense cold of short duration to the umbilicus will excite and stimulate intestinal activity in nervous and motor dysfunctions of the bowels causing constipation. The uterus may be stimulated to contract by short, sudden cold applications to the breast, and this is of use in delayed labor.

Hydropathic use of the secondary excitant effect

Usually, only cold applications are used for their secondary excitant effects since the secondary effect of heat is always atonic, or sedative. Heat, however, may be used in conjunction with cold to enhance the reaction, especially if the patient is sensitive to cold, or of poor vitality. Here, too, alternate hot and cold is used, but with each temperature applied longer, anywhere from 1–3 minutes.

GENERAL SECONDARY EXCITANT EFFECTS
General secondary excitant effects can produce a powerful systemic excitation where every nerve and cell is activated as well as many hormonal secretions. The intense cold application may be reinforced by percussion, as in a cold shower, giving intense excitation to the whole body. The effect may be restorative or tonic.

A single application of cold is restorative after physical or mental exhaustion. Muscular strength and mental alertness follow a short ice-cold shower or bath.

The tonic effect of cold is its most useful characteristic. It excites the entire system, increases circulation, nutrition, assimilation, and healing. Unlike coffee, which extracts energy from already depleted energy stores, leaving the body in a weakened state, cold water has only beneficial effects. The function of the brain and nervous system is stimulated and a sense of well-being follows a cold application, partly due to increased brain circulation. Ice pond plungers use this dramatic therapy to harden and strengthen their bodies for increased health and vigor.

In using the cold bath there are a few principles to keep constantly in mind. Like other great tonic agents, cold is a double-edged sword, capable of great benefit or harm. A patient I once saw in a totally devitalized and depressed state had heard of these tonic effects of cold applications and reasoned that if something was good, then twice as much must be that much better. He proceeded to take a 10–15-minute ice-cold bath 2–3 times each day. No wonder he felt devitalized. The best tonic effects are obtained by very cold and very short baths or douches once daily, followed by massage, friction rub, and exercise.

LOCAL SECONDARY EXCITANT EFFECTS
Local secondary excitant effects are the most often used hydropathic effects. The application of water of varying temperatures, duration, and pressure may affect the function of any organ of the body in whatever way desired. The skin may be cleansed, toned, and purged of impurities; the circulation of blood and lymph increased; and nerve and glandular structures normalized by sweating baths or

packs. Inhalations, sweat baths, and vapor baths may be used to clear congested mucous membranes and aid in expectoration. The kidneys may be stimulated by cold douches to the sternum or upper legs, or by application of a wet sheet trunk pack for 3–8 hours. The liver may be stimulated by cold or alternate hot and cold compresses or douches. Hot fomentations may help relieve gallbladder pain and dilate the ducts, allowing passage of stones. Gastric juices may be stimulated by cold douches over the stomach, or alternate hot and cold applications. In cases of amenorrhea, prolonged hot foot baths, hot sitz baths, or enemas may be used along with ice-cold douches to the thighs for 2–10 seconds and daily hot and cold sitz baths. Any pelvic congestion may be relieved by alternate hot and cold sitz baths and this treatment is used for the ovaries, uterus, fallopian tubes, bladder, and prostate. Hot footbaths with ice to the back of the neck will help relieve cerebral congestion and thus remove many headaches. The hot foot bath alone is a cure for insomnia. These and many more effects can be obtained easily with hydrotherapy.

Benefits of hydrotherapy

The benefit that a patient will receive from hydrotherapy depends on how strong a reaction is achieved. This depends on the patient's vital reserve, which must be carefully considered before vigorous treatments are prescribed, as no two people are alike. Aesculapius' disciple Antonius Musa attained fame by curing the emperor Augustus of chronic lung congestion and catarrh by using the cold bath. As a reward for this his statue was erected on the temple of Aesculapius. But lack of discrimination in the use of hydrotherapy led to his downfall. Being called upon to treat the emperor's nephew, a rather effeminate young man, he employed the same cold bath that worked so well for the athletic soldier and emperor, with the result that the youth was so prostrated that he soon died. Father Kneipp made a similar mistake. In treating the Pope for chronic rheumatism, he advised an ice-cold bath, with the result that on the very first treatment the Pope, then a frail and aged man unaccustomed to such heroic treatment, was in such pain that he cried for hours. Had the patient been a sturdy young peasant as Kneipp was accustomed to treating, rather than a feeble Italian gentleman, the prescription might have worked.

Several factors influence the degree and speed of a positive reaction to either heat or cold. The most important of these is the general vitality of the patient. Prolonged illness, fatigue, nervous exhaustion, and anemia may reduce the body's ability to react properly. Poor reactions sometimes occur in the very young, due to incompletely developed heat regulation, and in the very aged. In general, the more the temperature of the application differs from the body's temperature, the better will be the reaction. The reaction will also be directly proportional to the size of the area exposed. Sudden applications of short duration and high intensity give a better reaction than graduated or slowly applied applications.

The actual method of application can also influence the degree of reaction. Friction or pressure will enhance a reaction. Hot drinks taken during or after a treatment, as well as general exercise, will increase certain reactions. In some cases a warm application preceding a cold one will enhance its reactive effect. However, the prolonged application of either heat or cold may cause tissue damage and inhibit the natural reaction.

Once the basic concepts of hydrotherapy are understood (and I have given only a brief and incomplete summary here), they may be used to produce any of the following effects:

Anodyne—pain reliever
Antipyretic—lowers fever
Antispasmodic—reduces cramps
Anesthetic—local
Diaphoretic—increases perspiration
Diuretic—increases urine production
Emmenagogue—stimulates menstruation
Hypnotic—induces sleep
Purgative—causes bowel evacuation
Pyrogenic—causes temperature increase
Sedative—quieting and soothing effect to nervous system
Stimulant—exciting action
Tonic—increases physical or mental vigor

Hydropathic procedures

Following are just a few examples out of many developed by the founders of hydrotherapy and of hydropathic applications used successfully over the years. Those procedures mentioned in this book and which are beneficial and practical for home use are discussed below.

BATHS

Alternate hot and cold sitz bath
This frequently used bath may be applied with benefit in nearly any disorder of the lower abdomen or pelvic region, including menstrual disorders, diseases of the uterus, ovaries, or fallopian tubes, prostatitis, impotence, constipation, digestive disorders, and lumbar disc injuries.

Hydropathic institutions have specifically designed sitz baths, often like two water-filled armchairs, facing each other. One is filled with very hot water, the other with ice-cold water. The patient sits with his or her bottom in the hot water and feet in the cold water for 3 minutes, and then reverses, with the bottom in the ice-cold water and the feet in the hot water for 1-2 minutes. The patient alternates back and forth from hot to cold for three immersions in each temperature, and ends with the bottom in the cold. The patient finishes the bath by drying vigorously with a rough towel and exercising until sweating is produced.

Although these ready-made sitz baths are ideal, they are rarely available to the home patient. Simple home sitz baths may be improvised by using two large plastic tubs or galvanized washtubs. These must be large enough to accommodate the patient's bottom easily, and hold enough water to cover the person from the umbilicus to mid-thigh. The hot water temperature should be as warm as the body can comfortably bear and the cold must be *very* cold. In most areas this means that ice needs to be added to cold tap water and allowed to melt first to lower the water's temperature.

For maximum benefit these baths must be done from 1–4 times daily, depending on the patient's condition. The effect of this bath increases the circulation of blood and lymph to the pelvic region, removes internal congestion, and improves tissue vitality and nutrition.

Cold sitz bath

The patient sits in a container as described above, with cold water but no contrasting hot footbath. The duration should be short—from 30 seconds to 1 minute. This bath is used much less frequently than the alternate hot and cold sitz bath. This bath may be very useful in enuresis, with the duration of the cold gradually increased to 3–5 minutes. Friction rubbing with a loofa mitt may be administered with the cold sitz, rubbing the hips, back, and thighs vigorously to increase the body's reaction. This is a powerful tonic bath and may be continued 3–5 minutes daily. It is useful with bed-wetting, impotence, difficulty in conception, and uterine malposition.

Hot sitz bath

A hot sitz bath is the same as the cold sitz bath, except for the hot water, and is of longer duration—from 3–10 minutes. It is useful in relieving colic and spasm or pain due to menstrual cramps, low back pain, hemorrhoids, and intestinal disturbances.

Full-Immersion Bath

Full-immersion baths are similar to either hot or cold sitz baths except that the effect is more generalized since the entire body is covered with water.

Cold full bath

A cold full bath may be used as a tonic, but is less profound in effect than the cold plunge. Repeated cold plunges may be used to cause the temperature to rise, creating an artificial fever. In practice, the cold bath is not used frequently for anything other than its tonic effect.

Hot full bath

This is the common bath in most households, which is in many ways very unfortunate. A full hot bath should only be taken for short intervals of 2–10 minutes and for definite therapeutic purposes. Very hot full-immersion baths daily create debility, poor circulation, mental lethargy, physical weakness, and depression. The Japanese *furo* is a hot full-immersion bath and if prolonged will cause the same atonic effects. Short periods of heat need to be interspersed with ice-cold plunges to be of any use, and should end with a cold application if for general use and not specific therapeutic purposes. Hot baths may be beneficial if prolonged and taken at the time menstruation is expected in case of suppressed periods, or for dysmenorrhea as an antispasmodic. Other forms of colic benefit.

Hot full Epsom salts bath

This bath is similar to a full hot bath except that 1-1½ lb. (450-675 g) of Epsom salts are dissolved in the water. This bath is used for various therapeutic purposes and is very antispasmodic and cleansing. The bathwater should be as hot as the body can reasonably bear, and prolonged for 20 minutes. After the bath it is best to go to bed, cover up well, and sweat. After 3 hours or more of sweating the patient is sponged off with tepid water or given a tepid douche or bath.

Neutral or tepid full-immersion bath

A tepid bath is calmative and soothing if prolonged. It may last 30 minutes to 4 hours. Acute hysteria or mental disorders are relieved by this simple bath, as is insomnia. Generally, this bath is taken at 94-98°F (34-37°C). If a high fever is present no better bath may be used than this gently cooling application. To be effective for this purpose the bath must last at least 20 minutes or longer. Always remember, however, that fever is your body's friend and should not be indiscriminately or routinely reduced.

Local bath

Hot, cold, or alternate hot and cold water may be applied to any part of the body to elicit specific effects. The most frequently used is the alternate hot and cold bath. Simply obtain two containers larger than the part to be treated, and fill with hot and cold water. The method of application is simply to first immerse the part in hot, then cold water. The usual interval is 3 minutes in hot water to 1 minute in cold, although equal time in both temperatures may be used. Repeat this three times, always ending with cold water.

Sweating bath

The Turkish bath and Finnish sauna are essentially dry heat baths, while the Russian bath is that of moist heat. The bather sits on wooden benches until sweat is produced. Depending on the type of sauna, water is poured on hot stones to produce steam, or ice-cold water is poured periodically over the head and body, after which a masseur or partner will apply birch branches vigorously, all over the body, to increase the skin's action. The bath lasts 10-20 minutes and then a cold shower, cold plunge, or even a roll in the snow cools the body off and encourages a strong circulatory and nervous reaction.

This procedure is then repeated 1-3 times, with the individual remaining in the sauna 2-10 minutes after perspiration becomes noticeable. Saunas are used to increase circulation, skin function, respiration, and general vitality. They also stimulate the nervous and hormonal systems, and encourage mental relaxation and sleep. Cabinet baths are used in a similar way and allow the head to be cooled by wet compresses. This can usually be done with less severe bodily reactions.

COMPRESSES

Cold compress

The application of cold water, using 2-4 layers of cotton cloth. For home use cheesecloth folded to eight thicknesses, cotton diapers folded to four thicknesses, or toweling may be used. The effect depends on the temperature of the water and the length of application. Cold or ice-cold water may be used, depending on the need. Where prolonged cold applications are required, several compresses are used and alternated, one following the other with no resting interval. Intermittent cold compresses may be applied for 1-3 minutes, with an interval allowing a reaction to begin, followed by a reapplication of the compress. This is in essence similar in effect to alternate hot and cold water, since the value in a hydropathic application depends on a difference in temperature between the application and body. Continuous cold or ice compresses are used for pain relief or to prevent swelling in an acute injury. They also stop hemorrhages and reduce congestion in local applications—for example in sinusitis. Cold compresses are often used in conjunction with hot applications to aid further in the reaction desired. An example would be a cold compress to the back of the neck and a hot footbath at the same time for headaches and cerebral congestion.

Hot compress (fomentation)

Applied like a cold compress, using hot water and several thicknesses of cotton cloth or toweling. Thick compresses hold their heat better and are therefore usually more efficient. The compress may be covered with dry material or a towel to prevent heat loss. Where prolonged heat is needed the compress is replenished frequently, as with continuous cold compresses. Duration depends on the temperature of the compress and effect desired. Local heat is antispasmodic, pain relieving, and sedative. It dilates the local blood vessels and draws blood into the region. Take care not to apply heat too often or too continuously, which may cause damage to tissues and effusion of blood into the area, resulting in congestion.

Alternate hot and cold compresses

Tonic and curative, increasing blood flow and nutrition through a local area. They are used frequently in therapy, alternating hot and cold compresses at varying intervals, depending on the effect desired. The usual frequency is 3 minutes hot and 1-2 minutes cold. Alternate hot and cold compresses are often used just after the first 48 hours of an injury, until healing is complete.

PACKS

All packs are basically similar in design, having an inner wet cotton fabric covered by dry blanketing. They act by stimulating the body with cold for the positive reaction that later results. Among commonly used packs are the cold full-body wet sheet pack, trunk pack, abdominal pack, chest pack, and throat pack.

Full-body wet sheet (cold) pack

This pack has long been termed "the cold pack", which is misleading, since the end result is warmth. First, fold a sheet lengthwise and lay this across the upper end of the bed so that the top covers the lower one-third of a thin pillow, thus covering the upper one-half of the bed, except for a few inches at its upper end. Then spread a large double blanket so that it reaches from the lower edge of the pillow to well over the foot of the bed. The upper edge should leave at least 2 inches (5 cm) of sheeting exposed. One side of the blanket should extend at least 2 ft (61 cm) over the edge of the bed. Next, a thin linen sheet is soaked in ice-cold water and wrung out so that it is just wet and then spread out on the blanket so that its upper edge is 1–2 inches (2.5–5 cm) below the upper edge of the blanket. The patient lies on their back on the sheet so that the sheet extends 2–3 inches (5–7.5 cm) above the shoulders, and raises the arms above the head. The helper rapidly draws the sheet across the body and tucks it snugly underneath the side of the body. From the hips the sheet is wrapped around the leg on the same side, leaving the opposite leg uncovered. The arms are now lowered and the opposite side of the sheet is wrapped snugly over the arms and body, fully enveloping the entire body, except the head, within the sheet and in contact with it. The remaining sheet is tucked comfortably under the feet and lower legs. Next, the short end of the blanket is drawn across the body, tucked under the shoulder, side, and leg; followed by the long side, which is drawn tightly across the body and pinned. The lower end is tucked under the feet. The bottom folded sheet is then drawn across the body and tucked comfortably around the neck to prevent discomfort or irritation from the blanket.

No air draft should be present. If necessary, to produce the sensation of warmth, an extra blanket or two may be laid over the patient and tucked close to the head and shoulders. These may be removed later if needed. If the subject does not experience a sensation of warmth within 5 minutes, the pack must be removed, and after 10 minutes of brisk walking about while receiving friction massage, it may be reapplied, this time with a hot water bottle placed at the feet. In the case of nervous people or those who feel too restrained with the arms bound, they may be left out of the wet sheets, but still included in the blanket wrap.

In practice, the wet sheet pack is used with almost all acute diseases, especially conditions with fever or due to toxemia. The fever is not lowered by the pack; in fact it will be raised, but as a result of the pack if continued 3 hours or all night, the fever will have been aided in its work by increased elimination and thus be lowered due to decreased need. Wet sheet packs of short duration (3–5 minutes) repeated many times will lower the temperature rapidly. I rarely suggest it. Its major use is for elimination. After the pack, sponge the body well with tepid water, and dress. Do not reuse the sheet used for a prolonged pack without washing, since it contains many toxins.

Trunk pack

This procedure is the same as the full-body pack but is confined to the area from underneath the arms to mid-thigh. All that is needed in this case is a lower blanket extending from underneath the arms to mid-thigh. On top of this is placed a wet sheet 4 inches (10 cm) narrower so that when the pack is completed the blanket fully covers the sheet. Once the pack is pinned in place, the bedcovers are drawn over the entire body. This pack is somewhat more convenient than the full-body pack and easier for home use. It is used for the same purposes as the full-body pack.

Chest pack

This pack is similar to a short trunk pack, extending from the underarm to the umbilicus. The upper portions of the chest are included in this pack by using two pieces of sheeting cut 6–8 inches (15–20 cm) wide and 2½ to 3 ft (75–90 cm) long, and two additional towels.

Lay out the blanketing so that it will extend from underneath the arms to the umbilicus. Lay the towels in an X fashion at the top of the blanket so that 6 in. (15 cm) or more of the lower ends of the towels overlap the upper end of the blanket. Next, place the wet sheet and two smaller sheet pieces so that they fit well inside the blanketing and towels. The patient lies down on the sheets so that their head and neck are just above the crossing of the X-placed sheets. These are drawn across the chest, followed by the body sheet. The towels are then drawn across, followed by the body blanket, and pinned. The bedcovers are then drawn over the patient. Duration of the pack depends on the patient's condition. Usually, periods range from 3 hours to all night. This is an excellent method for all chest complaints.

Throat pack

This pack is usually used with abdomen or trunk packs. All that is needed is a thin strip of sheet, neck size, and a suitably sized towel. The sheet is soaked in ice-cold water, wrung out, and wrapped around the throat. This is then covered by the blanket layer and pinned. This may be worn for an hour or more and is very useful in tonsillitis.

INHALATIONS

Steam inhalations are often recommended for lung conditions, in conjunction with various herbs. One easy method is to place the suggested herbs in boiled water as if one were making tea. Let these sit for 2–3 minutes in the covered container. Remove the cover and place this steaming pot on a low table and drape a large towel over the pot and the patient's head so that the vapors are directed to the nose and mouth. The patient breathes in deeply for 5–15 minutes. Another method is to place two chairs back to front with the steaming pot on the front chair and the patient in the one behind. A large blanket is placed over all, creating a true inhalation tent. With children, another method is to place the chairs facing each other with the pot on one chair and the parent and child on the floor of the tent. This gives a less intense inhalation, but is much less suffocating and therefore more desirable with squeamish children.

THE ENEMA

During a cleansing fast when solid food is not taken, the bowels tend to cease functioning and their contents become more concentrated and hard. Unless this residue of waste matter is eliminated, harmful substances may be reabsorbed and reduce the effectiveness of any health regimen.

The enema should be taken only when fasting, or while on a semifast. Enemas and bowel irrigations are not recommended while on a normal or reduced diet.

Obtain an enema apparatus with a 1-2 quart ($\frac{1}{2}$-1 liter) container. The container is filled with warm (about body temperature) water or medicinal tea and placed or hung about 3 ft (1 m) from the floor. Adopt the knee–chest position, or lie on your left side on a towel in the bathroom, or near a toilet. Insert the nozzle into the rectum and allow the water to run in slowly by controlling the intake valve on the hose. When the pressure becomes too strong, or you feel it is becoming difficult to retain the water, stop the water intake and take a short rest; then continue. After the water has been drained off, take out the nozzle and turn on your back. Slowly massage the abdomen from lower left up to the ribs and across the abdomen to the right, with deep circular motions. Retain the water 5-10 minutes and then release the fluid into the toilet.

DOUCHES
A douche is a strong jet or spray of water directed locally or generally, like an ordinary shower. The only type of shower douche I routinely recommend for home use is the *alternate hot and cold shower*. This begins with a comfortably warm shower for 3 minutes, followed by a sudden change to cold for 1-2 minutes. Repeat the whole process for three cycles, ending with cold. Finish off with a brisk towel rub and some exercise.

MORNING DEW WALKS
An old tonic measure is to walk barefooted on the wet morning grass daily, year-round. It has the same effect as local cold foot baths and is very refreshing.

Simple though many of these hydropathic techniques may be, they are very effective aids in channeling the body's vital energies towards health.

PHYSIOTHERAPY AND MASSAGE

Naturopathic physicians use physiotherapy in their treatment of soft-tissue and connective-tissue disorders. These are used for various acute or chronic injuries. Some of the more commonly used physiotherapy devices are shortwave diathermy, microwave therapy, ultraviolet radiation, galvanism, iontophoresis, faradism, and ultrasound.

During my student years while observing therapy sessions at the office of a prominent naturopathic and osteopathic physician, I noticed that in his office, which he shared with other physicians, there were several physiotherapy apparatuses he never made use of the entire time I was at his treatment sessions. In an attempt to draw some information from him I asked what he thought of ultrasound and the other units in the office. His reply, "They are wonderful for practitioner who does not have hands," was characteristic of the pure osteopath.

While acknowledging that one of an osteopath's greatest attributes is trained hands, I have found in practice that certain physiotherapy modalities can greatly accelerate the healing process when properly used in conjunction with standard osteopathic soft-tissue techniques. When weeks of agonizing frictions across fibrocystic and calcified muscle fibers would otherwise be necessary, the use of ultrasound and frictions together might cut therapy time in half. Ultrasound in particular is very useful in removing calcified spurs that would normally require surgery.

Massage, per se, another form of physiotherapy, is not usually performed by the naturopath or osteopath in a busy office practice, although many practitioners recommend massage therapy and many have a massage therapist working in their office. As described in the section on Spinal Manipulation, a specific soft-tissue therapy, sometimes called the neuromuscular technique, is practiced by many osteopaths as an integral part of their therapy. Hydrotherapy, as described under that section, is another frequently used form of physiotherapy.

Spinal manipulation

BASIC HISTORY AND PHILOSOPHY

One of the main therapeutic techniques used by naturopaths as well as chiropractors and osteopaths is spinal manipulation. This method originated in ancient civilizations such as Egypt and Greece, many years before Christ. Hippocrates left detailed suggestions for spinal traction and manipulation. More recently a loosely knit group of lay "bonesetters" practiced widely in Europe and England in the early 1800s. Early in the 1870s a country doctor named Andrew Taylor Still from Virginia expounded the early philosophy of osteopathy. Still, disillusioned with drug therapy by the death of three of his children from spinal meningitis, sought new concepts of healing. Ultimately he became convinced that structural abnormalities affected the function and well-being of the body. In explaining this new science of "osteopathy" he evolved the "rule of the artery". This stated that the cause of disease was reduced blood circulation due to spinal abnormalities. Still saw osteopathy as a complete science and that all disease could be treated by it successfully without any other measures. Still's fervor was a bit exaggerated. Not only has the basic concept of osteopathy changed significantly over the past 100 years to include a more complete understanding of the actual modus operandi of disease and osteopathic therapy, but its scope is now generally considered more limited and it does not dismiss other forms of medicine.

In 1895 an unqualified practitioner from Iowa, Daniel David Palmer, expounded his philosophy of chiropractic. Palmer had overheard his deaf janitor saying that his hearing loss had coincided with a feeling that something in his neck had "gone". Palmer examined his neck, felt an unusual lump, performed a manipulation and the janitor reportedly regained his hearing. Out of this one adjustment grew chiropractic. Palmer developed a theory very similar to Still's, stressing that anatomical faults caused functional disturbances within the body. Palmer espoused "the rule of the nerve", stating that minor spinal displacements caused nerve irritation, which eventually led to disease.

As years have passed, the basic theories and philosophies of osteopathy and chiropractic have grown closer together as medical research and knowledge of spinal disorders has improved. It is now fairly well accepted by osteopaths, chiropractors, and naturopaths that spinal "lesions" (dysfunctions) or "subluxations" cause both changes in blood and nerve supply. Major differences, however, still exist between the two philosophies, which are reflected in both their methods of diagnosis and treatment. The basic concept that structure governs function is accepted by both schools. However, subtle differences of emphasis have led to large differences in actual practice.

The chiropractic philosophy states that "subluxations" impinge on structures (nerves, blood vessels, and lymphatics) passing through the intervertebral foramen, resulting in disease, and that "adjustment" of a subluxated vertebra removes this impingement, thereby restoring to diseased parts their normal innervation (and blood supply). The two major diagnostic techniques used to determine these "subluxations" are palpation and x-ray. Most chiropractors (however, not all, and in fact fewer as time goes by) routinely expose the patient to diagnostic x-ray to diagnose a subluxation. Others rely more on palpation of bony prominences such as the transverse processes of vertebrae to diagnose a positional abnormality. In either case the emphasis is usually on "position". Once this position is determined, manipulation is applied to correct the alignment and, theoretically, relieve the problem either locally or due to referred symptoms elsewhere in the body.

Osteopathy also concerns structural and mechanical faults as they affect the physiological processes, but defines these in relation to the spine as spinal "lesions" or "dysfunctions" rather than "subluxations". These lesions are "... impaired *mobility* in an intervertebral joint in which there may or may not be altered position relations of adjacent vertebrae."[16] The modern definition of the osteopathic or "somatic dysfunction" is a "dysfunction of the spine, joints, muscles and connective tissue and their related nerve, lymph and blood supply".

This concept stresses that the mobility and functional relationship of one bone to its neighbor, and their functional relationship with their muscle and connective tissue components is more important than its positional relationship. As a result of the basic concept of "mobility", osteopaths rarely employ x-rays, except to exclude pathological conditions. The key diagnostic technique used is called *mobility testing*, or *motion palpation*. With this technique each spinal segment is evaluated for proper mobility in all its planes of motion in relation to both the vertebrae above and those below. It is used for peripheral joint diagnosis, as well. Once a spinal lesion is diagnosed, osteopathic therapy is directed to this area to remove these restrictions and allow restoration of proper nervous, blood, and lymph supply, both locally and in referred areas elsewhere in the body. From the two basic philosophies, once again vast differences in actual treatment have evolved between osteopathy and chiropractic. Chiropractic, with its stress on "position", routinely and almost exclusively has used "chiropractic manipulation". This usually involves the use of short levers or direct contacts to bony prominences, with high-velocity, short-amplitude thrust to alter the position of the subluxation into alignment.

A historical distinction has been made in the past that osteopaths tend to use the principle of longer levers and indirect contact in their manipulations.

While this may have some historical fact, in reality actual techniques of many spinal manipulations of either chiropractors or osteopaths are the same or very similar. It is also fair to mention that there is an incredible variation, practitioner to practitioner, in both schools of healing, The main distinction, however, between a typical or traditional chiropractic and osteopathic treatment is that the osteopath routinely spends much time and energy working on the soft-tissue and connective tissue structures prior to actual osseous manipulation. This soft-tissue manipulation is considered even more essential to complete healing than the more dramatic "clicking" and "popping" elicited from osseous manipulation. Quoting Stoddard again, we find:

It is possible to restore normal alignment and yet not restore good function. Ideally we should attempt to restore both perfection of structure and harmonious function, but of the two the function is the more important. When we manipulate the spine, we are not so much concerned with putting a bone back into place as with removing any mechanical hindrances to the restoration of normal movements in the affected joints.[17]

In explanation, for example, it does little permanent good to repeatedly adjust a malpositioned or malfunctioning vertebra if the reason for its hindrance in function or position is a muscle or other connective tissue structure. As with pitching a tent, if the tent is found functionally distressed or malpositioned due to an improperly set guy line, it will do little good simply to realign the tent without first loosening or tightening the abnormal supports. Thus, in osteopathy a great deal of time is spent in normalizing the relationship of muscles, ligaments, tendons, fascia and joint capsules to their bony partners. Newer non-manipulative techniques of osteopathy called muscle energy techniques have evolved to restore normal joint function. These are very useful when traditional osteopathic manipulation is either contraindicated or the patient wishes or requires a more gentle approach.

Although I believe that traditional osteopathy is broader in concept than traditional chiropractic therapy, the difference between any two osteopaths or chiropractors can be immense, with some osteopaths more resembling chiropractors in practice, and vice versa.

Spinal manipulation is only one of the many modalities used by the traditional naturopath. No one method is sufficient in most cases to create real harmony within the body. It is in the intelligent use of all natural therapies, for the benefit of the patient, that the best form of medicine is to be found.

THE PRINCIPLES AS APPLIED IN PRACTICE

The first principle of osteopathy is not unique to this discipline at all. Just as Hippocrates stated, "vis medicatrix naturae" (only nature heals), Still reaffirmed that the greatest law governing the human body was its self-sufficiency and ability to heal itself if all hindrances were first removed. The second fundamental principle, as has already been stated, is that "structure governs function". The manner in which structure may affect the body was unclear during the birth of osteopathy. Still's "rule of the artery" and Palmer's "rule of the nerve" were early attempts to explain how spinal lesions or subluxations did their destructive work.

Early osteopaths and chiropractors assumed that alterations in spinal function placed direct pressure on either blood vessels or nerves, causing complete or partial blockage as they emerged from the intervertebral foramina. This has been proven untrue except in very severe trauma, or possibly in relation to lesions in the upper cervical region with their close association to vertebral arteries and veins which pass through the foramina on the transverse process. Actual dislocations, disc lesions, or pathological changes can produce such effects, but the spinal lesion or subluxation per se, which remains within the normal range of the vertebral segment, can never do so. What does occur, however, is indirect compression of other nerves or blood vessels due to irritation, inflammation, edema, metabolic by-product accumulation, and pH changes, leading to local and referred symptoms similar to actual compression. The key, therefore, to understanding spinal lesions is the soft-tissue components of the functional unit of the spinal column.

What occurs with a typical acute spinal lesion is swelling in response to improper body mechanics, or local, visceral, or peripheral trauma. This causes congestion, edema, decreased oxygen, increased carbon dioxide, and increased pH. This may lead to indirect nerve irritation or compression, causing pain, paresthesia, hyperesthesia, numbness, hypertonicity or hypotonicity, reflex vasoconstriction or vasodilation, and loss of muscle power or atrophy, depending on the nerve involved and the severity and length of the compression. The cause of a spinal lesion may be improper body mechanics causing abnormal strains on the spine or periarticular structures (muscles, tendons, ligaments, articular capsules, discs, etc.), or it may be due to local, visceral, or peripheral trauma.

The role of improper body mechanics is fairly easy to understand. Abnormal pressure exerted on the vertebral segment due to altered spinal curves causes local tissue changes in muscle, ligament, bones, and discs, which may result in compression or irritation of the closely associated spinal nerves, leading to altered conduction, and changes in the tissue or organs supplied. Compression of blood vessels (directly or indirectly), and vasoconstriction or dilation due to abnormal nervous impulses, can alter blood flow to tissues and organs, resulting in congestion or reduced blood flow.

Local trauma is also easy to understand as a cause of spinal lesions. This is due to the commonly occurring strained or twisted spine, or some severe local blow or fall. The immediate results are those of the typical spinal lesion, with acute symptoms of pain, edema, heat, muscle spasm, limited motion, and possibly referred or reflex symptoms. Chronic lesions show limited mobility and increased connective tissue, but less pain. Referred or reflex symptoms may or may not be apparent, but observed or unobserved degenerative changes are taking place and vitality is being reduced in the tissues and organs supplied from that vertebral nerve center.

Peripheral or visceral causes of spinal lesions is a subject usually only understood by practitioners of spinal therapy. Abnormal stimulation in a tissue or organ may cause contraction of the spinal muscles in 2–3 segments on the same side of the spine at levels that correspond to its nervous supply. Later this muscle spasm spreads and may set up the very conditions of a spinal lesion with indirect nerve compression which in turn sends abnormal impulses to the organ or tissue at fault, aggravating or perpetuating the original cause. Other more direct pathways may exist such as nerve irritation with subsequent neuritis.

What all of this means in simple terms is that an injury or "Somatic Dysfunction" not only elicits local and referred pain, but may also cause an alteration in the nerve, blood, or lymph supply to distant tissues and visceral organs, resulting in a disease state. Certainly this can be understood or accepted in relation to the nervous supply being directly altered to a muscle, causing pain, twitching, spasm, or even complete atrophy. The fact that spinal lesions can also profoundly affect internal organs should not seem too remarkable when we consider that their entire functioning is dependent on nervous impulses, either directly or through vasomotor nerves affecting their blood supply. There is plenty of evidence, both clinical and experimental, that the osteopathic "Somatic Dysfunction" or chiropractic "subluxation" causes physical, chemical, and tissue changes, not only in the local area, but also in the organs and viscera that receive their innervation from the same spinal segments. It is on this proven basis that spinal therapy is used to help treat internal complaints. I can remember quite well the first time I went for chiropractic therapy and listened with horror to other patients extolling the beneficial effects of chiropractic therapy for their asthma, sexual disorders, high blood pressure, their child's bed-wetting, and a whole host of other complaints. I congratulated myself that I was not so gullible as to believe such nonsense and that at least I had come for a back complaint, the proper realm of chiropractic, and would go away with something better than all this hocus-pocus. It was not until 15 years later, when I was literally forced into learning about osteopathy to attain my aim of becoming a naturopath, that I finally understood how accurate such assertions were.

The naturopathic approach to the use of osteopathy or other spinal manipulation is to employ this technique as one would any other tool of naturopathy. The aim of its use is to normalize nervous, blood, and lymph supply to diseased organs, or the body as a whole. This increases local nutrition, removes congestion, and raises general vitality so that healing may progress more rapidly. For those interested in pursuing this subject, I suggest Stoddard's two books, *Manual of Osteopathic Practice, and Manual of Osteopathic Technique*, and *Principles of Manuel Medicine (Second Edition)* by Philip E. Greenman, Williams & Wilkins 1996

HEALTH TOPICS OF SPECIAL INTEREST

POSSIBLE TOXIC EFFECTS OF SOME NUTRITIONAL AND BOTANICAL PREPARATIONS

Although some nutritional and botanical preparations can have toxic effects, the dosages required to produce such effects are usually far in excess of the normal prescriptive dose. As with nearly all substances the body is exposed to, even the seemingly most benign, excessive or prolonged use may produce undesirable, or even toxic effects. The criterion for determining how safe a nutrient, botanical medication, or even a drug is lies in how wide is the span between its pharmacologically effective dose and the dose where toxic effects are known to occur.

In general, nutritional supplement therapy and botanical medicine have a fairly wide range of safety between the normally prescribed dose and the dose at which known toxic effects can occur. In the press we periodically read of cases where a particular vitamin, mineral, or herb that may have been in use for many years has been found to cause undesirable, or even dangerous effects. Such reports can often be based on slanted research, placing a cloud of fear over an extremely useful substance.

An example of this occurred recently when the press covered widely the finding that vitamin B6 caused sensory neuropathy and ataxia in some patients. Immediately nearly every one of my patients on vitamin B6 therapy called with concerned questions about why I could have prescribed a medication that would paralyze them! Upon investigation of these stories, it has been found that the dose used to cause these toxic effects was from 2000–5000 milligrams (mg) daily of vitamin B6 for from 40 months at the 2000 mg per day level to as little as 2 months at the 5000 mg dose level. The recommended dietary allowance (RDA) for vitamin B6 is 2 mg daily. The usual therapeutic dose is between 50 and 250 mg daily. The dose required to cause these problems was 2500 times the RDA or between 8–100 times the doses used in therapy! It was later revealed that all the symptoms spontaneously disappeared when the subjects stopped taking such extreme doses of this vitamin.

Fortunately, such is the nature of naturopathy, we do not rely on the particular properties of just one herb to effect cures. We are skilled in the medicinal usage of many different herbs; a single herb has many therapeutically active constituents.

What is emerging in the literature, and often the focus of some slanted media reporting by the more commercial channels, is that some vitamins, minerals, botanical and other preparations have contraindicative effects with some pharmaceutical medicines. For example, if someone is on warfarin, then it may not necessarily be a wise thing just to start taking St John's wort (*Hypericum per-foratum*) without getting proper advice.

Now of course, this relational contraindication is precisely that; it has to do with the relative properties of the two medicines. And there are many known contraindications, and doubtless there are many more to be found out. But the whole thing here is one of perception. It is often sensationalized that, taking this instance, that therefore St John's wort may not be good for warfarin patients. It should be seen the other way around; warfarin is not good for those on *Hypericum*. After all, *Hypericum* has antithrombic effects, and no known dangerous side effects, unlike warfarin.

In this context it is interesting to note that many doctors still denigrate the value of herbal medicines, with arguments that they "don't work". Here we have an instance where *Hypericum* clearly works, and now that it "works", it becomes a problem for doctors!

Certainly vitamins, minerals, and botanical medications can have toxic effects, just as severe and as dangerous as drugs can if taken in excess. But please note, they do have wonderful beneficial and therapeutic effects, although many doctors are only just beginning to realize, or admit it. What is important to know, however is that the range of safety of most of these preparations is far wider than that of most drugs, and botanical extracts prescribed under the guidance of a trained herbalist or naturopath are certainly safe to use within recommended dosage controls, just as it should be.

The following survey of possible toxic effects of vitamins and botanicals, with some dose guidelines, may prove useful for reference, as you read the individual diseases in Part II. These toxic ranges do not apply to all individuals. It is possible for an individual to be more sensitive to a particular nutrient or botanical medication, just as it is possible for a person to be less sensitive to it. Some individuals may have an increased need for a particular nutrient due to an abnormality of their biochemistry.[18]

It is fairly common that a particular enzyme deficiency may require a particular nutrient far in excess of standard doses. In these patients, a higher than average dose is in reality the correct dose for their optimum health.[19] Other patients, who suffer from malabsorption, may in fact only be able to absorb a small percent of the oral doses given. In these cases, large doses taken orally may allow a standard dose to be absorbed internally. In this case, most of the nutrient is excreted, with only a small fraction actually having any therapeutic effect. Dose prescriptions must be chosen individually, keeping these and other factors in mind.

Vitamin toxicity

Bioflavonoids: Used to be called vitamin P (quercetin, rutin, hesperidin, citrin, and others such as oligomeric proanthocyanidins). Not toxic in doses up to 3000 mg daily and more.

Natural sources: Especially present in the skin of fruit and vegetables, flowers, berries, tea, and all plant sprouts, which may largely be missing in the western diet.

Biotin: No toxic effects have been reported. Therapeutic doses up to 5000 mcg daily.

Essential Fatty Acids (EFAs): While not often thought of as vitamins, the small chain fatty acids that make up the omega-3 (linolenic acid) and omega-6 (linoleic acid) groups are in reality vitamins. This is because the body cannot synthesize them, and has to obtain them from outside sources. Supplement diet to 3 g (2 tbsp) daily

Natural sources: Fish oil, cod liver oil, flaxseed oil, evening primrose oil, tofu, kelp, butternuts, nuts and seeds. Subject to loss through heat and light.

Folic acid: High doses (15 mg daily for months) may cause sleep disturbances, nausea, irritability, abnormal distension, anorexia, flatulence, and malaise. High doses mask a vitamin B12 deficiency and therefore recommended doses are 400 mcg as a standard dose, 800 mcg in pregnancy. High doses may be used as long as vitamin B12 status is adequate and no toxic symptoms are present. Doses more than 750 mcg ought to be accompanied with B12 supplementation, to avoid central nervous system symptoms as for B6.

P.A.B.A. (para amino benzoic acid): Sometimes called a contingent nutrient. Up to 1000 mg daily is generally OK, but can cause skin rash, nausea and fever in some sensitive individuals.

Natural sources: The B vitamins are generally found in whole (unrefined) grains (husks) e.g. rice, lentil, wheat, oats, etc., seed germ and kernels, nuts, yeast, soy, beans, peas, egg yolk.

Pangamic acid: Can be found in brewer's yeast, seeds and nuts, brown rice, and whole grain cereals. Natural sources of PABA include brewer's yeast, whole grain cereals, yoghurt, and liver.

Vitamin A: standard doses are from 10,000 to 25,000 IU (international units) daily. This vitamin is highly toxic if taken in excess. Main toxic effects are a transient hydrocephalus and vomiting. Chronic vitamin A toxicity can occur at supplemental levels at or above 50,000 IU daily, if taken for prolonged periods. The emulsified forms are best tolerated for higher dose levels. It is suggested that for long-term high vitamin A use that the patient take the supplement three weeks and then discontinue for one week to allow liver clearance.

Toxic effects include fatigue; lethargy; bone or joint pain; headaches; insomnia; restlessness; dry, rough, or scaly skin; loss of hair; loss of appetite; enlargement of liver and spleen; edema; and other cirrhotic-like changes; abnormal bone growth; and premature closure of epiphyseal plates.

Hypercarotenosis, or the toxic effects of large doses of carotene (vitamin A precursor found in foods such as carrots), has as its only toxic effect the yellowing of the skin. This is not known to cause any clinical symptoms and is reversible by reducing or stopping excess intake of carotene-containing foods or supplements.

Natural sources: Vitamin A is naturally present in cod liver oil, liver, parsley and other green herbs, carrots, fruit, green leafy vegetables like spinach, egg yolk, tomatoes.

Vitamin B complex: Vitamin B is a family of individual B-vitamins, with all sorts of synergies between members, some known, others yet to be discovered. A "multi-B" ought to include each member of this family.

Vitamin B1: Few toxic effects of this vitamin by mouth have been reported. Rare cases of anaphylactic shock occur from intramuscular or intravenous injection in hypersensitive individuals. Other symptoms include generalized urticaria, facial edema, wheezing, and difficulty breathing. Doses up to 125 mg daily are quite safe. Excess can cause anxiety and nervousness, sweating, fluid retention.

Vitamin B2 (riboflavin): Essentially non-toxic, doses up to 40 mg daily are fine.

Vitamin B3 (niacin, nicotinic acid, nicotinamide): Due to its vasodilating action, transient tingling or flushing sensations do occur at normally used doses. Other symptoms include nausea, gastric irritation, abnormal liver function, jaundice, elevated uric acid levels, and abnormal glucose tolerance. Excessive amounts over time might cause cold hands and feet, fatty liver, and an increase in heart rate and breathing rate

Vitamin B5 (pantothenic acid): In doses over 200 mg daily can create inflammation in joints; tends to be dose-related.

Vitamin B6 (pyridoxine): Toxicity of vitamin B6 has been considered extremely low until recently when transient sensory neuropathy and ataxia were reported at doses from 1200–2000 mg daily for extended periods of time. Usual doses range from 50–250 mg. Vitamin B6 is completely safe at these, or even twice these levels.

Vitamin B12 (cobalamin, cyanocobalamin): No toxic effects reported.

Vitamin B15: (pangamic acid): Amounts over 300 mg daily might cause drowsiness and mild skin flushing.

Vitamin B17: (amygdaline, laetrile): Contains cyanide in minute doses. The history of this B vitamin is an interesting one, and its potential as an anti-cancer agent requires further study. Especially concentrated in stone fruit kernels (e.g. apricot seed kernels).

Vitamin C (ascorbic acid, ascorbate): High doses (10 g or over) have been implicated in the formation of kidney stones. This has been disputed by some sources. Rebound scurvy has been reported from subjects suddenly withdrawing from very high doses of vitamin C. Diarrhea occurs at varying doses, seemingly dependent upon the body's need for this nutrient. Scurvy in newborns whose mothers took supplements, of high doses of vitamin C has been reported. This is not reported in the breast-fed infant. Usual doses range from 250 mg to 30 g or more daily. Given intravenously at 30–50 g daily in some cases, vitamin C is best taken in a buffered form rather than straight ascorbic acid, given its ability to disturb gastric function. Look for a form which contains other ascorbates such as sodium ascorbate, calcium ascorbate, magnesium ascorbate and others. Powdered form is best, without artificial flavoring. Ought to also contain bioflavonoids, synergists which occur with vitamin C in nature to protect vitamin C from oxidation, and ensure maximum vitamin C absorption.

Natural sources: Because vitamin C is unstable to heat (processing, cooking), light, and time, and because of modern practices in which fruit is picked while still unripe, and further because of increasing requirements given increases in physiological, emotional and biochemical stress, the traditional sources of vitamin C, fresh raw fruit and uncooked (salad) vegetables, can no longer be relied upon for vitamin C needs.

Vitamin D: Vitamin D, if ingested in excess, can cause excessive calcification of bones or elsewhere in the body (i.e. organs, especially kidneys) and may encourage kidney stone formation. Elevated serum calcium levels occur at high levels of intake. Vitamin D activity is enhanced by sunlight. In most people on a normal diet or with adequate sun exposure, vitamin D use is not usually warranted. Doses of 400–1000 IU may be used if no other vitamin D-fortified foods are used concurrently. Due to the fact that many nutritional supplements list vitamin D as an ingredient, it is possible for toxicity to occur, unless labels are read carefully. Intake of 2000–3000 IU daily may become toxic.

Vitamin E: Generally considered non-toxic. High levels (1200–1600 IU), if taken suddenly, have been reported to temporarily raise blood pressures. This later normalizes. Vitamin E may interfere with vitamin K activity, acting as an anti-coagulant in high levels. Vitamin E has also caused immune suppression at high levels. Usual doses range from 200–800 IU daily, with doses up to 2000 IU being used in some disorders.

Vitamin K: Used mostly in the newborn, to prevent hemorrhagic disease due to a prothrombin deficiency in the first few days of life. Also used as an adjunct to modify anti-coagulant therapy. Toxic effects include hemolytic anemia and kernicterus in infants.

Vitamin D (1, 25-dihydroxycholecalciferol): The therapeutic range is from 400–1600 IU daily. More than 4000 IU daily might cause nausea, diarrhea, excessive thirst, polyurea, and even kidney damage.

Natural sources: Vitamin D is synthesized in the body by the action of sunlight on the skin. It is richly present in fish liver oils, egg yolk, sprouts.

Vitamin E (tocopherol): All studies comparing the natural form (d-alpha tocopherol) with many other, artificial forms of tocopherol (DL-alpha tocopherol), demonstrate that d-alpha tocopherol is the only form you should supplement with, if you want effectiveness. Doses higher than 1600 mg daily may be counterproductive, and can cause fatigue, dermatitis, and allergy. Increase doses above 400 IU daily slowly to prevent blood pressure from increasing with use.

Natural sources: Unrefined soybean, wheat germ and corn oils, grains, raw nuts and seeds, eggs.

Choline: Therapeutic range is between 1 g and 20 g daily; excess can cause nausea, diarrhea, dizziness, excess salivation, anxiety. High doses cause a fishy body odor.

Natural sources: Beans, whole grains and cereals, lecithin, egg yolk, yeast, liver.

Inositol: Safe up to 0.5 mg/kg body weight. Might cause diarrhea.

Natural sources: Synthesized in the gut by floral bacteria and is also found in nuts and seeds, beans, grains, organ meats, and citrus fruits.

Carnitine: Neither requirement nor toxicity known.

Vitamin K (Phylloquinone—K1; menaquinone—K2; menadione—K3): Usually non-toxic up to 2 mg daily, but large doses have been associated with thrombosis, vomiting, porphyrinuria, kernicterus in infants

Natural sources: Synthesized in the gut by flora; other sources include soy beans, kelp, spinach, cabbage, broccoli, and liver.

Botanical toxicity

The use of herbs in the usual prescribed doses is generally quite safe. Many of the toxic effects of overdose that do occur are simply the body's action to rid itself of the substances through vomiting or diarrhea. *Some herbs, however, are extremely dangerous and have a very narrow range of safety.* Thorough knowledge of botanical medications and their possible toxic effects is essential before using these remedies. The following list of herbs and their common toxic effects is partial only, concentrating on the botanical preparations used medicinally that are most toxic, or those that have been mentioned frequently throughout this book. The toxic effects listed are not complete. For a detailed description of botanical toxicology, consult An *Introduction to the Toxicology of Common Botanical Medicinal Substances*, by Francis Brinker, pp. 1–123.

Aconite (*Aconitum napellus*): This herb is extremely toxic and has a very narrow range of safety. Its usual therapeutic dose of tincture is 1–8 drops, while toxic reactions may occur at only 10 drops. Fatal dose is 5 mL of tincture. Most frequently used in homeopathic dilutions, and as such is very safe. Toxic effects include nausea, vomiting, dizziness, tingling, burning, numbness, impaired speech, blurred vision, headache, anxiety, muscular weakness, low blood pressure, weak pulse, irregular heartbeat, chest pain, shallow breathing, excess perspiration, low body temperature, and death, due to respiratory failure or ventricular fibrillation.

Anemone pulsatilla: Toxic effects are abdominal pain, nausea, vomiting, burning in mouth or throat, cardiac arrhythmia, slow pulse, weakness, difficulty in breathing, paralysis, convulsions, coma.

Arnica montana: Topical use of the undiluted tincture can cause local irritation or eczema-type inflammation. Usual internal therapeutic dose is 1–10 drops of tincture. Toxic dose is 2 fl oz (60 mL) of tincture. Used internally mostly in diluted homeopathic potencies. Toxic effects (internal use): nausea, vomiting, diarrhea, muscular weakness, reduced pulse, cardiovascular collapse, convulsions, coma, and possibly death.

Artemisia santonica: Fatal dose is 2–5 grains for children, more for adult. *This herb has a very narrow safety margin.* Toxic effects: nausea, vomiting, diarrhea, cramps, vertigo, sweating, flushing of face, dilated pupils, reduced blood pressure, slowed pulse, reduced urine flow, convulsions, death by respiratory paralysis. May cause blindness or aphasia if taken over prolonged period.

Belladonna (*Atropa belladonna*): Very toxic. Normally used in homeopathic dilutions only and as such is safe for use. This remedy is a component of most over-the-counter teething mixtures. Toxic effects (due to atropine poisoning): nausea, diarrhea, vomiting, dry mouth, flushing, dilated pupils, rapid pulse, increased blood pressure, incoordination, speech impairment, visual impairment, hallucinations, coma, death.

Cactus grandiflorus: Its major action is as a cardiac stimulant. In excess may cause increased heartbeat, arrhythmias, headaches, vertigo, angina, cardiospasm, mental symptoms, and inflammation of the heart or pericardium.

Comfrey (*Symphytum officinale*): Hepatocellular adenomas in rats have developed after use of comfrey leaf in diet up to 8 percent of total intake or of root at 1 percent of diet for over a year. This dose is clearly above any reasonable intake, as normally prescribed. Care needs to be taken by those who consume large amounts of comfrey in the belief that its vitamin B12 content is high enough to be of significant nutritional value. One would need to eat 1–2 lb (550–1 kg) of comfrey leaves daily to get adequate vitamin B12 levels, and at this level toxicity may occur.

Foxglove (*Digitalis purpurea*): Contains many cardioactive glycosides that, when taken in excess, can cause an increase in ventricular irritability, ventricular tachycardia, and fibrillation, leading to death. Early symptoms include nausea, vomiting, appetite loss, visual abnormalities, drowsiness, and low blood pressure.

Indian snakeroot (*Rauwolfia serpentine*): The toxic effects are those of reserpine. These include diarrhea, abdominal cramps, sedation, pinpoint pupils, low blood pressure, and coma.

Lily-of-the-valley (*Convallaria majalis*): Contains many cardioactive glycosides that, if taken in excess, can cause cardiac arrhythmias, raised blood pressure, mental confusion, weakness, circulatory collapse, and death. Its toxic effects occur more rapidly than with digitalis.

Lobelia inflata: Toxic effects are due to lobeline; however, emesis normally occurs to prevent this. Toxic effects include nausea, vomiting, weakness, loss of consciousness, coma, and death.

May-apple or American mandrake (*Podophyllum peltatum*): Externally can cause severe ulceration and dermatitis. Internally may cause nausea, diarrhea, emesis and severe gastroenteritis, which may lead to death.

Pennyroyal (*Hedeoma pulegioides*): May cause liver damage. Standard dose is 2–10 drops oil. Toxic dose 4 mL.

Peruvian bark (*Cinchona ledgeriana*): Contains quinine and quinidine. If used for any prolonged or excessive doses, will cause the following toxic effects: nausea, vomiting, headache, tinnitus, deafness, visual disturbances, dilated pupils, abdominal pains, mental confusion, restlessness, weakness, delirium, and psychotic changes. If taken in pregnancy it is teratogenic, causing congenital visual and auditory damage.

Poke root (*Phytolacca decandra*): Berries from plant are very poisonous. Tincture is made from whole plant. Toxic effects: nausea, vomiting, diarrhea, gastrointestinal cramps, weakness, convulsions, reduced blood pressure, slowed pulse, coma, death due to respiratory paralysis.

Sassafras (*Sassafras albidum*): Tests have shown safrole, its main constituent, to cause cancer when injected under the skin in rats. This has not been observed via the normal oral route.

Squill (*Urginea scilla*): Toxic effects: nausea, vomiting, diarrhea, nephritis, cardiac arrhythmia, heart block, convulsions, death.

White bryony (*Bryonia alba*): Used most frequently in homeopathic dilutions. Toxic effects (of tincture): vomiting, diarrhea, bronchial irritation, cough, gastrointestinal upset, jaundice, weak shallow pulse, dizziness, headache, dilated pupils, temperature drop, collapse, death.

Wormseed (*Chenopodium anthelminticum*): Experiments show subcutaneous application causes cancer in rats. Other routes of entry as yet are not implicated. Other toxic effects include: nausea, vomiting, headache, tinnitus, reduced audio and visual acuity, sluggish bowels, ulcers, reduced blood pressure, paralysis, death.

Wormwood (*Artemisia absinthium*): Therapeutic dose of oil is 1–5 drops. Toxic dose is 15 mL of oil. Toxic effects: nausea, vomiting, unpleasant dreams, impotence, lack of vitality, headache, trembling, convulsions, death. Do not use in pregnancy (emmenagogue).

ANTIBIOTICS

Since the discovery of the first antibiotics in the late 1930s and early 1940s these "wonder drugs" have been used extensively in both hospital and outpatient care. Their incredible effectiveness in controlling or even destroying pathogenic bacteria has led to their widespread acceptance and use. Very few people question that, in case of infection, the obvious treatment is the use of antibiotics.

Infections that, a mere 70 years ago would have caused a great deal of suffering and even death, are now controlled effectively by antibiotics. Efficacy is not the question here. Safety, however, is.

A careful review of the known reactions and complications caused by the use of antibiotics is a sobering experience. In reading this information please bear in mind that antibiotic use is often essential to prevent organ damage or death. Antibiotics are wonderful tools if used sparingly and wisely; however, these drugs are a double-edged sword capable of great good and also great harm.

In terms of numbers, this planet could be described as being a bug's world. Millions and even billions of different species of bacteria, fungi, virus, protozoa and others, inhabit every nook and cranny, from polar regions to active volcanoes, the air, the oceans, the land. They were here prior to the entry of the animal and human species, and will doubtless be here long after we have gone. On and in everyone, there are trillions of bugs of many kinds. Golden staph, Streptococcus, Meningococcus, Pneumoniae, Tuberculosis, E. coli, etc. are present with us much of, if not all, the time.

All bugs have very important roles to play. They are all nature's little helpers; they act as biological agents of the ecosphere, constantly involved in recycling decaying matter, scavenging, and generally keeping the planet in sufficient health to maintain life. They know how to cultivate organically, they know what to do to maintain their own future, and they've been doing it since the dawn of life.

Within us, they perform the same sorts of duties they do on us and around us;

in fact, without them, we would die. For example, the bowel houses enormous quantities of these microscopic bacteria called "flora". In a healthy colon for example, there are between 100,000,000,000 and 1,000,000,000,000, of them, in every milliliter of bowel fluid. There are between 400 and 500 different species we know of residing along the length of the human digestive system, of which the best known are the *Lactobacillus acidophilus* and *Bifidobacterium bifidum*. In the healthy gut, they are all friendly, meant to be there; each has its place within this little "ecosystem", some live in the mucous lining, some on the right side, some on the left, others in the middle, some at one end, others at the other end. They communicate with us when there are imbalances, and play important roles in nutrition, digestion, including synthesis of valuable nutrients such as vitamin B5 and vitamin K, and production of valuable acids that actually nourish the enteral mucosa.

Flora also play a vital role in immune functioning, for example they produce natural antibiotics and anti-cancer substances. In a healthy intestinal environment, other opportunistic "bugs" cannot survive; our gut flora effectively deals with intruders, parasites, worms, etc., as a natural immunity to these things. They create "natural antibiotics" — substances which keep out unwanted microorganisms. They are involved in detoxification, and perform a host of other beneficial activities.

The practice of treating infection using antibiotics (and vaccines) is based on the idea that "bugs" cause disease. The commonly held "germ theory" developed largely from the work of Louis Pasteur, a microbiologist of the 19th century, who held that bugs (micro-organisms) which get into our system opportunistically, actually cause disease in our bodies. If we can stop these bugs getting in, or kill them as soon as they enter, we can essentially win the war, or so the theory goes.

Pierre Bechamp, his contemporary, held that the bugs are not themselves the *cause* of disease, but their opportunistic invasion is more the *effect* of a disease state. That is, they act in the same way within us as they do outside us, recycling, scavenging, etc. His idea was, that if the human (animal) organism is maintained in reasonable health, then imbalances of bugs will not occur, and disease will not occur. A healthy body will be able to maintain good health despite the bugs. We might well add … because of them.

Naturopathic philosophy favors the Bechampian model. It holds that God or Nature has created a body, replete with mechanisms to maintain health balances (homeostasis), and provided the animal lives in harmony with its natural environment, optimal health will be a natural concomitant.

And in the animal, plant and insect world, this is exactly what we see: balance and interdependence between the species. It could be argued that to the extent that the environment is polluted by man, imbalances have occurred which have brought stress, increased trauma and disease to the whole of the life-sphere.

Chemical warfare against our friends

The toxomolecular approach, developed on the Pasteurian model, opposes these presuppositions and suggests Nature (or God) got it wrong, that the bugs are in fact the enemy, and ought to be destroyed by all necessary means of chemical intervention discoverable. The dogma is: kill the bug, and get back to health.

The facts are, that even when we come into contact with a "contagious" germ, a large majority of people do not become infected, and even among those who do become infected, a large majority do not get sick. Even the dreaded poliovirus produces no symptoms whatsoever in over 90% of people who contact it. The notorious meningococcal bacterium which is involved in the deaths of some people each year, is present in up to 25% of the human population, and indeed most "killer bugs" are present in healthy human populations without producing any symptoms of disease. This would not, indeed, could not, be the case if the Pasteur germ theory were correct.

The role of bacteria in disease

Before exploring the fascinating and complex role of antibiotics as both savior and killer it is necessary to first understand the role of bacteria in disease.

When a susceptible person is exposed to a pathogenic bacteria (one which has the capacity to "cause" a disease), these bacteria can multiply and cause damage locally or systemically. The body's reaction to this intruder is to initiate a complicated series of defense measures. The end result of this interaction between the pathogenic bacteria and the body's defenses is termed an infection, the outcome of which is determined by several factors. These include the vitality of the individual's immune response, and the strength and numbers of the pathogenic bacteria. Human immune vitality is affected by hereditary factors, environmental factors, stress, activity level, diet, nutrition, mental attitude and other influences.

It is important to recognize that "the association of bacteria with human tissue does not necessarily constitute an infection nor is it necessarily a pressing indication for eradication of the organisms". As noted above, even so-called pathogenic bacteria are commonly found to colonize the body's skin and mucus membranes without causing the slightest bit of harm to the host.

Antibiotic over-prescription: a 20th-century mistake

The proper evaluation of when and if an antibiotic is safe or necessary is not as routine as we might assume by the frequency they are currently being prescribed. "Unfortunately, in many actual instances of the invasion and destruction of tissue which constitutes active infection, antibiotics are prescribed on purely clinical grounds without recourse to bacteriological evidence. On numerous occasions those infections are trivial and self-limiting. If antibiotics were free of toxicity, it would matter little how often they were misused. Sadly, analysis of the deaths (due to antibiotic sensitivity) reveals that the original disease treated with those drugs was sometimes minor and hardly in the category of high mortality".

63

Antibiotic toxicity

Antibiotics are not free of toxicity. In fact they can be extremely toxic, as we will see. It is in the best interests of the general population that antibiotics be seen for what they are ... extremely useful life-saving medications that unfortunately carry significant risk in their use and are substances that should be reserved for use only as a last resort in cases where no other therapy exists and the life or organ is in direct and obvious danger. Unfortunately this is not how antibiotics are commonly used today and some of the following reactions and complications are a direct result of their indiscriminate use.

By far the most obvious and severe reaction to antibiotic use is immediate anaphylactic shock. "Anaphylaxis and anaphylactoid reactions are abrupt, often life-threatening episodes, secondary to the liberation of certain chemical mediators, and their effects on target organs. The number of agents known to trigger such reactions is expanding, with the most common fatal reactions secondary to penicillin, iodinated contrast materials and hymenoptera stings. Limited studies point to upper airway obstruction and circulatory collapse as the cause of death". (*J. Emerg. Med.* 1983, 1(1): 83–95) Allergy and hypersensitivity reactions to antibiotics are particularly troublesome with penicillin and streptomycin. The topical applications of neomycin and other antibiotics increase the risk of inducing sensitization and allergic reactions. In a previously sensitized person these may be severe and life-threatening.

The skin seems to be particularly sensitive to allergic reactions to antibiotics. These hypersensitivity reactions vary in intensity and severity. Skin reactions that resolve spontaneously in a few days such as the common ampicillin rash which occurs in 5–10 percent of patient populations is not of great concern. However, other antibiotic skin reactions are more troublesome and some are life-threatening. Contact dermatitis can follow antibiotic eye drops and eye ointments, especially neomycin. In patients with chronic inflammatory ear disease, allergic patch testing demonstrated that 35% were due to antibiotic medication. Systemic contact dermatitis, termed "baboon syndrome", can occur causing diffuse skin redness and inflammation covering the entire buttocks, upper inner thighs, and axillae. Various allergy tests were performed on 245 patients suffering from chronic recurrent urticaria, with positive reactions to penicillin occurring in between 24–37 percent. The conclusion is "that these studies indicate that penicillin has an important role on the etiology and maintenance of chronic urticaria". Phototoxicity is a well-recognized problem of tetracycline therapy causing skin fragility, denudation and blister formation of sun-exposed skin. Even upon discontinuation of these antibiotics, the skin can remain fragile for up to seven months. A far more serious skin reaction to antibiotics is toxic epidermal necrolysis (Lyell's syndrome). In this reaction between 25–100% of the body's surface is covered with fluid-filled lesions. Death occurs in between 20–40% of cases. Another rare but possibly fatal skin reaction is penicillin-induced generalized post-inflammatory elastolysis. The following is a report in the literature of this severe and fatal reaction. "A 13-year-old boy received penicillin for influenza and otitis media. Within days of taking this medication, he developed recurrent edema of the face and a generalized urticarial eruption that waxed and waned. The salient and unusual features of this person's disease were: (a) a senile appearance of his face with flaccid folds and sagging of the skin; (b) dermatitis herpetiformis-like cutaneous lesions; and (c) gluten-sensitive enteropathy. Elastolysis increased in time and led to further deterioration of the patients' physical appearance. Six years later, the patient developed internal manifestations and died". (*Am. J. Dermapathology* 1983, 5(3): 267–76)

The ears are particularly sensitive to damage by medications. Today the number of potentially ototoxic substances is high, but the most important class is that of the aminoglycoside antibiotics. "The prevalence and severity of hearing impairment caused by these ototoxic drugs are surprisingly high. In 33.7% of these cases, the hearing impairment caused by ototoxic antibiotics was of severe degree and in 25.4% it was extremely severe. Because of the very poor speech intelligibility, most probably not only the spiral organ but the vestibulocochlear nerve and the higher auditory pathways are also affected by these antibiotics. In some cases, the severe distortion in sound perception cannot be compensated even by a hearing aid of the best quality, and lip-reading which was advised occasionally was without any result". (*Audiology* 1982, 21(2): 159–76) Until 1981 pediatricians commonly considered aminoglycoside antibiotics such as neomycin to be less ototoxic in neonates than in adults. However, evidence of abnormal hearing maturation and of anatomical damage of the cochlea has been found. Laboratory findings corroborate clinical findings that aminoglycoside antibiotics are more toxic in neonates than adults. Studies also show that even topically applied aminoglycoside antibiotics contained in eardrops may cause hearing loss. These findings underscore once again the special hazard for the inner ear that is associated with the clinical use of neomycin, regardless of the route of administration.

Two relatively common after-effects of antibiotic use are diarrhea and colitis. The incidence of diarrhea and colitis ranges from 12.5–22.2 percent of patients receiving antibiotic medication, according to a 19-month study of orthopedic inpatients at Guys Hospital in London. Pseudomembraneous colitis is a possibly lethal form of infective colitis that can occur following the use of a wide range of antibiotics. Despite recognition of this syndrome and withdrawal of antibiotics this condition can be impossible to reverse with death being the ultimate outcome. As a last resort in some cases great portions of the colon are removed surgically.

The incidence of pseudomembraneous colitis is considered a serious hazard in the elderly and may be caused by a wide range of antibiotics in common use including but not limited to ampicillin, penicillin, clindamycin, erythromycin and septrin. Arthritis can develop from cases of antibiotic induced colitis. Ulceration and mucosal damage can be caused by antibiotics elsewhere in the gastrointestinal tract. Ulcers occurring in the esophagus following oral antibiotic use are well documented. Malabsorption due to altered bacteria flora and vitamin deficiency due to blockage of vitamin production by the enteric flora is also a well-recognized result of antibiotic use.

Suprainfection

Suprainfection is another extremely disturbing occurrence attributable to the suppression of antibiotic-susceptible microorganisms that normally provide natural competition to prevent the unlimited multiplication of antibiotic resistant microorganisms. The administration of broad spectrum antibiotics, especially by mouth, may result in suprainfection with *Candida* and other yeast, filamentous fungi, coliform organisms, proteus or pseudomonas species". These organisms may then colonize and cause destructive damage in many sites throughout the body, even causing death in some cases.

The most recognized and researched form of suprainfection involves the previously discussed antibiotic related pseudomembraneous colitis. This condition is now known to be due to suprainfection by *Clostridium difficile*, which produces an enterotoxin, causing a potentially lethal outcome. The antibiotic treatment creates a susceptibility to this infection presumably by altering the normal barrier function of the colonic microflora.

Another form of suprainfection that is gaining medical recognition as a major problem associated with the use of antibiotics is *Candida albicans* overgrowth locally and systemically. Some forms of this *Candida* overgrowth are relatively benign, such as the common "yeast infection" many women have come to almost expect following a course of antibiotics. These yeast infections are fairly easy to treat in most cases. However, some women develop chronic or recurrent cases that are life-threatening. The most publicized of these infections involves the gastrointestinal tract. *Candida* has been known to colonize the mouth, esophagus, small intestine, large intestine, and anal region. Cases have been reported where tracheal obstruction and death was caused by a *Candida* fungus ball following the use of broad-spectrum antibiotics. When *Candida* colonizes and invades the mucus membranes of the small intestines it is suspected of causing an increased permeability of the wall (see Leaky Gut) allowing relatively large undigested protein molecules to pass directly into the bloodstream, where they may act as antigenic material initialing an immune allergy response. This may lead to allergic manifestations involving any target tissue or organ and be responsible for an extremely wide range of local and systemic pathology. In some cases this leakage of large food source protein molecules leads to the development of allergic response to a vast number of foods.

Internal organ damage

Some evidence exists that under certain conditions the *Candida* may mutate, losing their cell walls, and enter into the bloodstream. This presents great difficulty in therapy since Nystaten, the most frequently used antifungal agent is not absorbed into the blood but remains only in the gastrointestinal tract. Disseminated candidasis has been known to cause death due to multi-organ involvement. In a study of 109 fatal cases of systemic candidasis 88 percent of the patients had more than one deep organ affected, excluding mucosal lesions of the alimentary and respiratory tracts. Major organs involved in order of highest frequency use the lungs, spleen, kidneys, liver, heart and brain. A study of complete autopsies conducted in Kentucky during the period between 1964–73 revealed approximately 1% of the sample population had cerebral mycosis. In every one of these patients fungi were also seen in tissues outside the central nervous system. Cerebral candidasis was recognized only at autopsy in patients compromised by previous multiple antibiotic therapy.

The kidneys are highly susceptible to damage by drugs, and antibiotics are the most common drugs implicated in clinical reports of drug-induced nephrotoxicity. "Aminoglycoside antibiotics continue to be a mainstay of therapy in the clinical management of Gram-negative infections, but a major factor in the clinical use of aminoglycosides (ampicillin and others) is their nephrotoxicity. With Gram-negative organisms accounting for the majority of hospital-acquired infections, the occurrence of aminoglycoside-induced renal failure has become commonplace. Presently at least 10% of all cases of acute renal failure can be attributed to these antibiotics. Other classes of antibiotics including penicillin and sulphonamides also can cause kidney damage." (*Am. J. Kidney Dis.* 1982, 2(1): 5–29) The clinical manifestations attributed to these antibiotics include natural or spontaneous renal failure, renal colic, selective tubular defects, acute nephritic syndrome, hematuria, obstructive nephropathy. In the case of severe renal failure it may be necessary to utilize hemodialysis. The precise manner in which antibiotics damage kidney tissue is not as yet completely agreed upon. Virtually all antibiotics are excreted in part or in total by the kidneys. Proposed mechanisms of antibiotic-induced acute renal tubular necrosis involve either altering plasma membrane permeability or interference with cellular energy derived from mitochondria. Active enzyme systems in the kidney are also capable of activating drugs, which are concentrated by the action of kidneys, into reactive toxins. Drug-induced immunologic damage may occur in addition to direct action due to drug accumulation. Some antibiotics have been known to cause kidney damage by inducing the life-threatening autoimmune proteins of systemic lupus erythematosus.

The liver, the site of much drug detoxification and removal from the circulation via the bile, is another organ susceptible to damage from antibiotics. Chemically induced liver injury from antibiotic use has caused cholestatic jaundice, hepatitis and fatty infiltration of the liver.

Acute pancreatitis has recently been recognized as a separate iatrogenic disorder that may be caused by antibiotic use. Oxytetracydine and tetracycline can depress amylase and lipase activity. The impairment of digestive enzyme synthesis may cause a malabsorption syndrome, which may take months to normalize.

The immune system has been damaged in several ways by various classes of antibiotics. The previously mentioned induction of possibly fatal systemic lupus erythematosus is only one of the immune malfunctions caused by antibiotics that may be life-threatening. Fatal penicillin- and tetracycline-induced hemolytic anemia caused by the rapid destruction of red blood cells has been reported many times in the literature. It has also been reported that an immune mechanism similar to the well-recognized penicillin-induced immune hemolytic anemia may cause damage or destruction of blood platelets causing bleeding abnormalities, hemorrhages and an increased risk of thromboembolism. Also reported are neutropenia, thrombocytopenia and leukopenia as well as reduced phagocytosis by the cells of the reticuloendothelial system. It appears that penicillin and many other antibiotics reduce the effectiveness of the immune system and thus predispose to further infection.

Commonly used antibiotics can also cause various neurotoxic disorders. "Central nervous system toxicities include seizure disorders, encephalopathy, bulging fontanelles and neuropsychiatric symptoms. The abnormalities have been associated with the use of penicillins, cephalosporins, sulfonamides, tetracyclines, chloramphenicol, colistin, aminoglycosides, metronidazole, isoniazid, rifampin, ethionamide, cycloserine and dapsone. Cranial nerve toxicities, such as myopia, optic neuritis, deafness, vertigo and tinnitis have been associated with the use of erythromycin, sulfonamides, tetracyclines, chloramphenicol, colistin, aminoglycosides, vancomycin, isoniazid and ethambutol. Permanent peripheral nerve symptoms consisting or parasthesias, motor weakness and sensory impairment have been associated with the use of penicillins, sulfonamides, chloramphenicol, colistin, metronidazole, isoniazid, ethionan-dde and dapsone". (*Ann. Intern. Med.* 1984, 101(1): 92–104. Multifocal myodonus, encephalopathy, seizures, coma and death have been shown to remit from various antibiotics. These conditions have in some cases been resistant to all treatments.

A rare but possibly fatal complication of antibiotic use is acute bone marrow failure and aplastic anemia. This fatal condition has been caused by tetracycline, chloramphenicol, ampicillin, oxecillin, thiamphenicol and penicillin.

Antibiotics may also affect the heart and circulatory system. Cardiac toxicities due to antibiotics may cause drug-induced myocarditis and myocardial infarction.

Injection of antibiotics carries other serious dangers. Intravenous infusions of some antibiotics have been shown to cause phlebitis in up to 18% of patients after two days on therapy. The unintentional injection of an antibiotic into an artery, which may occur on occasion during a routine intramuscular injection, can have disastrous effects. Vascular occlusion gangrene has been reported several times in the literature. The following case report is typical of these reactions. "Irreversible ischemic gangrene of the upper limb developed in a one year old after an unintentional intra-arterial injection of procaine penicillin. The hand needed amputation." (*Aust. NZ J. Med.* 6(1): 71–3)

Similar reactions have also been caused by oral antibiotics as the following case report illustrates: "A nodular exanthema of the skin was observed in an 8-year-old girl. She had been treated with penicillin a few days ago because of a gastrointestinal infection. Continuation of penicillin treatment led to occlusion of larger arteries with gangrene of the forefoot". Generalized vasculitis with multisystem involvement also occurs with possibly fatal results. (*South. Med. J.* 1978, 71(8): 961–3)

Not only can antibiotics be toxic to those taking them, certain antibiotics are extremely damaging to the fetus. Tetracycline is a well-recognized teratogenic and embryo toxic agent linked to Diastrophic dwarfism. In this rare disorder the infant is dwarfed and the limbs are shortened. It is associated with marked joint abnormalities, limited movements and contractures. Dislocation in the hip or knee and kyphoscoliosis lead to progressive deformity.

The need for a change

The many toxic effects of antibiotics, only some of which have been covered here, illustrate clearly that these medications need to be used conservatively and with far more respect than seems to be the case at the present time. Rarely, if ever, does a physician sit down with his patient and give full disclosure of these possible hazards to antibiotics use. Many health complaints that routinely receive antibiotic therapy are easily treated with simple, safe and effective non-toxic approaches. A case in point is acne. Here we have a condition that naturopaths and holistically minded MDs manage quite well with dietary and life style changes and that shows a clear association with these easily identified factors. Yet the treatment of choice by most physicians is still oral antibiotics.

This might be acceptable if antibiotics were particularly effective in removing the problem and had no side-effects. However, the antibiotic class most frequently prescribed, the tetracyclines are far from non-toxic as we have already seen. In addition to the previous side effects noted, minocycline has been found to cause black pigmentation of the thyroid, sclera, bones, teeth, skin and nails and tetracycline can cause permanent staining of the teeth. The prolonged course of antibiotics used in the past for this condition, up to 12 years or longer in some cases, has profound effects on the body's normal ecology with possibly life-threatening complications. And all this for the treatment of a condition that was never a threat to life and is best treated through proper nutrition and dietary alteration. Recently topical antibiotics have come into vogue for the treatment of acne. These antibiotic lotions are certainly less toxic and avoid the possibility of adverse affects of systemic therapy. However, they still do not address the underlying cause of the condition, only its most obvious symptom. Bacteria do not cause acne, as any dermatologist must freely admit, so any therapy aimed at killing bacteria will be totally ineffective at removing the cause and thus will have no hope of curing the condition.

Acute otitis media is another condition that is responsible for a tremendous amount of needless antibiotic therapy. Often any patient who presents with pain in the ear and increased fluid behind the eardrum is prescribed antibiotics. The great bulk of these conditions are serous or secretary otitis, a non-bacterial condition for which antibiotics have no effect. In fact, quite the reverse; antibiotics seem to cause a lingering inflammation. Early antibiotic therapy in these cases may interfere with the development of local immunity and actually favor a recurrent syndrome.

Bacterial otitis media does occur, but is almost always the result of Eustachian tube dysfunction, a condition recognized to be caused by a primary catarrhal condition, often the result of improper diet or allergy. The bacteria then may proliferate within the stagnant serous fluid in the middle ear causing the typical acute symptoms of earache and fever. Certainly it is easier to prevent this condition or reverse it in early stages; however, even at this end-stage disorder with frank infection, antibiotic use is not usually required if proper holistic therapy is applied.

For many years, a large number of doctors routinely prescribed antibiotics in upper respiratory infections. "Antibiotic therapy has been shown to be of no value in the treatment of upper respiratory infections, either in shortening the course of the acute illness or in preventing the development of secondary bacterial infections. Patient expense, as well as the threat of adverse reactions, should prohibit the present practice by some of routinely prescribing tetracycline, erythromycin and ampicillin. Indiscriminate antibiotic therapy cannot substitute for proper diagnostic evaluation of the patient who may have either a bacterial or, far more likely, a viral illness," (*Pediatrics* 1975, 55(6): 552–6)

Antibiotics in the food chain

Antibiotic exposure may occur on a daily basis due to current farming and animal husbandry practices. After a short period of time, animals receiving antibiotics show a great share of antibiotic-resistant strains in the intestinal flora, in which also may be contained pathogenic strains. Through the excretions of the animals the resistant bacteria goes into the environment where it is now causing biological problems for creatures of the waterways, and may be taken up by humans. The resistant bacteria may be transferred to humans also by foods of animal origin such as meat, milk and eggs.

Bacterial mutations and antibiotic resistance

A final topic regarding antibiotics which is becoming recognized as a major internal and external ecological issue is the development of resistant strains of bacteria in human ecology. Resistance of a microorganism to an antibiotic is closely linked to the extent that antibiotics are used as medicine for man and domestic food source animals. Resistance may develop by selection of resistant strains which may develop by random mutation. Further, organisms resistant to one antibiotic may become resistant to another. This is termed cross-resistance.

A case in point is the emergence of a mutated enterococcal bacterium, vancomycin resistant enterococci (VRE), that is resistant to all pharmaceutical antibiotics. Normally, enterococci reside quite happily inside the gut and female genital tract. In diseased people (often in hospitals) enterococci can become opportunistic and cause heart valve or urinary tract infections. This bug actually thrives around antibiotics. The real potential for damage, however, has to do with the ability of bugs to so easily transmit genetic information to other bugs, such as golden staph.

The bugs have placed themselves in this war extremely well; they are mutating in ways we never dreamed were possible, and at rates which are alarming scientists. The overuse of antibiotics, both medically (probably by about 98%) and in meat and dairy production has led to bugs mutating to the point where they can threaten the existence of healthy people, a situation in the history of mankind that we have not seen before. Until now, if people died from infections, it was generally because of either poor health status to start with, or poor treatment choices, or both. But the situation is changing, and if it continues and we keep trying to destroy the bugs by chemical warfare rather than letting our bodies keep them in balance, we may see a risk to the human species from super bugs. This possibility is currently being discussed by the World Health Organization, which is concerned about antibiotic usage not just in medicine, but also in food production as well. Currently over 19,000 people are dying each year from antibiotic-resistant bacterial infestations, and the number is climbing dramatically. It could prove to be a pandemic of apocryphal proportions.

Conclusion

After a careful review of the adverse effects of antibiotics, it is obvious that we must re-evaluate their present widespread and often indiscriminate use in human and animal medicine. Unless we seek out other more ecological alternatives to infectious disease we may be setting the stage for large-scale epidemics of antibiotic-resistant diseases.

Until we begin to understand that the only truly effective antibiotic is a healthy and strong immune system and until we begin to direct our therapeutic efforts towards strengthening the body, not killing the germ, infectious disease will always remain a threat to humans, both in its effects, and in those of the medicines we use to control them.

WHEN DRUGS AND SURGERY ARE NECESSARY

The aim of naturopathy is to remove the cause of disease without harmful drugs or unnecessary surgery. Only when the actual causes of disease are removed can real health be present.

Many health problems can be cured with natural therapy. Abundant examples of this are given in this book. Still, there are times when the use of drugs or surgery may be necessary, even lifesaving. Obviously, mechanical injuries require a mechanical solution. If an arm or leg is fractured you need it placed in a cast, not a comfrey poultice; and it might even need to be surgically pinned. If the reason your child wets the bed is due to a congenitally abnormal genitourinary system, he or she needs reconstructive surgery and not sitz baths. If you have appendicitis you need surgery, not grape abdominal packs. Surgery, in its proper place, is the most admirable of medical achievements.

Some uses of drugs and surgery, both necessary and unnecessary, are the result of ignoring early signs and symptoms of disease. Tonsils that are greatly enlarged and severely scarred may cause enough distress to warrant removal on rare occasions, but may never reach such a state if the early symptoms of the disorder are heeded and treated properly. Appendicitis may develop into peritonitis, which is an acute surgical emergency by anyone's standards, but may never develop if the diet or the early digestive malfunctions are attended to promptly. Many surgical procedures, therefore, are necessary only because the individual has not listened to the disease's calling card until it is too late.

Drug therapy, like surgery, is also mostly preventable, in my opinion. A significant number of patients currently on high blood pressure medication for 5 years or less could be cured without drugs. However, the very life of some may totally depend on these drugs. Again, as with the case of surgery, the usual cause of this dependency was years and years of ignoring or improperly treating the first signs of high blood pressure or the diseased organ system that caused the blood pressure to rise. Insulin is lifesaving for a person with congenital or juvenile-onset diabetes, but many cases of adult-onset diabetes show early warnings that could and should have been attended to. With many chronic diseases the improper treatment of acute disease acts as the major factor in their development to the point where drugs are required.

Antibiotics fall into a separate and unique class of drugs. They are a double-edged sword, being essential in some stages of infection and at the same time detrimental in terms of human ecology (see Antibiotics). Nearly any infection anywhere in the body can develop to the point that the use of antibiotics is a wise course of action. This, however, usually occurs only if the earliest signs of infection are ignored, or if the individual's vital energy and immunological resistance are so depressed by poor diet or other factors that the body is no longer capable of self-cure rapidly enough.

72

The times when antibiotics are required must be carefully and seriously considered. If antibiotics are reserved for the few times in a person's life when an infection is actually life-threatening, or poses a serious threat to an organ system, their use is clearly justified. But these drugs are now employed for nearly every mild bacterial infection, and even for viral infections over which they have absolutely no effect. This reduces the future effectiveness of the antibiotic when it may really be required and favors development of antibiotic-resistant bacteria. By frequent use we are setting the stage for new plagues of antibiotic-resistant diseases.

The decision to use surgery, drugs, or antibiotics must be made as the very last resort, or if no other alternative exists. No general comprehensive guidelines, however, can be made as to when this point has come. Each case must be considered individually by a physician fully aware and proficient in natural alternatives as well as more orthodox methods. The central problem with the drug and surgical approach to disease is that it generally deals with the end of the disease spectrum and concentrates on localized manifestations only. Most processes have their origin long before drugs and surgery are required. We continually push the body towards catastrophe by ignoring or suppressing acute disease beginning in early childhood. If the language of disease had been heard and treated properly at these times there would be very little need at all for drugs or surgery in our lives.

The following chapters provide information concerning common diseases. Not all of this information applies to each person suffering from a particular disease. Each causative factor (etiological consideration) and therapeutic regimen must be considered separately, according to the individual.

By supplying this information in readily available form, my aim is to help people treat their own minor ailments in early stages. While minor disorders may safely be treated at home without supervision, any serious condition must be handled by a trained practitioner.

Use common sense. If you are dealing with a condition that is, or could become a serious health risk, consult a trained health professional you trust.

PART II

How to Use Natural Medicine

ACNE
(Seborrheic Dermatitis)

DEFINITION

An inflammatory condition of the skin where sebaceous glands are most numerous and active: on the face, neck, chest, and back.

SYMPTOMS

Characterized by blackheads, whiteheads, pustules, inflamed and infected nodules, sacs, and cysts. Infection occurs in the pilosebaceous follicle (hair follicle in the sebaceous gland). This may cause permanently dilated pores, obstruction of the pilosebaceous opening, and severe scarring.

ETIOLOGICAL CONSIDERATIONS— PRIMARY

• Puberty.
Androgenic hormones (e.g. testosterone) increase sebaceous gland activity, causing blocked pores.
• Diet.
Excess saturated fat (especially homogenized cow's milk); dairy products; meat; fried food; pastry; hydrogenated fats; excess sugar, which potentiates the effect of fats; refined carbohydrates; chocolate; cocoa; caffeine (cola, tea, coffee); salt; alcohol (see Hypoglycemia); improper liquids (carbonated beverages); lack of green vegetables.
• Nutritional deficiency or excess need for development.
Zinc (lack in diet, soil depletion; increased need for in puberty; rapid growth requires excess); malabsorption (hydrochloric acid deficiency reduces zinc absorption); vitamin B6 (individual excess need)—menstrually related deficiency common; B6 deficiency due to birth control medication (progesterone).
• Poor eliminations.
Bowel lesion (thinning) due to diet or stress; constipation; liver congestion or toxicity; overstressed kidney function; poor skin eliminations (incoordination of deep and superficial circulations)

ETIOLOGICAL CONSIDERATIONS— SECONDARY

• Food allergy.
• Cosmetics.
• Lack of exercise.
• Poor hygiene.
• Oral contraceptives.
• Steroids.
• Anti-epileptic drugs.
• Stress.
• Industrial pollutant exposure (e.g. petroleum products and machine oils).

DISCUSSION

Acne occurs most frequently in the teenage years when it affects 80% of all teenagers to some degree. This has been associated with an increase in androgenic (male) sex hormone activity which causes an increase in the sebaceous gland output, clogging the pores and allowing secondary bacterial infections to occur. The sebaceous glands, located at the base of hair follicles, produce lubricant oils for the skin. These hormone changes occur in both sexes. This can also be seen in cases of infantile acne just after birth, due to high levels of circulating sex hormones. Acne is rarely found in eunuchs. The incidence of teenage acne is so high as to be considered "normal" in developed nations. This fails to consider that not all populations experience such high rates of acne. One such population was the Canadian Inuit who, prior to 1950, had no incidence of acne. Later, as more modern foods, including sugar and refined carbohydrates, were introduced into their diets, acne became common.[20]

The main dietary offender in the modern diet is its high saturated fat content. A diet high in animal proteins, cheese, and milk causes abnormal development of the sebaceous glands, leading to acne. The modern teenage diet is a prescription for acne, with cheeseburgers, hot dogs, french fried potatoes, corn chips, potato chips, fried eggs, french toast, butter, milk shakes, milk, sugar, candy, cola, and chocolate.

Although meat (especially pork fat) and hydrogenated fats are detrimental, milk fat is often the main offender. We are the only species that feeds our young milk after weaning. The situation would probably be less serious if we gave our children mother's milk, but we give them cow's milk, with its excessive fat.

The link between diet and acne has long been recognized by both naturopathic physicians and the lay public. Every teenager knows that chocolate may aggravate acne. Other detrimental substances in the diet are coffee, tea, alcohol, and sugar. Sugar in particular facilitates the action of saturated fatty acids, making it the number two offender.

A second major cause of acne is an incoordination of the eliminations. This may include sluggish bowel and skin function, a toxic liver, or overstressed kidneys. When the eliminating organs become imbalanced, the superficial circulation becomes filled with toxic eliminants which then clog the superficial capillaries and small lymphatic vessels which feed the sebaceous glands and cause inflammation with secondary infection. This incoordination between deep and superficial circulation may also be due to spinal lesions which upset the cerebrospinal centers located in the ganglia of the automatic nervous system which control these circulations.

Another common finding is areas of the bowels that have thinned walls allowing leakage of toxins into the system. (See Psoriasis; Allergies and Food Intolerances for more details on this condition and leaky gut. Refer also to Constipation as it relates to incoordination of elimination.)

The habit of hot showers or baths is another factor that upsets skin function and causes an incoordination between deep and superficial circulation. Prolonged heat causes a vasodilation or a lax condition of the superficial blood vessels, leading to poor local circulation and congestion.

Certain dietary deficiencies have been associated with acne. Of these, vitamin B6, zinc, and essential fatty acids (EFA) are the most common. Vitamin B6 deficiency is common in acne related to the menstrual cycle, where acne is worse prior to or during menstruation and premenstrual symptoms of irritability and water retention are severe. Zinc is a common deficiency, especially during puberty with rapid growth, which requires an excess of this mineral. Zinc is deficient in most soils and therefore most foods.

TREATMENT

The orthodox treatment for acne is palliative rather than curative. The patient is usually told he or she will grow out of it and may be given antibiotics topically or orally if the condition is very severe. In some cases, if the acne occurs in an older female, oral estrogens are used. These treatments are not only ineffective, they are detrimental. Most teenagers grow out of their acne, but not before some scarring. Many never grow out of it and suffer acne lesions nearly all their lives.

Antibiotics are used to combat the secondary infections and often must be repeated every 3-6 months. This has a bad effect on the entire body by destroying friendly bacteria essential to our well-being (see Leaky Gut).

The skin is made from the inside out. It takes 20-30 days for the skin now being formed to reach the surface. It is obvious then that external treatments can do little to affect this developing skin. Acne is usually an internal problem, not an external one. A possible exception would be cosmetic acne due to excessive use of facial creams and lotions, which clog the pores and in some cases cause an allergic reaction or the acne caused by exposure to machine oils and petrochemicals. Poor hygiene will also affect the skin, but the majority of cases are caused by internal factors. True healing must come from within. This healing will take some time. Even if you begin today, the results will only start to show themselves in 20–30 days, usually more like 60. If any severe acne lesions are present, these will take even longer, due to the great damage that has already occurred in these areas. Perseverance and absolute adherence to the diet below are essential to get results.

Diet

Our main concern is to eliminate as many saturated fats as possible. Ideally the diet should contain no saturated fat, especially dairy products. We find it best to restrict the diet to *no saturated fat* for a reasonable length of time in the beginning, so that you can begin to see true results rapidly. If you can be motivated enough and convinced that this short-term, very strict diet will have some very long-term advantages, we advise 6–8 weeks of a no-saturated-fat diet. This includes plenty of non-citrus fruits, raw vegetable juice, salads, cooked vegetables, vegetable and seaweed soups, seeds and nuts in moderation, whole grains, and vegetarian proteins such as beans and tofu. Seaweeds are suggested for their high iodine content, as are pumpkin seeds for their zinc. All junk foods, fried foods, refined foods and carbonated drinks or alcohol are prohibited. A short *vegetable juice fast* of 1–7 or more days with enemas on days 1, 2, 3, 5, and 7 is useful to speed the healing process. These should be done every 2–4 weeks if possible. The diet that follows allows non-fat dairy products, but by no means suggest it. If possible, dairy products should be excluded from the diet until the skin is perfectly clear.

For best results we advise the elimination from the diet of all dairy products. However, some patients are very resistant to this idea. For dairy products to be included at all in the diet and still allow healing to occur it is essential that you understand more about the fat composition of available dairy products. The fat content of milk is fairly complex and must be understood if any milk products are to be added to the diet and favorable results still be achieved. The following summary should prove helpful:

Ice-cream	10% to 20% butterfat
Evaporated whole milk	8%+ butterfat
Whole milk	4% to 6% butterfat
Homogenized milk	4% butterfat
Evaporated low fat	4% butterfat
Low fat	2% butterfat
Nonfat, skim	0.5% butterfat
Dried skim	0.1% butterfat
Evaporated skim	0.25% buttermilk
True buttermilk	0.5% buttermilk
Dry curd cheese	0.5% buttermilk

Of these milk preparations only dried skim or evaporated skim have a low enough butterfat content to be consumed in moderation. Skim milk yoghurt is acceptable (but not advised) 1–2 times per week. Real buttermilk (butterfat removed) is acceptable on occasion. Dry curd cheese also is acceptable on occasion. No more than 6 fl oz (190 ml) of skim or buttermilk three times per week, 2 oz (60 g) powdered skim per day, or 1 cup daily of dry curd cheese is allowed. All cottage cheeses are too high in fat, as is butter. Margarine is generally made by hydrogenating unsaturated fats and making them partly saturated. Those fats are entirely unnatural to the body and should be avoided altogether whenever possible.

Commercial peanut butters also often have hydrogenated fats. Check all labels before purchasing. In general we restrict peanut butter and encourage other nut or seed butters such as almond, sunflower, or cashew. Peanuts are not nuts anyway—they are legumes.

Commercial breads usually contain about 1% saturated fat and must be avoided. Either buy well-labeled whole grain breads from reliable bakers or bake your own with cold pressed vegetable oils. Commercial baked goods often contain up to 20% fat and should be strictly avoided.

In later stages of this diet (and in some cases very early on) poultry in moderation and fish may be added, but never served fried. Cold water ocean fish (e.g. cod or salmon) is suggested as the best fish source.

Cold pressed unsaturated vegetable oils in the diet are acceptable in moderation, but never heated. It is suggested that you add 400 IU of vitamin E to a newly opened vegetable oil bottle to prevent rancidity and keep refrigerated. These should be used as salad dressings with lemon juice (the only citrus in the diet) or apple cider vinegar. Any herbs for taste are fine. Use plenty of onion and garlic.

Acne Diet

The following diet may be of some use as a basic guideline. Choose from the following:

Breakfast

Non-citrus fruit; non-citrus fruit plus skim yoghurt;* whole grain cereal (no sugar) with soy milk, skim milk, dried skim, or evaporated skim milk; poached eggs and whole wheat toast.*

Midmorning

Wholemeal pancakes:* vegetable juice (carrot, lettuce, nettle, and watercress). Potassium broth; herb tea.

Lunch

Fresh raw salad with plenty of green leafy vegetables, watercress, lettuce, cabbage, kale, chard, parsley, alfalfa sprouts, celery, onions, garlic, seaweed, sprouts, etc., with carrots and other combinations. Keep the salads varied and interesting. Salad dressing used should be based on cold pressed vegetable oil and lemon juice or apple cider vinegar. Garlic, various herbs, and honey may be used to add variety to the dressing. We suggest you obtain a good salad cookbook and experiment; tofu or soybeans;* A few nuts;* brown rice or millet.*

Midafternoon

As midmorning.

Supper

As lunch, or conservatively cooked (baked or steamed) vegetables, especially green and yellow vegetables. Carrots are also good. Use a wide variety.

- Tofu or soy protein, beans; fish (never fried);* turkey or chicken (never fried)*.
- Whole grains (especially brown rice and millet); dry curd cheese.*

Evening

As midmorning and midafternoon.
Drink 6–8 glasses of water each day.

Foods of Special Usefulness

Green vegetables; kelp; carrots; seaweeds; onions; fish (cold water ocean); garlic; whole grains; watercress; sprouts; dandelion greens; vegetable juices (carrot, lettuce, nettle, and watercress); nettles.

Physiotherapy

- Daily wash; warm water wash twice daily with mild calendula or castile soap. Alternate warm, then cold applications should follow.

---

*Asterisked foods are included depending on stage of diet or allergy. Remember, dairy is not advised but is included in this diet list for those patients who simply are unable to go dairy-free. If you really want to get rid of this condition, eliminate dairy completely.

- Ice applications directly on lesions has helped some.
- Hot steam or hot fomentations may help lesions mature.
- Ultraviolet (UV) applications daily are very useful. *Note:* Excess UV light can cause skin cancer. Use common sense and do not over-expose the skin. The exact amount of exposure that is safe depends on individual skin type.
- Lemon juice diluted in water may be applied externally for its antiseptic and astringent effect.
- Vitamin B6 cream locally in menstrual acne (100 mg vitamin B6 per g of ointment).
- Spinal manipulation—cervical and upper mid-course, weekly.
- Sun and air baths.
- Ocean bathing.
- Daily body brushing to entire body with loofah or soft bristle brush. (See Appendix I).
- Sulfur ointment (3-10%) topical.
- Dilute calendula tincture wash as antiseptic following maturation of lesions by hot fomentations.
- Tea tree oil, applied directly to infected pores or as a soap (antibiotic).

Therapeutic Agents

Vitamins and Minerals—Primary

- Vitamin A (micellized): high doses, 50,000-100,000 IU daily for several months in micellized (emulsified) form.
- Vitamin B6: 50-250 mg twice daily in menstrually related acne. B6 reduces the uptake of, and sensitivity to testosterone.
- Vitamin C: 250-1000 mg 3 times daily; antibiotic, antioxidant, stress reducer.
- Zinc: 25-45 mg 3 times daily. As effective as tetracyclines. Reduce dose if bowel upset occurs. Add 1-3 mg copper daily at higher doses. Selenium also may need to be increased 100 mcg daily at higher zinc levels.
- Vitamin B complex: 25-50 mg twice daily. If yeast allergy is diagnosed or suspected, use a non-yeast source.
- Vitamin E: 200-400 IU twice daily. Antioxidant.

Others—Primary

- Bioflavonoids especially quercetin: reduces inflammation.
- EPA (eicosapentaenoic acid—cold-water marine body oils): 1-3 capsules 2-3 times daily.
- Probiotics: 2 capsules 3 times daily (especially following use of antibiotics).
- Garlic: 2 capsules with meals.
- Lecithin (as concentrated phosphatidylcholine): 2 capsules 2-3 times daily.
- EFA (essential fatty acids): especially the omega-3s (e.g. flaxseed oil, evening primrose oil, black currant oil) 2-4 capsules 2-3 times daily, or 2 tsp daily minimum.
- Selenium: 200 mcg daily; antioxidant, improves tissue elasticity.
- Chlorophyll: (or some other green drink such as Spirulina): the more the better; detoxifies intestines.

Others—Secondary

- Glucose tolerance factor (GTF) yeast: to normalize blood sugar levels. Chromium is the effective agent, and is available in tablet form.
- Kelp: 2-4 tablets 2-3 times daily.
- Sulfur: 1-30 grains daily, or as homeopathic dilution. Larger doses may cause intestinal irritation and loose stools.
- L-cysteine: 500 mg daily. Contains sulfur, essential for skin maintenance.
- A topical cream of vitamin E, vitamin C, powdered comfrey (root, leaf), and calendula and tea tree oil will promote healing and reduce scarring in severe cases.
- Colloidal silver: use topically or orally as local or systemic antibiotic.

Botanicals—Primary

Echinacea: alterative (blood purifier),

anti-infective, bacteriostatic. Tincture: 15–60 drops (¼–1 tsp) diluted in water, 3–4 times daily.

Blue flag: excellent alterative; corrects imperfect lymphatic elimination; is glandular stimulant (especially thyroid).

Calendula: lymphatic tonic. Vulnerary to prevent scarring. Especially if skin is greasy.

Chaste tree: to balance out testosterone, reduces excess androgens (works at the pituitary level).

Oregon grape: alterative, activates lymphatic system. Tincture: 10–20 drops 3–4 times daily.

Burdock root: good alterative with skin disorders. Restores oil and sweat gland function; is antibacterial.

Aloe: local, topical use.

Botanicals—Secondary

Barberry.

Dandelion: detoxifies liver; cholagogue, depurative and alterative.

Red clover: alterative.

Sarsaparilla: alterative, diuretic.

Yellow dock: alterative, laxative (to increase bowel eliminations), depurative and diuretic.

Clivers, a good depurative in acne.

Therapeutic Suggestions

Remember this is primarily a dietary problem. Excess long-term use of many supplements should not be needed if you correct the diet and eliminations.

AGING

OLD AGE: ITS CAUSE AND PREVENTION

A Statement of Philosophy

Old age does not necessarily bring disease. There is nothing to suggest that the older we get, the more aches and pains we should have, or the less resistant we are to infections, or the more prone we become to heart failure or stroke. What sometimes suggests the above is when we look around and see a lot of sick, old people.

The question ought to be, what brings what? Does age bring disease, or does disease bring aging? What are the factors of aging? Sickness is caused by poor attention to health principles, not merely by the passing of time.

Many people experience longevity without any aches or pains, with heaps of vitality and energy. They have learned the lessons of good health, and live by the so-called laws of health. There are many models throughout the world of old folk enjoying perfect health, free of any aches or pains,

signs or symptoms, without any medication, not even an aspirin.

So do not accept the mediocrity of our chronically ill western civilization, in which the older you become the sicker you can expect to be. Rather, with age let wisdom come into her own; discover and practice the laws of good health and become less sick, more healthy.

Last century, a lot was said about achieving vitality in your mid-life, and sustaining it through into later life. Much of naturopathic practice focused on the basic "Seven Doctors" approach, that is, learning to live naturally within one's environment, with plenty of fresh air, sunshine, exercise, rest, eating healthy foods and drinking pure water, and being "happy" within one's heart. These are the essential ingredients of vitality and anti-aging. At the start of the 21st century we are more aware of the pollution of the planet, which can affect our vitality. One of the ways that pollution affects our health is called free radical damage to cells. Since early studies in the 1950s demonstrated that exposing laboratory animals to radiation aged them more rapidly than otherwise, focus on the aging process has been on free radicals, which are generated not only by radiation, but by environmental pollutants (chemicals in water, air, food, etc.), pharmaceutical drugs, as well as being normal by-products of cellular metabolism. It is now known that increased levels of free radicals in body tissues can be very detrimental to health and vitality and are implicated in the causes of many diseases, many of which are directly related to aging and longevity, such as cancer, arthritis, auto-immune diseases, senility and many more.

While this is but one theory of aging, (there are others discussed below), the free radical theory of aging provides a very practical framework for anti-aging strategies. The basics of naturopathy are still true, but we now have more of a focus. Today we live in an environment that exposes us to lots of free radicals. More and more antioxidants are being recognized. Many vitamins and minerals act as antioxidants in the body and slowly we are learning more about their specific activity. Most of the advice on longevity presented in the last 25 years of the 20th century was based on specific supplementation to provide nutrients that were found to be deficient in the typical devitalized western diet that acted to prevent or protect against the ever increasing free radical exposure and damage or provided support to a weakened or declining endocrine system. While there is strong evidence that this approach has been beneficial in prolonging health and sexual function it is obvious from a naturopathic perspective that this is not the only, or even best approach to these problems. Although you will find most of the nutrients and botanicals used currently to help prolong life are included in this chapter, and they are useful in some cases, especially where short-term goals are to be obtained, never lose sight of naturopathy and the truths it holds as the true foundation for long life.

With these reservations kept in mind, we would like to review some of the newest theories on aging and the specific nutrients now thought to be useful in preventing aging. Please remember that while some of these nutrients are found regularly in our food supply, and are therefore quite natural to the body, others are hormones produced by the body and the effect of long term ingested supplemental doses is still not well established. Therefore, their inclusion in your daily supplement regime should be undertaken with extreme caution and medical supervision.

Free Radical Theory of Aging

Probably the most publicized theory on aging, the free radical concept, first proposed by Denham Hamon of the University of Nebraska, suggests that many of the cellular changes that are age related are caused by oxygen radical damage. These "free radicals" have also been implicated in many degenerative disorders and disease states including cancer, cataracts, and degeneration of the brain and neurons. A free radical is a molecule with an unpaired and highly reactive electron. An oxygen-free radical is one of the byproducts of natural metabolism that is produced when cells change food and oxygen into energy. As these free radicals seek a mate for their lone electron, they take on an electron from another molecule, which then becomes unstable and in turn seeks another electron. In this way, a chain reaction occurs, causing a series of compounds, some of which are harmful to healthy tissues. The tissues most sensitive to this free radical chain reaction damage are proteins, cellular membranes, and nucleic acids. In particular, DNA and the DNA in mitochondria (energy producers) are affected. Many recent studies demonstrate a primary role of free radicals in the causation processes of the so-called diseases of old age, such as cancer, arthritis, diabetes, cardiovascular disease, impaired immunity, and brain aging and other degenerative conditions such as Alzheimer's and other dementias. As mentioned, this free radical production is a normal process, and naturally the body has its own defenses to protect it against this damage. These are termed antioxidants and are a normal part of a healthy diet or are produced naturally within the body. Included in this class are Vitamins A, beta-carotene, C and E as well as enzymes such as superoxide dismutase (SOD), glutathiaone peroxidase and catalase. The theory goes that these prevent most, but not all oxidative damage, and little by little cellular damage accumulates and is finally observed as the aging process of tissues and organ systems. Some people suffer accelerated free radical damage due to faulty diet deficient in naturally occurring antioxidants and others accumulate excess free radicals through a number of inappropriate lifestyle choices.

Supplemental antioxidant formulae are available from all health food stores that include most of the currently known nutrients with these properties. As clinical trials continue as to this protective role of antioxidants in the aging process, we do know that an optimal uptake of antioxidant nutrients will contribute to enhanced quality of life as well as longevity.

However, the supplementation approach of supplying extra antioxidants to help repair damage done by excessive free radical damage is not as effective as preventing free radical damage in the first place. Also, the suggested oral administration of antioxidants such as SOD (superoxide dismutase), which is normally produced endogenously, is not well supported in the literature. This is due to the belief that it is broken down in digestion and is therefore of little or no benefit in preventing cellular aging. The best approach to apply this knowledge to your longevity goals is threefold: to reduce cellular aging by consuming a diet high in naturally occurring antioxidants, to prevent accelerated aging by avoiding a diet and lifestyle that causes excess free radical damage, and to stimulate the body's natural production of SOD.

Glucose Cross-linking Theory of Aging

Elevated glucose levels, or blood sugar, can be a source of cellular deterioration as a result of a process called glycosylation or glycation, where glucose molecules attach to proteins binding together (cross-linking) and thus altering their biochemical and structural roles. This is a slow but steady process that seems to toughen tissue and cause some of the tissue deterioration commonly associated with aging. These cross-links, often termed advanced glycosylation end products (AGEs) are thought to harden connective tissue (collagen), arteries, the lens of the eye (cataracts), and reduce efficiency of the nerves and kidneys. In support of this theory it is observed that diabetics, who have raised glucose levels, show all of these tissue changes and have a greatly shortened life span. The body's normal defense against this process comes from the macrophages of the immune system. Specific AGE receptor macrophages actively seek out, engulf and break down AGEs and deliver them via the bloodstream to the kidneys for elimination.

This research clearly implicates modern western diets that are high in refined carbohydrates and refined sugars that cause rapid rises in blood sugar levels and thus favor AGE production and accumulation. To reduce AGE production a diet of whole grains is essential. It is also advisable to foster a healthy immune system to insure its active role in AGE elimination.

Accelerated DNA Damage/Reduced DNA Repair

As a part of normal cellular life, DNA undergoes continual damage. It is attacked by oxygen radicals, damaged by ultraviolet light and destroyed by many toxic agents, especially environmental chemicals and pharmaceutical or recreational drugs. DNA can suffer damage in the form of deletions, have sections destroyed, undergo mutation or have changes in the sequence of DNA bases that make up the genetic code. DNA damage accumulates throughout life and may be a major cause of aging. The accumulated DNA damage may lead to malfunctioning genes, proteins, cells, and eventually deteriorating function of tissues and organs.

The body once again has a limited ability to repair DNA damage and when this ability is compromised or the DNA damage is excessive, DNA related aging occurs.

Photoaging

It is now an accepted fact that excessive ultraviolet exposure damages and ages the skin. Photoaging damages collagen and elastin, the two proteins responsible for the elasticity of the skin. Other changes due to accelerated photoaging include damage to skin cells called keratinocytes, responsible for synthesizing keratin in the skin, and melanocytes, which are responsible for making melanin. These are killed by sunlight and then appear as dark spots or freckles in light skin. The exact cause of photoaging is yet unclear. It may be due to DNA damage or involve free radicals.

Heat Shock Proteins (HSPs)

These proteins are produced in the body as a response to various stresses, not only heat as the name implies. Included in these stresses are other factors like exposure to toxic substances such as drugs, chemicals or heavy metals, or extreme psychological stress.

Although incompletely understood, HSPs appear to be protective of age related damages. They are known to help the cell disassemble and dispose of damaged proteins and to aid in the production and transport of new proteins. In the adrenal cortex, and in other sites throughout the body, HSP production appears to be closely related to hormones released due to stress. HSP levels decline with age.

Hormones

Research into supplementation of a number of hormones known to decline with age has shown positive results in preventing and reversing many of the signs and symptoms of aging. While the research in this direction is very encouraging, it is important to remember that the long term effects or complications of supplementation of the hormones discussed here is as yet unclear and is still extremely controversial. As an example of this, even the commonly accepted use of estrogen replacement therapy for post menopausal women carries the possible risk of increasing the susceptibility to various cancers.

Growth Hormone

In a study performed in 1989 at the Veterans Administration Hospitals in Milwaukee and Chicago a small group of men aged 60 and over were given injections of recombinant human growth hormone (GH). This is a synthetic version of the hormone produced in the pituitary gland and plays an essential role in normal childhood growth and development. These men showed increased lean body mass, increased muscle, reduced excess body fat and thickened skin. GH is known to decline with age and is now thought to be closely related to the aging process.

Estrogen

Called the "female" hormone, estrogen levels decline with age, most rapidly after menopause. Produced mainly by the ovaries, but secondarily in the adrenal glands and adipose tissue, estrogen helps maintain bone density and maintains secondary sexual characteristics. Estrogen replacement therapy is used to help with the more troublesome symptoms often associated with menopause such as painful sexual activity due to reduced natural lubrication, flushing and osteoporosis. As stated above, estrogen replacement therapy is still controversial, carrying an increased risk to cancer.

Testosterone

Called the "male" hormone, testosterone is produced by the testes in men. Testosterone levels fall with age in men. Researchers are investigating its usefulness in later years to strengthen muscles and prevent frailty and disability in men; however, it appears also to increase risk to cancer, especially of the prostate if administered as a replacement therapy.

DHEA

DHEA, short for dehydroespiandrosterone, is a hormone produced by the adrenal glands. It acts as a relatively weak male hormone and as a precursor to testosterone and estrogen. DHEA supplementation is being researched for its possible effects on aging, including the decline in male testosterone levels, immune system decline and in the prevention of cancer and multiple sclerosis. DHEA is abundant in youth but declines by age 30. Very low levels are associated with some cancers, cardiovascular disease in men, and the institutionalized elderly. In animal studies, DHEA supplementation has had remarkable anti-aging effects. In humans, DHEA supplementation has been shown to favor lean body mass increase, fat reduction and increased ability to attain and maintain an erection at levels of 25 mg three times daily.

Melatonin

Produced by the pineal gland, melatonin responds to light and seems to help regulate biorhythms and seasonal changes in the body. It declines in aging and is thought to be one of the factors associated with sleep disorders among the elderly. It is used therapeutically to help restore normal sleep cycles.

Diet

If there is any subject with more conflicting "expert" advice than the proper diet for mankind, we have as yet to discover it. One of the reasons for this is the little understood fact that there isn't a single dietary approach good for everyone. In naturopathic practice, this fact becomes obvious with even a little clinical experience. It may seem logical, for example, that whole grains are an ideal source of energy, fiber and nutrients, and that everybody should regularly consume large amounts of them. But in reality, some people are simply not evolved to metabolize them, as in the case of gluten-sensitive individuals being intolerant to wheat and oats. It is commonly accepted, if not universally applied by those so informed, that raw vegetables are high in vitamin content, enzymes and fiber and are essential to good health and long life. But in reality, some people's digestive systems simply won't tolerate raw foods and they develop intestinal discomfort and diarrhea.

However, the above examples are the exceptions to the rule, and can be considered disease states, either congenital or acquired. To discover the basic rules of good nutrition, you need only to look to the past. Most ancient peoples were to some extent grain eaters and those grains were of an unrefined nature. Given the right choice of grains suited to your metabolism a diet composed of 40–50 percent whole and unrefined grains is ideal. Probably the worst blow to modern health has been the practice of refining grains, as much as we have come to crave them. As a direct result of this refining process, most diseases of modern civilization have resulted. Unfortunately, man's "staple" has become more of a giant nail in the coffin. Refined carbohydrate addiction now causes more disease than nearly any other negative health factor. Isn't it ironic that the one class of food most suited to provide long life and health has been so perverted to become our worst enemy?

The choice of proteins is less clear-cut than with grains. Many people feel vegetarianism is the logical answer and even many meat eaters feel secretly guilty of the habit. But how often have you seen vegetarians who look weak and frail? Although vegetarianism may be perfect for some, giving health and long life, often the opposite is the case. Some people thrive better on a meat diet. Obviously, the answer is based on individual metabolism. A dairy-sensitive person will derive only misery and disease from a diet high in milk products. However, dairy tolerant individuals derive great sustenance from fermented dairy products and the convenience of preserved dairy products in the form of cheese in moderation is a superb protein source. Some people simply cannot digest legumes and while it seldom kills them, those around them are sorely tempted to do so.

Animal protein, with its relatively high fat content has taken a beating in the press over the years. There is no question that modern meats are higher in fat than the-free-range meat our ancestors ate, and are often pumped full of dangerous antibiotics and hormones. But providing a decent source of meat or poultry can be obtained, there can be no question that we should be able to eat it regularly as our ancestors did. Of course, with the regular inclusion of meat in our diet we should also make sure that our activity level is adequate to metabolize it properly.

Seeds and nuts, in moderation, and obtained in the shell so that the oils have not gone rancid, are a good source of protein, fiber, intestinal lubricants and natural essential fatty acids.

Fish and fish oils are a well-recognized beneficial food and are universally accepted (except by vegetarians) to be healthy, life-prolonging foods, especially the cold-water fish high in omega-3 fatty acids.

The average person gets far too little of fresh raw or conservatively cooked vegetables. There is no better source or vitamins and minerals. Unfortunately, in our modern society, pesticides have systematically poisoned this great source of life prolonging nutrients, the residue of which remains within the food. There is no question that many of these pesticide residues, in sensitive individuals, can cause serious health problems. Furthermore, the huge incidence of cancer may be partly the result of these environmental toxins in our food and water. When possible, pesticide-free vegetables should be obtained for maximum health benefit and reduced health risk. Another problem with store-bought vegetables is that they are often grown in mineral-deficient soil and these deficiencies are passed on to our food. Organic sources are best if available, or home grown if you have the time and space.

Fruits are accepted by most people as healthy and nourishing and with the same provision as above, excluding harmful pesticides, this is generally true. Those individuals with sugar sensitivity, usually created by the habitual consumption of refined carbohydrates from an early age, must restrict or entirely eliminate this otherwise delightfully pleasurable food source or pay the price of chronic hypoglycemia and its constant strain on the endocrine system. Skin-sensitive or digestive-sensitive individuals may also need to limit this food source (especially citrus fruits) until better harmony exists within their system.

The subject of dietary oils is ongoing and seemingly never ending. Each decade we see new "magic" oils enter the food chain with supposed health giving or cardio-protective functions. The bad boy "saturated fat" continues to be flogged from all directions until most people secretly fear a heart attack directly following the consumption of a hot buttered baked potato and a 250 g steak. History and population studies show olive oil to be relatively safe, in moderation, and beneficial to liver and gall bladder function. We feel relatively safe with its use, especially unheated in salad dressing, and flaxseed oil is of particular benefit in the civilized nations to help correct the essential fatty acid imbalances that are so prevalent as a result of our faulty diet habits. The only obvious statement about oil consumption in the western world is that less is better; at least of the type of oils and fats commonly consumed, and fried foods are just simply not good for you at all.

Consumers are led to believe that margarine will actually be beneficial to their health. We feel far safer eating and recommending good old-fashioned butter, in moderation, than any of these modern fabrications. If a person would simply avoid oils as much as possible, with the exception of a little olive oil, and have at least small amounts of seeds and nuts regularly, the rest of dietary fats occurring naturally in our dairy and meats would cause no problems, given adequate physical activity to properly metabolize and use them

If there is any one truth to be said about nutrition, it simply is that nearly everybody is consuming too much. Too much meat, too much dairy, too much oil, too much sweets, too much of almost everything. Even when you can find a person who really does eat the right things, it is usually just too much of that.

Thin people usually live longer than obese people. Just look around. How many 300-pound people do know who are 100 … or even 65 years old? If you want a chance at long life, eat right, but eat less. You should fast occasionally. Be a little hungry. It's good for you.

Exercise

As important as diet is to your health, it's not enough just to eat correctly to live long. Of equal importance to diet is adequate exercise. One of the most cherished books in our library is *Old Age: Its Cause and Prevention* by Sanford Bennett.

Mr Bennett was given only months to live at the age of 52 in the year 1892. He was an old man at 50, with not much time left. He decided it was about time to change his life. There was so little left if he didn't, and the results were simply amazing. The pic-

tures of him at 72 could easily be confused for a 40-year-old, except for the gray hair. His was a body Adonis would be proud of.

How did Mr Bennett do it? In its day, it was called "physical culture". Sanford devised a home exercise program, one that could even be done in bed, which strengthened and toned every muscle and tissue in his body.

There is no great secret here, or shouldn't be. Every few years we see newspaper articles where progressive therapeutic exercise programs (i.e. gentle gym work) are found to benefit the aged. These are always reported as if it's something new and a spectacular finding. We just have to pick up Sanford's book and chuckle. Old Sanford knew how to regain youth a long, long time ago.

Back in Sanford's day, routine daily exercise was less available in the diverse forms we have today. Now even most small metropolitan areas have decent gyms and various exercise classes in abundance to fit nearly anyone's needs. We usually recommend that patients join a gym if possible, when it suits their temperament, and gradually and safely increase their workouts and aerobic activity. It is often useful for them to get personal training advice, at least at first, to help familiarize them with the equipment and to help prevent injury.

In our last office, we had a fully equipped gym for patients' use so we could supervise their workouts and a fitness trainer was employed to help them safely progress. we saw remarkable results. One patient aged 90 years, came to us first with the aid of a fixed walker. It took him nearly 20 minutes just to make his way through the office back to the gym. Within 3 months, he threw his walker away!

We also recommend yoga as a superb method of health and strength maintenance. Whatever exercise program you choose make sure it includes provisions for muscle toning, flexibility and cardiovascular stimulation. Some form of aerobic training should be included to get the blood moving rapidly and clear the arteries. This can be anything that gets you breathing heavily for 20–30 minutes. You might try vigorous walking, a stepping machine, a rowing machine, calisthenics, *anything* really, but at least *something*.

Sanford's unique exercise program for muscle toning is included for those who are either unable to find a gym or travel in your work frequently. There are lots of other exercise systems that don't require a large amount of equipment. If you ever find Sanford's book in a rare or collectors' bookstore, you should buy it. He has many useful insights and advice to keep you young and healthy. There is another useful book on exercise, *Fit for Business* by Harry Hodge and Rob Rowland-Smith.

Breathing Fresh Air

A wise sage was once asked the secret to long life. He replied, "Just keep breathing!" Many of you may think that's a joke, but actually it's true. Most of us are shallow breathers. We sit, we type, we talk, and an unfortunately large number of us smoke. Maybe our modern world has unconsciously taught us to take small shallow breaths. Maybe city life and all its pollution teach us bad traits but they are traits we must break, if we want a long life. Get out in nature as much as you can. Take the morning air as deeply as you can. Get up, raise your arms high, and expand those lungs. Whole systems of yoga are based on breath. At least do what should come naturally.

Be Happy—Have Fun

In the words of the Blues artist, Duke Tumato, "Work is good, but it's not *that* good. When the work is through, it's time for me and you to get loose!"

We shouldn't need to be told, but it is vitally important to our health to have fun. We need to keep our working life, with all its pressures, in balance with a good social life. Don't become a workaholic or an obsessive

parent. Leave some quality time for yourself. Do whatever it is that makes you enjoy yourself. Don't be afraid to get out and have a few drinks if that's what it takes for you to really let go. Most people have enough vitality to handle small amounts of alcohol without doing long lasting damage, and it really is important to relax and let your hair down a bit. We have all heard of the wise advice "Everything is moderation". With that in mind, we would like to advise a little "Excess in moderation". As the Duke advises, "Let's get loose!"

Create Long Life

The mind is the maker. If you want to attain the grand age of 100, decide to do so now. Set your goal and believe in it. The old vaudevillian George Burns was the finest example of this concept. When asked on his 80th birthday how long he thought he would live, he replied, "I'm already booked for a show on my 100th birthday, so I can't go before then." George made that booking. He died two months later.

Learn to Love

If the mind is the maker, it is the heart that sustains the mind and body. Without the help of love and contentment, all the dieting, exercise, breathing and mind control will be like loose change in a pocket full of holes. Love is the single most important elixir to long life. You can find it anywhere and everywhere. Each cell of your body vibrates with your love, and in love disease can find no home.

How to Take the First Step

Ensuring a healthy, vital older age must begin right now, if it already hasn't. Here are the steps you need to take.
Step 1. Have your present health assessed by a naturopath interested in and familiar

with anti-aging strategies. You need to know where you are right now, in terms of medical, dietary, work, stress, relationships, and lifestyle practices. The assessment will also review past health history such as immune system weakness (influenza, etc.), fatigue, allergy, gut function, cardiovascular, family history and other health parameters. The importance of this cannot be underestimated. What you have experienced in the past is a key to why you are where you are today, and is predictive of where you will be in later years, unless you make some changes.

Step 2. Based on that information, the changes you may need to make can be identified, a multi-stage plan of implementation devised (even big change is easy if it is structured around small steps), and you can start getting to where you want to be right now.

Step 3. Anti-aging medicine is about prevention. Most, if not all, of the so-called diseases of old age can, and must be prevented if you want vitality, a clear mind and painless body however long you live. Arthritis, osteoporosis, cancers, heart and circulation problems, diabetes and dementia do not happen by chance. Whether they are "in your genes" such that you are susceptible to a particular disease or not, is quite irrelevant; these diseases often occur because one does not take steps to prevent them. Getting diseases is not "the luck of the draw", and avoiding diseases is not luck either. It can happen if you are prepared to take the necessary steps.

Step 4. We all need objective advice, and we all need a measure of guidance and motivation in whatever we attempt to do. Good health is no different. Unfortunately most doctors do not teach their patients good health, but simply prescribe drugs. As a group, doctors themselves are one of the sickest sub-sets within the affluent populations of the world. Either they do not know what is good health, or they are not very good at applying it. Of course not all medical practitioners are unaware of naturopathic healing principles and if you are lucky enough to have such a physician in your area his advice and help will be invaluable to

you. Naturopaths specialize in this type of knowledge and advice and it will be well worth your time and money to gain their insight and guidance.

Step 5. When should I start? Whenever you sense your own mortality. It is sometimes said that good health is (often) wasted on the young; they simply do not appreciate it. But there comes a time when the inexhaustible fountain of youthful vitality starts to crumble. Often it is in the so-called crisis years of your 40s or 50s. But you are not too young even in your 30s to start some preventative strategies, and make minor and/or major changes if need be. You are never too old to make important gains in good health. While it is true that the older we are the harder it is to make changes, we often have people in their 60s, 70s, 80s and more, who want to discover a greater potential for health than they already have.

Step 6. Reversing disease pathways is an integral part of anti-aging medicine, and is part and parcel of prevention strategy as well. Just because the medical system is not interested in reversing arthritis, or diabetes, or the processes of cancer, does not mean it cannot be done. It is best to act decisively when such processes are just becoming evident. Don't go for the "quick fix" (the drugs), as there is no cure with drugs, just symptom palliation. The sooner one heeds the signs, and acts to deal with the causes, the better the outcomes.

If processes have been happening for a long time, it generally takes a longer time to achieve the desired outcome of change than if the processes are only recent. But that is not always the case ... some people who have had severe even crippling arthritis for 10 or 15 years walk out arthritis-free after 3 months being on their program of change. Expected outcomes must be qualified by any pathology present at this time, such as existing organ, nerve or bone damage, and only time will tell just how far you can reverse any stage of a disease process.

The good news is, it doesn't cost much at all. What it takes is information, wisdom, and motivation, and that is what you pay for.

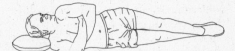

The extra benefit to you in lifestyle, happiness, and vitality improvement is up to you.

There are a lot of products being released claiming to be indispensable to anti-aging, almost like the "missing ingredient" for that miracle cure to aging you've always dreamed of. As clinicians, we are interested in new products. But good health, vitality and longevity has not (to date) come in the shape of a pill, and we cannot see a time when it will. We advise a relaxed attitude about the new wave of products. Spend your time and money first on the basics, the vitamins, minerals, herbal medicines, organic food and fresh, pure water, and allow time to demonstrate if there is a relative value and efficacy of the newer products.

OLD AGE PREVENTION EXERCISES

From *Old Age: Its Cause and Prevention*, by Sanford Bennett

1 Resistance Exercises for Back of Neck

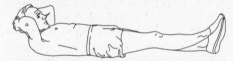

Begin on your back. With hands clasped behind the head, raise your head off the pillow and then press backwards while resisting this movement with the arms. Allow the head movement to be slightly stronger than the arm resistance. Repeat exercise 5 times the first week and increase by 2 repetitions a week until 25 repetitions are reached. This exercise develops all of the muscles of the back of the neck.

2 Development of Throat and Neck Muscles

Begin in the side lying position. Turn your chin as far as possible towards the upper shoulder. Begin with 5 repetitions and gradually work up to 50 daily. Do on both sides. This exercise will develop the muscles on the side of the neck, and the throat muscles under the chin.

3 Development of Throat Muscles

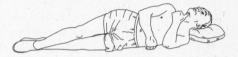

Begin in the side lying position. Place your thumb on the throat immediately under the chin in the position shown in the illustration. If you lie on the right side, use your right thumb. Alternately bring your head backwards and then forwards towards your chest using resistance from your thumb. This exercise will develop and firm the muscles of the throat. Begin with 10 repetitions and gradually work up to 50 repetitions.

4 Muscles of the Throat

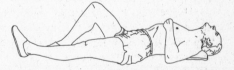

Begin lying on your back with a small pillow under the shoulders. Allow the neck to extend backwards as far as comfortable and slowly flex it forwards attempting to touch the chest with your chin. Do not lift your head off the table. Begin this exercise slowly. If dizziness occurs, reduce the amount of extension (backward bending) at first or consult a physician to make sure this exercise is safe for you. Begin with 5 or 10 repetitions and gradually increase to 100 repetitions. This exercise will firm the muscles under the chin and remove "double chin" problems or "loose jowls".

5 Muscles of the Neck and Abdomen

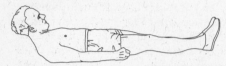

Begin lying on your back with no pillow under your head. Slowly raise your head off the table or bed and look towards your feet. Slowly lower your head and repeat 5 times initially. Increase to 50 times. This exercise strengthens the muscles of the neck and abdomen.

6 Lower Abdominals

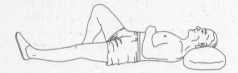

Begin lying on your back, bend one knee and draw it upwards and inwards, lifting up the hip on the same side. Slowly return to neutral position and repeat with opposite leg.

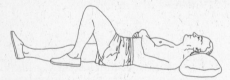

Begin with 5 repetitions on each leg and gradually increase to 25. This exercise strengthens lower oblique abdominals and will help remove the typical "pot belly" and will help in the treatment of constipation.

7 Percussion Abdominals

Begin lying on your back with a small pillow under your head. Lift your head and look towards your toes. Using balled fist strike your abdomen 25 times using a light rapid

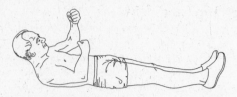

stroke. Alternately raise and lower your head while continuing the percussion. Gradually increase the number of strokes to 100 or more and their intensity. This is an excellent method to strengthen the abdominal muscles and incidentally to help cure poor digestion.

8 Loin Muscles

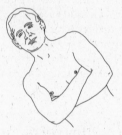

Begin lying on your back with your head on a small pillow. Fold your arms across your chest and raise your head and shoulders slightly so they clear the pillow. Bend the upper part of the body as far to one side as possible, and then alternate to the other side.

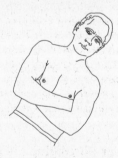

Begin with 5 to each direction and gradually increase to 25. This exercise will develop the muscles of the side of the lower back, buttocks, outer upper leg muscles and abdominals. This exercise can also be done standing if you wish.

9 Hips and Loins

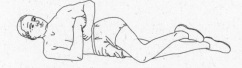

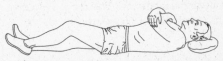

Begin in the side lying position with two small pillows or one large pillow under your head. With a bent knee, move your upper hip forwards and with bent upper arm simultaneously move your upper arm backwards, then return to neutral position. You may choose to resist the upper arm movement with your lower hand as illustrated, or allow the upper arm freedom to encourage better counter rotation of the upper torso. Do 5 repetitions on both sides and gradually increase to 10 repetitions per side. This exercise gives a spinal twist to help maintain mobility and gives strength and flexibility to the upper hip muscles, lower back and mid to upper back muscles, as well as the abdominals.

10 Muscles of the Sides

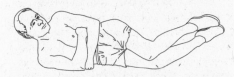

Begin lying on your side with two small pillows or one large pillow under your head. Fold arms across chest. Raise head, upper torso and lower legs simultaneously. Begin with 3 repetitions and gradually increase to 6 or 7. Take care with this exercise, as it is strenuous. This exercise will strengthen all the muscles of the side of the torso and legs.

11 Shoulder Shrugging

Begin lying on your back with a small pillow under your head. Grasp the left elbow with the right hand and the right elbow with the left hand exerting a gentle outward and upward pressure on both shoulders. From this position, do shoulder shrugs. The lateral strain and tensed condition of the muscles, combined with the up and down movement of the shoulders is a very effective method of developing that part of the body. Begin with 5 repetitions and gradually increase to 25 repetitions.

12 Shoulder Blade Muscles

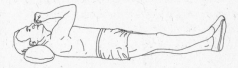

Begin lying on your back with a small pillow under your head. Bend elbow and then strike elbow across chest, moving the elbow and shoulder and keeping the hand close to your face. This will develop the muscle covering the shoulder blades. Begin with 5 repetitions and work up to 20 repetitions.

13 Muscles Covering Shoulder Blades

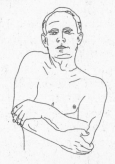

Begin on your back with arms crossed across your chest holding opposite elbows. Alternately raise your shoulders upward and forward as far as possible. This works muscles of the upper trapezius and shoulder blade region. Begin with 5 repetitions and gradually increase to 50 repetitions.

14 Single Arm Pulling Exercise for Shoulder and Back

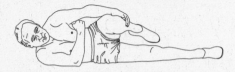

Begin lying on your back with two small pillows or one large pillow under your neck. Bend the upper leg and grab the lower leg just above the ankle. Pull with your arm with full extension, holding the strain for 4–6 seconds. Slowly release. Repeat 10 times initially and gradually increase to 25 repetitions. Do on both sides. This exercise will work muscles across the top of the shoulders and upper back.

15 Two Arm Pulling Exercise for Shoulder and Back

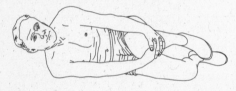

Begin lying on your side with two small pillows or one large pillow under your head. Bend upper leg and clasp both hands over the knee. Exert full strength, hold for 4–6 seconds and slowly relax. Repeat 10 times initially and gradually increase to 25 repetitions. Do on both sides. This exercise works the back and shoulder muscles as well as the buttocks.

16 Bar Exercise on Back, Two Arms

For this exercise, you will need a bar firmly attached across the headboard. Hardwood 1½ inches (4 cm) in diameter will suffice, mounted at a height that is comfortable. Begin lying on your back with a small pillow under your head. Grasp the bar with both hands and pull towards the feet with full

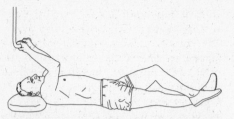

strength but not enough to move your body. Maintain tension for 4–6 seconds and slowly relax. Repeat 5 times initially and gradually increase to 25 repetitions. This exercise develops arms, shoulders and upper chest and back.

17 Bar Exercise on Side, One Arm

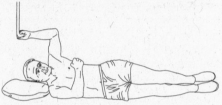

Begin lying on your side with pillow supporting head. Grasp the upper bed cross bar used in the previous exercise with the hand of your upper arm. Exert a strong pull towards your feet, hold for 4–6 seconds and slowly relax. Begin with 5 repetitions and increase to 25 repetitions. This exercise works arm, shoulders and muscles below the armpit.

18 Striking Exercises with or without Dumbbells

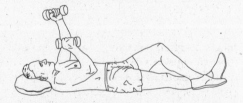

Begin on your back with head supported by a small pillow. Using 2–4 pound (1–2 kg) weights, perform fast "striking" motions upwards. Begin with 10 strikes and increase to 50 or more as your condition improves. This exercise is for arm development. In addition to this exercise, you may wish to extend your arms slowly at right angles from your sides and slowly raise them again. Repeat 10 times and increase to 25. When at the sides you may also rotate your hands back and forth to revolve the shoulder joints and keep them mobile. Often it is helpful to lay a thick folded blanket or pillow between your shoulders to allow more of an outward motion in this exercise. This will develop the chest muscles.

19 Developing Arms by Dumbbell Movements with Massage

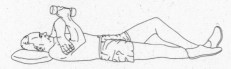

Begin on your back with pillow under your head. Use weights between 2-4 pounds (1-2 kg) while performing slow movements upwards (forwards) with your arm. Massage both biceps and triceps. This exercise will safely and rapidly strengthen both these muscle groups.

20 Resistance Forearm Exercise

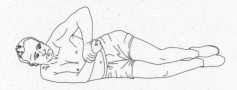

Begin lying on your side with head supported by pillows. Bend your lower arm to just less than a right angle. Grasp the lower arm wrist with the opposite hand. Exert downward pressure slowly with increasing pressure. Hold for 4-6 seconds and slowly relax. Repeat 5 times and gradually increase to 15. Repeat exercise with opposite arm.

This exercise strengthens both upper arm and forearm.

21 Resistance Triceps

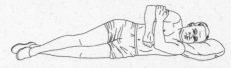

Begin lying on the side, head supported by pillows. Bend the upper arm at a right angle and using the lower arm grasp just above the elbow of the upper arm. Pull backwards with the upper arm, at the same time resisting the pull by the firm grasp and downward pull of the lower arm and hand. Begin with 5 repetitions and increase to 20. As with all the other exercises, begin slowly and end each action slowly to prevent injury. This exercise works the shoulder and triceps.

22 Arm Twisting Exercises

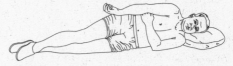

Begin lying on your side with head supported by pillows. With arm extended to side, clench fist and tense the muscles of the upper arm. Slowly twist your arm as far as it will go in both directions. Begin with 5 repetitions and gradually work up to 25. It is amazing how much development of the upper arms this little exercise will provide. Repeat with the other arm.

23 Resistance Arm Movement

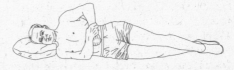

Begin lying on your side, head supported by pillows. Grasp the upper wrist with the lower hand. Pull upward with the upper arm and resist with the lower arm. Hold for 4-6 seconds. Perform exercise 10 times initially and increase to 20. Then rotate the wrist 180° so you grasp the inside of your upper wrist and perform the exercise again as above to work a different set of muscles. Do both exercises with both arms.

24 Climbing Muscles of Legs

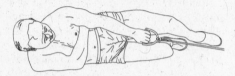

Attach to the foot of the bed a cord 1½ feet (46 cm) long terminating in a standard pulley handle. Begin lying on your side with head supported by pillows. Grasp the handle with the upper hand and press firmly against the footboard of the bed with the ball or your foot, knee bent at 45°. Hold for 4-6 seconds and release slowly. Begin with 10 repetitions and gradually increase to 25 with each leg.

25 Using the Lifting Board

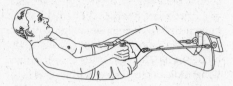

For this exercise, you need to make a simple apparatus. This device called by Sanford a "lifting board" is needed. Use a hardwood base 15 inches (38 cm) in length and 4 inches (10 cm) wide. One inch (2.5 cm) thick will suffice. Use two strong eyebolts mounted through drilled holes (eye screws could be pulled loose). Attach ropes 18 inches long and attach pulley weight handles as pictured. To do the exercise, begin in lying position on your back with a pillow under your head. Grasp the pulley handles with both hands and gradually increase pressure using legs, arms and back. Hold for 4-6 seconds and relax. Begin with 5 repetitions and increase to 15 or 20. Take care with this exercise especially where known disc problems exist. This exercise strengthens the legs, shoulders, and back.

ALCOHOLISM

DEFINITION

Habitual alcoholic consumption to the point where it interferes with the performance of daily responsibilities.

SYMPTOMS

Late symptoms include blackouts, dizziness, slurred speech, incoordination, nervousness, irritability, tremors, heart disease, liver disease, increased cholesterol, high blood pressure, and blood sugar disorders.

ETIOLOGICAL CONSIDERATIONS

• Hypoglycemia
• Diet
  Refined foods; sugar; vitamin and mineral deficiency; excess coffee
• Psychological
• Stress
• Heredity

DISCUSSION

The commonly held view of alcoholics as psychologically sick or simply lazy and irresponsible may be incorrect. There is a growing body of evidence indicating that some cases of alcoholism may be the result of a nutritional disorder.[21] For years it has been recognized that a large number (95%) of alcoholics suffer from hypoglycemia (low blood sugar). They also show multiple nutritional deficiencies. The usual explanation of these associated nutritional disorders is that as alcohol is consumed in preference to food (as is the case with most alcoholics) deficiency and hypoglycemia will obviously result. However, there is much evidence suggesting that many of the nutritional disorders, especially hypoglycemia, precede alcoholism.[22] In fact, it appears that hypoglycemia may be the *cause* of alcoholism and not its result.[23]

An interesting experiment to suggest this view was performed on rats. One group of rats was fed a refined carbohydrate diet typical of most hypoglycemics. Another group was fed on unrefined carbohydrates and supplemental vitamins. The last group was fed unrefined carbohydrates and high protein, a diet commonly used to prevent or treat hypoglycemia. Each group was supplied with two drinking sources—water and alcohol. The group fed refined carbohydrates, a diet known to cause low blood sugar, slowly began to prefer the alcohol over the water until they shunned the water almost completely. The low protein group drank a little alcohol, while the third group eating unrefined carbohydrates and high protein avoided the alcohol. Another study showed that rats fed a reasonably good diet but fed sufficient sugar also began to drink alcohol.

These studies clearly show that if hypoglycemia is allowed to develop, ideal conditions then exist for the development of alcoholism. This should not be too surprising when we consider that alcohol is probably the ultimate refined carbohydrate. Alcohol gives an even quicker blood sugar rise than sucrose. If the person is a social drinker, or has been exposed to alcohol enough for the body to recognize the very rapid blood sugar rise from alcohol, a craving even greater than sugar craving

becomes established under the right conditions.

The original causes of drinking may be social, but once the body establishes an alcoholic dependency (a *physiological* need to consume alcohol to maintain blood sugar levels) the person has stepped into a vicious circle. He or she drinks to relieve standard hypoglycemic symptoms of depression, tension, irritability, tiredness, inability to think, and so on. The alcohol gives a blood sugar boost which acts as positive reinforcement, conveying relaxation, increased energy, and in general a reversal of the unpleasant hypoglycemic sensations. Over a period of time the typical alcoholic displaces what little nutritious food he or she may still consume in favor of alcohol, until the diet is even lower in protein and nutrients, further setting the stage for more hypoglycemia and therefore alcoholism.

The same progression can occur for a person who takes his or her first drinks due to true psychological problems. Long after the original psychological cause is gone, the physiological alcoholic addiction remains. Most naturopaths agree, however, that an alcoholic addiction is very rare on a proper diet. Malnutrition usually precedes alcoholism and is aggravated by it.

TREATMENT

Diet

Initially it is best to stabilize the person on the typical *hypoglycemic diet* to provide a stable blood sugar level. If possible a diet composed of 50% whole grains with absolutely no refined carbohydrates or fruit is the best course of action. Include plenty of raw and conservatively cooked vegetables and adequate protein. Protein snacks every two hours are useful to keep blood sugar levels under control. Be sure to avoid those vegetables that cause rapid blood sugar elevations such as carrots This normalizes the blood sugar and stops the physiological alcoholic addiction. To help break the psychological addiction and make inroads against the firmly established positive associations of drinking, Alcoholics Anonymous is a very useful program.

Therapeutic Agents

Vitamins and Minerals—Primary

Vitamin A: 25,000 IU twice daily. Use emulsified form for better absorption.

Vitamin B complex: 50 mg 3 times daily; intramuscular injections 1–3 times per week; nervous system nutrient, liver support.

Vitamin B1: deficiency is extremely common in alcoholism. The final stages of beriberi are similar to late alcoholism. 100–3000 mg daily.

Vitamin B3: 100–200 mg twice daily (up to 5–20 g given in some cases). This helps reduce alcohol craving. Increase dose slowly.

Vitamin B5: 50–100 mg 2–3 times daily. Helps reduce effects of stress and aids in alcohol detoxification.

Vitamin B12: 250–1000 mcg daily. Use sublingual form or injectable.

Vitamin C: 1000–5000 IU 3–6 times daily (or more). Detoxifies; anti-stress agent. 20–30 g daily intravenously to reduce withdrawal symptoms.

Vitamin E: 400 IU twice daily.

Zinc: 25–50 mg 1–2 times daily. Zinc deficiency is very common in chronic alcoholism.

Chromium: 200 mcg daily. Helps reduce hypoglycemia.

Selenium: 200 mcg daily. Helps protect against alcohol-induced liver damage.

N,N-dimethylglycine (DMG): 50–100 mg daily.

Vitamins and Minerals—Secondary

Vitamin D: 400–1000 IU or plenty of sunshine.

Calcium: 800–1500 mg daily. Antispasmodic, sedative.

Magnesium: 400–800 mg daily.

Folic acid: 800 mcg daily.

Others—Primary

Brewer's yeast: 1 tsp 3 times daily. High in GTF chromium to help normalize blood sugar levels.

L-glutamine (a non-essential amino acid): 2–4 g daily. Provides brain cells with an energy source, reduces alcoholic craving, and decreases harmful poisoning effects of alcohol. Glutamine has glucogenic properties.

Glutathione: protects the liver from damage and reduces alcohol craving.

L-methionine: 1000 mg daily. Works with glutathione to protect the liver from damage.

L-cysteine: 500 mg once or twice daily. Aids in liver regeneration.

GLA (gamma-linolenic acid): alcohol is an enzyme blocking factor in the metabolism of essential fatty acids. EPA (eicosapentaenoic acid), may also be useful.

Free-form amino acid complex: 500 mg 2–3 times daily. Aids in liver regeneration and reduces withdrawal symptoms.

Tyrosine: adrenalin precursor, reduces withdrawal symptoms (use with vitamin B3).

DL-phenylalanine (reduces withdrawal symptoms) doses of 1500 mg daily or more may be indicated.

Others—Secondary

Digestive enzymes: blood glucose level stabilization; digestive enzyme support.

Raw adrenal tablets: anti-stress, adrenal support.

Raw liver tablets.

Probiotics.

Botanicals—Primary

St Mary's thistle: protects and restores liver structure and function.

St John's wort: CNS relaxant.

Siberian ginseng: adaptogenic, adrenal support.

Valerian: a calming nervine/sedative.

Dandelion: useful in the repair of the liver.

Botanicals—Secondary

Angelica induces distaste for alcohol.

Chelendonium: for liver repair.

May-apple, or American mandrake: highly toxic; use only with experienced advice.

Hops: a mild nervine/sedative.

See also Hypoglycemia for herbs.

Useful Prescriptions

1 drop oil of eucalyptus, $\frac{1}{2}$ drop oil of turpentine, $\frac{1}{2}$ drop compound tincture of benzoin Place in 00 capsule. 1–2 times daily. Makes person nauseous if alcohol is taken.

ALLERGIES AND FOOD INTOLERANCES

DEFINITION

The body's adverse reactions of any variety to otherwise normal stimuli.

SYMPTOMS

Allergies can do just about anything to almost any part of the body. Common symptoms are runny nose, watery eyes, ear infections, sinusitis, rhinitis, tonsillitis, asthma, headaches, gastrointestinal complaints, nausea, vomiting, cramps, colitis, flatulence, constipation, edema, menstrual disorders, palpitations, hypoglycemia, obesity, emotional disturbances, learning disability, mental deficiency, schizophrenia, hyperactivity, skin rashes, eczema, psoriasis, hives, ulcers, neuritis, arthritis, phlebitis, epilepsy, and others.

ETIOLOGICAL CONSIDERATIONS—PRIMARY

- Drugs
  Vaccines and drug reactions (especially antibiotics)
- Improper weaning
- Adrenal exhaustion
- Alcohol; coffee/tea (caffeine); drugs; hypoglycemia; stress
- Stress
  Adrenal exhaustion; vitamin deficiency (B complex and C); hypoglycemia

- Diet
  Hypoglycemia; sugar; refined carbohydrates; deficiency; veganism; food intolerance (e.g. milk, wheat and egg); green vegetable deficiency; fried foods
- Leaky gut syndrome
  Increased permeability of intestines to large protein molecules due to a thinning of the bowel walls (see Leaky Gut).
- Heredity
  Immune deficiencies (e.g. gamma A-globulin, or IgA); defective enzyme structure; poor pancreatic function
- Inhalant sensitivity (i.e. dust, mold, pollen, grasses, animal hair)
- Chemicals: severe exposure
- Poor eliminations
- Liver disorders
- Severe viral infection (e.g. mononucleosis, flu, hepatitis), causing immune system disturbance

ETIOLOGICAL CONSIDERATIONS— SECONDARY

- Digestive enzyme deficiency: incompletely digested foods are irritant, toxic, allergenic.
- Acidosis: due to pancreatic enzyme deficiency and allergic reaction itself.
- Food additives, preservatives, colorings, etc.

- Heavy metal poisoning; aluminum cooking utensils; chlorinated water.
- Radiation.
- Psychosomatic.
- Spinal lesions, especially in neck and upper thoracic region.
- *Candida albicans* intestinal and systemic infection.
- Free radical oxidative damage.
- Antioxidant insufficiency.

DISCUSSION

What we usually are dealing with in cases of allergy is a hyperallergic system, not a system with an allergy or two. This can easily be seen in the typical allergy patient who finds himself or herself first allergic to one thing, only later to develop more allergies as time goes by. We have seen patients who claimed food allergies to nearly everything except potato chips and cola! Another interesting fact is that allergies may be inconsistent, being worse on some days and almost absent on others. This reflects variations in the individual's reaction, due to factors other than mere exposure.

The difference in many cases between a normal reaction and an abnormal reaction to otherwise normal elements in the environment is weak and overstressed adrenal glands. This is not the only cause as we shall see later, but certainly is a major factor. Overstressed adrenals may be due to an improper diet of sugar and refined carbohydrates, alcohol, or coffee, all of which put an excess burden on these glands. Hypoglycemia, a result of such a diet, is closely associated with most cases of allergies. Prolonged psychological stress also stimulates and depletes the adrenal glands. This creates a vicious cycle of stress, adrenal exhaustion, and allergy, which in turn usually creates some degree of stress, and so on.

A very common history reported by many allergy patients clearly shows this allergy–stress relationship. As a child, many symptoms of allergy were present. These disappeared sometime in the teens or earlier.

For years the patient was symptom-free, until the onset of a severely stressful incident or period of life such as a divorce (or marriage), death of a loved one, stressful job, difficult child, or other similar situation. Shortly after this, severe, often different, allergic symptoms return.

Here's how it works. The body has an amazing ability to *adapt*, or get "used to" repeated exposures to a particular (potential) allergen, in order to initially survive it. It does this by adjusting to a new set point, increasing output of enzyme detoxification systems and immune enhancement. Initial exposure often produces "alarm" (acute) symptoms, such as indigestion, nausea, headache, flu-like symptoms, before the body "masks" (i.e. moves the immune, metabolic and detoxification systems to a new set point), and symptoms become less severe and often disappear. Much of drug medication has this effect, of "treating" (masking) the symptoms; the effect is much like sticking a band-aid over the red light indicator which warns of low oil in the vehicle. Deliberate masking in this way only further exacerbates the problem. The second stage of masking is signaled by consequent development of more severe difficulties and is really maladaptation. This phase occurs with prolonged exposure to the inciters, and this phase is pathologic, with tissue changes occurring as there is a gradual depletion of essential nutrients.

Eventually, be it minutes, days, or years depending on the nature of the chemical exposure and an individual's capacity to detoxify, the body's defense mechanisms will break down and fail altogether, and end-organ failure and fixed-name disease will inevitably occur, such as diseases of heart, blood vessel, lung, gastrointestinal, genitourinary, or any of a host of other tissues and systems.

Toxicity, which initially may have been limited to one particular area of the body (e.g. the blood/brain barrier or peripheral cellular membranes of the skin, lung, nasal mucosa, intestinal mucosa) once having damaged a barrier, or depleted the nutrient fuels (such as magnesium, zinc, all B vitamins, amino acid or fatty acid) of the enzyme or coenzyme defenses, will *spread* to other tissue and organs. This is known as spreading phenomenon. Immune or pharmacological releasing mechanisms such as serotonin, kinin, or vasoactive amines may become so damaged that they are then triggered by many non-toxic (e.g. food) substances in addition to the specific one or several substances to which the initial reaction occurred. It is well substantiated that antigen recognition sites may be disturbed or destroyed by pollutant overload. Hormone deregulation (feedback mechanisms) may occur, allowing still greater dysfunction and sensitivity.

A *switch phenomenon* may also occur, in which a set of symptoms affecting one end-organ response can change to another. For example, transient brain dysfunction can be followed by arthralgia, followed by diarrhea, followed by cardiac arrhythmia. This phenomenon frequently occurs when symptom-suppressing medication therapy is used over a period of time. For example a patient may have their sinusitis cleared by medication (e.g. cortisone), but since the cause has not been eliminated, they may later develop arthralgia and eventually arthritis; or their colitis may clear up but then they will have cystitis later. This tells us that initially treating the cause effectively can curtail a lifelong progression of illness and premature death.

The final aspect involved is the concept of *biochemical individuality*. A person's uniqueness is dependent on at least three factors: genetics (which at present we cannot alter, although it is an area of current research); the state of a foetus's nutritional health and toxic body burden during gestation (which only the prospective parents can alter, e.g. sperm and ova health, and gestational health); and an individual's toxic body load in relation to his nutritional state at the time of exposure (which we can all modulate).

Biochemical individuality has to do with the differing quantities of proteins, carbohydrates, fats, enzymes, vitamins, minerals and immune and enzyme detoxification parameters. It accounts for the fact that while a group of individuals may be exposed to the same allergens, one person may develop arthritis, another sinusitis, another diarrhea, cystitis, asthma, dermatitis or psoriasis, and another may remain apparently unaffected. An example is of two women both working for a relatively short period in a photographic development lab, one developed symptoms of MS, the other chronic fatigue syndrome (CFS), within a relatively short time (approx. 6 months).

Another common cause of allergies, especially in the form of chronic skin rashes, is the use of vaccines and other drugs. A common history obtained from those with chronic eczema or psoriasis is single or repeated vaccinations followed closely by the onset of allergy. This is probably due to a similar mechanism of thymus gland destruction as found with massive chemical exposure, of severe viral diseases such as mononucleosis, hepatitis, or influenza. Certain cells, called T-regulatory cells, are produced by the thymus gland and help suppress formation of excess antibodies (and thus reduce allergic reactions). These cells are easily destroyed by many vaccines, some drugs, massive chemical exposure, severe viral infections, and radiation. The thymus plays a pivotal role with most allergies. Antibiotics are notorious for allergic skin reactions that can be most difficult to resolve. In some cases, however, the roots of allergy are not so easily traced, but a history of repeated vaccination is always suspect. Once a foreign protein is introduced into the bloodstream, some degree of allergic reaction, depending on individual variables, is probable.

Certain foods may act as the primary cause of allergies. These cause different reactions in the body than the common inhalants and other topical allergens. For example, the body may, due to inherited tendencies, have a gluten intolerance causing malabsorption of any grain that contains this protein. The intestines become irritated and lose their normal villi necessary for proper absorption. This thinning of the bowel's walls allows toxic substances to be absorbed into the bloodstream, which may cause allergic symptoms far from the original disorder to complicate the local intestinal complaint. Thus we see how a single digestive incompatibility may lead to multiple allergic symptoms.

Milk intolerance is also a very common problem. Some individuals from birth lack the enzyme (lactase) to digest milk sugar, while others lose this enzyme later in life. Up to 85% of Oriental people are deficient in lactase by adult life, while up to 85% of the Caucasian population retain adequate levels for normal digestion. If lactase levels are too low or absent, milk cannot be digested and it ferments, causing diarrhea, constipation, gas, abdominal pain, and many other systemic allergic reactions. The protein in milk may also cause problems.

Part of the problem with these two main food groups, wheat and milk, stems from improper weaning. The infant's intestine is much more permeable than the adult's. Large proteins or protein fragments can be absorbed directly into the blood. If protein-containing foods such as milk, wheat, or eggs are introduced into the diet too early, these protein components can set the stage for life-long allergy. Breast milk seems to protect against this foreign protein absorption into the blood by sealing the intestinal mucosa and making it less permeable. Most children are either not breast-fed, or are breast-fed for too short a period and then weaned to pasteurized, homogenized, cow's milk, possibly containing antibiotics and pesticides. If breast-feeding were continued for a minimum of 9-12 months and the child then weaned to raw goat's milk, which is closer in constitution to mother's milk, fewer allergies (and allergists!) would exist.[24]

Wheat also is added to the average infant's diet much too early. Digestive enzymes necessary for proper starch digestion are not even present until 4-6 months. We usually advise adding wheat cereal grains as one of the last, not first elements of the diet, somewhere around the first birthday. This most definitely includes breads and crackers, no matter how wholesome. We find that the children with the most colds and allergies generally eat the most starches. Children who are breast-fed eat less starches and get plenty of fruit and vegetables, and are generally very healthy during their first year of life.

Eggs are the third major food allergen and should not be given until the child is about 8-12 months old, and then no more than one poached egg should be consumed every other day, to prevent allergies in the early years.

The general procedure of weaning is also a major cause of undetected allergy. Many parents indiscriminately add foods to their young infant's diet without carefully observing for any adverse reactions. In our practice we have seen 3-month-old infants with chronic eczema, whose parents already routinely fed the child a "normal diet", which for them was cow's milk, fried sausage, fried eggs, fried potatoes, hamburgers, potato chips, candy, and Coca-Cola! It is essential that the first foods given to an infant be as close to their natural state as possible, either raw or conservatively steamed, in a small amount only, and separate from any other foods. This should be done for a period of 2-3 days at one meal, to observe for a rash or any other adverse reaction. If no reaction occurs, increasing amounts may be given and then may be combined with other tested and compatible foods. It is a really good idea to keep a detailed weaning diary so you can record when you first introduced foods to the infant, and keep a record of any adverse reactions.

Sometimes an allergic reaction will be noticed to otherwise healthful foods such as broccoli or cabbage. In these cases discontinue these foods for 6-8 weeks and try again. If the child repeatedly reacts, he or she may indeed have specific food intolerance. More likely than not, however, the second or third try will be met with success. Specific food allergies are very rare when foods are introduced properly.

We emphasize the necessity for proper weaning since it is far easier to pinpoint a reaction earlier, than later on when a full diet has been introduced. In some cases it then becomes impossible to detect the offending food without reweaning the infant—a painful process for both infant and mother.

Liver congestion and toxemia due to improper diet may also be a factor in allergies. If this is coupled with digestive enzyme deficiency or other causes of incomplete digestion, the allergic reaction is enhanced. Undigested foods usually stimulate an increase in histamine which may initiate an allergic reaction by the cells. The liver normally detoxifies histamine, but a damaged or toxic liver may do so inefficiently, causing the histamine to build up in the system, initiating a reaction. Antihistamines used as allergy medication may further cause liver damage, reducing the body's ability to detoxify histamine.

Another factor of increasing importance in the last 70 years is the widespread use of chemicals, pesticides, and other additives to the food supply. Evolution naturally adapts us to our environment; however, the pace of this exposure to foreign substances has been so rapid that evolution has been unable to keep pace. A dramatic increase in various allergic reactions has been the result.

Candida albicans (yeast) infection of the digestive system has been implicated in some stubborn cases of allergies. The yeast proliferates and irritates the intestinal mucosa, causing it to become inflamed and more permeable, allowing foreign proteins to enter into the blood. A history of antibiotic use or the birth control pill is suggestive.

It has been estimated that 80% of allergy sufferers have increased permeability of gut mucosa, or leaky gut, and treatment must aim to repair the pathology (see Leaky Gut).

TREATMENT

The object of naturopathic therapy in this case is to strengthen the entire system, especially the overburdened adrenal glands. If specific allergens exist, they may need to be avoided where possible, to allow the system time to repair itself and establish equilibrium. If an isolated food that causes a reaction can be discovered, it will need to be eliminated. Often, however, after prolonged therapy, these may once again be added to the diet, at least in moderation.

Allergy Diagnosis

Several methods exist to diagnose individual allergies. Unfortunately none of these is sufficient on its own to distinguish all allergies. In fact all of them put together still are not sufficient to identify all allergies. Any test can yield false positives and false negatives. However, at least they can give us a good idea of the allergens mediated by the allergy systems we now know about.

Radioallergosorbent Test (RAST Test)

This test is a method to identify specific antibodies in the blood to certain foods or other substances. The problem with the RAST test is that a person must already have a good idea of what his or her allergies may be. It can get fairly expensive pretty quickly to have substances tested at random. Usually, common foods are tested such as wheat, milk, eggs, yeast, and citrus; however, any food can be the problem. We also test for any favorite foods, since these frequently used items are the most likely to be the problem. Most good laboratories do RAST testing. The RAST test is very selective and will only show up as positive IgE-mediated allergies. Many false negative reactions therefore occur. The foods tested must have been eaten in the three days prior to the test for best results.

Cytotoxic Allergy Test

This test exposes the white blood cells to a sample of the suspected food or substance to observe for a specific reaction. This test is more convenient than the RAST test since a battery of 38–40 tests of common foods are routinely tested for at a cost of $100–$120. Any other specific foods, inhalants, food dyes, or chemicals may be tested for by request. Cytotoxic tests are less routinely available than the RAST, but can usually be found at large medical centers. Many false positives, however, occur with this test, and there is some question about its reliability. It is subject to error in interpretation.

Unfortunately, results from the RAST and cytotoxic tests rarely ever are the same. Thus, a positive reaction to wheat on the cytotoxic test may end up negative on the RAST. This does not mean that one test is more or less valid, but that we are dealing with two out of several systems of allergic response. Allergists feel that several as yet undiscovered systems exist, which hopefully will soon be discovered.

Pulse Test

This test, originated by Dr Arthur Coca, may be attempted in full as outlined in his book, *The Pulse Test*, or the modified approach may be used to test for single allergens. This is a very good technique in conjunction with the two previous diagnostic tests and may help to confirm both. The basic concept of the pulse test is that foods that cause an allergic reaction also cause the pulse to rise suddenly. To do this test take a resting pulse. This will usually be somewhere between 50–70 beats per second. Consume the food group you wish to test and take your pulse 15 minutes later. If you are allergic your pulse will rise by at least 10 beats per second. Only test one food group daily. This is the simplest and most reliable allergy test we have found.

Testing the Suspected Allergen

Once a potential allergen, whether a food for some other substance, has been identified, the only reliable way to verify the hypothesis is to test the substance by totally excluding it from your external and/or internal environment for a period of about 21 days. During this time, the body

will desensitize to it, and then you can expose yourself to an appropriate amount of it, and your body will send you very clear signals, if indeed there is a positive reaction.

The following are some common signs and symptoms associated with a positive allergic response:
- Gastrointestinal: stomach pain, bloating, wind, diarrhea, constipation.
- Skin: rash.
- Respiratory: wheezing, excess mucus, asthma attack.
- Central nervous system: headache, irritability, hyperactivity.

Elimination Diets and Fasts

One approach is to eliminate suspected foods for 7–21 days to see if symptoms are removed. This is only rarely successful, since most people respond to several unsuspected foods. The better approach is to fast for 5 days and then add foods individually to the diet to test for reaction via the pulse test or by eating only one food item for several days to test for negative reactions. Many reactions take 5 days to settle down and 3–5 days to begin again, so this can be a very difficult procedure. It is, however, the best procedure to diagnose food allergy accurately.

Food rotation diets are extremely useful in reducing the allergy load, allowing a supplement program to have maximum effect. Grains, proteins, and other suspected foods are arranged in the diet so that their consumption is not repeated more frequently than every 4–5 days.

The typical skin patch test is of some use.

Once an attempt to isolate specific allergens is complete, these items are removed from the diet. The next stage of therapy involves the actual process of healing the body. As previously mentioned, the allergic reaction, and along with this the specific allergens, are usually only the symptoms of a deep-seated disorder. The next step is to soothe the hyper allergic system.

Diet

Periods of vegetable juice fasting in any acute phase of an allergic reaction are very useful. Such fasts are also essential to eliminate toxins and establish equilibrium within the body. The fast may be anywhere from 3-21 days with supervision. Use organically grown vegetables only. Carrot is usually the base ingredient with other vegetables added for variety.

Raw food vegetarian diets are beneficial for varying periods of time, alternated with either the vegetable juice fast or the full hypoglycemia diet (minus any allergic foods). Low blood sugar is a consistent causative or coexistent factor in most allergic patients. (See Hypoglycemia for more details on this aspect of allergic reactions.) All foods or juices should be obtained unsprayed from reliable organically grown sources. Many times a "food allergy" is in reality a chemical, pesticide, or color additive allergy.

In severe cases it is often necessary to follow vegetable juice or better yet, water fasting with the introduction of single food meals on a rotation basis. Unsuspected foods are introduced into the diet with the patient eating only one food type per meal and not consuming the same food again for at least 4 days. The body is thus able to rest from repeated allergic reactions and heal itself using the appropriate nutrients. Once the body has become less reactive, combination meals of the tested foods are introduced and the diet is continually expanded. Any food that causes an allergic reaction is eliminated until later in the healing process, until ultimately the individual is free of all or most allergic reactions.

Physiotherapy

- Meditation twice daily.
- Relaxation exercises twice daily.
- Spinal manipulation 1-2 times per week.

Therapeutic Agents

Caution: Before any major supplementation program is implemented, it is important to identify major suspected allergens (being the cause of the problems), and eliminate exposure to them, or else supplementation will at best tend to be simply palliative, providing mere symptomatic relief.

Vitamins and Minerals— Primary

Vitamin A with beta-carotene: 10,000-75,000 IU daily or more for short terms in acute cases. Emulsified forms are best in high doses. Very useful in conditions involving the respiratory system or the skin. Supports immune function.

Vitamin B complex: 25-50 mg 3 times daily (essential in adrenal function).

Vitamin B6: 100-250 mg or more in acute cases, 3 times daily (essential in adrenal function).

Vitamin B12: 200-300 mcg 2-3 times daily. Use sublingual form or injections.

Pantothenic acid: 100-500 mg twice daily (antihistamine, essential in cortisone production).

Vitamin C with bioflavinoids: 500-1000 mg 3 times daily, or up to bowel tolerance (essential to adrenal function; antioxidant, anti-allergy, detoxifies histamine).

Vitamin E: 200-400 IU 1-2 times daily (antioxidant).

Glutamine: to repair leaky gut.

Selenium: 20 mcg daily (anti-inflammatory with chemical allergies and allergic toxemia).

Zinc: 15-45 mg 3 times daily (immune support).

Vitamins and Minerals— Secondary

Calcium: 400-800 mg daily.

Magnesium: 200-400 mg daily.

Calcium, magnesium, and potassium: as bicarbonate buffers.

Manganese: 2-5 mg 2-3 times per week.

Others—Primary

Probiotics: to correct Candida overgrowth and restore bowel flora ecology. One of the principal roles of flora is to protect against allergic reactions.

Raw adrenal tablets: 1-2 tablets 3 times daily.

Raw thymus tablets: immune system support. 2-6 tablets 2-3 times daily.

Quercetin: 500 mg once or twice daily. Enhances immune function. Take with 100 mg of bromelain to enhance absorption.

Coenzyme Q10: 100 mg daily. Improves immune function and cellular oxygenation.

Others—Secondary

L-cysteine and L-tyrosine: 500 mg daily. Useful with respiratory allergies.

Bee pollen: (locally produced is best) richer source of amino acids than animal protein; rich in omega-3 EFAs.

Germanium: 50 mg daily. Stimulates the immune response.

Biotin: with Candida infestation: 200 mcg 3 times daily.

Castor oil: 5 drops in the morning on empty stomach.

Comb honey: chew ½ tsp twice daily; especially therapeutic if local comb honey is used.

Pancreatic enzymes: 1-2 tablets. Take with meals.

Evening primrose oil: especially with eczema or other skin disorders.

Garlic: 2 capsules 3 times daily.

Hydrochloric acid: if hydrochloric acid deficiency has been proven, take 5-60 grains with meals.

Kelp: 2-4 tablets 3 times daily.

EPA (eicosapentaenoic acid): may be useful in hypersensitivity reactions such as asthma, allergic rhinitis, or the panallergic patient.

Botanicals

Prescribed according to individual symptoms and general needs. The protocols will address improving elimination, digestion, immune function, and liver function, as well as treating the symptoms of the particular allergy. The following herbs will be of some assistance.

Ephedra (ma-huang): asthma, nasal and lung congestion.

St Mary's thistle: cholagogue.

Goldenseal: cholagogue.

Goldenseal: trophorestorative to mucous membranes.

Echinacea: immunostimulant.

Picrorrhiza: immunostimulant.

Clivers: eliminative and decongestant.

Golden rod: eliminative and decongestant.

Poke root: eliminative and decongestant (highly toxic, see page 60).

Albizzia: anti-allergic.

Oats: adrenal tonic and adaptogen.

Ginseng: adrenal tonic and adaptogen.

Licorice: adrenal tonic and adaptogen.

Gentian: digestive stimulant.

It should be noted that echinacea is most useful as a preventive, and that better herbs can be selected to actually treat aspects of specific allergic reactions.

Therapeutic Suggestions

Due to the extremely diverse nature of the allergic response, the nutritional supplement program must be individually tailored, depending on the organ or tissue groups affected.

More vitamin A will be required, for example, with an allergic manifestation affecting the lungs' mucous membranes or skin. Extremely high doses may be required when malabsorption of fats is present in steatorrhea. Use the micellized form in these cases. Any level taken over 50,000 IU daily should be monitored closely with blood tests. Use any dose of vitamin A over 50,000 IU daily with medical supervision only.

The B complex group is particularly essential in reversing an allergic tendency. High levels of B6, B12, and pantothenic acid are almost always required with an additional balanced B complex. In some cases these may need to be given by intramuscular injection in the initial stages.

Vitamin C at bowel tolerance doses is also essential. In cases of severe reactions, it may be given intravenously in doses of 5-20 g with 500-1000 mg calcium (as calcium gluconate) and 250-500 mg magnesium (as magnesium sulfate).

Vitamin E is an excellent antioxidant and should be a regular part of any program.

Zinc acts as an autoimmunity factor, working with vitamins A and E.

Selenium is of particular usefulness with any chemical allergies or sensitivities, especially if given with kelp.

Where pancreatic digestive deficiency exists, pancreatic digestive enzymes and free amino acid powder supplements are useful to reduce the absorption of undigested anti-genic proteins and also to increase the amino acid pool necessary for protein synthesis, to help encourage proper immune and digestive enzyme function. Raw thymus taken three or four times daily in the early stages of therapy helps boost immune function. In cases of intestinal *Candida albicans* overgrowth causing multiple allergy symptoms, Lactobacillus (probiotics) and biotin therapy is sometimes very effective. Other cases require nystatin for up to 3-6 months to rid the system of this yeast. Proper internal ecology is then restored through proper diet and the avoidance of birth control pills and antibiotic therapy when possible.

ANEMIA

DEFINITION

Anemia literally means "without blood", and is a deficiency of red blood cells, or the presence of abnormal red blood cells due either to reduced production, abnormal production, excess destruction, or blood loss.

SYMPTOMS

Pallor, tiredness, dizziness, headaches, depression, slow healing, loss of sex drive, bruising, nervousness, shortness of breath, and palpitation.

ETIOLOGICAL CONSIDERATIONS—PRIMARY

- Iron deficiency (hypochromic) Malabsorption (caffeine, coffee, chocolate, etc.) reduces ability to absorb iron; post-hemorrhagic (heavy menstruation, ulcers, hemorrhoids, fissure, etc.); sideroblastic (failure to utilize iron).
- Vitamin B12 or folic acid deficiency (megaloblastic)

Nutritional (vegans: no animal products)—lack of vitamin B12; lack of green vegetables—lack of folic acid); Addisonian, pernicious; drugs, insecticides (may destroy bone marrow); gastrointestinal (stomach removal, hydrochloric acid deficiency); intrinsic factor deficiency.
- Colitis, malabsorption, food allergy, etc.; bleeding ulcers.
- Heredity: hemolytic, sickle cell, thalassemia or autoimmune anemia.
- Repeated pregnancies.
- Old age: poor absorption; poor dentures leading to lack of green vegetable consumption.
- Infancy: iron deficiency after 6 months; vitamin E deficiency in pregnancy and early life; iron deficiency (on cow's milk diet); vitamin C deficiency.
- Puberty: rapid growth of muscle (myoglobin) leading to iron deficiency.
- Abnormal bacterial flora.
- Chlorine in drinking water destroys gut flora (as do a lot of other things); blind loop syndrome; improper diet leading to change in bacterial flora.
- Cellular obstruction to nutrients causing poor utilization.

ETIOLOGICAL CONSIDERATIONS— SECONDARY

Vitamin C deficiency: scurvy; vitamin C deficiency withdrawal in newborns from mothers on high vitamin C doses.
Vitamin E deficiency.
Vitamin B6 deficiency.
Thyroid and liver disorders (e.g. myxedema anemia, cirrhosis).
Bone marrow disease.
Zinc-induced copper deficiency anemia.
Excess onion/garlic use.
Alcoholism.
Marathoner's anemia.
Infectious diseases (malaria and others).
Autoimmune diseases (rheumatoid arthritis, lupus and others)
Reduced exposure to sun; intestinal parasites.
Lead toxicity.

DISCUSSION

Anemia can be caused by a very wide variety of conditions, as seen by the long list of etiologic considerations. The most significant and common forms of anemia are those related to diet. It is to these that we wish to confine this discussion.

Most people equate anemia with *iron deficiency.* This is encouraged by commercials for products such as Geritol (a product high in supplemental iron), which promote this product almost as a cure-all for any condition that produces tiredness. While iron deficiency anemia is fairly common for women in the childbearing years due to frequent loss of iron-containing hemoglobin in the menstrual flow, it is less likely to be the cause of anemia in the elderly who are the prime target for these advertisements.

In fact, due to years of consuming excess iron in supplement form, many elderly persons actually develop severe iron *excesses*. Extreme iron overdose can cause the dangerous condition known as siderosis, resulting in damage to the liver, pancreas,

and heart; and cause a form of arthritis.

Iron deficiency should be tested for prior to medication. It is to be suspected in infancy, puberty, pregnancy, females with heavy periods, and any other condition causing sudden or chronic blood loss, such as a chronic bleeding ulcer. Iron absorption is reduced by the consumption of coffee, tea, edetic acid (EDTA), or excess soy protein.

Vitamin B12 deficiency anemia is becoming an increasing concern. Pernicious anemia, a rare condition, is due to intrinsic factor deficiency, essential for vitamin B12 absorption. This must be corrected by vitamin B12 injections. Another form of B12 deficiency caused by restricted diet is less rare. Vegans (people who abstain from all animal protein and animal products, including eggs and dairy products) may find themselves creating a vitamin B12 deficiency with its insidious effects. Vitamin B12 deficiency takes 6-10 years to become apparent, but once manifest the damage is permanent. It produces nerve destruction similar to multiple sclerosis, with sensations of pins and needles, sore muscles, neuritis, stiff spine, difficulty in walking, and paralysis.

Vitamin B12 is found almost exclusively in animal products, with the exception of traces in comfrey, kelp, sunflower seeds, raw wheat germ, and grapes. Even in these the vitamin B12 is often the result of fermentation such as that found on grapes. Any fermented foods also contain significant amounts of vitamin B12, and it is with these sources that the informed vegan supplements his or her diet. The amount available in vegetable sources, however, is minute. One would need to eat 1-2 lb. of comfrey daily to get adequate vitamin B12. Brewer's yeast as naturally found is deficient in vitamin B12, and if this is to be used as a reliable source, B12 must have been added and will be so marked on the package. Seed yoghurts, unboiled miso, seaweed, kelp, sunflower seeds, and grapes should be eaten frequently.

Arguments are heard that vitamin B12 may be made by the bacteria of the small intestine and that these precautions are unnecessary. There are several considerations that must be kept in mind. It is true that a healthy bacterial flora will synthesize vitamin B12 in some people, and it is also true that a vegan diet, being high in vegetables and fiber foods, will generally favor a healthy floral colony. It has been suggested by some researchers, however, that not all vegans develop this vitamin B12 synthesizing ability. The reasons for this are not entirely clear. It is probable that the problem stems from the drastic and sudden way in which many vegans have changed their diet. In many cases, for their entire lives and for the entire lives of each of their ancestors, the food eaten had some animal origin. Through the process of natural evolution, the capability to synthesize the body's own B12 was irrelevant as a survival factor, therefore was not favored genetic material. A further complication is that the folic acid found very prominently in the raw green vegetables so prevalent in a vegan's diet will mask the effects of vitamin B12 deficiency until very late, when the damage is already extreme.

Whatever the cause, the fact is that no person can be absolutely certain that his or her own vitamin B12 production is active or adequate enough to prevent vitamin B12 deficiency anemia without the precaution of eating vitamin B12 source foods. If individuals wish to restrict their diets for whatever reason, be it religious, humanitarian, or health, they must become more and more aware of what special attention the body may need to prevent deficiency. We suggest all vegans take a B12 supplement daily.

Folic acid deficiency is most commonly caused by a diet deficient in raw green vegetables and foods, which contains insufficient vitamin C to aid absorption. Vitamin C is also a factor in the absorption of essential minerals, including iron and vitamin B12, and helps conserve vitamin E.

Vitamin E is essential in blood building. Deficiency of this vitamin is often a factor in pregnancy; babies born of vitamin E deficient mothers, and who are given prolonged feedings of cow's milk, can become deficient in vitamin E and iron.

For those on very high zinc supplementation, copper stores may be depleted since the zinc and copper ratio is interrelated. Copper is an essential ingredient in an enzyme necessary for iron to be oxidized into a form capable of being incorporated into the hemoglobin molecule. Thus a zinc excess may produce a copper deficiency, leading to the production of an iron non-responsive anemia correctable by copper supplementation.

One final but little-mentioned aspect of anemia is cellular obstruction. All the nutrients in the world are useless if they never reach the cells. This is the reason, contrary to established ideas, why many naturopaths routinely fast some anemic patients. Instead of hemoglobin levels falling even further during a fast, they are found to rise markedly, thus improving the condition. The reason for this is that the fast stimulates the blood-forming tissues to function more effectively. Obviously, this must be done in selected cases where cellular obstruction is the primary cause and not, for instance, in a true case of vitamin B12 or iron deficiency.

TREATMENT

Diet

Foods Rich in Iron
Meat, liver from organically raised cattle, fish, egg yolks, blackstrap molasses, dark-green vegetables (e.g. lettuce, spinach, alfalfa, asparagus, cabbage, broccoli, parsley, celery, kale, cucumbers, leeks, and watercress), dried fruit (e.g. apricots, raisins, figs, dates, peaches, prunes, and pears), cherries, berries, bananas, grapes, apples, beets, carrots, yams, legumes, whole grains, rice, wheat, black cherry juice, grape juice, plus many others.

Foods Rich in Vitamin B12
Meat, fish, eggs, dairy products, comfrey,

bitter almonds, and the seeds in stone fruits* (vitamin B12 is synthesized from vitamin B17 in this case) such as apple seeds, apricots, prunes, etc., fermented foods such as yoghurt, seed yoghurt, grapes and miso, wheat, sunflower seeds, seaweed, brewer's yeast with vitamin B12 added, and Spirulina.

Foods Rich in Folic Acid
Dark green vegetables, liver, yeast, lentils, beans, grains, and Spirulina.

General Anti-Anemia Foods
- Vegetarian food sources: green vegetables, especially alfalfa, cabbage, chard, watercress, kale, parsley, spinach, comfrey, dandelion leaves, green onions, lettuce, cucumbers, leeks, nettles, beet tops, turnip greens, asparagus, Spirulina.
- Other vegetables: onions, beets, carrots, legumes (lentils, black beans, etc.), yams, potatoes with skin.
- Fruits: dried apricots, figs, raisins, dates, grapes, bananas, plums, oranges, and grapefruits.
- Nuts: almonds, hazelnuts, sunflower seeds, sesame seeds.
- Other special vegetarian sources: wheat germ, whole grains, blackstrap molasses, brewer's yeast, miso, kernels of stone fruits (e.g. apricots, prunes), apple seeds, seed yoghurts.
- Lacto-vegetarian food sources: yoghurt, milk, kefir, eggs, cheese, cottage cheese.
- Herbal teas: dandelion leaf, comfrey, yellow dock, raspberry, and fenugreek.
- Non-vegetarian food sources: liver, muscle meats, organ meats, eggs (especially egg yolk), fish.

Anti-Anemia Diet
The following diet may be useful as a guideline:

On Rising
1 tbsp blackstrap molasses in hot water, orange juice, or grapefruit juice.

Breakfast
1. Yoghurt, fruit, almonds, sunflower seeds, hazelnuts, wheat germ, and honey.
2. Stewed dried fruits, plain or with yoghurt and wheat germ.
3. Muesli (granola) or oatmeal and milk.
4. Eggs (not fried) and whole-wheat toast.

Midmorning
Dandelion leaf tea, comfrey leaf tea, parsley tea, yellow dock tea, raspberry tea, fenugreek tea, or any combination of the above.

Lunch
1. A raw salad, primarily green, including any of the following: alfalfa sprouts, lettuce, cabbage, spinach, watercress, green onions, cucumber, parsley, beet tops, asparagus, kale, chard, other green vegetables, carrots, beets, and sunflower seeds.
2. Baked yam or potato in jacket if desired, or
   Cottage cheese or other cheese.

Midafternoon
Same as midmorning.

Supper
Choose from the following:
1. Conservatively cooked vegetables, whole grain and fish, liver, organ meat, or muscle meat.
2. Miso soup with vegetables, seaweed and/or fish.
3. Egg or cheese vegetarian savory.

Physiotherapy

- Sun and sea baths.
- Outdoor exercise.

---

*Note: Seeds in stone fruits contain cyanide compounds that can be toxic and even fatal if taken in excess. Never eat more than 6–8 apricot, prune, or peach pits or more than 10–12 apple seeds daily, and best under supervision.

Fasting

- Beet juice.
- Red grape juice.

Therapeutic Agents

Vitamins and Minerals—Primary

Vitamin B complex: 50 mg 3 times daily.
Vitamin B12: 25 mcg to 1 mg daily.
Folic acid: 400 mcg to 5 mg daily (especially needed in anemia of pregnancy).
Vitamin C: 500-1000 mg 3-4 times daily. Enhances hemoglobin production and folic acid usage and increases iron and vitamin B12 absorption; conserves vitamin E.
Vitamin B12 and folic acid: 1 mg once per week intramuscularly.
Iron chelate or ferrous gluconate, fumarate or phosphate: 20-50 mg daily when iron deficiency has been diagnosed.
Vitamin E: 800-1200 IU daily.

Vitamins and Minerals—Secondary

Vitamin B6.
Calcium: 800 mg daily.
Copper: 3-5 mg daily or 1 mg per every 10-15 mg of zinc taken.
Trace minerals: (e.g. Celtic salt)

Zinc orotate: sickle cell disorder.

Others—Primary

Organic raw liver tablets: 2-4 tablets 3 times daily.
Apple cider vinegar: acts like vitamin C as a reducing agent to increase absorption of iron.
Blackstrap molasses: source of iron.
Brewer's yeast: 1 tsp 3 times daily (source of B complex).
Intrinsic factor (raw stomach tablets).
Probiotics: especially indicated, to give the flora every chance to manufacture B12 naturally.
Hydrochloric acid: where hydrochloric acid deficiency has been diagnosed, take with meals.

Others—Secondary

Chlorophyll.
Pancreatic enzymes: 1-2 tablets with meals in cases of poor assimilation.
Protein supplements.
Wheat germ.

Therapeutic Suggestions

Complete blood tests are essential to help differentiate the type of anemia and therefore the nutritional supplements required.

ARTHRITIS

DEFINITIONS

Osteoarthritis (OA): local or generalized degeneration of the articular cartilage and the formation of bony "lips and spurs" (osteophytes) at the edges of joints. An exaggeration of the normal aging process.
Rheumatoid arthritis (RA): an inflammatory disease involving the synovial membranes and the periarticular structures. Localized bone atrophy and rarification of the involved bone is common, with associated muscle atrophy.

SYMPTOMS

Osteoarthritis: onset is gradual, with progressive pain and joint enlargement. No constitutional symptoms are present. May involve single or multiple joints, but does not migrate from joint to joint.

Rheumatoid arthritis: onset is abrupt or insidious. Synovial membrane thickens and joint swells with redness and tenderness. Symmetrical joint involvement is common. May migrate from joint to joint. Constitutional symptoms present. Joint deformity with contracture. Subcutaneous nodules commonly found.

ETIOLOGICAL CONSIDERATIONS—PRIMARY

- Poor eliminations and inadequate assimilations
  Poor digestion; hyperacidity/hypoacidity; enzyme deficiency; sluggish bowels; poor skin, kidney, gallbladder, and liver activity; poor circulation (blood, lymph); toxemia; spinal imbalances causing reflex conditions as above, leading to accumulated toxins, which cause an inflammatory reaction
- Chemical imbalances and dietary deficiency
  Diet: excess meat and soda drinks (phosphorus/calcium ratio upset); excess refined carbohydrates, sweets; raw vegetable deficiency; excess acid-forming foods: excess coffee; excess phytic acid (bread) binding calcium; excess salt
- Multiple vitamin and mineral deficiencies, e.g. copper deficiency—RA
- Excess copper blood levels (copper pipes, low iron) may increase copper levels in joints; lack of zinc and manganese increases copper levels
- Excess vitamin D; lack of sulfur
- Excess irritants (coffee, tea, salt, spices, alcohol)
- Food allergy: gluten intolerance; intolerance to foods in nightshade family (tomatoes, potatoes, etc.); isolated food allergy
- Psychological factors
  Being inflexible, stuck, unwilling to change; long-held resentments; worry; envy, fear; anxiety, depression, deep shock
- Autoimmunity (RA)

Rheumatoid factor found in blood of at least 50% of patients with RA
- Excess wear and tear (OA)
  Joint trauma; excess weight bearing (obesity); overuse

ETIOLOGICAL CONSIDERATIONS— SECONDARY

Glandular imbalances (esp. adrenals); post-immunization arthralgia (German measles); lack of exercise; menopause; protozoa infection; sexual excess; anemia associated; chronic infections (e.g. tonsils and gallbladder); tonsillectomy; chronic fatigue; muscular tension, fibrositis; water allergy (locally irritant water supply)

DISCUSSION

Of all the diseases that affect humanity, arthritis, in its multitude of forms, is one of the most debilitating and widespread. Orthodox treatments have proven unsatisfactory and completely unable to cure these disorders. The reason is simple. Due to the complex etiology and constitutional nature of most forms of arthritis, only individualized therapy has any hope of removing the cause. There is no one quick and easy cure, no magic pill, and no miracle diets suited for all. With arthritis, as with most degenerative diseases, there are as many different approaches as there are patients, and each one is unique.

Only when all the causative factors are recognized and corrected can true healing take place. Arthritis is a process, and at the very least, the process can be stopped so that you don't get any worse. The process can often be reversed and the arthritis is then cured. That is the desired outcome of naturopathic arthritis treatment. Often the improvement is slow, although very often it can be rapid as well. It *always* involves lifestyle changes, which may not be easy.

This implies that the only type of arthritis patient who can ever hope for real improvement must have a real desire for health and the persistence and patience to obtain it at all cost. The rewards, however, are worth the effort. The dream of a body free of pain can only be fully understood by one who lives day and night with severe arthritis.

As to the orthodox approach to arthritis, we have never met or heard of a single arthritic patient who received drug therapy who did not become progressively worse. Although aspirin, which is advised in most cases of painful osteoarthritis or rheumatoid arthritis, does help relieve the immediate pain, it certainly is no cure.

In addition to its other side effects, as well as reactivating or causing ulcers, aspirin lowers vitamin C levels (essential in the health of connective tissue, useful as a detoxifying agent, and needed for proper adrenal function), damages connective tissue, causes an increase in uric acid levels (a cause of gouty arthritis), depletes the adrenal glands, and in toxic doses will cause salicylism, leading to paralysis of the respiratory center as well as central vasomotor paralysis. If taken over a prolonged period of time, aspirin can mimic other diseases such as Ménière's syndrome and cause severe respiratory distress and mental confusion. Most health authorities now agree that if the present FDA regulations existed when aspirin was first produced, it would now be a prescription drug only.

Self-induced aspirin toxicity is very common. Although no physician would ever prescribe aspirin in doses that could become toxic, the fact is that patients often take more of this medication than suggested. This is particularly the case with some elderly patients who suffer from poor memory and cannot remember if they took their pain medication three or thirteen times in daily. For many with pain, anything that gives some relief 3 times daily might be better 6–10 times daily. One last word on aspirin. As one doctor put it, "Do you really think you have arthritis because of an aspirin deficiency?"

Cortisone is another prescribed drug for arthritis, especially rheumatoid arthritis. Compared to this drug aspirin is an essential vitamin! We consider cortisone one of the most deceptive and dangerous drugs ever produced. Its well-known anti-inflammatory effects hide its insidious side effects. Cortisone depresses the immunological system so dramatically that even minor infections can become life threatening. It directly depresses the function of the adrenal gland, the gland that is so often the cause of the disorder in the first place. Cortisone causes calcium depletion, resulting in osteoporosis, another major cause of arthritis. It also aggravates peptic ulcers and in overdose will induce Cushing's syndrome with its symptoms of obesity, muscle wasting and weakness, poor wound healing, bruising, high blood pressure, diabetes, psychiatric disturbance; with balding, excess body hair, and menstrual disorders in the female. In short, cortisone is a very dangerous drug and its use should be reserved for life-threatening diseases only. The common medical opinions that "diet has nothing to do with arthritis" and that "you will have to live with it" are simply not acceptable, nor are they true. Only when the individualized concept of disease causation is understood will the true cause and cure of arthritis at long last be recognized.

TREATMENT

Diet

Therapy must begin by identifying which of the etiologic factors interact to cause the abnormality. While no two arthritic patients are alike, it is usually not very difficult to pinpoint the major problem areas. Diet, as with many other degenerative or autoimmune disorders, stands out as the major detrimental influence. Many sufferers of both osteoarthritis and rheumatoid arthritis have dietary patterns that are clearly a problem.

Heavy meat consumption is a common finding. Meat contains anywhere from

20-50 times more phosphorus than calcium. This stimulates the parathyroid glands, responsible for the mobilization of calcium from bones. This extra calcium is then deposited around the joints, explaining the common finding in arthritis of less dense bones with calcium buildup around the articulations. This one factor alone may be the reason why vegetarians have less of an incidence of osteoarthritis than meat eaters. A good vegetarian diet will have a much better phosphorus-to-calcium ratio. Another source of excess phosphorus in the diet is soft drinks. It may seem odd that a condition such as osteoarthritis characterized by calcium deposits would be benefited by calcium and magnesium supplements, but the average diet clearly shows us why.

Another aspect of concern in the average diet is an excess of refined carbohydrates and sweets. Not only are these foods robbed of many of their naturally occurring vitamins and minerals, the relative ratios of many minerals are completely altered. As we have seen in many other conditions in this book, not only are the absolute values of vitamins and minerals important to human health, but also their ratios and interactions. Vitamin E, magnesium, vitamin B complex, and essential fibers are removed by the refining of whole grains. These are all very important in the prevention and cure of many degenerative conditions, arthritis included.

Refined carbohydrates, especially sugar, contribute to a generalized acid condition of the body, especially when accompanied by a diet low in fresh vegetables. Fresh vegetables are a protective factor against arthritic changes, whereas processed vegetables can actually aggravate the condition. Once again we find that essential mineral balances are upset in the processing. One example is the sodium and potassium ratio. Fresh vegetables usually have a higher potassium-to-sodium ratio than when canned. The amount of salt in the diet has increased dramatically over the past 70 years. Coffee is another common problem. In fact, so many facets of the average arthritic's diet are negative health factors that all of them cannot be mentioned here. A complete individual dietary appraisal is necessary to eliminate any possible health risks. The question of food allergy must also be investigated, especially in rheumatoid arthritis.

It must be remembered that arthritis is a degenerative and possibly an autoimmune disease taking years to develop. Subtle dietary changes are rarely successful in reversing the problem. More heroic therapy is required. The following dietary manipulations will gradually help establish equilibrium, if applied diligently and coupled with a good nutritional supplement program.

Raw Vegetable Juice Fasting
This is the fastest method of attaining results with RA. OA will also respond to this regimen. The fasting period depends on the patient and the condition, and may range from 7–21 days or longer, under close supervision.

The following liquids are especially useful: carrot and celery juice; potassium broth; chlorophyll drink; alfalfa mint or seed tea; watercress, celery, and parsley juice.

Raw Non-Citrus Vegetarian Diet
This initial diet may follow the fasting period and should last 2–4 weeks or longer. The bulk of the diet is raw green vegetables, with no animal proteins whatsoever. All stimulants such as coffee, tea, alcohol, nicotine, or sweets are forbidden.

Food allergy tests (cytotoxic, RAST, pulse tests) should be performed prior to dietary treatments, to disclose any hidden food sensitivity.

The following foods have been found beneficial in the majority of arthritic patients with both RA and OA: green vegetables; carrots; seaweeds; Spirulina; watercress; avocado; parsley; bananas; celery; pecans; okra; potassium broth; kale; wheat grass juice; alfalfa sprouts; whey; kelp; cod liver oil drinks; soy milk; apple cider vinegar and honey; soy; papaya; soy products; dandelion coffee; distilled water; seeds; millet;

garlic, onions; brown rice; wheat germ; egg yolks; figs plus molasses; raw goat's yoghurt; cherries (gout).

The following should be strictly avoided: citrus; fried foods; dairy products (goat products OK in some cases); drinks with meals; wheat; meat; refined carbohydrates, sugar, etc.; alcohol; salt; foods of the nightshade family (tomatoes, eggplants, potatoes, peppers, tobacco).

Members of the Solanaceae family, are related to deadly nightshade (belladonna), thus their common grouping as "nightshade" foods. Some people show a strong reaction to this food group. As with other severe food sensitivities, even minute doses in the diet can be a problem for these hypersensitive people. Care must be taken to avoid hidden nightshades found in prepared foods. For example, potato flour thickeners are used in a wide variety of products, including surprising ones such as some yoghurts. Capsicum also shows up hidden in foods such as pink-colored cheeses or herbal teas. Tomatoes are used in a large variety of prepared foods. Only strict avoidance will be of benefit to those truly sensitive to this food group.

Physiotherapy

Daily Massage Formulas

- Peanut oil: 2 fl oz (60 mL), olive oil: 2 fl oz (60 mL), lanolin: 1 tsp.
- Peanut oil.
- Olive oil: 2 fl oz (60 mL), peanut oil: 2 fl oz (60 mL), oil of pine needles: $\frac{1}{2}$ fl oz (15 mL), oil of sassafras root: $\frac{1}{2}$ fl oz (15 mL), liquefied lanolin: 1 fl oz (30 mL).

Hydrotherapy

1. Hot and cold showers (alternate): to stimulate general circulation and act as a general tonic.
2. Hot and cold compresses (alternate): local use.
3. Hot compress (pain relief).

4. Hot Epsom salts baths or local bath or compress (see Appendix I).
5. Cabinet bath with or without Atomodine fumes.
6. Sauna baths.
7. Paraffin bath: local: 4 parts paraffin, 1 part mineral oil. Heat to 125–130°F (51–54°C), or let cool until thin film forms. Dip part repeatedly until $\frac{1}{4}$ inch (6 mm) thick, or paint on larger areas.

Eliminations

Correct eliminations using as many of the following as possible:

- Castor oil packs (see Appendix I); anti-constipation foods; Epsom salts baths.
- Hot and cold showers; skin brush and salt rub; sea bathing; sun bathing; trunk packs.
- Mineral spring baths; hot sand baths; seaweed baths; sulfur baths (sulfur hot springs).
- Sweat baths; wet grass walks.

Others

Ultrasound; cabbage leaf poultices, in acute cases; comfrey leaf poultice; joint mobilization; infrared heat; flowers of sulfur in socks daily; counter-irritant therapy.

Therapeutic Agents

Vitamins and Minerals—Primary

- Glucosamine: clinical trials have shown glucosamine salts (a substrate of proteoglycans which is 75% of cartilage structure), are an effective and safe treatment to reduce joint pain and swelling, and improve range of movement. This supplement is an absolute must in all cases of arthritis. It is very effective, but must be taken regularly. Powder or capsule forms are available. The usual dose is 1 tsp or two capsules taken 3 times daily.
- Shark or bovine cartilage: contains chondroitin sulfate, an important substance

needed for mucopolysaccharide synthesis, integral to healthy cartilage. Some people find the shark cartilage to have a fishy aftertaste, which they find objectionable and some find it upsets the stomach. Various quality of shark cartilage is available. Some of the cheaper brands have residue of other fish material other than the cartilage, which may be the source of the adverse smell or gastric irritation. Should you wish, you can also find glucosamine power or capsules in combination with chondroitin to avoid this problem.

- Vitamin C and bioflavonoids: 1000–2000 mg 3–4 times daily, or larger doses, up to bowel tolerance. Increases natural cortisone production; anti-inflammatory; aids adrenals. Bioflavonoids, especially quercetin, inhibit histamine release from mast cells, reduce the swelling, and are antioxidant. Large doses of vitamin C may aggravate some cases; so take care to evaluate its effect separately from other medications. Try ascorbate form of this vitamin if this is a problem.

- Niacinamide: 200–1000 mg 2–4 times daily. Increases joint mobility by up to 85% if taken daily for 3–4 weeks. It is used for osteoarthritis and some rheumatoid arthritis. If nausea occurs at these doses this may be a toxic reaction and the dose should be reduced by one half or stopped completely.

- Vitamin E: 400 IU 1–2 times daily; antioxidant; anti-inflammatory.

- Selenium: 50–200 mcg daily work in synergy with vitamin E. (Selenium has also been found useful in cases of Osgood-Schlatter disease of the knees. Standard dose is 250 mcg of sodium selenite daily, along with 800 IU vitamin E daily for 1 month, later reducing to 400 IU daily; vitamin C: 3–6 g daily; B complex: 25–50 mg 1–2 times daily; zinc: 15–25 mg 2–3 times daily; calcium: 800–1000 mg daily; magnesium: 400–500 mg daily, and a diet high in raw vegetables).

- Copper: high doses used with medical supervision only. Copper aspirinate (for RA)—anti-inflammatory and SOD (superoxide dismutase) activation.

- Boron: 3 mg daily. Trace mineral needed for healthy bone.

- Silica: a source of silicon needed for bone formation and the repair of connective tissue.

Vitamins and Minerals— Secondary

Vitamin A: 25,000–100,000 IU daily.

Vitamin B complex: 50 mg 2–3 times daily.

Pantothenic acid: 250–500 mg 2–3 times daily.

Vitamin B6: 100–250 mg 2–3 times daily. Especially indicated for females on birth control pills and those with carpal tunnel syndrome and non-articular rheumatism.

Vitamin B12: 1000 mcg intramuscular injection once per week, or in some cases daily for 7–14 days. Useful with heel spurs and other osteoarthritic joint disorders. Use 1 mL daily until pain subsides.

Folate: reduces the need for NSAIDs.

Calcium: 800–1000 mg daily.

Calcium pantothenate: 2 g daily in RA.

Magnesium: 400–800 mg daily.

Manganese: superoxide dismutase activation.

Taurine: (500 mg 3 times daily) to improve chemical detoxification, and gastric acid production.

Trace minerals.

Tryptophan: some arthritics respond to $1\frac{1}{2}$ g daily.

Zinc: 25–50 mg 1–2 times daily, SOD activation. Especially indicated in psoriatic arthritis.

Others—Primary

- Bromelain enzyme: 2 tablets 3 times daily, taken on an empty stomach only. Most containers of bromelain will be marked to take with food. The reason for this is that the most common use of bromelain is as a digestive enzyme, not as an anti-inflammatory. To use as an anti-inflammatory it is essential to take it only on an empty stomach. Be aware that mixed meals of protein and fat can take up to five hours to digest, so it is not all that easy for most people to find the right time to take this supplement. First thing in the morning is always a good time. Allow at least one half hour after taking this supplement before eating, or more if possible. Just before lunch, supper or bedtime are also usually good times if you don't snack between meals. This is a very useful supplement, so it is worth the effort to take it effectively. You will also find it useful for all types of tendonitis (e.g. tennis elbow). Decreases soft tissue swelling, inflammation and pain. Induces formation of prostaglandin E.

- Essential fatty acids: 2–4 capsules 3 times daily. These down-regulate prostaglandin and leukotrienne pathways of inflammation.
- Evening primrose oil: source of essential fatty acids to reduce inflammation and joint pain. Helps in the production of anti-inflammatory prostaglandins.
- Coenzyme Q10: 60 mg daily. Helps in the repair of connective tissue and improves oxygenation of tissue.
- Hydrochloric acid: if hydrochloric acid deficiency has been proven, take with meals. Hypochlorhydria is very common in rheumatoid arthritis patients.
- SOD (superoxide dismutase): in injectible form it has proven useful in RA, gout, and other inflammatory joint disorders. It has been used as such in veterinary medicine for years. The affected joint is injected once weekly; enhancing zinc, copper, and manganese orally stimulates the body's production of native SOD. Even with questions over its effectiveness orally, we have still found that reliable superoxide dismutase oral tablets have proven effective in some cases.
- DMg (dimethylglycine): 125 mg twice daily. Helps prevent damage to the joints.
- Grape seed extract (pycnogenol): a powerful antioxidant and anti-inflammatory. Strengthens connective tissue.

Protects and repairs damage from free radicals.

Others—Secondary

Alfalfa tablets (6–10), plus tea, 3 times daily.

Atomodine or 636 (Cayce products).

Apple cider vinegar.

Bee pollen.

Bone meal.

Brewer's yeast: 1 tsp 2–3 times daily.

Cod-liver oil capsules: 3–4 capsules 3 times daily.

DL phenylalanine: analgesic; 300 mg 3 times daily.

L-cysteine: 500 mg once or twice daily. A sulfur-containing amino acid needed for collagen repair.

Germanium: 100–150 mg 2–3 times daily. Antioxidant, helps reduce inflammation and pain.

Green-lipped mussel tablets: may help some people with RA.

Kelp: 2–4 tablets 3 times daily.

Lecithin (as concentrated phosphatidyl choline): 1–2 capsules 3 times daily.

Molasses plus eggs: sulfur source.

Raw adrenal tablets: anti-stress.

Raw thymus tablets: immune system support.

Wheat germ concentrate.

Botanicals—Primary

Ginger: an excellent anti-inflammatory.

St John's wort: works through the central nervous system to reduce pain, and promotes detoxification through the cytochrome P450 liver pathways.

Devil's claw: anti-inflammatory, analgesic action similar to phenylbutazone. Reduces uric acid levels.

Feverfew: anodyne (can be given as a simplex).

Ginkgo biloba: inhibits PAF.

Guaiacum: pain modulator, and anti-inflammatory.

Botanicals—Secondary

Autumn crocus: for gout (contains colchicine).

Bee sting: homeopathic dilutions used for inflammation and edema.

Bryony: low homeopathic dilutions for pain aggravated by movement.

Burdock: alterative.

Celery: stalk eaten in abundance; seeds used as medicine.

Poison ivy: homeopathic dilutions used for rheumatic pain and inflammation improved by motion.

Prickly ash: circulatory stimulant, anodyne.

St James wort: use as topical lotion.

White willow.

Wintergreen oil: used as topical 10–20% solution. Antirheumatic, local irritant; contains methyl salicylate.

Yucca.

ASTHMA, BRONCHIAL

DEFINITION

Asthma is a disease of inflammation of the airways, causing constriction of the bronchi and bronchioles, increased mucus secretion, and manifesting as recurrent paroxysms of difficult breathing and wheezing.

SYMPTOMS

Difficult breathing, sense of choking, wheezing, coughing, difficulty in exhalation, causing use of accessory muscles of respiration. (The use of intercostal muscles and the pectoralis minor requires the patient to brace the shoulders by sitting upright and grasping the side of bed or chair.) Eventually can cause "barrel chest" formation. Expectoration usually ends spasm; attack worse lying down.

ETIOLOGICAL CONSIDERATIONS—PRIMARY

- Improper weaning
- Diet
  Excess carbohydrates and sweets; excess dairy products; difficult-to-digest foods; overeating
- Allergy
  Wheat; dairy products; inhalants; other
- Food additive sensitivity
  Sodium metabisulfite; tartrazine; acetyl-salicylic acid; sulfur dioxide; sodium benzoate and others
- Hypoglycemia (associated with many allergies and adrenal gland malfunction)
- Constipation
- Emotional (e.g. insecurity, fear, over-protective mother)
- Suppressive treatment (improper therapy for previous colds, bronchitis, and eczema.); repeated antibiotics; steroids
- Environmental pollution
- Free radical damage
  Improper cooking oils
- Leaky gut syndrome

ETIOLOGICAL CONSIDERATIONS— SECONDARY

Spinal (cervical and thoracic); birth trauma; lesions in larynx and/or bronchi due to previous acute infections; glandular imbalance (adrenal); poor circulation; hydrochloric acid deficiency; infection by parasites such as Ascaris.

DISCUSSION

Asthma is an abnormal, chronic (or episodic) inflammation of the airways tissue, the bronchial epithelium. This abnormal inflammation causes muscle spasm (constriction) of the airways making it difficult to breathe, especially to breathe out. It should be stated that asthma is a specific diagnosis; it has to do with a limited capacity to breathe out; it cannot be diagnosed simply because there might be a little wheeziness, or excess mucus. Furthermore, it cannot be diagnosed (as often it is) simply by giving an anti-asthma drug, and seeing if it "helps".

Causes, as Distinct from Triggers

There is the idea that chronic exposure to certain triggers turns an otherwise healthy individual into an asthmatic. This commonly held notion is wrong; it is an assumptive hypothesis that has unthinkingly been accepted into medical ethos. Evidence of this is in the fact that the usual medical treatment does not cure asthma.

Distinction must be made between having asthma attacks, and being asthmatic. Some triggers (e.g. pollen, dust-mites, moulds and yeasts, viruses, strong odours, exercise in cold air, cigarette smoke, animal danders) will cause attack symptoms in the asthmatic, but not in the non-asthmatic person. The real question ought to be: what creates the characteristic inflammation, the susceptible internal environment in some individuals in the first place? Why is it that 100 people can all be exposed to the same triggers and only some (the "asthmatics") show a disordered response?

Time for a Rethink

Despite all the attempts by researchers, rheumatologists, and asthma foundations, the situation is getting worse, rapidly. In the early 1900s, Sir William Osler wrote, "Asthma is not a life-threatening disease." What has contributed to the increasing morbidity and mortality rates over the past century to change this state of affairs? Certainly the external environment has become more pol-luted with large amounts of sulfur dioxide from petrol refineries and coal-fired power stations, higher levels of sulfites from petrol fumes and in general, a much greater airborne chemical load from over 70,000 chemicals in production today. Cigarette smoking has increased significantly. And we are eating more junk foods that are highly processed and contain harmful chemical additives. The dietary changes have favored a hyper-acidic internal environment promoting inflammation and hypersensitivity of bronchial tissue.

There are specific connections, which are clearly established in the medical literature, between:

- Poor weaning and early dietary practices lead to lowered immunity.
- Lowered immunity leads to infections, especially of the respiratory tract, such as middle ear infections (otitis media), colds and influenza.
- These infections are then routinely treated with antibiotics.
- Antibiotics damage flora populations which protect bronchial and gut tissue.
- Damaged bronchial and gut tissue allows further immune system degradation, which in turn causes all the known symptoms of asthma.

The Role of Weaning and Early Childhood Diet

There is a lot of evidence that poor weaning practices, such as infant and early childhood diets based on animal products, e.g. milk and other dairy products, red meat, chicken, and wheat products, is one significant risk factor in many cases (if not most) of asthma. Such a diet can cause inflammation anywhere in the body, including the airways.

Animal products are naturally high in arachidonic acid and other potent mediators of inflammation. These mediators create inflammation responses in epithelial tissue, such as those that line the airways (and skin). Such inflammation responses in airway tissues can cause production of

119

excess mucus (the body's attempt to stabilize the inflammation and eliminate the excess arachidonic acid and other inflammatory agents). Dairy milk peptide beta-somorphine-7 (a protein structure) causes airways inflammation and histamine release from mast cells lining the airways in humans causing excess mucus production.

The problem is exacerbated when one understands that during the slaughtering of animals, the beasts are subjected to stress. The organs of these animals (mainly the adrenal glands) secrete large amounts of stress hormones, notably adrenalin, into their bloodstream and their tissues. These elevated stress hormones remain present in the meat eaten by us. These hormones are also mediators of inflammation in our bodies.

When meat is cooked, fats and oils are often heated to temperatures where the oils change their molecular structures, and powerful "free radical" molecules are formed. Hydrogenated vegetable oils, which are present in margarine, contain large amounts of these free radicals. These free radicals also cause inflammation in our body, which further exacerbates the problem. They also weaken the body's immune system, making it less able to deal with the processes of extra-inflammation occurring.

Another problem with the typical western diet is that the ratio between the omega-3 fatty acids (the so-called "good oil" because it is anti-inflammatory in the body) and the omega-6s and other fats and oils (e.g. saturated fats which are inflammatory in the body) has altered a lot over the last 100 years, as our diets and lifestyles have changed

The organs of digestion in an infant are not properly developed until at least 12 months of age. Giving an infant such foods as noted above means a lot more of these mediators of inflammation are going to be absorbed straight into the bloodstream than would otherwise enter once the gastro-intestinal tissues and organs are mature. The effect of *any* impartially digested protein fragments thus in the bloodstream, can be to cause immune confusion. There is an abnormal production of inflammatory mediators (e.g. LTs, PGs, kinins and others), and autoantibodies, which will attack susceptible tissue, such as bronchial (airways) tissue. So poor weaning practices (especially those which encourage young mothers to wean their infants onto animal formula products and animal proteins before 12 months of age) lie as a primary culprit in this matter of childhood infections.

Role of the Immune System

In a healthy individual, the body's natural defenses can handle asthma-triggering assaults. But in the immune-compromised person, the body's natural immune functions become overwhelmed and sluggish, creating a susceptibility to the triggers. A history of chronic colds and bronchitis (symptomatic of a lowered immune state) is usually reported by asthma sufferers prior to their disorder.

Infants and young children who have a history of colds and infections, for example respiratory tract infections such as middle ear infections (otitis media), demonstrate a history of repeated antibiotic usage as well. The effects of even just one course of antibiotics can be devastating to bronchial as well as gastrointestinal flora, the flora that is designed by nature as primary protectant of those tissues. Many of the antibiotics prescribed are known to cause asthma in certain individuals. There is no doubt that exposure to antibiotics during manufacture can cause asthma (called "occupational asthma"). It could also be considered equally, if not *more* harmful, to ingest a substance such as a drug, than to breathe air contaminated with its dust.

Dr Lisa Landymore-Lim notes, "An association between antibiotic exposure and asthma is accepted by the medical profession and the Department of Social Security in the UK and the Health Department of Australia. However, general practitioners and the general public are either apparently unaware of this association, or have not drawn what we consider to be a logical conclusion; that exposure to antibiotics for medicinal purposes may actually *cause* asthma." (i.e. make an otherwise healthy person into an asthmatic, not merely act as a trigger).[25]

Medical literature is replete with cases of children who have been treated for eczema with steroids, who end up suffering from asthma later on. The relationship of continuity between the "external" skin and the "internal" skin (airways and gut epithelium) is often overlooked. Apart from the fact that eczema itself is a sign of allergy, the routine suppression of symptoms of eczema may well be causatively implicated in asthma (and gut problems also). While the relationship between the liver and (external) skin has been acknowledged, the relationship between the liver and (internal) bronchial epithelium is less acknowledged in current medical research, but surely exists for the same reasons.

These are compelling reasons enough, let alone risking damage to gut tissue causing leaky gut, to abhor the common medical practice of profligate antibiotic prescription.

The Role of Antibiotics

With the over-prescription of antibiotics, and consuming meats such as chicken, pork and lot-fed beef which commonly contain antibiotic residues, what we are seeing today is chronic damage being done to the bronchial and intestinal tissues of a generation of young children (see Leaky Gut). In the light of the foregoing, recent attention is being given to leaky gut as a cause of asthma. Bacterial endotoxins such as lipopolysaccharides, as well as other toxic metabolites of digestion and excretion, and opportunistic *Candida albicans* which can become systemic, can be (re)absorbed across semi-permeable gut membranes and into circulation, triggering

immune sensitivity and overload, with activation of T-lymphocytes and macrophages releasing cytokines (e.g. IgE, TNF). These cytokines in turn activate bronchial eosinophils and mast cells to release inflammatory substances such as histamine, nitric oxide, products of arachidonic metabolism such as leukotrienes and prostaglandins, as well as proteolytic and glycolytic enzymes, PAF (platelet activating factor), and substance P released from afferent nerve endings. All these inflammatory mediators are associated with the hyperreactivity of the airways, as evidenced by bronchial smooth muscle spasm, micro vascular leakage leading to mucosal edema and mucus secretion, all characteristic of asthma. Asthma is sometimes called "leaky gut of the lungs". Two things can be meant by this: that asthma is one manifestation of the leaky gastrointestinal tissues, and that bronchial tissue itself can become leaky, which sets up a whole vicious cycle of inflammation.

Another possible involvement is the vagus nerve: irritation and inflammation of the colon caused by food allergy/hypersensitivity causes reflex irritation and inflammation of the bronchial mucosa.

TREATMENT

Diet

Testing the Allergy Hypothesis

The food allergy hypothesis is best tested by eliminating dairy and dairy-containing products and wheat and wheat derived products absolutely from the diet for 3 weeks. During this elimination phase, favorable changes will be noticed within the respiratory tract. The levels of mucus and wheezing will diminish as the body desensitizes to the allergen. Then a challenge is made, exposing the body to the suspected allergen after a length of time will create very clear signs and symptoms. Follow the elimination–challenge program as outlined below.

Step 1

You have been on a program that has excluded the potential allergens from your body for 21 days (minimum). During this time, the body will have "desensitized" and will now be able to tell you in a very clear way if indeed there is an allergy to the suspect foods.

Step 2

Test for wheat

(Record date and times)

Have several pure wheat cereal biscuits (use non-dairy milk, e.g. soy, rice, oat) for breakfast and a wheat-based bread for lunch.

Note: Allow 3 days between each test or part of a test.

Test for dairy

(Record date and times)

Day 1: yoghurt

Day 4: butter

Day 7: white cheese

Day 10: yellow cheese

Day 13: milk

What to Look For

Some common signs and symptoms of allergy:

- Gastrointestinal: stomach pain, bloating, wind, diarrhea, and constipation.
- Skin: rash.
- Respiratory: wheezing, excess mucus, and asthma attack.
- CNS: headache, irritability, hyperactivity.

    Write down any specific or vague symptoms, noting time and duration of symptoms. Don't be surprised if simply a glass of milk creates a lot of mucus in just a few hours. There could even be an asthma attack, although since the respiratory tract will be much less inflamed, it is unlikely.

    If the elimination–challenge testing proves positive, you will need to avoid foods containing the allergen in all its forms. For example, if it is dairy, exclude dairy milk, ice-cream, cheese, butter and yoghurt, and dairy products used in biscuits, cakes, breads, etc. Find out what alternatives you can use for this time. Clearly, to allow healing, you must exclude all forms of dairy and/or wheat

from the diet, until such time as a rechallenge proves negative (maybe 12 months).

Benefits of a Vegetarian Diet

Studies from as early as 1985[26] have shown a 92% improvement in one year of asthma attacks when patients are placed on vegetarian diets. Now even a 10–15% improvement would have been significant. In our clinic about 70–75% of asthma *is* food-related, *and* asthma can reverse when foods are properly addressed. In more than 90% of cases poor food choices aggravate asthma, and good food choices will alleviate it.

Program a change to a largely vegetarian diet (which can include deep-sea fish, but not chicken) and make the change over a 3-month period for all the family (everyone will benefit, and parents must lead by example). Use large amounts of anti-inflammatory herbs in your cooking, such as garlic, onion, ginger, turmeric, chilli peppers; and include the "good oils" (high in omega-3s, which are also anti-inflammatory) such as flaxseed oil and marine oils such as cod liver, salmon, sardine in the diet.

Preventing Childhood Asthma

Prevention is still better than cure! Take proper, naturopathic advice as to weaning: the best method is to breast-feed for at least 12 months, then introduce infants to fresh, organic (chemical-free) fruit and vegetables first (which contain much less complex molecules than protein molecules of milk or soy). Once the immature digestive system has gotten used to these, small amounts of more complex molecules may be added, *from vegetarian sources* such as soy milk, rice milk, oat milk or some nut milks.

Do not rush into animal products or wheat products (e.g. enriched breads, breakfast cereals) until the child is at least 2 years old. Remember, meat and dairy are not the only proteins. Children do not need these products to survive or thrive, either for calcium or protein. A balanced vegetarian diet will give them all the nutrients they need, without all the downsides animal products bring. Unless you are willing to find a source of meat uncontaminated with antibiotics or hormones, this is the best way to protect you child against asthma and many other allergies.

Also, learn how to honour the body's natural immune system. Learn how to treat the usual childhood coughs and colds, influenza and fevers, sore throats and infections naturally, without resorting to antibiotics or other drugs.

Diet

Sweets; refined foods; dairy; excess carbohydrates; additives; sulfites; alcohol, tea, or other non-food irritants; very hot or very cold foods

Periods of fruit juice or vegetable juice fasting or at least an all-fruit diet (see Appendix I) are necessary to help restore balance. Children may find it difficult to fast, but very easy to go on a 3–5-day all-fruit diet. The specific mucus-cleansing diet (see Appendix I) regimen with onions and citrus is useful in nearly all cases, and should be employed during any acute episodes.

Alternatively, the modified carrot mono diet is sometimes found more appealing and almost as effective in the severe acute case. On this diet the patient drinks an abundance of carrot juice and eats raw carrots if desired between meals, with a large plate of three-fourths cooked carrots to one-fourth cooked onions at mealtimes. After this, stage 2 of the diet below should form the basis for the general diet for the first 2 months. As improvement is seen by the use of frequent fasting, mucus-cleansing diets, and an allergy-free vegetarian diet, along with physiotherapy, spinal manipulation, exercise, nutritional supplements, and botanical remedies, the diet may be slowly and carefully expanded. If

hypoglycemia is a factor, protein levels may need to be increased (see Hypoglycemia).

We have seen young children with mild to moderate asthma attacks lasting weeks and unrelieved by drugs, respond within 24–48 hours and be symptom-free in less than 1 week on this regimen.*

The following is a sample diet that has proved very useful in these cases.

Asthma Diet Regimen

Begin treatment with one of the following diets, depending on your doctor's advice.

Stage 1
Liquid Diet (3–7 days) No solid food is to be taken.
On Rising
Herb teas such as chamomile, alfalfa, mint, linden flower, etc., or a glass of fresh fruit juice from fully ripened (and if possible) unsprayed and organic grapefruit, grapes, papaya, oranges, apples, guavas, or any other fresh fruit.

Breakfast
Hot vegetable broth (potassium broth, see Appendix I).

Midmorning
Any herb tea, fruit juice, or fresh vegetable juice (not tomato juice).

Lunch
Potassium broth (hot vegetable broth).

Midafternoon
Any herb tea, fresh fruit or vegetable juice (not tomato juice).

Supper
Potassium broth (hot vegetable broth).
An enema should be taken on days 1, 2, 3, 5, and 7.

---

*Note: Severe asthma attacks can be life threatening. *Seek medical attention* to stabilize the attack. Naturopathic care may then be sought to resolve the underlying cause.

All-Fruit Diet (3–7–10 days)

On Rising
Herb tea or grapefruit juice.

Breakfast
Any fresh fruit (organic).

Midmorning
Herb tea or fruit juice.

Lunch
Any fresh fruit.

Midafternoon
Herb tea or fruit juice.

Supper
Any fresh fruit.
Note: One type of fruit per meal. No bananas.

Carrot Mono Diet (Modified)

On Rising
Carrot juice.

Breakfast
Carrots.

Midmorning
Carrot juice.

Lunch
Large plate of boiled or steamed carrots and onions.

Midafternoon
As midmorning.

Supper
As lunch.

Evening
Carrot juice.

Mucus-Cleansing Diet (3–7–10 days)
Breakfast
Citrus fruit (especially grapefruit).

Midmorning
Herb tea, fresh fruit juice, or fresh vegetable juice (carrot).

Lunch
A large plate of boiled or steamed onions; a little soy sauce may be used to flavor, but no salt. An orange for dessert if desired.

Midafternoon
Potassium broth, or as midmorning.

Supper
Same as lunch.

Evening
Potassium broth, or as midmorning.
Take 2 garlic capsules with lunch and supper.

Stage 2
Breakfast
Any fresh fruit, raw or stewed; or stewed or baked apple with soaked or simmered raisins.

Lunch
A large, varied raw salad composed of vegetables that grow mostly above ground, in the ratio 3:1 below (e.g. lettuce, cabbage, celery, watercress, cucumber), plus carrots. Also have a large plate of boiled or steamed onions with soy sauce or nut cream. A few walnuts, almonds, or hazelnuts may be added to the salad. Tofu may be added to meal.

Evening
Same as lunch, or a vegetarian protein meal (excluding eggs and cheese) plus steamed or baked vegetables. Fresh or stewed fruit if desired as dessert.

Later in regimen: lean meat, fish, or poultry (not fried) with vegetables.
When thirsty, choose from fruit juice, vegetable juice, potassium broth, or herb teas. Take 2 garlic capsules with meals. Always include raw onions in the salad meals.
See Allergies and Food Intolerances for an alternative approach.

Physiotherapy

Exercises

- Blow up balloons; blow out candles; outdoor singing.

- Stand before open window with hands behind head. Pull elbows in front and have them touch. As inhalation begins, arms are flexed outward and backward. Exhale as they return forward. Breathe slowly and deeply with full exhalation.
- Diaphragm breathing: on back, begin slow progression of abdominal diaphragm breathing to lower costals, then to upper chest. Counter pressure on ribs may help localize the breathing effort to diaphragm and lower costal area. Exhale normally.
- Sitting with back supported, right arm across chest, bend to right inhaling, to left exhaling, with hand helping. Then switch hands and reverse.
- Sitting with hands on ribs, inhale and then exhale while leaning forward with pressure exerted on ribs by hands. Progress to hands above head on inhalation, bending forward until chest reaches the knees on exhalation. This may also be done in puffs and pushes rather than continuous exhalation (after only one inhalation). This is a very useful exercise in loosening mucus.
- During an attack, blow through a straw into water and then inhale fresh air, or if available, oxygen.
- Relaxation exercises.

Note: In these exercises it is the *exhalation* that is to be stressed, not deep inhalation. The diaphragmatic breathing is to teach the proper progression of breathing. No excessive deep inhalation breaths are required.

Other Treatment

- Neuromuscular: deep muscle massage between ribs, along spine, and along diaphragm.
- Spinal manipulation: cervical and thoracic manipulation weekly for 6-8 weeks. Rest and repeat cycle as needed.
- Outdoor exercises: swimming is one of the best activities for asthmatics.
- Massage: between shoulder blades (acute cases).

Hydrotherapy

Chronic: hot Epsom salts baths twice per week (see Appendix I); alternate hot/cold showers daily; chest packs nightly.

Acute: hot chest compresses plus hot foot bath; hot foot bath with mustard and lobelia plus ice to back of head; hot fomentations with olbas oil; warm bath for 45 minutes with relaxation and diaphragmatic breathing.

Therapeutic Agents

Water is an important part of good health. Lung tissue requires water to form surfactants which coats the inside of bronchioles, to ensure these tiny air sacs do not collapse. Many asthmatics do not drink enough water. You can't count coffee or tea or alcohol, as these and even some herbal teas are diuretic; that is they weigh negatively on hydration balance. Particular requirements will vary with age, exercise, climate, occupation, and dietary habits.

Vitamins and Minerals— Primary

Vitamin A: 10,000 IU 2-4 times daily in acute cases for children; 25,000 IU 2-4 times daily in acute cases for adults. Mucous membrane integrity, immune system support.

Vitamin B complex: 25 mg 3 times daily for children, 50 mg 3 times daily for adults.

Vitamin C: antihistamine. Stimulates natural adrenalin production; antioxidant, promotes vasodilative PGE2, detoxifies nitrogen oxides (e.g. from vehicle emissions). 1000 mg 3-8 times daily or to bowel tolerance.

Bioflavonoids (e.g. rutin, quercetin): inhibits histamine, cyclooxygenase, TNF and PAF activity; inhibits eosinophil activation; reduces bronchial edema.

Vitamin E: 400-1200 IU daily.

Vitamin B6: antihistamine. 100-250 mg 2-3 times daily.

Vitamins and Minerals—Secondary

Vitamin B3: antihistamine.

Vitamin B12: some cases benefit from 1-3 mg intramuscularly daily for 1 month, then reduce dose to 3 times per week until stabilized. Maintain dose at level needed to control.

Calcium: 400-1000 mg daily. In acute cases, take more at frequent intervals.

Magnesium: 200-800 mg daily. Bronchial smooth muscle relaxant.

Manganese: 5 mg twice per week.

Zinc: 15-25 mg 2-3 times daily for immune support.

Others—Primary

Coenzyme Q10: anti-inflammatory as it inhibits histamine, improves cellular respiration of airways cells.

Essential fatty acids: (especially omega-3s), as anti-inflammatory in airways, anti-allergy. High doses.

Flaxseed oil: valuable source of dietary essential fatty acids.

Garlic capsules: 2 with meals.

Glutathione: antioxidant, important for surfactant; low levels in asthmatics.

Probiotics.

Lipoic acid: 50-100 mg daily. Detoxifies peroxynitrite (nitric oxide), which is a major mediator of airways inflammation and subsequent constriction of airways.

Honey/onion syrup: (see Appendix I).

Others—Secondary

Apple cider vinegar: aids calcium absorption.

Atomodine or 636 (Cayce product): with doctor's prescription.

Bee pollen: preventive for inhalant allergies.

Chlorophyll.

Digestive enzymes.

Kelp: 1-2 tablets 2-3 times daily.

Raw adrenal: 1 tablet 2-3 times daily, or every 15 minutes in acute cases; anti-stress, anti-allergic nutrient.

Raw thymus: 1-2 tablets 3-6 times daily; immune support.

Raw comb honey.

Selenium: anti-inflammatory especially in lipoxygenase pathway of arachidonic acid.

Trace minerals.

See also Allergies and Food Intolerances.

Botanicals—Primary

Asthma weed: useful in most asthmas. 25 drops of tincture in a small amount of water 2-4 times daily.

Albizzia: especially if onset is less than 2 years; anti-allergenic, stabilizes mast cells.

Lobelia: antispasmodic, bronchodilator, expectorant, emetic, mucolytic agent. Use in severe cases. 10-15 drops tincture, 3-4 times daily, or in acute attack a once only dose of 30-45 drops. Larger doses become emetic and possibly toxic.

Ma-huang: bronchodilator; contains ephedrine. Useful in emergencies for extreme difficulty of breathing.

Garlic syrup: expectorant, mucus solvent. Dice garlic and cover with 1 tsp honey. Allow to sit 4-8 hours, then mash and strain. $^1/_4$-$^1/_2$ tsp 2-4 times daily or more frequently in acute episodes. Hot garlic tea is also useful.

Botanicals—Secondary

Cayenne.

Coltsfoot: demulcent, mild expectorant.

Galphimia glauca.

Ginkgo biloba: inhibits PAF.

Grindelia: expectorant and antispasmodic.

Licorice: expectorant, demulcent.

Magnolia.

Mullein: can be used as tea, or the leaves may be smoked for asthma relief.

Picrorrhiza: inhibits histamine production.

Scutellaria.

Skunk cabbage: expectorant, mild sedative, antispasmodic. 15-60 drops of tincture.

Tylophera.

Useful Prescription

Kloss antispasmodic: tinctures of: lobelia, 1 part; skullcap, 1 part; skunk cabbage, 1 part; gum myrrh, 1 part; black cohosh, 1 part; cayenne, $\frac{1}{2}$ part. Take 10-15 drops 2-3 times daily. In acute cases, a one-time dose of 1 tsp.

Therapeutic Suggestions

Due to the chronic nature of this complaint, many supplements are required. As with other disorders of the respiratory system, high doses of vitamin A are required. Those with fat absorption problems should use the micellized forms. In acute phases vitamin A may be taken four or even six times daily. Care must be taken, however, to monitor for vitamin A toxicity when it is used at high doses for any prolonged period of time.

Vitamin B6 helps as an antihistamine when taken in conjunction with a balanced B complex. Vitamin C is always prescribed at as high a dose as the bowels will tolerate. Other medications routinely prescribed are vitamin E, calcium, magnesium, and zinc. Calcium is prescribed as often as every half hour in acute attacks. Iodine-containing medications such as kelp, Atomodine, or 636 are often found useful, but never taken coincidentally, to avoid iodine excess. Kelp is more frequently prescribed, but often a series with Atomodine will be a more effective glandular stimulant.

Doses must be individually prescribed with iodine, but a typical course will be 1 drop daily for 3 days; 1 drop twice daily for 3 days; 1 drop three times daily for 3 days, and then followed with at least 1 week of no iodine medication prior to a second course at the same or a lower dose.

Garlic capsules, although fairly antisocial, are very useful as mucus solvents. Raw adrenal tablets should always be on hand in case of acute reactions. Take 1-2 tablets up to every half hour for a few hours, along with the calcium supplement. Raw thymus should be given several times to enhance immune function.

The most useful botanicals are asthma weed, lobelia, and ma-huang, but these are banned in some places, e.g. Australia.

ATHLETE'S FOOT

DEFINITION AND SYMPTOMS

A fungus infection of the foot caused by *Trichophyton rubrum*, *T. mentagrophytes*, and *Epidermophyton floccosum*. These fungi invade the outer layers of the skin, especially between the third and fourth interdigital spaces. The lesions are macerated areas with scaling borders. The area between the toes may become dry, scaly, itchy, cracked, bleeding, and very tender. Various bacteria may also settle in this area, causing a weeping, malodorous type of athlete's foot that can be very painful.

ETIOLOGICAL CONSIDERATIONS

- Immune deficiency
- Warmth, moisture, and maceration (e.g. from exercise, tight shoes, moist socks, perspiration)
- Diet (excess sugar, hypoglycemia, protein deficiency)

DISCUSSION

These fungal infections are very common among athletes who may have their feet exposed to warmth and moisture over prolonged periods of time. The toes commonly affected are the third, fourth, and fifth. These interdigital spaces are so close that perspiration does not evaporate readily, providing an ideal medium for fungus growth on the dead layers of skin. Secondary bacterial infections may occur that will not respond to antifungal treatments.

TREATMENT

Prevention is the best form of treatment. Always take care to dry between toes after showers, and change socks after exercise or sweating. Wear less constricting shoes when not exercising, or go without shoes if possible, for prolonged periods daily. Keep feet exposed to fresh air as much as possible. If you have a tendency to athlete's foot, it may be useful to apply powder between the toes to assure a dry, moisture-free surface. If you remove the environment for fungus development, it cannot take hold. Some people, however, have a reduced resistance to fungus infections of all kinds, and a detailed investigation of their diet and lifestyle patterns may help reveal the cause of this reduced immunity. Some cases are due to a diet high in sugar or fruit and some may result from very low-protein diets or immune depression.

Therapeutic Agents

Vitamins and Minerals
Vitamin A: 25 mg twice daily. Stimulates immune system. Aids in maintenance and repair of skin.
Vitamin E: 400 IU daily. Helps promote healthy skin. Antioxidant.
Vitamin C: 1000–3000 mg 2–3 times daily. Helps improve immune function.

Zinc: 25 mg twice daily. Stimulates immune system and inhibits growth of fungus.

Others
Garlic: 2 capsules 2–3 times daily. Antifungal.
Probiotics: helps normalize internal and external bio-flora.
Essential fatty acids: aids in the healing of skin disorders.

Primary Applications

- Castor oil: 1 part; Peruvian balsam, 1 part; tea tree oil, 1 part. Apply 4–6 times daily. May also be useful for secondary bacterial infection.
- Colloidal silver: applied topically. Acts as a powerful antiseptic to destroy fungus.
- Tea tree oil: very effective as a powerful antifungal. May be dabbed on neat or soak feet in solution of 2 tsp tea tree oil in two cups of very warm water in a shallow bowl for 30 minutes daily. Best treatment for nail fungus (will take six weeks).
- Vinegar foot wash: wash feet and between toes with dilute or straight vinegar 3–4 times daily.

Others
Urine therapy: collect urine from first morning, stand in a shallow bowl, and soak affected parts, repeat over 5 mornings.
Mutton tallow applications.
Boric acid soak: 1 tbsp per quart (liter) of water. Soak feet 10–20 minutes 3 times daily.
Ultraviolet light exposure and fresh air.
Vitamin E (topical use).

BALDNESS OR HAIR LOSS

DEFINITION

Partial or complete loss of hair on the scalp.

SYMPTOMS

Thinning of hair over entire scalp; total loss of hair uniformly or male pattern loss.

ETIOLOGICAL CONSIDERATIONS—PRIMARY

- Excess male hormone (thickening of galea aponeurotica)
- Glandular imbalance
  Thyroid (hypothyroid); diabetes; pituitary; adrenal
- Heredity
- Poor local circulation
- Pregnancy or menopause
- Improper hair treatment: shampoo
  Strong alkalis or acids; hair dyes; hair dryers
- Radiation/chemotherapy
- Skin disorders
  Seborrhea; excess secretions; dandruff

ETIOLOGICAL CONSIDERATIONS— SECONDARY

Single or multiple nutritional deficiencies (vitamin B complex; biotin; inositol; para-aminobenzoic acid (PABA); vitamin B6; folic acid); contraceptive pill (B6 loss); stress; overwork; severe fevers; heavy metal poisoning; refined diet; anemia; alcohol; nicotine

DISCUSSION

Hair health depends on the amount and quality of its circulation. If the blood and lymph supply to any given hair follicle is cut off, it will die. What occurs in baldness is exactly this process. Whatever the causative factors, the end result is a reduction of the circulation and hair follicle death. This may be the result of hormonal factors, as in male pattern baldness. In this instance the galea aponeurotica membrane in the scalp becomes thickened and inelastic. The scalp becomes tight and thick, cutting off circulation. In seborrhea and dandruff the follicles are clogged and suffocated by excess oily secretions and accumulated dead cells. The end result, once again, is reduced circulation and hair death.

Many nutritional deficiencies have been found associated with balding. Most of these are part of the vitamin B complex. It is well known that severe malnutrition will cause hair loss. While this extreme of poor nutrition is rare, subclinical vitamin B complex deficiencies are extremely common. Our entire modern society seems to threaten consumption of an adequate B complex supply. The refining of whole grain removes a valuable source of many B vitamins, as does overcooking vegetables in boiling water. Being water-soluble, B vitamins are lost in cooking water. In addition, the ordinary diet usually lacks raw green vegetables, a major source of many B vitamins. Even if intake of B complex is adequate, these vitamins are often utilized excessively to digest concentrated carbohydrates such as sugar, white bread, or other refined grains whose own B vitamins have been stripped away in the refining process. This robs the body of valuable vitamins needed for other purposes.

Hypoglycemia, so common in modern civilization, also requires an excess of B complex to support adrenal function. Any factor, be it hypoglycemia or even simple stress that causes the adrenal glands to work overtime, will deplete the B complex group.

Stress not only depletes B complex as stated above, but also acts directly to reduce blood circulation to the scalp. The hormonal system is particularly susceptible to emotions and may affect hair growth. A sudden shock has often been found to precede sudden hair loss or even complete baldness. Sluggish thyroid function is a common finding in many cases of hair loss.

At certain times a sudden loss of hair is considered normal. During the last few months of pregnancy or for 3–4 months post-partum, many women will lose a significant amount of hair. This process usually reverses itself within 6 months after the baby is born. Sudden hair loss is also common following severe illness or high fevers. The hair usually regrows normally.

A major cause of baldness not previously mentioned is improper hair treatment. Strong shampoos, hair dyes, or hot hair dryers may damage the hair and hair follicles. If caught early enough this type of hair loss may be reversed.

The normal lifetime of a single hair is anywhere from 2–6 years. It is then replaced by a new hair. In the typical case of balding, we find a larger proportion than normal of shorter, thinner, younger hair. Progressively the follicles produce fine baby-like hairs with a short life span and then, in time, cease to function altogether. Hairs found in cuttings of short to moderate-length hair should show blunt ends due to previous haircuts. If a large proportion show the thin, pointed ends of new hair growth, the balding process may have begun.

Once the hair follicle itself has died, no new hair growth is possible. The fine hair growth found so commonly on a balding head, however, can many times be reversed so that normal hair once again is produced. In some cases, even when no hair growth is present, new hair growth can be stimulated. These cases, however, are less common. We have seen several remarkable cases where the follicles did not appear to be producing any hair, and still the patient regained hair development with vigorous therapy.

One case stands out in our practice of an elderly Japanese woman who was 80% bald due to diffuse hair thinning. She had dyed her hair black for over 30 years and this was suggested as the possible cause. After 2 months of vigorous application of the treatments below, and no hair dye, all she had to show was a head still 80% bald, but now very gray. When we saw her 3 months later, however, to our great surprise she not only had begun to grow new hair, but the new hair was black! With continued treatment for a further 2-month period, she had regained 80% of a normal head of hair and threw away her wig. The new hairs that grew were all black while those that never had fallen were still gray. Needless to say, the patient was very happy with her new head of hair, even though it never got quite as thick as it had been when she was younger.

TREATMENT

Therapy in all cases must be vigorous. Haphazard or occasional therapy will have little or no effect.

Diet

Foods eaten should obviously all be of the best possible nutritional value. Eat only unrefined wholesome food. Certain groups of foods are found especially useful. Sulfur foods, silicon foods, and iodine foods are very beneficial. Eat plenty of onions, horseradish, garlic, egg yolks (not white), watercress, mustard greens, radishes, alfalfa, celery, lettuce, raw greens, carrots, sea foods, kelp, sunflower seeds, pumpkin seeds, seed sprouts, and other whole grains, wheat germ, lecithin, and brewer's yeast. In addition, the diet found under Anemia may be useful.

Physiotherapy

- Scalp massage: massage scalp each day vigorously with fingertips or an electric vibrator for 20–30 minutes. (*Note:* These vigorous applications will cause an excessive amount of hair to fall in the first 2–4 weeks. This should not cause alarm. These hairs were weak and unhealthy and will be replaced with strong, healthy hair.)

- Hair brushing: use only a natural bristle brush. Brush hair twice daily, making sure to stimulate the scalp with each stroke.
- Crude oil scalp massage: twice weekly massage unrefined, undiluted Pennsylvania grade crude oil (Crudoleum—Cayce product) into the scalp vigorously with the fingertips and then massage the entire scalp for 30 minutes with an electric vibrator.
- Pure grain alcohol rinse (20% solution with a few drops of pine oil)—Cayce. After massaging the scalp with the crude oil, product rinse with this alcohol and pine oil solution.
- Shampoo only with a mild olive oil shampoo (Cayce product).
- Alternate hot and cold head sprays: during the shower, alternate first warm then cold water to the scalp—3–4 times, always ending with the cold.
- Upside-down exercises: do head stands, slant board exercises, hang from hips or knees, or any other exercises that stimulate blood flow to the scalp and brain. One nice way to do this is the back swing, which is a device to hang from the feet. Another available product is gravity inversion boots, also used to hang from the feet. This is not to be done by those with high blood pressure or other circulatory disorders.

The essence of therapy for hair loss in most cases revolves around the above local treatments. A good individually prescribed nutritional program is also useful. Emphasis should be placed on nutritional adequacy, good digestion and assimilation, and glandular stimulation.

The following rather broad list may help in your choices. These nutrients have not been decisively linked to baldness, but are general in their use, to increase vitality.

Therapeutic Agents

Vitamins and Minerals—Primary

EFA (essential fatty acids): flaxseed oil is a good dietary choice.

Vitamin B complex: 50 mg 2–3 times daily.

Vitamin B6: 50 mg twice daily. Used in female hair loss.

Niacin (niacinamide): 50 mg twice daily. Take at doses needed to give a strong flushing sensation. Enhances peripheral circulation. May be used to increase blood flow to scalp.

Vitamin E: 400 IU twice daily.

Multimineral supplements.

Biotin: 5 mg 2–3 times daily

Zinc: 25–50 mg twice daily

Vitamin A: 10,000–50,000 IU daily.

Vitamin C complex.

Copper: 3 mg daily. Needed in conjunction with zinc for hair growth.

Others—Primary

Atomodine or 636 (Cayce product): iodine, to be used on doctor's prescription.

Kelp: 500 mg daily. A good source of iodine and trace minerals.

Silica: the botanical horsetail is a good source.

Coenzyme Q10: 60 mg daily. Improves scalp circulation.

Dimethylglycine: 100 mg daily. Improves scalp circulation.

Brewer's yeast: as a food supplement to supply B complex.

Others—Secondary

Cysteine.

Inositol/choline.

Pancreatic enzymes: take with meals where poor absorption may be causing nutritional malabsorption.

Lecithin.

Raw thyroid: where thyroid disorders are the cause.

Therapeutic Suggestions

Iodine-containing supplements such as kelp, Atomodine, and 636 are used fairly routinely as thyroid stimulants. Where this is not contraindicated, we usually choose 636 for its tonic qualities. The dose of iodine in it is fairly low (1 drop per tsp) and it is taken for 10 days, then stopped for 5–10 days, prior to repeating the prescription.

BED SORES
(Pressure Sores)

DEFINITION AND SYMPTOMS

Ischemic necrosis and ulceration of tissue, especially over bony prominences, due to pressure from prolonged confinement to bed, or from a splint or cast.

ETIOLOGICAL CONSIDERATIONS—PRIMARY

- Nutritional deficiency
- Poor circulation
- Infrequently changed positions
- Poorly made beds

ETIOLOGICAL CONSIDERATIONS—SECONDARY

- Prolonged fever
- Emaciation
- Obesity
- Old age
- Paralysis
- Diabetes
- Anemia

DISCUSSION

Bed sores are a common problem among elderly, weak, or emaciated patients, and for anyone who must remain in one position or be confined to bed due to illness or orthopedic problems. Areas most affected are the overly bony prominences such as the sacrum, hip, heels, elbows, shoulder blades, and back of head.

TREATMENT

Prevention of bed sores is much easier than treatment. The bed must be kept clean and the sheets without wrinkles. Sheepskin bed covers help disperse weight more evenly, as do air or water mattresses. The patient must be turned regularly and observed for any redness (first stage). Regular massage to increase circulation is useful, as is exposure to sunlight. The following therapies are useful to help remove an established bed sore.

Diet

Plenty of greens and carrot juice three times daily.

Physiotherapy

Sugar or honey poultice applied continuously; ultraviolet exposure; colloidal silver (applied topically three times daily); goldenseal (mix powder with honey and vitamin E to a paste and apply to sores); tea tree oil (mix with aloe vera and apply to sores).

Therapeutic Agents

Vitamins and Minerals—Primary

Vitamin C: to bowel tolerance. Begin at 2-6 g daily and increase 2 g daily until loose bowels occur. Reduce dose 2 g and maintain. Vitamin C intravenously will speed healing.

Zinc: 25-50 mg 2-3 times daily.

Vitamin A (with beta-carotene): 50,000-100,000 IU daily. (See warning under Vitamin Toxicity, page 56.)

Vitamin B complex: 50 mg 1-2 times daily.

Vitamin B12: 2000 mcg daily.

Vitamin E: 400 IU once or twice daily.

Calcium and magnesium: a ratio of 2:1. 2000 mg calcium and 1000 mg magnesium daily.

Others

Kelp: 500 mg twice daily.

Garlic: 2 capsules 3 times daily.

BED-WETTING
(Enuresis)

DEFINITION

The involuntary loss of urine that may occur beyond the age when urinary bladder control is usually acquired (around age 3-4).

SYMPTOMS

Involuntary loss of urine, especially while sleeping.

ETIOLOGICAL CONSIDERATIONS

- Urinary tract disorders
- Obstruction to urinary tract; urethral stricture or stenosis; ectopic urethral insertion into bladder; immature bladder, lack of neuromuscular development and control, small bladder with reduced capacity.
- Diet
- Food allergy; excess sugar; excess liquids; excess spices; excess salt
- Excess irritants, chemicals, pesticides, strong spices, etc.
- Hypoglycemia
- Diabetes
- Spinal lesions
- Psychological

DISCUSSION

Development of bladder control is gradual. Usually a child will be able to stay dry by day during the second year of life and stay dry at night late in the third year of life, with only occasional accidents. By age $3\frac{1}{2}$, 75% of all children have acquired bladder control both day and night. By age 5, over 90% have bladder control. The incidence of bed-wetting continues to fall so that by age 15 less than 1% still suffer from enuresis. The frequency of bed-wetting is still fairly high up until the fifth year due to immaturity of the bladder and neuromuscular system.

Organic causes of bed-wetting usually involve the genitourinary system. These include conditions such as chronic infection, urethral stricture or stenosis, obstruction, and ectopic urethral insertion into the bladder. Only 3% or less of all children with enuresis have an organic cause to their condition. The incidence of organic causes becomes much more frequent in the older groups, where up to 75% of all adolescents who suffer enuresis *do* have an organic cause. Organic lesions are more common among long-term primary enuretics (those who have never gained bladder control). They also usually suffer loss of urine during the day.

The most commonly accepted finding with young children with enuresis is that they have very small bladders. Not only do they wet the bed, but they also have frequency of urine all day long. Their bladders simply do not have the capacity to hold all the urine formed at night and enuresis results.

Some authorities feel that part of the problem in enuresis is due to a deeper than usual state of sleep. This has been associated with hypoglycemia, which can give a deep coma-like sleep. This deep state does not allow the part of our brain responsible for social awareness to receive the signal of a full bladder.

Other cases are linked to dietary factors. Hypoglycemia has already been mentioned, but food allergy has also been found as a causative factor in some children. Dairy allergy is always the first suspect. Any food may cause an allergic reaction, and any part of the body may be affected. Some respond with a stuffy nose, others have itchy eyes or skin rashes, and some become enuretics. Once these food allergies are traced down using the cytotoxic test, RAST test, or pulse test and eliminated, the enuresis disappears. Other foods are also suspected, perhaps not as pure allergens but rather as irritants. These include strong spices, salt, sugar, pesticides, and chemicals.

Probably the most important cause of enuresis, which is so often neglected, is spinal lesions. These may be caused by birth trauma or any one of the serious falls that all children seem to take so frequently. These lesions may disrupt the normal flow of both nerve impulses and circulation to the bladder. This is such a common finding that all children suffering enuresis should receive a spinal examination as part of a complete history and comprehensive physical examination.

The psychological causes of bed-wetting are fairly well understood. They are also more common in secondary enuretics (those who gained bladder control and then lost it) over age 5. One common finding is that an older child will develop enuresis on the arrival of a second child. This is a method to gain attention, or a desire to return to an earlier stage of development with more parental care. Other emotions causing enuresis are fear, anxiety, resentment, and the desire to "get even" with the parent for some reason.

Psychological causes are found frequently in children of split marriages or those in institutions. Too-rapid or strict toilet training may actually cause enuresis (also, too little attention to toilet training may lead to bed-wetting. After the age of 4 toilet training becomes very difficult). Anxiety due to parental disapproval or teasing children may slow the learning process. Punishment will usually make the situation worse rather than better.

TREATMENT

It is important to remember that all children do not develop bladder control early. A child should not be suspected of enuresis unless, in spite of steady, consistent but gentle attempts at toilet training, persistent bed-wetting occurs after age 4. During treatment, the aim should be to make the child feel secure and understood, and that with a little help cure is expected. He or she should know that bed-wetting is not normal or desirable, but not made to feel guilty. He or she must be encouraged to make their needs known by day. The child's urine volume should be measured several times to determine the bladder's capacity. If 8–10 fl oz (250–300 mL) can be passed, the problem is not a small bladder.

Liquid intake should be stopped after 3–4 p.m., including all drinks, fruits, or soups. The bladder should then be fully emptied before going to bed. The child should be on his or her back while a story is read for half an hour. Then the bladder is emptied once again. A towel may be tied around the waist so that a large knot protrudes from the back. This will prevent the child from comfortably sleeping on the back. This position has been found to be the worst for enuretics. The parent must then wake the child just before going to bed or at 10 p.m. and possibly again in 3 hours.

Hypnotism has been found to be very useful in these cases. Mild forms of positive suggestions may be all that is needed. As the child is just falling asleep, tell him in a soft, reassuring, and positive tone that when he needs to urinate he will awake all by himself and go to the bathroom and urinate all by himself, and return to his nice dry bed. Tell him that each time he does this it will make it that much easier to do it again the next time until before he knows it his bed it will be dry every night. Tell him also that when he awakes in a dry bed he will feel very happy. This procedure must be repeated every night. Never include any mention of *not* wetting the bed or any other suggestion that is negative. Suggest only the positive behavior that you wish him to develop. If you wish you may also consult a trained hypnotist for more complete self-hypnotic instructions.

Ask the child to keep a record of the dry nights and reward him for a high weekly score. Do not punish or in any way consider wet nights. Reward only the positive.

Exercises

Bladder Stretching
If the urine output and bladder volume is reduced but the frequency is high, the child may be suffering from a small bladder. Bladder capacity may be stretched by giving an excess amount of liquids during the day and asking the child to refrain from urinating as long as possible. Tell him that if he has an accident he should not be embarrassed. Explain what you are doing. You must also expect an increase in the frequency of bed-wetting during this bladder-stretching procedure. When the bladder can void 8–10 fl oz (250–350 mL), bed-wetting will usually cease.

Kegal Exercise
This exercise is performed by using the voluntary muscles to slow down and stop urine flow. During each urination stop the flow several times and hold 1–2 seconds. This is a very effective method. Once the child has learned which muscles to contract he or she should be instructed to do the Kegal exercise at other times throughout the day as well.

Physiotherapy

Cold Sitz Bath or Alternate Hot and Cold Sitz Baths
These are essential to tone the bladder and associated organs. They stimulate both circulation of blood and lymph as well as nervous flow to these areas. A further benefit is the strengthening of both voluntary and involuntary muscles in the pelvic region.

Begin the bath with just cool and add colder water progressively until the temperature is as cold as the child will bear without undue complaint. The object is to stay immersed from hips to midthigh in very cold water for up to 5 minutes.

The duration of the sitz bath should begin with short immersions, gradually increasing the treatment time to the maximum of 5 minutes. If the child is willing, it is more therapeutic to immerse directly into very cold water rather than decrease the temperature gradually. Repeat this cold sitz bath 1–2 times daily for several months or longer, as needed. Follow the bath by vigorously drying with a rough towel until the child feels warm. (Note: If the cold sitz bath is too severe for your child, try the alternate hot and cold sitz, remaining in the hot water 1 minute and the cold water for 2–3 minutes, Repeat three times, ending with cold water.)

Spinal Manipulation

Weekly lumbar, lumbar/sacral, and sacroiliac manipulation is helpful in some cases.

Therapeutic Agents

Vitamins and Minerals

- Vitamin A: 5000–10,000 IU 1–2 times daily. Helps to normalize bladder muscle function.
- Magnesium: 100 mg twice daily. Helps reduce muscular spasm of the bladder.
- Calcium: 200–300 mg 1–2 times daily. Tranquilizes.
- Vitamin B complex: 25–50 mg daily.
- Vitamin E: 100–200 IU 1–2 times daily.

Others

- Cranberry juice: 1 glass 3 times daily.
- Celery.
- Raw bran: before bed.

Botanicals

Bearberry: excellent urinary tonic.
Cornsilk: urinary antiseptic.
Cranesbill: urinary astringent.
Witch hazel: urinary astringent.
Goldenseal.
Cinnamon.
Crataeva: a Chinese urinary tract herb.
High bush cranberry, or cramp bark.
Queen of the meadow: kidney involvement.
St John's wort.

Therapeutic Suggestion

The single most effective tonic for the bladder is the alternate hot and cold sitz baths. These should be accompanied by specific nutritional therapy according to the needs of the patient. Homeopathic medication is a useful approach.

BEHAVIORAL DISORDERS, DEPRESSION, STRESS

DEFINITION AND SYMPTOMS

Feelings of sadness and hopelessness resulting in reduced desire for socialization or communication. Fear, anger, and guilt may be internalized and directed inward upon the self.

ETIOLOGICAL CONSIDERATIONS

- Nutritional deficiency
  B complex; vitamin B3
- Hypoglycemia
- Endocrine imbalances

DISCUSSION

When no recognizable situational or psychologically based cause can be found, it is often very useful to look towards nutrition for an answer. The link between nutrition and behavior has been recognized for centuries. From the earliest days of the discovery of the B complex vitamins, it has been observed that deficiency of these nutrients often led to various emotional problems. More recently, many physicians have suggested that diet may play a role in hyperactivity, schizophrenia, and a whole host of other behavioral disorders.

Nutritional deficiency can be caused by consumption of nutrient-deficient foods, or be the result of improper absorption, transport, or metabolism. Not only may nutritional deficiency lead to emotional disorders and stress syndrome, but conversely prolonged stress or severe depression may result in the rapid use of many nutrients beyond the body's normal supply. It is therefore very common for a stressful situation to result in a nutritional deficiency state, even with a normally adequate supply from the diet.

An interesting example of this stress-induced vitamin deficiency state is the now-recognized vitamin B3 dependency found among former POWs, who lived for long periods under stress and nutritional deficiency. After returning to a normal diet and normal stress, it was discovered that a large percentage of these victims could only maintain proper mental and physical health with daily megadoses of vitamin B3. It appears that stress, or long-term severe deficiency of a single nutrient, vitamin B3 in this case, has led to a permanent excess need for this nutrient for the remainder of that person's life. Evidence with zinc deprivation in rats has shown some dependency and reduced immune function for up to three generations. It would not be too surprising to find similar conditions of vitamin or mineral dependency induced by severe dependency in past generations, gestation, or early life. This may help explain some psychological similarities between parents and children.

Other causes of emotional disorders are also caused by diet, but along different avenues. Hypoglycemia and diabetes are certainly well-recognized sources of emotional lability and depression. Any sudden drop in the blood sugar level will lead to lethargy and depressive tendencies. Allergy is a less frequently thought of as a cause of depression or emotional imbalance, but can be a very real factor. Hyperactivity states due to food additives and sugar is just one of many examples of this type of reaction. Literally any food or food component can be the cause of abnormal emotional states.

Heavy metal toxicity is another frequent cause of emotional disorders. Mercury, cadmium, and lead toxicity are well-documented sources of mental problems.

Endocrine imbalances often affect the emotions. Everyone is familiar with the frequent references to the menstrual cycle and emotional swings. Hypothyroidism also may be a cause of lethargy and depression. Many of these endocrine-related emotional disorders can be corrected through proper nutrition.

TREATMENT

All cases of depression or emotional problems should first be evaluated for blood sugar abnormalities, food allergy, or endocrine imbalance. If hypoglycemia, hypothyroidism, or diabetes tendencies are discovered, the diet regimens in those sections should be used. Care should be taken to remove as many artificial food additives or chemicals as possible from the diet. Foods suspected of containing heavy metals such as swordfish, tuna, or canned foods, should also be eliminated. Sugar, alcohol, coffee, smoking, and any unnecessary drugs should be discontinued. Occupational sources of toxins must be removed. See Allergies and Food Intolerances for details on their diagnoses and therapy.

Vitamins and Minerals— Primary

Obviously, we are discussing a wide range of disorders and only specific supplementation will be of benefit. The following list, however, represents the most commonly used nutrients for these emotional problems:

Vitamin B1: 200–1000 mg daily.
Intramuscular injection may be needed in individual cases.

Vitamin B3: megadoses are often needed for B3-dependent symptoms; 3–9 g daily.

Vitamin B6: pyridoxine dependency symptoms need megadoses. 250–500 mg daily or more are needed, especially where edema exists, or if related to menstrual cycle.

Vitamin B12: 1 mg intramuscularly per week.

Vitamin B complex: 50 mg twice daily.

Folic acid: 400 mcg up to 10 g daily.

Vitamin C: any stressful condition requires bowel tolerance doses.

Calcium/magnesium: in a 2:1 ratio. If there is a relatively high dietary (and supplemented) calcium intake, a relative deficiency of magnesium can cause anxiety, mood swings, depression, and fatigue.

Multiminerals.

Vitamins and Minerals— Primary

Iron; magnesium (400–2000 mg daily to reduce stress factors); manganese; zinc.

Botanicals

Botanicals are emerging as the most effective therapeutic agents

St John's wort: antidepressant.

Bacopa monniera: nervine tonic.

Damiana: antidepressant.

Kava kava: nervine sedative.

Oats: nutritive for the CNS.

Passion flower.

Schisandra: antidepressant, adaptogenic.

Siberian ginseng: adrenal tonic, adaptogen.

Skullcap: CNS tonic, sedative, spasmolytic.

Valerian: sedative.

Withania: nervine sedative.

Others

DL-phenylalanine: 250 mg 3 times daily; or if not effective (with depression), or if it aggravates condition, use tyrosine, 100 mg per kg of body weight.

Desiccated thyroid: dose as per that prescribed by physician.

Lithium: 2–3 mg daily.

L-tryptophan: 1500 mg twice daily.

L-glutamine: 500 mg, 3 times daily.

Probiotics.

Phosphatidyl serine: (capsule form) a naturally occurring fat, in every body cell, concentrated in the brain (cell membranes of neurons). Lowers stress hormones, increases alpha-waves 15–20%, relieves depression. Stimulates memory of faces and facts. 100–300 mg daily.

BODY ODOR

DEFINITION AND SYMPTOMS

The secretion of foul-smelling perspiration.

ETIOLOGICAL CONSIDERATIONS—PRIMARY

- Excess saturated fats:
  Meat; dairy products; hydrogenated fats; fried foods
- Improper diet:
  Zinc deficiency; essential fatty acids deficiency; green vegetable deficiency; excess sweets and refined carbohydrates
- Toxemia
- Soap and water deficiency

ETIOLOGICAL CONSIDERATIONS— SECONDARY

Bacteria; liver disorder; systemic disease; fungus; chemicals; kidney disorder

DISCUSSION

Millions of dollars are spent annually in the development and usage of underarm deodorants and antiperspirants. These not only ignore the basic cause of body odor, but in some cases can be detrimental to your health. Offensive body odor may have two basic causes—external or internal.

The external cause of offensive body

odor is obviously an acute soap and water deficiency. The oily secretions of sweat accumulate and provide an ideal medium for the growth of bacteria, the accepted cause of this type of body odor. Fungus infections may also contribute to body odor.

Internal causes of offensive body odor are, in general, ignored or simply not understood. The skin acts as a major organ of elimination, releasing toxins through the skin. In certain areas such as under the arms this secretion is most noticeable. However, the entire body sweats. If there is an excessive amount of toxic substance in the body that exceeds the capacity of the digestive system, liver, or kidneys to deal with, it must then exit via the skin. Such toxic substances accumulate due to liver disease or congestion, poor eliminations, kidney disease, uremia, pneumonia, acute rheumatism, scurvy, other systemic diseases, and improper diet.

Improper diet, probably the most ignored cause of foul body odor, is also the number one factor in most cases of internal origin. The main offender is excess saturated animal fats or hydrogenated fats. This not only leads to liver toxicity but causes the sebaceous glands to work excessively, producing a greater media for bacterial infection. When a wet sheet body pack is applied overnight to a toxic, heavy meat eater, the sheet will become both stained and offensive smelling, due to the eliminated poisons in the sweat.

Some cases are due to an unsaturated fat *deficiency* rather than saturated fat excess. These may coincide. Zinc deficiency is also recognized as a causative factor in many cases.

TREATMENT

The only real long-term improvement will come from good hygiene, internal cleansing, elimination, and proper diet.

Diet

Various regimens will be effective. The aim of each is to address the major cause for each person. The following have proven useful:

1. 12–14-day elimination diet
Days 1–3
Fruit juice fast with an enema nightly.

Days 4–6
Fresh fruit and fruit juices only.

Days 7–12
Breakfast
Fresh fruit.

Midmorning
Fruit or vegetable juice.

Lunch
Raw salad.

Midafternoon
Same as morning, or potassium broth.

Supper
Same as lunch, or 3-4 steamed vegetables with lemon juice and unsaturated oil.

Evening
Same as afternoon.

2. Prolonged fruit or vegetable juice fasting for 7–21 days

3. Raw foods diet for 2–6 months

4. Vegetarian diets (no dairy products)

5. Liver-cleansing diet (see Gallbladder Disease)

6. Mucus-cleansing diet (see Appendix I)
The best approach is to begin with either the 12-14-day elimination regimen, or prolonged fasting, and then adopt the vegetarian diet until symptoms are cleared. Several periods of elimination diets or fasting may be required over a 2-4-month period. If, at

the end of this procedure, you desire animal products, they may be introduced 5 days a week, with 2 days remaining vegetarian. Red meat (especially pork) is not recommended. Fish is the preferred animal product, then properly raised turkey or wild turkey and chicken. Wild meats contain less fat and are therefore more desirable.

Physiotherapy

- Epsom salts baths: these are useful for body odor due either to internal or external causes. Put 1-1½ lb (450-675 g) of Epsom salts into a hot tub and soak for 15-20 minutes. Finish with a cold spray. Repeat daily the first week, then reduce to 2-3 times per week until the body odor is normal.
- "Salt glow": mix 1 lb (450 g) fine salt in enough water to make a slurry. Begin with a warm shower and then with water off rub salt all over the body firmly. Finish with a cold shower. Your skin will "glow" for hours.
- Alternate hot and cold showers: daily to maintain proper skin function.
- Wet sheet trunk packs: these should be applied nightly during fast and 1-2 times per week for 4-6 weeks.

Therapeutic Agents

Vitamins and Minerals

Zinc: 30-50 mg 2-3 times daily.
Magnesium: 400-800 mg daily.

Others

Chlorophyll: 2-4 tablets 3 times daily.
Essential fatty acids: 4 capsules 3 times daily.
Lecithin: 2-3 tbsp granules 1-2 times daily; or 2-4 capsules taken 2-3 times daily.
Silica (6 ×): 4 tablets daily; also homeopathic, e.g. 30C.

Botanicals

Burdock: alterative, diaphoretic. Helps restore oil and sweat gland function.
Coneflower: alterative, blood purifier.
Oregon grape root: alterative.
Yellow dock: alterative.

Therapeutic Suggestion

Zinc, chlorophyll, and EFA are always prescribed in high doses. The botanicals may be of some use as blood purifiers and as general tonics.

BOILS, FURUNCLES, AND CARBUNCLES

DEFINITION

Boils and furuncles: an acute inflammation and infection of a sebaceous gland, hair follicle, or subcutaneous layer of the skin. *Staphylococcus* infection is most common. *Carbuncles*: a group of adjacent furuncles with extension of inflammation and infection into the subcutaneous layers of the skin.

ETIOLOGICAL CONSIDERATIONS—PRIMARY

- Toxemia
- Constipation
- Improper diet:
  Excess saturated fats; excess hydrogenated fats; excess sweets, refined carbohydrates; excess chocolate; protein deficiency; acid-forming diet; unsaturated fatty acid deficiency

- Immune depression (and use of immunosuppressive drugs)

ETIOLOGICAL CONSIDERATIONS— SECONDARY

Allergy; diabetes; liver congestion; glandular imbalance; poor skin function; excess sebaceous gland activity; local irritation

DISCUSSION

Even a relatively healthy person may experience a boil or two on rare occasions due to local irritation by a splinter or other foreign object. Systemic or repeated boils, however, are always a sign of internal disorder.

The most common cause of recurrent boils is toxemia. This may be due to reduced function of other organs of elimination and detoxification such as found in constipation or congestion of the liver; or it may be due to an excess burden being placed on these organs that cannot be met. Such congestion occurs on an improper diet with excess saturated fats. The overconsumption of meat, pork, eggs, milk, cheese, butter, or other saturated fats congests the liver, thickens the blood, slows circulation, and increases sebaceous gland activity. Similar mechanisms apply to boils as they do in acne (see Acne).

The overconsumption of sweets and refined carbohydrates is also associated with recurrent boils. Although mechanisms similar to those of Staphylococcus infections are found (see Staphylococcal Infection), the character of systemic or recurrent boils is different from those of the typical *Staphylococcus* infection. This may seem paradoxical since both conditions show infections with *Staphylococcus* bacteria. Boils in general differ from a typical *Staphylococcus* infection in that the lesions are more clearly bordered, generally deeper, involving hair follicles or glands, and far less infectious. They are also less likely to be quickly thwarted with external measures alone.

In most cases of systemic or recurrent boils we find glandular disturbances similar, once again, to those found under Acne. Diabetes or food allergy should also be considered as a possible cause in isolated cases.

TREATMENT

Boils are usually the result of self-cleansing and self-repairing efforts of the body to regain equilibrium. As such it is important in our treatment to understand the body's aim and assist in making this cleansing more efficient and complete.

Diet

Nearly any diet that encourages internal cleansing will be effective. However, the raw vegetable juice fast seems to be the most effective, followed closely by the citrus juice fast in cases where excess fruit has not been the usual pattern. Either of these diets may be continued anywhere from 7–21 days or even longer with care and supervision. Shorter fasts may be used and repeated frequently until the desired result is obtained.

Either of these fasts may then be followed by an all raw diet with an abundance of green vegetables, vegetable juices, seaweed, sprouted beans, seeds and grains, and a little fruit. Until the condition has totally cleared, we suggest adhering to a low-saturated-fat diet (see Acne).

Other diets of use in some circumstances are the liver-cleansing diet, apple mono diet, and the mucus-cleansing diet (see Appendix I).

Physiotherapy

Local Applications—Primary
Ice placed directly on a boil in its early
  stages will usually abort its
  development. However, for systemic

141

boils it is better to encourage eliminations.

Flaxseed poultice (with slippery elm powder, comfrey powder and a few drops of tea tree oil): grind flaxseeds and boil to porridge-like consistency; apply as poultice. Helps mature lesions.

Clay poultice.

Colloidal silver: apply topically three or 4 times daily. Promotes healing. A natural antibiotic and disinfectant.

Chlorophyll poultice.

Cooked hot onion or garlic poultice.

Green papaya poultice.

Hot Epsom salts compress: dissolve Epsom salts in hot water and apply as a compress all night.

Tincture of green soap wash: followed by hydrogen peroxide application.

Tea tree oil: apply 4-6 times daily, after green soap and hydrogen peroxide.

Local Applications—Secondary

Aloe; dilute calendula tincture wash as an antiseptic; ultraviolet exposure in careful doses; vitamin E (200-400 IU twice daily); sugar or honey application for deep, ulcerated sores.

General

Hot Epsom salts baths: repeat daily at first, and then 3-4 times per week (see Appendix I).

"Salt glow": (see Appendix I).

Alternate hot/cold showers: as a general systemic tonic. Regularizes deep and superficial circulation.

Therapeutic Agents

Vitamins and Minerals—Primary

Vitamin A: 50,000-100,000 IU daily for 2-4 weeks. Immune support. (See warning under Vitamin Toxicity, page 56.)

Vitamin C: 1000-6000 IU daily or more. Antibiotic, antioxidant, immune support.

Vitamin E: 400-1000 IU daily.

Zinc: 30-50 mg 2-3 times daily.

Vitamins and Minerals—Secondary

Vitamin B complex: 25-50 mg 3 times daily

Vitamin B12.

Folic acid.

Others—Primary

Garlic: 2 capsules 3 times daily. Very effective natural antibiotic.

Chlorophyll: 1 tbsp three or 4 times daily. Local and internal detoxifier.

Bromelain: take 2 tablets 3 times daily on an empty stomach. A proteolytic enzyme which aids to reduce inflammation of soft tissues after trauma and speed healing and cleansing of damaged tissues.

Atomodine: (Cayce product).

Others—Secondary

Kelp (not with Atomodine): 2 tablets 3 times daily.

Propolis (a resinous beeswax): antibiotic. 5-15 drops tincture, 3-4 times per day.

Raw spleen tablets: immune support.

Raw thymus tablets: 2 tablets 4 times daily. Immune support.

Coenzyme Q10: aids in oxygenation of tissues and is a stimulant to immune function.

Botanicals—Primary

Burdock: alterative. 20-40 drops tincture, 3-4 times daily.

Coneflower: blood purifier, specific for systemic boils. 15-30 drops tincture, 3-4 times daily.

Oregon grape root: alterative. Used in skin conditions due to impure blood.

Botanicals—Secondary

Blue flag: lymphatic, depurative.

Calendula: antibiotic.

Red clover.

Yellow dock.

Therapeutic Suggestions

Immune function supports are useful, including vitamin A, B complex, vitamin C, vitamin E, zinc, and thymus. Garlic is essentially used as a mild antibiotic systemically along with propolis. Some cases benefit with some glandular stimulation using kelp or Atomodine 1–2 drops daily for 1 week. Of the botanicals, echinacea stands out as the most effective. Burdock and Oregon grape also are used frequently, in addition. Liver cleansing and liver cleansing herbs are needed in some chronic cases.

BRONCHITIS

DEFINITION

Inflammation of the bronchial tree. May be acute or chronic.

SYMPTOMS

Acute

Symptoms of acute upper respiratory infection; slight fever; cough (dry or productive); mucopurulent secretions; flu-like symptoms, which may lead to bronchopneumonia; chest pain and reduced respiratory excursion

Chronic

Cough; sputum; difficulty in breathing; wheezing; asthmatic episodes; recurrences of pulmonary infection; respiratory failure; exhaustion

ETIOLOGICAL CONSIDERATIONS—PRIMARY

- Diet
  Excess carbohydrates; acid-forming diet; excess dairy products; vitamin A deficiency
- Suppressive treatments of previous health problems
  Improper treatments of common colds; improper treatment of asthma and emphysema and allergy
- Antibiotic use
- Lowered resistance (immune deficiency)
- Exposure, fatigue, malnutrition
- Poor eliminations
- Irritants
  Occupational inhalants; cigarette smoke; pollution; passive smoke damage
- Inadequate circulation
  Lack of outdoor exercise; lack of demanding physical exercise; shallow breathing
- Spinal: C7 to T4, kyphoscoliosis (spinal curvature)

ETIOLOGICAL CONSIDERATIONS— SECONDARY

Frequent colds (viral, with secondary bacterial invasions); foci of infection: tooth or sinus infection acting as reservoir; bronchial constriction; stomach trouble; constipation; chronic catarrh

DISCUSSION

Chronic bronchitis is usually preceded by a series of colds and acute bronchitis. If these two conditions were treated properly, no chronic condition would develop. The most common cause of any chronic lung condition is suppressive treatments for the common cold. These simple eliminations should be allowed to run their course. They act as safety valves to prevent more serious disease from developing from the excessive accumulation of toxic waste within the system. At the first sign of any acute illness, all solid food intake should be halted immediately, and a fruit juice fast, or vegetable juice fast (depending on the condition and patient) should begin. If this were common practice, chronic bronchitis would be rare and restricted to those exposed to lung irritants or cigarette smoke.

Chronic bronchitis is often associated with emphysema. They frequently coexist and are very difficult to differentiate in many cases. In chronic bronchitis, the bronchi become thick and inelastic. The mucus becomes thick and dry and the normal cilia action (little hairs that help remove waste and bacteria) is reduced by degeneration, leading to retained mucus. This acts as an ideal medium for infection. As mucus accumulates, the total available oxygen exchange area of the lung is reduced, leading to dyspnea (difficult breathing). Smoking has a similar action on cilia and reduces their motility.

Coughing in these instances is beneficial. This reflex action aids in removing mucus and waste that the cilia are unable to move further. The cough reflex should therefore not be indiscriminately suppressed. Rather, the causes of excess mucus production and retention should be corrected and the cough will then disappear.

Improper diet and poor eliminations are major causes of excess mucus production. This results in accumulated irritants in the gastrointestinal, lymph, and blood systems. These toxins produce inflammatory changes in the respiratory system.

Spinal abnormalities also predispose the lungs to disease. Kyphoscoliotic changes reduce lung excursion and are a factor in mucus accumulation and downgraded vitality. This also is influenced by decreased lymph, blood, and nervous flow to these tissues. The areas from C7 to T4 are the most commonly involved, causing inflammatory and congestive changes in the lungs and bronchi.

TREATMENT

There is no quick cure for chronic bronchitis. The causes must first be removed and then the entire respiratory system revital-

ized. Much attention must also be spent on normalizing eliminations by improving skin and bowel function. Certain herbal preparations have proven useful to help clear the lungs of excess mucus and heal their delicate linings. These herbs should be used in conjunction with other systematic therapies. Too many people rely on herbal therapies in much the same way as most depend on drug therapy. The only true healing comes from within. These external agents should only be used as a temporary aid to help stimulate the body to action.

Diet

The following diets are of use in these cases, and it important to drink lots of water, as the inflamed mucous membranes require water for secretion.

Mucus-Cleansing Diet
See Appendix I for details.
For more detailed diet advice with mucus conditions refer to the chapter on Asthma.

Physiotherapy

Steam Inhalations
Pine needles, olbas oil, eucalyptus, and elecampane (for asthma-like symptoms). Add the above inhalants to a pot of boiled water. These may be either the herb or oil form. Make a tent over two chairs with a large towel or blanket. Place steaming pot of herbs under tent and inhale fumes for 5–15 minutes. Alternatively, you can simply place the pot on a table or chair and drape a towel over your head and the pot. Inhale deeply. Repeat 3–6 times daily.

Hot Fomentations, Compresses, and Poultices to Chest
Use any of the following:
- Simple hot fomentations, followed with cold.
- Hot ginger fomentation with or without mustard.

- Lobelia hot fomentation for spasmodic cough.
- Lobelia, pleurisy root, and mullein hot fomentation.
- Camphoderm (Cayce product): mutton tallow, spirits of camphor, spirits of gum turpentine.

Rub into chest and apply a hot compress.

Postural Drainage and Percussion (Following Hot Chest Fomentations)

Lie with upper torso hanging over a bed and have someone pound with a flat hand over the entire back. Any mucus brought up should be expectorated into a bowl placed near the head. This will help clear the lungs of excess mucus and facilitate healing.

Hydrotherapy

Any of the following will help:
- Saunas—2-3 times per week, to sweat; chest packs (see Hydrotherapy, page 36).
- Cold wet sheet cross packs over chest, or cold wet sheet simple chest pack. Apply nightly in severe bronchitis.
- Alternate hot and cold showers to stimulate respiration and circulation.

Breathing Exercises

- Blow up balloons: increase force of exhalation.
- Diaphragmatic breathing: begin to breathe by causing the stomach to protrude, followed by the chest. Exhale naturally. It sometimes helps to learn this technique by having someone place the hands over the upper three or four ribs to prevent the chest from rising first. This is important to learn in lung complaints such as bronchitis and asthma. Avoid mouth breathing.

Others
- Spinal manipulation: respiratory excursion must be increased to clear lungs and restore normal diaphragm movements.
- Outdoor exercises: swimming is an excellent exercise for those with lung disorders.

Therapeutic Agents

Vitamins and Minerals—Primary

Vitamin A: essential for lung health. High doses of micellized A, 25,000 IU 2-3 times daily, or more in acute cases (up to 6 times daily for several weeks). (See warning under Vitamin Toxicity, page 56.)

Beta-carotene: 10,000 IU 3 times daily. Essential for lung tissue health and repair.

Vitamin C (with bioflavinoids): 1000 mg 3-6 times daily or more; in acute cases up to bowel tolerance. Enhances immune function and is an antihistamine.

Vitamin E: 400 IU once or twice daily. Helps in the healing of tissues. Antioxidant and improves oxygenation of tissues.

Zinc: 15-25 mg 1-3 times daily. Aids in tissue repair.

Vitamins and Minerals— Secondary

Vitamin B complex: 25-50 mg three times daily.

Vitamin B6: 100-250 mg 1-2 times daily.

Calcium and magnesium: 1000 mg calcium and 500 mg magnesium.

Others

Garlic: 2 capsules 3 times daily. Acts as antibiotic and expectorant.

Raw thymus tablets: 2 tablets 3-4 times daily or equivalent of 1000 mg daily. Enhances immune function.

Colloidal silver: a natural antibiotic; can promote faster healing.

Quercetin: 500 mg daily. A useful antihistamine in allergic bronchitis cases.

Coenzyme Q10: 60 mg daily. Helps improve breathing and circulation.

Honey/onion syrup (see Appendix I): 1 tsp every 1-2 hours in acute cases; 4 times daily in chronic cases.

N-acetylcysteine: 500 mg twice daily. Helps to reduce the viscosity of mucus.

Botanicals

Refer also to asthma herbs. Selection of an appropriate herbal remedy will depend on the case history, but the following represent commonly used and useful herbs.

Bloodroot: expectorant, bronchial membrane stimulant.

Coltsfoot: demulcent. Soothes irritated bronchial mucous membranes. Use as warm infusion.

Ginger: warming, anti-inflammatory.

Elecampane.

Asthma weed: asthma-like condition with restricted breathing.

Gum plant: expectorant, antispasmodic. Used for dry, harsh, and unproductive cough. 10-20 drops tincture 2-3 times daily.

Goldenseal: specific for toning mucous membranes, trophorestorative, anti-catarrhal.

Horehound.

Hyssop: for asthma-like condition, with cough.

Ipecac: 5-15 drops tincture, 2-3 times daily for violent, spasmodic cough.

Lobelia: expectorant, antispasmodic; useful in spasmodic coughs. 10-15 drops tincture 2-4 times daily.

Mullein: soothing, anti-catarrhal, also as a tea.

Onion syrup with wild cherry, horehound, and licorice.

Squill: expectorant for dry, bronchial cough. 5-20 drops tincture 2-3 times daily.

Pleurisy root: expectorant, diaphoretic.

Sundew: antispasmodic, expectorant.

Thyme: spasmolytic, antibacterial, antitussive.

Wild cherry bark: (antitussive) for irritable cough.

Therapeutic Suggestions

High doses of vitamin A supplements are usually very effective with lung complaints. Take care to monitor serum vitamin A levels to prevent toxicity. Where high vitamin A is needed, however, higher levels can usually be better tolerated. Vitamin B complex and extra vitamin B, are useful, as well as vitamin C, to bowel tolerance. Garlic acts as a wonderful mucus solvent, and should be taken in as many ways as possible (e.g. capsules, food, condiment, garlic syrup and foot poultice). Onion syrup is also very useful and less offensive. Raw thymus as an immune stimulant is very helpful, as well.

BURNS

DEFINITION

Tissue damage of skin or mucous membranes in response to heat, chemical or radiation injury.

SYMPTOMS

Burns are classified as *first-degree*, when there is only superficial involvement of the outer layer of the epidermis. The area is pink but blanches white on pressure. Depending on treatment, may or may not blister.

A *second-degree* burn involves the entire epithelium, including glandular structures and hair follicles. Blistering and scar formation occurs.

Third-degree burns involve the full thickness of skin with extensive tissue damage. Areas may be oozing, or in severe cases (*fourth-degree* burn) may be dry and charred.

ETIOLOGICAL CONSIDERATIONS

- Heat
  Open fires; hot liquid; ultraviolet rays and sun lamps
- Chemicals
  Topical; inhalation
- Electricity
- Radiation

DISCUSSION

The rapid and proper treatment of burns is essential to prevent or reduce blistering, scar formation, or contracture of skin. First-degree burns may be treated safely at home. *However, extensive second- or third-degree burns always need to be treated under medical supervision.* These injuries can lead to severe loss of fluids and electrolytes with shock and even death as a possibility. If possible, obtain the services of a doctor familiar with or willing to try the simple measures outlined under the treatment section. Severe burns respond remarkably to these measures. Any extensive second- or third-degree burns should always be treated with medical supervision to prevent scarring and disfigurement.

TREATMENT

There are a vast number of home remedies or first aid for burns. Of this large variety, however, several stand out as the most effective. They are simple, readily available, and reliable. Most have slowly graduated from the "folk remedy" status to at least the fringe of standard orthodox practice.

Hydrotherapy

The simplest, most effective measure with any burn is to immerse the area in cold water immediately after the injury and until all pain has subsided. With a first-degree burn this will often prevent a blister formation. In more severe burns it will minimize tissue damage. If the burn is severe and transport to a hospital necessary, either continue soaking the area if possible, or gently wrap the area with wet sheets and apply water at frequent intervals over this sheeting.

Oil Applications

Just after the injury has been soaked in water, apply a strong concentration of vitamin E. This may be applied to a small area by puncturing a 400 IU capsule and gently covering the burn; or it may be sprayed on with an oil atomizer for larger areas. This needs to be repeated every 1–4 hours. Vitamin E has been found extremely beneficial, even in third-degree burns, to promote early healing and prevent scar formation. Vitamin E is used externally with great success with all types of burns. High doses of vitamin E should also be taken internally at 800–1600 IU daily.

Vitamin C

Between vitamin E applications a 1–3% solution of vitamin C should be sprayed every 2–4 hours. This reduces pain, accelerates healing, reduces the chance of infection, and decreases local swelling. Vitamin C may also be taken as an injection in severe burns, in megadoses. In all burns vitamin C should be taken orally up to 1000 mg every hour. These three applications make the best therapy for burns. Severe burns require nutritional supplementation to speed healing.

Vitamins and Minerals—Primary

Vitamin A: up to 100,000 IU daily for three weeks. Test liver function for toxic effects, however severe burns cause an excess need for this vitamin and toxicity is rare. Reduce dose to 50,000 IU for a further three weeks. Consider allowing one week between doses to clear liver if needed. Emulsified form is less toxic. Essential for healing of epithelial tissues.

Beta-carotene: 30,000 IU daily. A precursor to vitamin A and a powerful antioxidant. Found in yellow/orange foods (e.g. carrots), so also include these in diet in large amounts.

Vitamin B Complex: 50 mg balanced mix twice daily. Aids in repair to the skin.

Vitamin B12: 1000 mcg twice daily. As sublingual form or IM injection daily. Essential for cell reformation and protein synthesis.

Vitamin C (with bioflavinoids): 1000–3000 mg taken every two hours to bowel tolerance or up to a maximum of 30,000 mg daily. Use intravenous vitamin C in severe burns. Promotes healing of burns by aiding in the formation of collagen. Also an antioxidant.

Vitamin E: 400 IU twice daily or up to 1600 IU in severe cases. Helps in faster healing and to prevent scarring. May be applied externally also to prevent scarring.

Zinc: 50 mg twice daily. Aids in healing of skin.

Vitamins and Minerals— Secondary

Calcium and magnesium: 500 mg 3 times daily of calcium and half as much of magnesium.

Selenium: 200 mcg daily. To improve tissue elasticity.

Others

Coenzyme Q10: 100 mg daily. To increase circulation and aid in healing.

Essential fatty acids (e.g. flaxseed oil): to speed healing.

Chlorophyll.

Cod-liver oil: 2–4 capsules 2–3 times daily.

Raw adrenal tablets: 1 tablet 3 times daily with second- or third-degree burns.

Germanium: 200 mg daily. Speeds healing and circulation.

Aloe: obtain fresh aloe and apply the gelatinous inner contents of the cactus leaves to sunburn and other minor burns. Bottled gel may also be obtained from most health food stores, but is less effective.

Aloe gel and propolis: this combines the soothing and anti-inflammatory effect of aloe with the antibiotic nature of propolis. Comfrey poultice: steep comfrey leaves or boil root and apply to burn as a continuous compress.

Comfrey and wheatgrass poultice.

Comfrey, wheat germ, or vitamin E oil and honey poultice: this classic poultice combines the beneficial effects of three well-known applications, each individually proven beneficial with burns.

Honey, or honey plus herbs: apply and cover with gauze (comfrey, marshmallow, calendula.).

Honey, propolis, and zinc oxide.

Calendula succus compress: $1/4$ dilution applied to gauze.

Witch hazel (non-alcoholic, dilute).

Bicarbonate of soda plus water: for acid burns flush immediately with water or water plus bicarbonate.

Essential fatty acids (EFA) ointment.

Chlorophyll ointment.

BURSITIS

DEFINITION

Acute or chronic bursitis: inflammation of a bursa (a fluid-filled cavity, especially common where tendons pass near bones).

SYMPTOMS

Pain, tenderness, reduced mobility, swelling, redness, possible fever, muscle weakness.

ETIOLOGICAL CONSIDERATIONS—PRIMARY

- Direct trauma
- Microtrauma (overuse)
  Sports; work; housework
- Poor diet
- Meat excess; lack of green vegetables;
  excess alcohol; excess coffee
- Stress

ETIOLOGICAL CONSIDERATIONS— SECONDARY

Metabolic disturbance; toxemia; infection; gout; allergy

DISCUSSION

Although most people think of the shoulder (subdeltoid) when bursitis is mentioned, bursitis may affect a number of joints throughout the body. Other fairly common sites are the hip (iliopsoas), ischia (so-called tailor's or weaver's bottom), prepatellar (housemaid's knee), retrocalcaneal (Achilles), olecranon (miner's elbow), semimembranosis (behind knee), trochanteric (bunion), or radiohumeral (tennis elbow). Bursae exist at areas of friction in the body, usually between tendon and bone, acting as cushioning barriers to tissue damage. The two most common causes of bursitis are direct trauma and microtrauma. Direct trauma, such as a severe blow to the shoulder, causes the bursa to swell, leading to pain on motion and reduced mobility. This type of bursitis, if well rested after the initial injury, will usually resolve easily within a short period of time. If aggravated and used too soon after the initial injury, this acute bursitis may become chronic, lingering for years.

Microtrauma as a cause of bursitis is the use of the joint and muscles in an "ordinary" activity repeated frequently, such as found in the action of screwdriving or tennis, with rotation (supination) of the forearm against resistance. A similar trauma may occur to the shoulder with repeated hammering. All these actions are within the normal range of expected activity for the body, but many repetitions over a prolonged period of time ultimately cause irritation and inflammation of the bursa and later the joint itself if the bursa communicates directly with the joint as it does with the shoulder. Repeated small blows in the area of the bursa, such as the pushing or stamping on a lever as in some industrial occupations, or repeated kneeling, as in housemaid's knee, will also cause bursitis. Even prolonged or repeated carrying of a heavy purse or shopping bag can initiate bursitis.

Once bursitis has developed there is a tendency for the periarticular structures to become thickened and fibrotic. If the effusion or swelling has been severe, adhesions may form to limit mobility further, causing pain and recurrent swelling.

Much confusion exists regarding bursitis among patients, since many physicians use the term fairly loosely. The label of "bursitis" of the shoulder may be used to mean arthritis, a tear in the periosteum at the insertion of the supraspinatus muscle, calcification of the supraspinatus muscle, pain from the third costovertebral joint, other partial muscle tears, or true subacromial/subdeltoid bursitis.

One commonly neglected aspect of bursitis is the possibility that if the nutritional state had been more adequate the same amount of trauma may not have resulted in any symptoms whatsoever. Certainly, high levels of vitamin C are known to help protect against connective tissue injuries. Apart from athletic injuries resulting in bursitis, the average person we see with bursitis is on a poor, vitamin-deficient diet. Not surprisingly, then, we find the nutritional approach to therapy essential to allow other local therapies to function best.

An interesting consideration with bursitis and other inflammatory conditions is that some people are particularly prone to inflammatory reactions. Two people of similar age and build will respond quite differently to an episode of trauma or repeated microtraumas. One may show only minor symptoms lasting a short period of time, while the other may develop a bursitis that causes discomfort for years, perhaps decades. The difference in these two is that the latter is an inflammatory condition, even before the traumatic incident. We believe the causes of this predisposition are usually dietary or stress-related. Cases of bursitis very rare among those who are on a highly nutritious, alkaline (more vegetarian) diet with few obvious irritants, such as coffee, alcohol, refined sugars, salt, and strong spices. This applies to all diseases but particularly to inflammatory conditions such as bursitis, arthritis, gastritis, and colitis. Stress plays an obvious role in these conditions, working along a variety of negative pathways.

TREATMENT

Since the average case of bursitis is caused by trauma or repeated use as in tennis, angling, baseball, cricket, hammering, or other activities with repeated actions, these are strictly forbidden until full healing is complete. The only cause of chronic bursitis is improper care of acute bursitis, and the best part of this cure is rest. Cases of slow-to-heal bursitis need careful dietary evaluation to find areas that cause inflammation within the system. A strict vegetarian, and preferably vegan diet, is very helpful in stubborn cases. When the patient is unwilling to comply with such a drastic change, we suggest four glasses of carrot juice daily and at least one solely salad meal daily. Periodic fasting or all vegetable days will also help speed recovery. Alcohol is a main offender, as is coffee, and these need to be eliminated until all pain and inflammation are gone for at least two months.

Acute

- Ice compress: when the first symptoms appear, apply cold compresses, leaving

them on for 20–40 minutes. Repeat this application every 3 waking hours for the first 2 days.
- Restraint: fix the joint in a resting position and do not use actively. In the case of a shoulder, use a sling if this is necessary to prevent the shoulder's use.
- Passive mobilization (see below) is necessary several times daily.
- Ultrasound: treatments daily after the first 48 hours for 1 week, then 4 times per week the second week.
- Alternate hot and cold compresses: after 48 hours of ice-cold applications use ultrasound and alternate hot and cold applications, or use heat followed by joint mobilization ending with cold applications.

Chronic

- Heat compresses.
- Alternate hot and cold compresses.
- Ultrasound 4–5 times weekly.

Exercises

Passive mobilization, or movement of the injured joint with the help of another person, should be done after the first 48 hours 2–6 times each day, to the full range of motion *without* the assistance of the patient's muscles. This speeds healing and reduces the possibility of adhesions forming. Machines for this purpose, to mobilize without muscle assistance, have had success in healing joint and soft tissue injuries.

Once all or most of the pain and swelling has subsided, non-muscle-assisted exercises can begin:
1. Arm swing (1): stoop to 90° angle from waist and let arms hang freely, then gently swing arms front and back and then side to side. Do not use shoulder muscles in this action. Then gently swing arms in small circles in both directions, gradually increasing the diameter of the circle as each day progresses.

2. Toe touch: bend forward at waist and touch toes repeatedly.
3. Bed exercise: lie in bed and slowly raise arm from the shoulder out from side to point of pain and back.

Begin the following muscle-assisted exercises once the previous two exercises are easily performed without much pain.

1. Wall creep: stand 1 ft (30 cm) from wall with hands on wall at whatever level is comfortable, say, waist high. Slowly creep your hands up the wall by pulling your fingers forward and back like a spider. Stop when you reach the level where pain increases. Repeat exercises 4–5 times daily. Mark this level on the wall and over the next few weeks try to exceed this level progressively, going higher until arms can go completely overhead.
2. Arm swing (2): stand erect and swing arms across body repeatedly in a gentle action. Swing arms in gradually larger swings front to back until full-circle swings can be easily and painlessly made.
3. Apron tie: repeat tying and untying an apron.
4. Collar button-up: attempt to button and unbutton a real or imaginary button behind the collar, repeatedly.
5. The pickpocket: repeatedly attempt to remove a billfold from the back pocket.
6. Pulley exercises: arrange a pulley on the wall with a strong rope about 8 to 10 ft (2.5–3 m) long running through. Attach a handle to both ends, or attach through a firm rubber ball with a large knot. If possible, arrange the pulley so that its height from the floor may be freely adjusted. Sit on the floor or on a stool with back to pulley. Begin with pulley close to floor and pull with the injured arm on the rope against the resistance provided from the good arm which is holding onto the opposite end of the rope. Two-pound weights may be used instead. Repeat several times and then raise the pulley 6 inches (15 cm). Repeat these exercises until a height is reached

that causes mild to moderate pain. Do not overdo. The object is to increase both the strength and mobility of the shoulder slowly. Repeat, sitting facing the pulley. Ready-made pulley exercise units are available at most sports departments. Increase weights slowly.

7. Stick, rope, ball, and door techniques: this simple technique substitutes for the previous one and is more portable. Attach a wooden handle to one end of a 4–6 ft (1.2–1.8 m) rope and attach the other end through a firm rubber ball with a large knot. The ball end is then slipped behind the door and the door closed so that the rope may be secured at literally any position along the door's perimeter. Stand with back to door, with rope in the near-floor level. Gradually pull the rope against the resistance for 3–6 seconds, and relax. Repeat 2–3 times, then repeat at higher levels along the door frame. Stop at the level you feel pain and repeat, facing the door.

Poultices

- Green cabbage leaf poultice. Apply to tender, swollen bursa nightly.
- Comfrey leaf poultice.
- Apple cider vinegar and salt compress: prepare a saturated solution of iodized salt dissolved in hot water and add an equal amount of cider vinegar. Saturate a compress and apply hot for 10–15 minutes twice daily. Helps with tissue damage, fibrositis, and calcification.
- Castor oil packs.
- Hot Epsom salts packs (with no swelling).
- Ice compress (with swelling).

Physiotherapy

- Peanut oil massage.
- Ultrasound therapy daily for first 2 weeks; reduce to 3 times per week for the next 2 weeks.

- Positive galvanism to bursa with magnesium sulfate or oil of wintergreen.
- Shoulder mobilization and manipulation to break adhesions in chronic cases.

Therapeutic Agents

Vitamins and Minerals—Primary

Vitamin A: 10,000-25,000 IU 2-3 times daily. To aid tissue repair and immune function.

Vitamin B12: intramuscular. 1000 mcg once per week.

Vitamin C with bioflavinoids: 1000 mg 6-12 times daily, or to bowel tolerance. Reduces inflammation.

Vitamin E: 400 IU twice daily. Anti-inflammatory

Zinc: 50 mg daily. Aids tissue repair.

Calcium: 800-1000 mg daily. For proper connective tissue repair.

Magnesium: 400-500 mg daily. For proper connective tissue repair.

Vitamins and Minerals—Secondary

Vitamin B complex: 50 mg 3 times daily.

Vitamin B6: 250-500 mg daily.

Pantothenic acid: 250-500 mg twice daily.

Selenium: 200 mcg daily.

Other—Primary

Bromelain: anti-inflammatory, 2-4 tablets 3-4 times daily. Taken only on an empty stomach. Very effective with bursitis. These high doses may cause some gastrointestinal upset in some people. Use with care if history of ulcers.

Glucosamine and chondroitin: 1 tsp of powder or two capsules 3 times daily. Helps to heal connective tissue.

Other—Secondary

Atomodine or other iodine source.

Raw adrenal tablets.

DL-phenylalanine: 500-1000 mg 2-3 times daily. For pain relief.

Coenzyme Q10: 60 mg daily. To improve circulation.

Botanicals

Bryony: pain with motion. 5 drops tincture 2-3 times daily, or used as homeopathic dilution.

Comfrey: use as strong infusion, decoction, or tincture, 2-3 times daily for 1-3 months as therapeutic trial.

CANCER

Despite better diagnostic equipment and earlier diagnoses, the causes and cures of cancer seem to be still quite elusive from a medical viewpoint.

Cancer is viewed medically as the manifestation of the abnormal, uncontrolled growth of body cells and tissue causing lesions (neoplasms), which can spread (infiltration, metastasis) to other parts of the body and cause obstruction of vital functions, which can prove fatal. The medical approach is to attack the lesion, and to use surgery, chemotherapy and radiation therapy to get rid of the lesion.

Up until the 1960s, surgery was the primary medical approach to cancer, the idea being that if cancer is a lesion, it can be cut out. This approach has limited success, as the cancer usually makes a reappearance somewhere else later.

The availability of a variety of new drug agents in the 1960s gave rise to chemotherapy. Variables included dose, schedule, combination of drugs and sequential therapy. This led to successful treatment first of acute lymphocytic leukemia, then Hodgkin's disease and non-Hodgkin's lymphoma, testicular cancer and some of the childhood solid tumors.

By the 1970s, the focus had changed to adjuvant therapy (use of drugs after surgery or radiation therapy), because it became evident that microscopic tumors are much more easily eradicated by chemicals than are large ones. This reduced mortality by 25% for pre-menopausal patients with breast cancer, and some 60–70% in patients with esteogenic sarcoma.

In the 1980s neoadjuvant chemotherapy was developed in an effort to reduce tumor size and render more operable selected solid tumors. The introduction of tumor necrosing factor (TNF), interferons (If), and hematopoietins was the result of a better understanding of the biochemical aspects of cancer such as the role of oncogenes and oncogene products such as growth factors in the maintenance of malignant phenotypes.

However, in the most common cancers such as breast cancer, the survival statistics have changed very little since the 1950s. Why is it that cancer still represents an often fearful threat to vitality and longevity, and seems to be on the increase?

Put simply, drugs which have the potential to damage cancer cells (cytotoxic drugs) also have the potential to damage healthy tissue. The big problem for the chemists is target cell specificity. Drugs can directly damage normal cellular DNA, causing secondary malignancy. Most commonly, secondary tumors include a range of acute leukemias, non-Hodgkin's lymphomas, and others.

Chemotherapeutics recognises a 3-stage response:
- Phase 1: tumor regression.
- Phase 2: stable decrease/no detectable tumor.
- Phase 3: tumor progression.

If cytotoxic drugs are continued during Phase 2, natural immune defenses are further weakened. If the tumor starts to grow again (Phase 3) the second course of drugs is usually less effective, because there is little or no immunity to manipulate. This phase sees

susceptibility to non-specific infections or activation of latent viral oncogenesis.

In addition, chemotherapy is a sufficient stressor to induce malnutrition (induces poor appetite, nausea, vomiting, etc.); malnourishment (e.g. low serum levels of vitamin A and E) results in poor response to chemotherapy anyway. More than 40% of cancer patients die from malnutrition (catechia). It may be as simple as creating too much of a load on the body's defense systems, in which the internal environment becomes overwhelmed, toxic, acidic, and polluted.

Evidence suggests that the best time to give chemotherapy is between 12 midnight and 4 am, as immune natural killer (NK) cells are less active then, and less damaged by the chemotherapy.

Radiation therapy, whether as a primary or adjunctive therapy, has the potential to damage healthy tissue, and is known to cause massive free radical damage throughout the body, itself a cause of cancer.

A New Model

The last 40 years of cancer research has not brought us much closer to understanding what causes cancer, let alone curing it.

In 1952 Dr Ernst T. Krebs, Jr., a biochemist in San Francisco, hypothesized and clinically demonstrated that cancer, like scurvy and pellagra, is not caused by some mysterious bacterium, virus or toxin, but is a deficiency disease caused by a lack of a certain compound belonging to the nitriloside family (vitamin B17—laetrile). This compound occurs in over 1200 different plants throughout the world, and especially prevalent in the seeds of stone fruits such as apricot, cherry, plum, nectarine, peach, also in the bitter almond, maize, sorghum, millet, cassava, linseed, apple seeds and many other foods and grasses, all of which have been generally deleted from the average western diet.

His work was rejected by his peers, and this is discussed in *World Without Cancer* by G. Edward Griffin. Of course, we do not suggest that B17 is the whole answer, but the clinical work of Krebs, Jr. and the model of cancer being a nutrient-deficiency disease, did deserve much greater attention than it got, and new studies ought to be done on this compound.

Not much scientific investment has been put into the nutritional aspects of cancer. And yet naturopaths the world over, as well as some outstanding scientists and doctors who have risked everything by going out on this limb, have demonstrated clinically that success in treating cancer (remission, reversal, cure) lies down this path. This approach involves changing the internal environment to one in which cancer cannot survive and the body's own defense systems can get back on top.

Schipper, H. and coworkers write in *The Lancet* 348, 1149–51, 1996 suggesting the old models of cancer which view the neoplastic lesion as the disease, are not correct. Oncology treatments are based on these models (surgery, chemotherapy, radiotherapy), in which the aim is to eradicate every last cancer cell. Schipper and his team see cancer as a process. This model suggests that cancer is aberrance in the control of cellular behavior in an otherwise normal cell. New approaches to therapy ought to aim at the reinstitution of normal regulatory processes, he says.

Naturopaths have always approached cancer treatments using this paradigm. What we see here is science asking, "Might not the naturopathic model of understanding the disease and treatment of the disease (which has outstanding clinical success) in fact be the correct one?"

Cancer, a Biochemical Abnormality

From studies of cancer at a cellular level, we now know that mineral deficiencies (e.g. magnesium, zinc, germanium, selenium and others) and vitamin deficiencies (vitamins A, B, C and bioflavonoids, D, and E) all have a role in maintaining normal cell behavior.

Cancer patients demonstrate deficiencies of these nutrients. At tissue level, inflammatory mediators play a huge part in creating an environment for cancer cells to grow from metastasis, and cancer patient histories illustrate this fact.

Cellular energetics is the study of how cells maintain vitality, and are able to function properly. When cells lack essential nutrients with which to function properly, they become inefficient energy producers. When the Krebs cycle and electron transport chain becomes impaired, there is the potential for mitochondrial DNA damage and neoplasm. Mitochondrial DNA more readily mutates than does nuclear DNA, and does so in response to intracellular toxin build-up and radiation exposure. Many cancer patients demonstrate a history of fatigue prior to any cancer diagnosis, and this is consistent with the nutrient deficiency model that naturopaths have always believed.

TREATMENT

The primary role of treatment ought to focus on cellular, tissue and organ detoxification by restoring the toxin removal systems of the body to optimal performance; in denying the body those things which predispose it to biochemical stress, such as environmental toxins and food chemicals, pharmaceutical and recreational chemicals, foods which create internal acidity, and by reducing exposure to external stress (see Stress). This will mean different things to different people of course, but naturopathic experience over the past 100 years demonstrates that a vegetarian diet, with attention to all the essential nutrients, coupled with a less stressful lifestyle, is protective against, and even curative of, cancer.

Vitamins

• Vitamin A: best as beta-carotene up to 100,000 IU (5500 IU = 10 mg) (quenches singlet oxygen, thus protecting body fat and lipid membranes). (See warning under Vitamin Toxicity, page 56.)

- B-complex.
- Niacin (B3): anti-fatigue; normalizes sugar metabolism.
- B17 (amygdalin): 5 g/kg body weight, IV
- B12 and B9: methyl group donors (cancer cells are under-methylated, leading to proliferation)
- Vitamin C: oral (to bowel tolerance), and IV (30 g per week).
  Potent antioxidant, immunostimulant. Inhibits DNA, RNA and protein synthesis in neoplastic blood cells and squamous cells.
  Antithrombotic activity (anti-platelet).
- Flavonoids: (potent antioxidants)
  Inhibit rouleaux formation (e.g. in leukemia, myelomas).
  Inhibit lipo-oxygenase inflammatory pathways.
  Inhibit mast cell release of histamine.
  Inhibit abnormal platelet adhesion.
  Protect vitamin C and adrenalin from oxidation.
  Reduce capillary permeability.
  Increase macrophage strength (proteolysis).
- Vitamin D: inhibits cancer cell proliferation (episome production) especially in melanoma, breast and bone cancers, and leukemia.
- Vitamin E: (1200 IU)—especially with estrogen-dependent cancers.
  Inhibits estrogen.
  PAF inhibitor.
  Enhances humoral and cell-mediated immunity.
  Augments phagocytic activity.
  Reduces lipid peroxidation associated especially with chemotherapy (bleomycin, doxorubicin) and radiation treatment.
  Human epidemiological studies have demonstrated that high blood levels of vitamin E are associated with a decreased cancer risk.

Minerals

- Selenium (200–400 mcg daily) May be specifically contra-indicated in leukemias, and myeloproliferative cancers.
- Magnesium: important regulator of intracellular DNA copying (binds phosphates).
- Zinc: promotes natural enzyme systems involved in liver detoxification pathways, protein metabolism, lymphocytic integrity, PAF inhibitor, DNA replication regulator and DNA repairs.
- Organic Germanium: carrier of oxygen to tumor cells which causes lysis.

Essential Fatty Acids

- GLA/EFA: these oil vitamins down-regulate the arachidonic acid cascade, as they are anti-inflammatory, and anti-PAF; they also prevent and reverse chromosomal damage; they activate macrophages, and regulate cyclic adenosine monophosphate. Flaxseed oil, evening primrose oil, fish oil, 2 tbsp daily.

Amino Acids

- Glutathione.
- Arginine: a precursor to nitric oxide (NO), which kills tumors. 2–4 g daily.
- Glutamine: reduces damage and promotes repair of bowel (e.g. as in leaky gut).
- Taurine: improves cellular electrical potential, and stabilizes the sodium ATPase pump.
- Methionine: detoxifies estrogen (methylation) thus reducing excess.

Other

- Digestive enzymes: between meals, and with meals; essential supplementation.
- Glucosamine: impairs metabolism of nucleotides in cancerous tissue.

155

- Enzymes: e.g. pancreatic, bromelain, papain.
- Probiotics: bowel flora produce anti-cancer compounds, and deserve priority attention
- Bovine cartilage: anti-angiogenic, anti-proliferative (contains all the water soluble components of hyaline cartilage, predominantly proteoglycans or glycosaminoglycans) effective in cancers of the cervix, kidney, lung, ovary, pancreas, prostate.
- Melatonin: inhibits estrogen activity.

Foods

- Kelp: iodine inhibits estrogen; especially for breast cancers.
- Papaw: (green, with seeds and skin) can make up into a soy smoothie. Half a papaw daily.
- Bitter melon.
- Spirulina, barley green, wheat grass, chlorella, etc.: (chlorophyll, an oxygen transporter; high in magnesium, cleanses the blood, etc.).
- Juices: (home made, e.g. beet, wheat grass, pineapple). Isoprenoids (active in fresh raw vegetables, fruit and cereals) actively suppress human cancer cells; gamma-tocotrienol and beta-ionone slow the growth of leukemia, breast cancer and colon cancer cells.
- Green tea: (antioxidant rich, contains epigallocatechin-3 gallate EGCG) up to 10 cups daily.
- Ginger tea: (anti-inflammatory)
- Lecithin: (build up intake to 1 tbsp each 2nd day) and/or raw egg yolk.
- Ginger, onion, garlic.
- Soy products: down-regulate oncogenes with protease inhibitors (contain genistein and isoflavones which compete at estrogen sites; especially significant in estrogen-dependent tumors e.g. breast, cervical, prostate).
- Coenzyme Q10: a primary cellular regenerator increasing energy output (increases the phagocytotic activity of macrophages, IgG)

- Psyllium husks: lowers blood pressure; as a bulk fiber, and food for bowel flora, it is an anti-colon-cancer agent, etc.
- Barley flour: contains twice the amount of insoluble fiber as wheat flour, and CSIRO trials in Australia demonstrate prophylaxis against colon cancer.
- Beet juice: $1/3$ cup (100 mL) daily—raw is preferred), can add a little ginger, a clove of garlic, celery and carrot juice as well.
- Cherries: contain monoterpine perillyl alcohol (can lead to tumor cell death).
- Wheatgrass, green vegetables, mangoes: all contain abscisic acid, an anti-cancer agent which destroys the growth hormone cancer cells make.
- Lipoic acid: antioxidant.
- Niacin (B3).
- Cytochrome C.
- Beet juice: contains an active ingredient which has the capacity to increase respiration of cancer cells by up to 350%, making them less malignant.

Preventing metastasis

- Ensure adequate nutrients for surfactant production in lungs: lecithin, egg yolk, water
- Strengthen body's immune system (NK, phagocytes, etc.).
- Healthy blood means oxygen and nutrient transport throughout the body (cancer cells favor anaerobic environments).
- "Thin the blood" (reduced viscosity of blood and lymph, means optimal hydration). Anticoagulant therapy with warfarin and other coumarins (vitamin K antagonists) reduce the incidence of metastases. Bromelain improves fibrinolytic activity; rutin inhibits rouleaux formation.
- Pancreatic enzymatic defenses (modify hormone receptor sites on cancer cells, meaning these cells are less responsive to growth).
- Reduce systemic inflammation: especially important after surgery, radiation.

- Make platelets less sticky: flaxseed and fish oil supplementation; antiplatelet aggregation herbs include coleus, ginger, *Salvia miltiorrhiza*, dong quai, garlic.

Preventing Angiogenesis

Angiogenesis is the process of blood vessel development, which can supply a tumor with nutrient.
- Prostaglandins, PAF, lactic acid, histamine, and leukotrienne-B4 all stimulate angiogenesis. Therefore, inhibiting these inflammatory factors is important.
- Mucopolysaccharides (proteoglycans, glycoproteins), e.g. as derived from shark cartilage or bovine trachea.
- Genistein is a phytoestrogen found in soy foods, and is also anti-angiogenic.

Improving Oxygenation to the Body

Tumors thrive within an anaerobic (oxygen deficient) environment. Improving oxygenation to the system (including to the tumor itself) improves the overall functioning of the immune system, and can actually reduce the size of tumors.
- Check iron levels; exercise; deep breathing; circulatory stimulants; vasodilator herbs.
- Niacin improves tumor oxygenation.
- Organic germanium.

Repairing Damage to Immune System from Medical Treatment

- Potent multivitamin, especially vitamin C and bioflavonoids (to bowel tolerance).
- Multimineral, reducing inflammation.
- Detoxification program.
- Anti-stress program.
- Sunshine, fresh air, simple foods, lots of water, laughter.

Reducing Catechia

(Malnourishment itself kills about 40% of cancer patients)
- Grazing (5–6 small meals daily).
- Fish (no red meat).
- Omega-3 oils only—2 tsp daily (e.g. flaxseed, fish oils).
- Acetyl-l carnitine (improves the efficiency of burning of fat for energy, i.e. uses less fat).
- Glutamine.
- Digestive enzymes (2 or 3 with meals).
- Probiotics.

Herbal medications

Here are some things we know from research into the anti-cancer properties of herbs.
- Schisandra: more potent than vitamin E against lipid peroxidation, and increases activity in the liver of antioxidant enzymes such as superoxide dismutase (SOD).
- Baical skullcap.
- Chaste tree: best taken at 7 a.m. and 4 p.m. In estrogen-dependent cancers, (e.g. breast, uterine, and prostate), it is important to down-regulate the production of prolactin PRL by the anterior pituitary, as PRL seems to be a potent modulator of the disease. *Vitex agnus castus* has been demonstrated as PRL suppressive and promoted natural progesterone synthesis over a 3-month period, with no side effects.
- Adaptogens: licorice, goldenseal, schisandra, ginseng (both Panax and Siberian), withania.
- Immune stimulants: goldenseal, astragalus, licorice, St John's wort, echinacea, pau d'arco, poke root, Oregon grape, ginger, picrorrhiza.

Other Botanicals

Red clover: anti-tumor.
Pau d'arco: anti-tumor.

Cat's claw: anti-tumor, anti-leukemia.

Mistletoe.

Ginkgo biloba: inhibitor of PAF.

Feverfew: reduces hyaluronidase.

Ginger: systemic anti-inflammatory.

Astragalus: increases NK cell activity, and increases WBC count.

Bupleurum.

Rosy or Madagascan periwinkle, from which vinblastine (anti-Hodgkin's) and vincristine (anti-leukemia) are extracted.

Bloodroot: anti-tumor.

Essiac formula, as developed and used with historical success by Canadian doctor Rene Caisse. Special formulation containing burdock root, sheep sorrel, rhubarb root, and slippery elm powder.

Adjunctive Anti-Cancer Practices

General Dietary Guidelines

- Strictly vegetarian diet (only concession: cold-water fish, e.g. tuna, salmon, sardines).
- Mostly (80%) raw foods (organic—ideal), rich in enzymes, vitamins, minerals.
- Limit food intake to grazing over a 6 hours period daily (from a light 8 a.m. breakfast to 2 p.m. lunch. At other times, juices, miso, broths, teas, water, etc.
- Avoid boiling, microwaving, frying, chargrilling, barbecue—these practices devitalize food, destroying the necessary enzymes and heat-sensitive vitamins.
- Avoid processed foods and simple sugars (nutrient-poor, cause pancreatic impairment and hypoglycemia, acidic in tissue, use stored nutrients in metabolism and excretion).
- Check for allergies, sensitivities.
- Avoid toxic stimulants: nicotine, caffeine, alcohol (except a little red wine), drugs
- Ensure proper hydration (e.g. no other salt but Celtic salt, water, fresh juices, miso, broths, herbal and green teas).

- Fasting (variations, e.g. juice: 10–12 fresh juices daily).

Foods with Anti-Carcinogenic Properties

- Raw yoghurt (acidophilus).
- Most vegetables but especially cabbage, beet, broccoli, shallots, ginger, onion, garlic, mint and parsley, sprouted grains (e.g. wheat, mung) Most fruit but especially pawpaw, or papaya (green and ripe—high in digestive enzymes), pineapple, apple, berries.

Other

Stress Management

Studies have indicated that stress plays a large part in causing cancer. Stress acidifies the internal environment, and compromises nutrient digestion and absorption, so it is imperative that stress is managed properly (see Stress). It is important the cancer patient has a strong support base, one that includes regular support meetings with other cancer patients. And most importantly, one must learn not to be afraid.

"Spontaneous Remissions"

Orthodox oncology does not concentrate on the many cases of so-called "spontaneous remission". Attention is directed at "treating the sick". Disease reversal and cure is never "spontaneous" in the sense that is sometimes implied, that is, "without cause", any more than the disease process itself is without cause or spontaneous. It is one thing to say, "We might not know or understand why something happens."; it is quite another to imply something is without cause. Nature works very predictably on the cellular as well as the universal level; there is always cause and effect.

There is no secret cure for cancer; there is cure, but it is not secret. Cure lies in reversing the processes which have lead to the manifestation in the first place, on every level of being from the physical to the emotional and psycho-spiritual.

Cancer is not a death sentence. The worst thing perhaps that a doctor can do is to say "you've got 6 months" or something such. A mind focused on recovery and hope is a powerful tool in dispelling disease, and clinical experience shows that is especially so with recovery from cancer. In this context we recommend the work of Larry Dossey, Meaning and Medicine (1991: Bantam Books, NY) and many other books which explore the healing potential of the mind–body connection.

Stress Management and Healing Techniques
- Thymic pummeling.
- "Laughter, the best medicine".
- Exercise.
- Colon cleansing (e.g. enemas, colonic irrigation).
- Dry body brushing/cold shower.
- Epsom salts baths/sauna.
- Meditation, yoga.
- Visualization techniques.
- Support group meetings.

Therapeutic Suggestion

Reversing causative processes leading to cancer must be a holistic affair, and often involves changes not only in the way we live physically, but in how we think about things, and indeed, challenges our spirituality as well.
See also Skin Cancer.

CATARACTS

DEFINITION

Developmental or degenerative opacity of the lens.

SYMPTOMS

Progressive and painless loss of vision.

ETIOLOGICAL CONSIDERATIONS—PRIMARY

- Diet
  Excess milk; excess cholesterol; galactose intolerance (milk sugar intolerance commonly found in children); fatty acid intolerances; protein deficiency; deficient nutrition (general, single, or multiple); excess sugar (activates sorbitol pathway); sorbitol (commonly used sweetener for diabetics); vitamin C deficiency; vitamin B2 deficiency
- Diabetes (sorbitol accumulation in lens)
- Free radical damage (antioxidants are useful to prevent this)

ETIOLOGICAL CONSIDERATIONS— SECONDARY

Improper calcium metabolism; hormone imbalance; liver disease; toxemia; mercury toxicity (free radical damage); drugs; heavy metal toxicity; irradiation; trauma; eyestrain; spinal (cervical and upper thoracic); stress and adrenal exhaustion; poor eliminations; deficient local circulation

DISCUSSION

The common opinion among most cataract patients and physicians is that cataracts are an accepted fact of growing old. Cataracts are so common in the over 60s group that they are considered almost normal. The usual procedure up until recently was to wait until the cataract had "matured" sufficiently to be surgically removed. Newer procedures, however, are able to deal with cataracts at relatively early stages. We can expect future surgical developments to be even more advanced.

Unfortunately, very little research has attempted to link cataract development with dietary habits. We feel that it is along these lines that the cause and prevention of cataracts will most probably be found. Research has already linked some cataracts to the consumption of milk sugar. This has been found experimentally in rats and also lactose-sensitive infants. Some researchers feel that excess milk and saturated fat predispose to cataracts. Excess sugar may also affect this picture by potentiating the effects of saturated fats in the body.

Extreme nutritional deficiencies of protein or vitamin C have also been linked to some cataracts, along with improper calcium metabolism, hormone imbalance, liver disease, diabetes, and many drugs.

Toxemia is felt to be a factor in many cases. This is often difficult to prove, but a general toxic devitalized condition is a common finding in many with cataracts. Spinal lesions also are routinely found in the upper cervical region, causing alterations in blood and nervous supply, which can affect the health and integrity of the tissues involved.

Cataracts may also form due to sorbitol accumulation in the lens of the eye. In diabetics (and to a lesser extent hypoglycemics), blood sugar elevations cause the cells of the lens to absorb large amounts of glucose. This is then converted to sorbitol, an insoluble storage form of sugar, which crystallizes out in the eye, forming a cataract.

TREATMENT

Proper prevention and treatment for cataracts lie in general tonic therapy, where all negative health factors are eliminated, and general vitality is increased to the maximum point for that individual. The actual specifics of therapy differ from person to person.

Diet

Unless the patient is extremely emaciated it is always wise to begin with a 7-day fruit juice and vegetable juice fast. This should be composed of juices from organically grown fruits and vegetables, taken throughout the day whenever the patient is thirsty. No two different juices are to be taken at any one meal. Warm water enemas are to be taken on days 1, 2, 3, 5, and 7. The following vegetable juices or combinations of these are useful: carrot, beet, celery, parsley, watercress, spinach.

This diet should then be followed with 1–2 days of a transitional diet of raw fruits and then on to a 7-14-day raw foods diet, composed of fresh fruit and fruit juice, vegetable juice and raw salads, sprouts, seaweed, seeds and nuts. This regimen will help cleanse the system of toxins, encourage better eliminations, and supply an abundance of high-quality "live" foods with all their vitamins, minerals, and enzymes. It also gives the body a rest from the toxic effects of animal proteins.

This diet is followed by a good general diet emphasizing more raw foods, seafoods rather than meats, and fewer dairy products. The following is an example:

On Rising:
Hot water and lemon juice.

Breakfast:
Choose from: fresh fruit; fruit smoothie; fresh or stewed fruit, nuts, honey, and a little low-fat yoghurt; whole grain cereal.

Midmorning:
Fresh vegetable juice.

Lunch:
Always a large mixed raw salad, with plenty of greens (keep the vegetables varied).

Salads should be tasty and interesting. Include avocado, cooked beans, sprouted beans, artichoke hearts, olives, etc., for variety. If still hungry, choose from the following: wholemeal vegetarian sandwich; tofu; baked potato; any other wholesome vegetarian main dish.

Midafternoon:
As midmorning.

Supper:
Salad as lunch or cooked vegetarian protein main meal; whole grains; conservatively cooked vegetables and seaweed; fish (not shellfish).
Note: Absolutely no tea, coffee, sugar, alcohol, or smoking is permitted during any of these diets.
These diets may be alternated repeatedly to encourage further detoxification and increase general vitality. In cases where hypoglycemia or diabetes is a factor, refer to detailed treatment regimens under those headings. Blood sugar regulation is of primary concern with cataracts.

Physiotherapy

The following suggestions may be of use to increase circulation and enhance local nutrition to the eyes.
- Alternate hot and cold showers to stimulate circulation and proper hormonal balance
- Alternate hot and cold sprays to head.
- Warm castor oil eye packs.
- Cold eye baths: blink eyes open and closed for 2-5 minutes into a container of ice-cold water twice daily.
- Neck exercises.
- Bates eye exercises (These are found in *The Art of Seeing*, by Aldous Huxley, Chatto and Windus, London, 1974).
- Endonasal technique (see Appendix I).
- Spinal manipulation to cervical and upper thoracic region, 1-2 times per week for 6 weeks; rest 2 weeks and repeat.

- Sauna baths (weekly).
- Local applications.
- Cineraria eyedrops: 1 drop 2-3 times daily in affected eye.
- Castor oil eyedrops: 1 drop twice daily.
- Honey eyedrops: 1 drop twice daily.

Therapeutic Agents

Vitamins and Minerals— Primary
- Vitamin C: 2-30 g daily (in high doses, increase both magnesium and vitamin B6 to prevent possibility of increased calcium excretion).
- Bioflavonoids: inhibits enzyme aldose reductase which is responsible for conversion of glucose to sorbitol; used to prevent diabetic cataracts.

Vitamins and Minerals— Secondary
Vitamin A (micellized): 25,000 IU twice daily.
Vitamin B complex: 50 mg 3 times daily.
Vitamin B2: 15-50 mg twice daily (prevention).
Niacin.
Pantothenic acid.
Vitamin B6: 50-100 mg twice daily.
Vitamin E: 400-800 IU 1-2 times daily (antioxidant).
Calcium and magnesium.
Inositol.
Lipoic acid.
Selenium: 200 mcg daily (prevents mercury-induced free radical damage).

Others
Atomodine or 636 (Cayce product).
Chlorophyll.
Cystein.
Lecithin.
Methionine.

Botanicals
Cineraria eyedrops: 1 drop 2-3 times daily.

Therapeutic Suggestions

Therapies for cataracts are general and certainly not well proven. They are mostly tonic therapies. This does not mean, however, that they may not be effective. The true beauty of a systemic rather than a local approach is that the cases due to systemic causes will be dealt with. Good evidence does exist to place some blame on blood sugar abnormalities, as in diabetic cataracts, and any therapy that helps control blood glucose levels has a good chance of at least preventing further cataract formation, and possibly reversing it. We do not suggest that any cataract patient ignore the advice of his or her ophthalmologist, but do encourage a complete nutritional and structural investigation.

The most tried and tested botanical application is cineraria drops, and these should be given a 2–6 month trial.

CATARRH

DEFINITION

Chronic excess mucus production affecting tissues, organs, and ducts lined by mucous membranes.

SYMPTOMS

Sinusitis, headaches, runny nose, post-nasal drip, sore throat, gastritis, digestive disorders, appendicitis, salpingitis, glue ear syndrome, eustachitis, cystitis, gallbladder disease, prostatitis.

ETIOLOGICAL CONSIDERATIONS—PRIMARY

- Improper diet
  Excess carbohydrates (especially refined); excess dairy products; excess saturated fats, fried foods; green vegetable deficiency; overeating
- Poor eliminations
  Skin; liver; bowels
- Stomach derangement
  Salt; spicy foods; poor food combinations; acidic foods; stress; hydrochloric acid deficiency, digestive enzyme deficiency
- Allergies

ETIOLOGICAL CONSIDERATIONS— SECONDARY

Toxicity; local irritation (smog, fumes, chemicals, allergens); lack of exercise; poor circulation

DISCUSSION

The term "catarrh" will be more familiar to English readers. In the United States it is not used much. What we are speaking about when we use this term is excess mucus production. Most people think of excess mucus in terms of runny noses and sinusitis. Nasal catarrh certainly is a common complaint, however, certainly not the only place in the body where excess mucus may become a problem.

First of all, it is important to appreciate that mucus is a natural and normal secretion of the body. In usual small amounts it lubricates and protects the delicate mucous membranes wherever they are found throughout the body. If, however, this mucus accumulates or is produced excessively, the condition of catarrh is created, which interferes with the normal action of the tissues or organs affected. In addition to the common upper respiratory or nasal catarrh, excess mucus may interfere with the ears, stomach, intestinal tract, Fallopian tubes, ducts, or any other mucous membrane-lined part of the body. Often these conditions are treated repeatedly with antibiotics, which fail to give relief, since any bacterial infection, if present at all, is merely a result of the internal congestion or inflammation caused by the catarrhal condition, and not its cause. We often see "ear infections" treated with repeated drug prescriptions, when in truth the situation can only be relieved when the cause of the body's excess mucus production is corrected. Similar situations frequently occur with salpingitis, which is very important to resolve rapidly for a woman desiring pregnancy.

There are many dietary causes of catarrh. The most frequent problem is an extremely unbalanced diet, with excessive consumption of carbohydrates. Any carbohydrate, even the best unrefined whole wheat bread, if consumed in excess, will tend to create an increase in mucus production. This situation is much more pronounced if the excess is of a refined, devitalized nature such as white bread, white rice, or sugar. If such foods are not more than compensated for by a high vegetable intake, their acidic and mucus-forming nature predominates. One of the most common problems we see in practice is mucus-clogged infants and children who eat mostly starches and very little vegetables, causing chronic or recurrent colds and earaches.

Milk and other dairy products are well-known mucus producers. Sometimes it is difficult to determine if their mucus-forming characteristics are due to a simple excess, their abnormal and adulterated state (pasteurized, homogenized, and containing many toxic chemicals, pesticides, and hormones), digestive enzyme deficiency (lactose), or a true allergy. As with all things, people respond quite differently to dairy products in their diet. Some seem very well adapted to dairy products, never showing any sensitivity whatsoever. Others find they can only tolerate small amounts before experiencing difficulties. Often we find people who cannot tolerate dairy products from cows, but who can handle goat's products. Others can only eat fermented dairy products, while a much larger percentage cannot cope with any dairy substances whatsoever. Orientals are particularly sensitive to dairy products, with up to 85% of adults lacking the digestive enzyme lactase necessary to digest lactose, the sugar found in milk.

Any specific allergy or food intolerance may result in a catarrhal condition. The most common food allergies are wheat, yeast, eggs, and dairy products, but literally any food may present a problem.

Another major cause of both general and local catarrhal conditions falls under the classification of "irritants". Local irritants include fumes, smoke, foreign objects, chemicals, drugs, spicy foods, salt, pepper, alcohol, and even poor food combinations. Any factor that irritates a mucous membrane will stimulate excess mucus secretion. An imbalance in the digestive system is a common finding with excess mucus secretion. Gastric catarrh is usually the primary condition in catarrhal conditions elsewhere in the body. Once the digestive organs become inflamed, proper digestion is impossible. If the inflammation reaches the state where toxins seep through the irritated, and in some places thinned mucosa, the stage is set for systemic disease. If the organs of elimination are not working efficiently, or are overburdened by this toxic and irritant excess, a catarrhal condition will develop.

Lack of exercise and poor circulation work together to cause local and systemic congestion, which sets the stage for local accumulation of normal toxic products of metabolism, leading to irritation and ultimately mucus formation.

TREATMENT

Diet

In the initial stages of any catarrhal condition, wherever its location, it is wise first to eliminate foods most frequently associated with excess mucus production. We routinely eliminate all wheat, yeast, dairy products, and eggs for the first 1-2 months, or until progress permits their experimental addition. Obviously excluded from the diet are all refined carbohydrates, sugar, alcohol, coffee, tea, salt, pepper, strong spices, junk foods, and tobacco.

Various elimination regimens are effective with catarrhal conditions throughout the body. Some locations respond better to one or another particular juice, fruit, or vegetable. Citrus fruit (grapefruit and lemon) juices are very useful in some mucus conditions. They are eliminative and help break up congestion. They are not usually employed in cystitis, acute gastritis, or where citrus is known to cause unpleasant symptoms such as sour stomach, rash, etc. An apple juice fast or apple mono diet is well suited for mucus elimination. It is eliminative, but gentle on the stomach and does not usually cause any problems.

Vegetable juice fast (carrot or carrot/beet with or without green vegetables) is usually easily handled by most people. Its effect, however, is much slower, but very gentle and pleasant. Vegetable juices are eliminative, but also act to nourish and rebuild tissues.

The classic onion mucus-cleansing diet as found under Asthma is extremely useful to clear congested mucus conditions. It is excellent for catarrh of the ears, nose, sinuses, throat, and Fallopian tubes.

The "master cleanser diet", as popularized by Stanley Burroughs, which advises lemon or lime juice, maple syrup, and cayenne pepper, has some limited value in instances of deep-seated catarrh.

It must be remembered that cayenne pepper is, in itself, a strong irritant, and much of the mucus eliminated was produced as a result of this property. It certainly is not well suited to stomach complaints. Often it is useful in "getting the mucus flowing" in deep-seated chronic conditions.

No general procedural instructions can be given. The individual regimen depends on the patient and the complaint. Usually the regimen will begin with some type of fast for varying periods of 3-21 days, followed by a raw foods diet, with only vegetarian proteins, and absolutely no starch or dairy products. Once it is decided to expand the diet, the first grains added are brown rice and millet. Once dairy substances are to be reintroduced, if at all, goat's yoghurt is added first and then goat's cheese if desired. Dairy foods are minimized in the diet for some time. Whole wheat may then be added experimentally, first unyeasted, and later as home-baked yeast breads. Eggs are also added in poached form. Often several periods of fasting and raw diets are needed to eliminate the condition. If allergy is still suspected, food allergy tests should be performed. Attention must be directed at all times to establishing and maintaining proper bowel function.

Physiotherapy

- Outdoor exercise.
- Swimming (particularly ocean bathing)
- "Salt glow" (1-2 times per week; see Appendix I).
- Body brush daily (see Appendix I).
- Colonics.
- Alternate hot and cold showers.
- Alternate hot and cold compresses locally to site.

Therapeutic Agents

Vitamins and Minerals
- Vitamin A: 10,000-25,000 IU 1-3 times daily or more in some cases. Dries excessive mucus production.
- Vitamin C: 500-1000 mg 3-6 times daily. Use a buffered form (such as sodium and/or calcium ascorbate form) in gastritis.
- Zinc: 25-50 mg 1-2 times daily.
- Vitamin B complex (non-yeast): 25-50 mg 1-2 times daily.

Others

- Digestive enzymes: between meals (especially bromelain) to break up mucus.
- Garlic: 2 capsules 3 times daily; not in gastritis.
- Honey/onion syrup: (see Appendix I): 1 tsp 3–6 times daily.
- Thymus tablets: 1–2 tablets 3–6 times daily.
- Quercetin: inhibits PAF, is anti-inflammatory.
- n-acetyl-cysteine: is mucolytic.

Botanicals

Clivers and poke root: lymphatic decongestants.
Comfrey.
Eyebright: especially when mucus is clear, runny.
Goldenseal: specific for mucous membranes, especially indicated where thick, tenacious yellowy mucus is present.
Mullein: anti-catarrhal, especially in the lower respiratory tract.
Slippery elm.
See also individual topics.

CELIAC DISEASE

DEFINITION

A chronic malabsorption syndrome due to gluten intolerance.

SYMPTOMS

Failure to thrive; weight loss; loss of appetite; vomiting in some cases; diarrhea; stools bulky, pale, frothy, foul-smelling, floating; dermatitis; abdominal distention and pain; weakness; anemia; possibly fatal in infants.

ETIOLOGICAL CONSIDERATIONS—PRIMARY

- Gluten intolerance
- Improper weaning

ETIOLOGICAL CONSIDERATIONS— SECONDARY

- Vitamin B6 deficiency
- Stress
- Other food allergy
- Digestive enzyme deficiency

DISCUSSION

Celiac disease may manifest itself very dramatically, causing severe malnutrition and wasting, or else it may act insidiously to downgrade general health and vitality over a number of years. Classic forms of the disorder begin early in life, just as soon as cereal grains containing gluten protein are introduced. In this case the infant fails to thrive, muscular structures begin to waste, especially in the gluteal region, and the abdomen protrudes markedly due to intestinal fermentation. Fat absorption is reduced and fat-soluble vitamin deficiency is common. Other necessary nutrients pass out with the frequent stools.

Adult-onset celiac disease may date from childhood, but with only mild or unnoticed symptoms that gradually progress for multiple reasons.

Gluten is a protein found in wheat, oats, rye, barley, and other grains related to wheat. It can cause severe intestinal irritation and a flattening of the jejunal mucosa, obliterating the small finger-like villi necessary for proper absorption in the small intestine.

The two main causes of celiac disease are strict gluten intolerance, which may be caused by enzyme deficiency, or other

165

metabolic fault, and improper weaning. Although we know of no solid evidence implicating celiac disease with the early weaning of infants to cereal grains, we suspect this as the single most important factor in most patients. We acknowledge that some infants may have a true gluten intolerance for biochemical reasons, but this is the minority. The introduction of cereal grains before the body's enzymes can digest them can only set the stage for celiac disease by causing gastric irritation, antibody reaction, and intestinal thinning. This seems obvious, since the average infant is approximately 4 months old at the onset of the disorder, a full 2 months before the body has even developed the digestive ability to handle concentrated carbohydrates. Add to this the frequency with which these foods are usually given in the diet and we see how simple irritation can later lead to permanent reaction. The foods mostly commonly found allergic are those given the earliest and most frequently.

Celiac disease may also be complicated by other food allergies such as milk sugar intolerance or yeast. Breast-feeding is a protective factor and may help prevent future food sensitivities.

Associated with celiac disease are several quite serious health problems. Researchers have found a significant percentage of schizophrenics and victims of multiple sclerosis who suffer from a gluten reaction. This may be caused by the malabsorption of vitamins (B3 and B6 deficiency are closely associated with schizophrenia) or fat-soluble substances (essential fatty acids found in seeds or nuts are deficient in multiple sclerosis patients).

TREATMENT

Diet

Therapy is based on instituting a totally gluten-free diet. This can be quite a change for most households and is not easy. Most patients exclude gluten grains permanently, while others are later able to add them in moderation.

It is essential in the early stages of therapy to exclude all grains that contain gluten. This effectively excludes everything except brown rice, millet, and corn. The greatest difficulty of this regimen is in excluding the convenience of sandwiches. These may be substituted for by several soft corn tortillas. Brown rice cakes make a convenient carrier for nut butters and other spreads. Puffed rice, corn, or millet cereals are also available at most health food stores. Another difficulty is in making sure that wheat or wheat flour has not been added to any prepackaged products consumed at home or in a restaurant. Gluten-containing grains are found in a wide variety of restaurant and commercially prepared foods, such as ice cream, candies, salad dressings, luncheon meats, soups, sauces, and even condiments. Great care must be taken to pay attention to all ingredients, especially when eating at restaurants. Read labels religiously. Even an incredibly small amount of gluten in the early stages of the disease can initiate a reaction lasting up to 5 days, so you can see how important it is to be sure gluten is totally excluded.

Some celiacs obtain gluten-free flour for baking. We do not advise this since these products are refined and vitamin-deficient. It is better to exclude these grains once and for all and be done with it. The rest of the diet must be composed only of highly nutritious vegetables, fruits, proteins, and non-gluten grains.

Physiotherapy

- Castor oil packs: (see Appendix I)
  Since the bowel condition resembles that found in psoriasis (and to which it may often be associated) We advise a similar regimen of abdominal packs (see Psoriasis).
- Spinal manipulation: 1–2 times per week; midthoracic to lumbar.
- Meditation and relaxation exercises.

Therapeutic Agents

Vitamins and Minerals—Primary

- Vitamin A (micellized): 10,000–25,000 IU 2–3 times daily or more. Fat-soluble vitamin need is increased.
- Vitamin C (buffered): 500–1000 mg 3–10 times daily, depending on how well it is tolerated.
- Vitamin D: fat-soluble vitamin; malabsorption requires extra D. 400–800 IU daily.
- Vitamin E: 100–400 IU twice daily. Fat-soluble vitamins are essential due to malabsorption.
- Vitamin K: malabsorption of fat-soluble vitamins is common in these cases.
- Vitamin B complex (liquid): 25–50 mg twice daily. Intramuscular injection of B12, folic acid, and B complex, 1–2 times per week.

Vitamins and Minerals—Secondary

Calcium: 800–1000 mg daily.
Magnesium: 400–500 mg daily.
Zinc: 25 mg twice daily.

Others—Primary

- Probiotics: (especially *Lactobacillus acidophilus*, and *L. bulgaricus* which act especially in the small intestine).
- Free form amino acid complex: to supply easily available protein.
- Acetyl-L-carnitine.
- Glutamine (to repair leaky gut).
- EFA (essential fatty acids): 2–4 capsules 3 times daily or flaxseed oil as dietary source.

Others—Secondary

- Chlorophyll.
- Lecithin.
- Mucopolysaccharides.
- Pancreatic enzymes.

Botanicals

Slippery elm: soothes inflamed mucosa. $^1/_4$–$^1/_2$ tsp in warm water 4 times daily.
Goldenseal: trophorestorative, specific for mucous membranes.
Albizzia: anti-allergy.
Alfalfa: nutrient tonic.
Chamomile: carminative.
Comfrey: use as infusion.
Licorice: soothing.

Therapeutic Suggestions

The intestine of a patient with celiac disease is extremely thinned and the stomach is irritable. In early stages nutritional supplements may be very poorly tolerated. Try to begin the therapy with a fast of 3–5 days, to give the digestive system a chance to rest. Use, as much as possible, intramuscular vitamin injections for the first few weeks and then wean to liquid forms and emulsified forms whenever available.

Due to the prolonged malabsorption, nutritional deficiency is broad-based. Emphasis should be placed on vitamins A, D, E (fat-soluble), essential fatty acids, B complex, vitamin C, calcium, magnesium, iron, and zinc, but any other nutrient may have become deficient in a prolonged case.

CERVICAL DYSPLASIA

DEFINITION AND SYMPTOMS

Abnormal cell development of the cervix. As a rule no obvious symptoms exist. Diagnosis is by Pap smear.

DISCUSSION AND TREATMENT

Thirty to 50% of women with cervical dysplasia later progress to cervical cancer. If there is an abnormality on a Pap smear, a biopsy may be needed to confirm the Pap test and help in clarifying the precise stage. Abnormal Pap smears alert the patient and physician to a problem, and help prevent precancerous lesions from progressing into cancer by allowing the doctor adequate time to perform conization, cautery, or cryosurgery, thus preventing a further and more serious problem from developing.

Abnormal Pap smears that do not as yet indicate precancerous or cancerous lesions can usually be reversed with natural therapy. This includes dietary changes to exclude all negative health factors such as coffee, tea, sugar, salt, alcohol, excess animal-based protein, and any unrefined, fried or overcooked foods. The patient is placed on a 6-month regimen of raw and cooked vegetables, seeds, nuts, beans, whole grains, and low-fat yoghurt (if no dairy allergy exists). Fish is also allowed several times weekly. No other animal-based protein is allowed. Carrot juice, or other fresh vegetable juice combination, should be taken twice daily. Supplement regimens are instituted according to case history and physical indications, but must always include the following:

Vitamins and Minerals
- Folic acid: 5–10 mg daily.
- Vitamin B12: 1 mg intramuscularly 1–2 times per week.
- Vitamin A: 25,000–100,000 IU daily. (See warning under Vitamin Toxicity, page 56.)
- Vitamin C: to bowel tolerance.

Alternate hot and cold sitz baths are very useful if done 2–3 times daily, to increase local circulation and nutrition. In some cases the vaginal depletion pack is also used. Periodic follow-up Pap smears are used to monitor results of treatment.

Botanicals
Red clover.
Calendula.
Violet leaves: anti-cancer.
Raspberry leaves.
Burdock: anti-cancer.
Sarsaparilla.
Poke root (highly toxic, see page 60).
Damiana: hormone balancer.
Final word of advice: Do not rush into conization without obtaining a second biopsy and opinion later.

CHILDHOOD DISEASES

CHICKEN POX, MEASLES, MUMPS, WHOOPING COUGH

DEFINITION AND SYMPTOMS

Chicken pox: a common acute childhood disease caused by a virus. It is characterized by crops of thin-walled vesicles which erupt and crust. Each lesion lasts 2–4 days, leaving a pink scar which later disappears. Pock marks may remain. The disease is usually mild.

Measles: an acute viral infection common in children from 6 months to 5 years. It begins with cold-like symptoms and also includes cough, conjunctivitis, and photophobia (avoidance of light). The fever falls after 1 or 2 days, then rises suddenly by day 5 or 6. Associated with this rise is a blotchy rash first appearing on the forehead and behind the ears and rapidly spreading to the trunk. This gradually fades in 3–4 days and the dead skin is then lost. During the first signs of the rash, symptoms are at a peak, with a strong fever and bronchitis.

Complications include otitis media, loss of hearing, bronchopneumonia, and rarely encephalomyelitis, with later convulsions and rarely death.

Mumps: an acute viral infection characterized by mild fever, malaise and sore throat, with swollen parotid glands, swelling either unilaterally or bilaterally. It may last 2 or 3 days, or weeks. Fever usually lasts only a few days. Complications are rare before puberty, and involve swelling of ovaries or testicles, which may affect reproductive ability.

Whooping cough: an acute bacterial disease characterized by a severe paroxysmal cough. The organism grows on the trachea and bronchi, producing an endotoxin which sensitizes nerve endings in the respiratory tract, and may have toxic effects in the central nervous system. Symptoms begin with a mild fever, cold-like symptoms, and a cough which gradually becomes more severe, with a prolonged series of expirations, followed by a sudden "whooping" inspiration. This may also induce vomiting. Paroxysms are usually worse at night. The disease lasts 2–4+ weeks. Complications include convulsions, hemorrhage from the nose or into conjunctiva or into brain, and bronchopneumonia. Rarely, death occurs.

ETIOLOGICAL CONSIDERATIONS

- Normal childhood diseases.
- Improper diet.
- Suppressive treatment of other conditions.
- Toxicity.
- Complications due to improper treatment.

DISCUSSION

These common childhood diseases are contracted by nearly all children, but to varying degrees. Some children show little or no symptoms and the result is that the condition is passed off as a mild cold or cough. Other children, however, suffer and are permanently damaged by complications. It is this individual difference in resistance and vitality that is the single most important factor in our understanding acute disease. Even Louis Pasteur, the father of the germ theory of disease, began to better understand the true nature of disease when he stressed, "The germ is nothing; it is the soil that matters." Germs are not the most important factor in causing disease; the environment must be suitable for them to flourish.

The fact is that germs and viruses are always in our midst. The body normally is capable of maintaining a proper balance of these invaders, both the friendly and the not-so-friendly. The body's self-defense mechanisms attack and remove any dangerous foreign invaders before they may take hold. Its secretions form protective boundaries, its glands act as filters, and the cell walls act as effective barriers. The entire cell, tissue, organ, and body "vitality" is our constant protector. If the "vitality" is maintained, all is well, peace prevails, and health reigns. If, however, we let our defenses starve through poor nutrition and deficiency, poor circulation or lack of oxygen, trouble begins. If we further clog our tissues with too many toxins or change the pH (acid/alkaline balance) of the secretions, the "soil" of our body changes, becoming a favorable environment for infection.

There is no single factor that predisposes our children to disease, but rather a multitude of assaults on their bodies. The role of early gut flora balance is a primary consideration, and many factors including cesarean delivery, poor flora balance in the lactating mother, antibiotic treatments, poor weaning practices, and more. Diet certainly takes the most blame. Excess milk and carbohydrates are the two most obvious offenders. Most people are now aware that white bread, refined cereals, and sugar are not an optimum diet, but even excess unrefined carbohydrates can alter the body's secretions.

Most children do not suffer from a single vitamin deficiency as much as from a "green vegetable" deficiency. We wean our children too soon and too much to starches and complex proteins without understanding that the cleansing and balancing effect of vegetables is absolutely essential for good health. Too often we see sick children whose mothers say, "He just won't eat vegetables." To this we must ask "And whose fault is that?" Dietary habits are just that—habits. You can quite easily get a baby to eat vegetables if that is what he is weaned to. It is easy to give the child a wheat cracker or a bottle of milk to keep him quiet, but certainly not the best choice, healthwise.

A well-fed child will usually be strong enough to deal with infection in a successful way. Well-nourished children either do not catch common childhood diseases, contract only mild cases, or develop strong, healthy reactions that are short in duration, leaving the child feeling none the worse for the experience. It is much more healthy, for example, in measles, to develop a high fever, short in duration, with sweats and good rash formation, than to have a lower fever, little perspiration, and a slowly developed rash. In the first instance, the child is more likely to be over and done with his or her complaint and out playing, while the latter is still being treated for otitis media or bronchopneumonia.

TREATMENT

The treatment of many of the common childhood diseases is fairly basic. The first priority is a liquid diet in the acute stages (with the later introduction of fruits and vegetables). Even breast-feeding is contraindicated as the child is thirsty, not hungry.

The fever should not be suppressed, but moderated according to the needs of the patient, with gentle hydrotherapy. The establishment of perspiration with the fever is essential. Bowels must be kept open and herbal laxatives or enemas may be needed. Various herbal medications are useful at different stages in most of the diseases. Do not forget the role of probiotics, and their capacity to effect specific antiviral activity. Below are a few suggestions useful in each of the complaints.

Chicken Pox

The only real concern with chicken pox is pock scarring. This may be minimized by several simple baths and applications. And, of course, avoid scratching.

Hydrotherapy

- Tepid baths: with starch; baking soda; apple cider vinegar; oatmeal.
- Applications: burdock, goldenseal, and yellow dock tea—dab areas frequently. Calamine lotion: $1/3$ part vinegar, $1/3$ part water—dab area then powder.
- Hot baths: to bring out latent rash.

Botanicals
Dwarf nettle: to bring out latent rash. Nettle.

Vitamins and Minerals— Primary
- Vitamin A: 10,000–25,000 IU 2-3 times daily depending on age and severity of case.
- Beta-carotene: 5000–15,000 IU daily. Dilute carrot juice is an acceptable addition to diet. Both vitamin A and beta-carotene speed healing of skin and enhance immune function.
- Vitamin C: take to bowel tolerance. Helps reduce fever and stimulate the immune function.
- Vitamin E: 200–800 mg daily depending on age. Increases oxygenation of tissues and promotes healing of skin.

Vitamins and Minerals— Primary
Zinc: enhances immune function.

Other

Raw thymus tablets: 1-4 tablets every 1-2 hours depending on the age of child. Stimulates the production of T-lymphocytes produced by the thymus gland which are essential for immune function.

Fruit juice, vegetable juice (carrot).

Clear vegetable soups.

Propolis.

Measles

This disease needs to be treated a little more vigorously than other diseases. Complications may occur because of nutritional deficiency, suppressive treatments, or overfeeding during the disease.

Vitamins and Minerals—Primary

- Vitamin C: 100-500 mg every two hours depending on the age, or up to bowel tolerance. Acts as an antiviral and enhances natural immune response.
- Vitamin A: 10,000-50,000 mg daily. Enhances immune function. (See warning under Vitamin Toxicity, page 56.)
- Vitamin B complex: 25-50 mg dose, balanced mix, 2-3 times daily. Aids in healing and immune response.
- Vitamin E: 200-800 IU daily. Enhances immune function.
- Zinc: 10-15 mg every 3-4 hours in the form of zinc lozenges. Enhances immune function and is locally antiviral.

Others

Raw thymus tablets: 1-2 tablets every two hours. Stimulates the immune reaction.

Hydrotherapy

- Tepid baths and applications for itch, as with chicken pox.
- Hot baths to bring out latent rash.
- Hot foot baths.
- Hot ginger chest poultice.
- Steam baths (not packs) to sweat.

Botanicals

Burdock, plus echinacea and goldenseal.

Dwarf nettle: for slow, poorly developed rash.

Garlic.

Garlic foot compresses (see Whooping Cough below).

Lobelia.

Honey/onion syrup (see Appendix I)

Pleurisy root and ginger tea.

Wild clover plus sundew: for cough.

Yarrow and pleurisy root tea: to sweat.

Chamomile tea: to settle the system, if hyperactive or irritated.

Sundew: useful in cough of measles or whooping cough. 15-20 drops tincture 3-4 times per day.

Goldenseal tea and boric acid: for painful eyes. Make a strong tea as stock mixture. Take 1 tsp of tea, add to $1/2$ cup (125 mL) of water. To this add 2 to 3 drops of boric acid. Flush eyes every 2-4 hours.

Diet

Fruit juice, lemon juice, citrus juices, vegetable juice, and vitamins A and C to bowel tolerance (vitamin C intravenously in severe cases).

Mumps

This disease usually looks much more severe than it really is. The only complications occur during puberty, when swelling of the ovaries or testes can occur, which may cause sterility. The general principles of treatment are those of any other fever, with plenty of fluids and bed rest during the acute phase.

Vitamins and Minerals—Primary

Vitamin C: 100-500 mg every two hours depending on the age, or up to bowel tolerance. Acts as an antiviral and to enhance natural immune response.

Vitamin A: 10,000-50,000 mg daily.

171

Enhances immune function. (See warning under Vitamin Toxicity, page 56.)

Vitamin E: 200–800 IU daily. Enhances immune function.

Zinc: 10–15 mg every 3–4 hours in the form of zinc lozenges. Enhances immune function and is locally antiviral.

Others

Probiotics (*Lactobacillus bifidus*): helps inhibit growth of virus and bacteria by establishing normal bioflora.

Fomentation

(For relief of pain and swelling)

Poke root: 1 part

Lobelia: 1 part

Mullein: 3 parts

Botanicals

Coneflower: enhances immune function; helps cleanse blood and lymph.

Poke root: for hard, painful glandular enlargements (highly toxic, see page 60).

Pulsatilla: for ovaritis or orchitis.

Whooping Cough

Of the common childhood diseases, whooping cough deserves the most attention. Unfortunately, there is no guarantee that with vaccination you get prevention, as in many of the cases the child with whooping cough is fully "up to date" with vaccines. The cough of even a mild case of whooping cough may be extremely disturbing, especially for the parents, but fortunately the disease is usually mild, and can be treated at home. However, we advise you to obtain professional naturopathic advice which will focus attention on the particular individual's requirements. For more difficult cases, and with proper naturopathic treatment in an inpatient facility, the disorder may be brought under control and leave the child no worse for wear. Treatments must be vigorous and unrelenting to get best results.

Diet

A light diet is essential. Overfeeding during the whooping cough prolongs the disease and causes complications. In the breast-fed overfeeding is also a problem. The child is thirsty, not hungry. Once the disorder has been diagnosed or is suspected, a full fruit juice fast should be started. Citrus juices are especially useful. This may be followed with a diet of fruit juice, vegetable juices (carrot), and clear broth vegetable soup. Later, fruit may be added. Vitamin A and C should be administered in large doses.

Applications

- Garlic foot compress (see Appendix I): mash garlic and apply ¼ inch (6 mm) thick between gauze. Oil soles of feet with olive oil to prevent blistering and apply poultice; then secure with bandage and cover with a sock. Apply all night and 1–2 times daily if possible for 1–2 hours each time. This is a very useful application.
- Hot fomentations of strong ginger and garlic tea, followed by Camphoderm (Cayce product) applications. Repeat every 2 hours.

Spinal Manipulation and Physiotherapy

Adjust cervical upper and midthoracic region daily, followed by a deep neuromuscular massage with olive oil, olbas, and myrrh over entire area (or rub 20% grain alcohol across shoulders, neck, and diaphragm area.)

Inhalations

Use olbas oil steam inhalations with a little extra eucalyptus and pine needle oil.

Therapeutic Agents

Vitamins and Minerals

- Vitamin A: 10,000 IU 2–6 times daily. Enhances immune function. (See warning under Vitamin Toxicity, page 56.)
- Vitamin C: 250–1000 mg up to every hour, or to bowel tolerance. Intravenously in severe cases. Enhances immune function.
- Thymus: 2 tablets 4–6 times daily. Enhances immune function.

Botanicals—Primary

Coneflower: enhances immune function. Helps cleanse blood and lymph.

Sundew: 15–20 drops 3–4 times daily, for spasmodic cough.

Thyme: antispasmodic.

Goldenseal: has specificity for mucous membranes, is anti-catarrhal and antiseptic.

Hyssop: expectorant.

Wild cherry bark: antitussive.

Marshmallow: soothes the respiratory tract.

Lobelia: antispasmodic, expectorant. Used for whooping cough with difficult expectoration.

Botanicals—Secondary

Black currant leaves: strong tea of leaves; take 1 cup (250 mL) 3–4 times daily.

Ephedra (ma-huang): bronchodilator.

Glycothymoline: 5–15 drops daily.

Ipecac: 5–10 drops in water 3 times daily.

Senna: laxative; as needed.

Syrup of squill: 3–5 drops 3–4 times daily.

Others

Garlic syrup.

Onion syrup (raw): place a sliced onion in a bowl with 1 tbsp honey. Cover the bowl overnight. In the morning mash and strain. 1 tsp every 1–2 hours.

Onion syrup (cooked): mix 1 lb diced onions with 2 fl oz (60 mL) honey and 2 pints (1 liter) water. Simmer 1–3 hours. 2 tbsp every 1–2 hours.

Propolis: chew frequently; take 2 capsules 3 times daily.

See Bronchitis for expectorant, sedative, and antispasmodic herbs.

COLDS, COUGHS, AND SORE THROATS

DEFINITION AND SYMPTOMS

Common knowledge.

ETIOLOGICAL CONSIDERATIONS

- Diet
  Excess acid-forming, mucus-forming foods; excess carbohydrates; excess dairy products; excess sweets; overeating; fried foods; irritants (spices, coffee, tea, alcohol, smoking, etc.)
- Toxicity
- Improper diet; stress, lack of sleep; poor eliminations
- Spinal
- Reduced nerve, blood, and lymph supply
- Allergy (See Allergies and Food Intolerances)
- Lack of flora/flora imbalance
- Suppressive treatments for previous acute disorders
- Strep throat (requires antibiotic therapy)

DISCUSSION

The common cold is probably the most poorly understood health complaint. Most of us look upon a recurrent cold as an irritating nuisance, caused by some virus going around, and direct all our efforts to eliminate, by any means possible and in as short a time as possible, the various uncomfortable symptoms. At the local drugstore we find a bewildering arsenal of weapons to wipe out this enemy, the common cold—antipyretics, antihistamines, decongestants, sedatives, and many more. This is the treatment given us in childhood, recommended daily on TV, and what our doctors recommend. How strange it must sound to hear that this is the worst possible of all courses to follow!

The common cold is not an infection that leaps out and attacks an innocent, unsuspecting passerby. It is not a disease whose symptoms are best suppressed or shut off like one would a leaky faucet. A cold is not even a disease. It is rather the cure of disease.

The most important thing to understand about a cold is that the multitude of symptoms usually present are actions, not reactions, by the body in an attempt to establish internal equilibrium. The body's defense mechanisms are working fast and furiously to re-establish balance. If this can be seen to be true, then to suppress these actions by the body is not a reasonable course of action.

The original causes of the imbalance that the body is attempting to correct may be multiple.

Improper diet is the single most influential factor. An excess of dairy products and carbohydrates (especially refined carbohydrates) will cause an increase in the amount and quality of mucus formed by the body. Body fluids become more viscous and acidic. Other factors causing acidity are coffee, tea, spices, salt, alcohol, smoking, lack of exercise, and stress.

Toxicity is a second major factor. This is a fairly loose term, which implies that something detrimental has accumulated within the body. This may be due to simple excess consumption of normal food elements beyond the body's capacity to deal with effectively. Excess animal fats will certainly cause the liver to work overtime on their

metabolism. Other substances are less benign. Blatantly toxic pesticides, food colorings, hormones, heavy metals, and preservatives are found routinely in the average diet. These must be detoxified by the liver or stored in the tissues. The same is true of toxins caused by excess alcohol or drug use. Couple all the above factors with poor eliminations due to constipation and lack of demanding exercise, smoking, vitamin deficiency, and environmental air and water pollution, and it is easy to see how the body's vitality and ability to maintain inner balance become vitiated.

It is this multitude of factors that the body is trying desperately to counterbalance. Once toxic levels reach an unacceptable level, the body acts to clear the crippling debris. It opens all channels of eliminations and pours forth poisons from all available avenues. The nose begins to run and the excess mucus stimulates both sneezing and coughing to help expel the blockage. Sometimes vomiting and diarrhea are also present to purge the stomach and intestine. Fever increases the general speed of metabolism and circulation, and promotes perspiration to rid the body of toxins and to help burn up and destroy any secondary bacteria or virus that may have taken hold in the more favorable environment created by downgraded health.

If the body is acting out of an innate intelligence (as it must be since we do not direct our body's heartbeat or other life-sustaining activities), then it is reasonable that we encourage, not discourage, its healing actions. Instead of suppressing our cold by the use of drugs, we must stimulate and aid the body's actions.

In a healthy individual a cold needs little or no encouragement. Since general vitality is high to begin with, all one needs to do is, *almost* as the TV advertisement says, "Rest, drink plenty of fluids, and *don't* take aspirin." The body will do the rest. It is simply doing a "spring cleaning" of all the toxic accumulations stockpiled routinely and almost unavoidably in our modern world. Certainly, everyone must breathe and even our very air, in most cases, has become somewhat toxic. In an otherwise healthy individual a cold will be moderately intense, short-lived, and if treated properly, will leave the individual feeling in good health after it is over.

The cold of a healthy individual contrasts sharply with the cold of a sickly person. Rather than the one or two quickly resolving eliminations that are common and acceptable per year, these sickly persons will suffer for weeks with the acute stage and may keep a cough for up to 2 or 3 months. The end result of such an episode is a feeling of weakness and fatigue, which may become chronic. This occurs for two reasons. The first is that the cold usually is treated with drugs, or at least not treated properly (i.e. with fasting, fluids, rest, and gentle herbs, if needed). The second is that due to the severity of the internal congestion and toxicity usually due to chronic self-poisoning and suppression of previous attempts by the body to heal itself, the body is acting out of desperation, rather than desire.

An analogy can be found comparing the normally cleansing effort undertaken each spring with the effort needed after a flood or hurricane. In the latter instance great resources are needed, and in the case of the sickly person these may simply be unavailable. This is the reason these colds are much more sluggish and prolonged, and also the reason these people often need external assistance to aid the body in its attempts at equilibrium. These aids should not be drugs, which are no real aid at all, but simple, gentle measures such as fasting, hydrotherapy, spinal manipulation, and herbs.

The real danger of a cold if handled improperly is not only its prolonged nature, but the possibility of complications such as pneumonia. If colds are actively suppressed the body eventually loses its ability to release internal toxins safely. The end result is the development of chronic disease many years later such as bronchitis, emphysema, and other serious diseases possibly unrelated directly to the respiratory tract.

Often we hear the proud announcement "I *never* get colds" from individuals who show absolute disregard for their health by improper diet, excessive drinking and smoking, and excesses of all kinds. They are, in fact, too sick to have a cold! This is precisely the individual who is prone to chronic disease, heart attack, cancer, and the rest of the so-called degenerative diseases. A cold is your friend and ally. Don't try to fight it off.

A final note on sore throats. Group A beta-hemolytic streptococci can have serious complications that can damage the heart. Always have a throat swab done on any *serious* sore throat, especially if it is accompanied by infected white patches on the throat cavity. Antibiotics should be used for any diagnosed strep throat condition, followed by a course of probiotics.

TREATMENT

The proper treatment of colds is to encourage eliminations through all channels so that eliminations through only one channel do not become excessive.

Diet

Liquid fasting is the best diet during a cold. The following fluids have been found most useful: citrus (grapefruit); hot water, lemon, and honey; potassium broth; hot water, apple cider vinegar, and honey; medicinal herbal teas

In some cases prolonged juice fasting will actually *lengthen* the cold process too long. An overly prolonged elimination is not always in the best interests of the body. In these cases the fruit juice diet may be discontinued after 3–7 days and the patient placed on *cooked* vegetables. This will usually moderate the elimination and help establish normal equilibrium.

Another method useful in cases of severe mucus congestion with sinus congestion or excess chest involvement is the mucus-cleansing diet (see Appendix I). This involves eating oranges or grapefruit for breakfast, a large plate of boiled or steamed onions for lunch and supper, and an orange as dessert. Medicinal herbal teas are taken between meals and either carrot or citrus juices whenever thirsty.

Physiotherapy

- Hot Epsom salts baths plus sweating teas: take 1-2 lb (500 g-1 kg) Epsom salts and dissolve in a hot tub. While soaking, consume 2-3 cups of hot pleurisy root tea. Immediately after the bath get into bed and cover with plenty of blankets. The object is to sweat profusely.
- Trunk packs: each evening apply a full cold trunk pack (see Hydrotherapy, page 36). The object is to stimulate skin elimination and induce perspiration. Leave this on at least 3 hours or all night.
- Hot mustard foot bath: to increase eliminations and reduce congestion in head and sinuses.
- Salt water nasal douche: to open sinuses.
- Hot ginger chest compress: followed by application of Camphoderm (Cayce product) or olbas.
- Inhalations: eucalyptus, pine needle, cloves, and thyme. To prepare: in 2 pints (1 liter) of boiled water place eucalyptus leaves or oil, pine needles or oil, cloves, and thyme. Make an inhalation tent by draping a large towel over the uncovered pot and your head. If treating a child, place him or her on your lap and hold tightly around abdomen (with arms well away from child's teeth!). An infant will naturally protest vigorously and will sputter and cry deeply. This is good as it gets the fumes well into the lungs. Another approach is to make a tent by using two chairs and one or two very large beach towels or a light blanket. This gives more room and is often more acceptable to young children. Repeat application every 2 hours.
- Olbas inhalant.
- Gargles (sore throat): hot water and salt; hot water, lemon juice, and honey.
- Goldenseal, myrrh, and water; sage tea; sage, cayenne, and honey; bayberry bark decoction
- Compresses: cool compresses to reduce fever as needed (see Fever); apple cider vinegar compresses or rubs (fever control); ice-cold throat compress: apply and leave on 1-3 hours or all night, for sore throat; alternate hot and ice-cold throat compress; hot lobelia and hops throat compress for throat pain.
- Spinal manipulation.
- Sweat baths.
- Saunas in pine and eucalyptus steam.

Therapeutic Agents

Vitamins and Minerals

- Vitamin A: high doses are needed in upper respiratory conditions. This should be in the form of emulsified vitamin A. Adult doses may be 25,000 IU 4-6 times daily for 1-2 weeks. (This is a toxic dose if taken for several months, but completely safe for short periods.) Children's dose: ages 3 months to 1 year—4000 IU 2-4 times daily for 1-2 weeks; ages 1-6 years—10,000 IU 2-4 times daily. Again, this is a toxic level if prolonged, but entirely safe and sometimes required in acute respiratory complaints for 1-2-week periods. Vitamin A is essential for the health of the mucous membranes and increases cilia action to expel mucus.
- Beta-carotene: 10,000 IU twice daily. a precursor to vitamin A. Boost immune function and helps heal skin and mucus membranes.
- Vitamin C with bioflavinoids: at least to bowel tolerance. Adult—1000-2000 mg 4-8 times daily; child—300 mg 4-8 times daily. Infant—100-250 mg 4-8 times daily. Helps the body defend against viral infections by improving the immune response.
- Zinc: (in gluconate or acetate with glycine, because the citrate and tartrate forms are ineffectual). Dissolve in the

mouth. Improves immune function.
- Pantothenic acid: antihistamine.

Others—Primary
- Bioflavonoids, especially quercetin.
- Coenzyme Q10: increases macrophage activity, and improves cellular energetics.
- Garlic: 2 capsules with meals.
- Raw thymus tablets: 2 every hour. Stimulates immunological system.

Others—Secondary
- Chlorophyll.
- Lysine.
- Propolis: 2 capsules with meals, or for sore throat chew small amount of raw propolis hourly.
- Raw adrenal tablets.

Botanicals
Boneset: for achy feelings.
Coltsfoot: for cough.
Cayenne: warming, circulatory stimulant.
Echinacea: increases macrophage numbers.
Elder blossom: for colds.
Eucalyptus: for congestion. Use as inhalant.
Ginger root: useful as tea or hot chest compress (use infusion).
Goldenseal: antimicrobial; useful in staph, strep (with antibiotics), and thrush; use with myrrh for sore throat. Use tinctures as throat swab; dilute for gargle.
Gum plant: for cough.
Licorice: for cough; demulcent, expectorant.
Marigold: use tincture for throat swab.
Ma-huang: for cough, bronchodilator.
Mullein: for cough.
Mustard.
Peppermint: hot tea for sweating.
Pleurisy root: for sweating.
Siberian ginseng: adaptogenic, and increases energy levels.
Squill: for cough.
Sundew: for cough.
Wild cherry bark: for cough; sedative expectorant.
Wild clover: for cough.
White pine: expectorant.
Yarrow.

Useful Prescriptions
- Honey/onion syrup (see Appendix I): 1 tsp per hour.
- Garlic syrup.
- Mother Earth cough syrup (Cayce product): wild cherry bark, horehound, rhubarb.
- Wild ginger.
- Honey.
- Mustard chest plaster: 1 part mustard, 4 parts flour, white of egg or 1 tsp olive oil. Add water to form thin paste. Place between cloth and apply to oil-covered chest.

Botanicals for specific types of cough
Dosage ought to reflect the acuteness of the situation, so small amounts, more frequently is recommended.

Upper respiratory tract (throat) coughs
Demulcent: mullein; licorice; marshmallow.
Antiseptic: thyme; elecampane; goldenseal/ Indian barberry (berberine); myrrh; can add 2–3 drops of eucalyptus or tea tree oil.
Anti-inflammatory skullcap; ginger; white willow bark (salicylic acid); licorice.
Anti-catarrhal: goldenseal (esp. thick, tenacious, yellow mucus); eyebright (runny, watery mucus); sage.
Mix appropriate dose in some warm water and gargle, then swallow.

Lower Respiratory Tract (Lung) Coughs
Demulcent: as above.
Expectorant: sundew; grindelia; ginger (if cold).
Anti-catarrhal: goldenseal; sage; mullein.
Spasmolytic: thyme; licorice.
Antitussive: wild cherry; thyme (mild); pleurisy root (also diaphoretic, expectorant).

Hard, Croupy Cough
Spasmolytic: wild cherry bark; thyme; sundew; black cohosh.
Soften phlegm: elecampane.

Bath oil: thyme is good.

Herbal teas: mullein, anise seed, with honey.

Whooping Cough

Antispasmodic: sundew (specific); thyme.

Antiseptic: goldenseal.

Anticatarrhal: mullein, goldenseal esp. if copious mucus (also tones mucous membranes).

Expectorant: thyme, fennel, hyssop; elecampane.

Antitussive: wild cherry bark (esp. if tracheitis).

Watery Cough

Diaphoretics: pleurisy root, lime flowers, yarrow, aniseed; fennel; ginger; prickly ash (to warm up the system).

Mucolytic herbs (e.g. garlic): can be made into a paste (with flaxseed or olive oil) and bound onto soles overnight.

Sample Formulation

Ginger: 5 mL; licorice: 15 mL; mullein: 20 mL; elder flower: 10 mL; thyme: 10 mL.

Wild cherry bark: 15 mL; horseradish: 10 mL; echinacea: 10 mL; euphorbia: 5 mL.

COLD SORES
(Herpes Simplex
of the Face and Mouth)

DEFINITION AND SYMPTOMS

An infectious viral disease caused by herpes simplex (*Herpesvirus hominis*) and characterized by thin-walled vesicles which have a tendency to recur in the same area, usually at the junction of skin and mucous membranes such as the border of the mouth. They may also affect the gums, mouth, or conjunctiva.

ETIOLOGICAL CONSIDERATIONS

* Stress
* Immune deficiency
* Diet
* Local irritation

DISCUSSION

Some people have regular outbreaks of cold sores, while others seem relatively immune, even when exposed. Those susceptible often find stress is a major factor in instigating an outbreak. Some women notice a relationship between their menstrual cycle and outbreaks. Local irritants, such as excess ultraviolet exposure or acidic foods, can instigate an outbreak. Dietary factors often are related. It is a common finding that a cold sore outbreak will follow episodes of drinking or improper diet. The common denominator seems to be a condition of immune deficiency related to stress or dietary indiscretions, with local irritation as an instigating factor.

TREATMENT

Diet

Avoid foods containing arginine (e.g. chocolate, peanuts, almonds, cashews, pecans, peas, garlic, wheat).

Physiotherapy

* Thymus ointment: apply 6 times daily.
* L-lysine ointment: apply 6 times daily.

- Ice application: apply ice at first sign of tingling for 15–20 minutes; repeat frequently throughout the day. Apply vitamin E between applications.
- Zinc: 0.025% (topical).
- Myrrh tincture (topical).
- Hydrastis (goldenseal) tincture (topical). Alternate with aloe vera.
- Colloidal silver: apply topically.

Therapeutic Agents

Vitamins and Minerals
- Vitamin A: 50,000–100,000 IU daily in acute stages. (See warning under Vitamin Toxicity, page 56.)
- Vitamin B complex: 50 mg dose 1–3 times daily.

- Niacinamide: 500–1000 mg daily.
- Pantothenic acid: 250–500 mg daily.
- Vitamin B12: 1 mg intramuscularly daily in acute stages.
- Vitamin C and bioflavonoids: 1000 mg of vitamin C every 2 hours.
- Zinc: 25–50 mg 1–3 times daily.

Other
- L-lysine: 2–4 g daily.
- Lactobacillus (probiotics): 1 tsp 4–6 times daily.

Botanicals
Cayenne: circulatory stimulant.
Echinacea: immune stimulant.
St John's wort: antiviral (especially against enveloped viruses), also a CNS sedative.
Valerian: if anxiety is present.

COLITIS
(Spastic Colitis, Ulcerative Colitis, Irritable Colon, Mucous Colitis)

DEFINITION

Ulcerative colitis: a chronic, inflammatory disease of the colon characterized by ulcer formation, with passage of blood and mucus.
Spastic colitis, irritable colon, mucous colitis: a chronic motor disorder of the colon, characterized by pain, constipation, diarrhea, or alternating episodes of each.

SYMPTOMS

Ulcerative colitis: attacks of bloody diarrhea, cramps, blood in stool, and mucus. May be symptom-free between episodes.
Spastic colitis: abdominal pain, abdominal distension, cramps, gas, constipation, diarrhea, mucus, but no blood in stool.

ETIOLOGICAL CONSIDERATIONS

- Food allergy
  Additives; dairy; lactose; gluten intolerance
- Previous antibiotics
- Emotional stress
  Overwork; anxiety; irregular habits; lack of sleep; hurried lifestyle; frustration
- Primary intestinal flu episode common
- Diet
  Refined diet (fiber deficiency); sugar, coffee, spices, irritants, salt; fried foods
- Chronic constipation (irritating residue adhering to walls of intestine)
- Aluminum cookware
- Hurried meals
- Abuse of laxatives
- Intestinal parasites

DISCUSSION

The occurrence of colitis almost exclusively in civilized nations places it in the class of so-called "civilized diseases". This stems from its main causes, which are dietary and lifestyle. A refined diet, with its fiber-deficient foods, causes habitual constipation which eventually leaves toxic residues adhering to the intestinal lining. These toxic substances lead to irritation, inflammation, and eventually ulceration of the delicate membranes. This in turn causes a lymphatic disturbance due to local irritation and the absorption of these toxic forces into the lymphatic channels. The chronic use of laxatives to correct poor eliminations further irritates these membranes and by the action of the law of dual effect, causes reciprocal bowel statis after their initial stimulating action is completed.

The emotions also have a direct effect on the digestive system. Both motor and secretory functions of the gastrointestinal tract are influenced by the autonomic nervous system. It is stimulated by the parasympathetic and inhibited by the sympathetic nervous system. Any strong emotion, stress, or anxiety will be interpreted by the body more or less as an emergency situation, with the result that the sympathetic nervous system takes control. Among its actions is diverting energy away from digestive functions and instituting defense actions. The digestive result of these actions is a slowing or stopping of all digestive activities, including peristaltic action. This causes constipation.

Occasionally, if the stress or sympathetic action is particularly strong, the result may be quite the opposite, with a powerful and expulsive peristaltic action causing sudden diarrhea. Thus we see the commonly occurring symptoms of alternate constipation and diarrhea, so frequently seen in colitis.

Many cases of colitis follow an acute bout of intestinal flu. This is more common in ulcerative colitis. This initial irritation may then be very difficult to heal if the body is already downgraded in health and vitality by poor diet and any of the other possible causative factors. Food allergy, especially to milk or wheat, is commonly the main cause of the intestinal irritation and when the offending substance is removed from the diet healing commences immediately.

Naturopathy has traditionally been very effective with the treatment of all gastrointestinal problems, and colitis is no exception.

TREATMENT

Diet

Roughage is the key consideration in the dietary regimen. Roughage does not cause colitis, as many seem to believe who place patients on permanent low-fiber diets in an attempt to cure the condition. A high-fiber diet is the best prevention and cure. However, it is true that in the initial stages a bland, low-fiber diet is often necessary due to bowel irritation and devitalization. Later, a high-fiber diet is instituted to complete the healing process and prevent recurrence.

In most cases an initial period of liquid fasting is the treatment of choice. The length of the regimen depends on the ability of the patient to abstain from solid food, and the general health picture, vitality, weight, etc.

The following liquids are especially useful for the fasting period of from 3–14 days: carrot juice; apple juice; slippery elm tea (warm, not hot); comfrey tea (warm, not hot).

An enema is to be taken nightly on days 1, 2, 3, and every other night thereafter during the liquid fast (or less, at the discretion of the physician). This fast should be broken slowly, adding ripe mashed banana with slippery elm powder, unsweetened apple sauce or baked apple (no skin).

An alternate initial plan beneficial in some cases is to begin with a mono diet of raw grated apples plus apple pectin and slippery elm powder 3–4 times daily, with apple juice between meals. Some patients respond best on a strict well-cooked brown rice diet for up to 10 days.

After either of these initial phases, a bland diet follows, composed of carrot juice, stewed or baked apple, apple sauce, raw grated apple (eaten alone), ripe bananas, avocado, yams, sweet or white potatoes, and a few steamed vegetables such as carrots, parsnips, or squash. Meals must be kept as simple as possible. As improvement becomes apparent, further steamed vegetables are added, and well-masticated cooked brown rice, and if no soy allergy exists, tofu, and steamed fish. At this point the gradual introduction of raw and high-fiber foods is the goal. The first aim is the introduction of a salad for lunch. Raw grated carrots are best to begin with, and slowly all other raw vegetables are added until a large salad is well tolerated.

At this point cure is at the doorstep. The only further hurdle is to experiment with the common allergic foods—dairy products and wheat. It is best to begin with goat's yoghurt. If this is well tolerated for a week, other dairy foods may be tried, such as low-fat cottage cheese. Wheat should be tried last. Should any of these foods cause any adverse reaction whatever, they should immediately be stopped and tests performed for food allergy and lactose or gluten intolerance. Dairy allergy is very common in cases of colitis.

The final diet should be meat-free for several months. Fried foods are absolutely forbidden.

Hydrotherapy

- Cold compress: apply over abdomen to reduce inflammation.
- Colon irrigation: use a few drops of glycothymoline to remove adherent fecal waste. This may be done in special cases 1–6 times in a series of 1–2 times per week, and then stopped and normal bowel movements established through diet.

Spinal Manipulation

Thoracic and lumbar.

Psychological Factors

Since colitis is so frequently influenced by the emotions, all patients should pursue a program of relaxation therapy and meditation. The lifestyle must be altered so that the patient may learn how to relax. All activities must be analyzed and any that evoke stress, destructive emotions, or require a hurried pace must be avoided or dealt with differently. Activities may not need changing, only the attitude. Even the best of foods will become indigestible when the mind and emotions are in turmoil.

Therapeutic Agents

Vitamins and Minerals

- Multivitamins: given intramuscularly daily in early part of therapy. Malabsorption of many basic nutrients requires broad-based supplementation.
- Vitamin A: 25,000 IU 1–4 times daily in micellized form. (See warning under Vitamin Toxicity, page 56.) All fat-soluble vitamins are needed due to poor absorption and fast transit times.
- Vitamin B complex: liquid B complex is best, taken 1–3 times daily. Yeast-free sources are needed if yeast allergy exists. Intramuscular injection of B complex with high doses of BI, (1 mL daily for 10–14 days) are essential in the first few weeks of therapy.
- Calcium pantothenate: 200–1000 mg daily.
- Vitamin C (buffered): take in powdered form diluted in water. 1–2 g 3–4 times daily, or more if well tolerated. Intravenous injections of vitamin C may be very useful in early stages.
- Vitamin E: 400 IU 2–4 times daily (prevents scarring and encourages healing). Some cases require much higher doses. Malabsorption requires large doses to insure adequate supply on a cellular level.
- Calcium: 800–1000 mg daily.
- Magnesium: 400–500 mg daily.
- Zinc: 25–50 mg 1–2 times daily.

Others—Primary

- Glutamine: 500 mg twice daily. To heal leaky gut.
- Probiotics: are essential.
- Proteolytic enzymes: helps reduce inflammation. Aids digestion.
- Bromelain: 1-2 tablets just after meals, or other source if this is not well tolerated.
- Psyllium powder/husks: 1 tbsp with water before meals in later stages of diet; not to be used in cases where wheat allergy exists, or if aggravation occurs.
- Free amino acid complex: as per label 3 times daily between meals. To supply essential building blocks for protein synthesis. Essential for tissue maintenance and repair. Needed do to poor long-term absorption.
- Essential fatty acids: as per label or use flaxseed oil. Malabsorption problems require supplementation.
- Glucosamine: as per label (usually two capsules 3 times daily or one tsp 3 times daily diluted in 20% non-citrus juice. Helps in the formation of mucus secretions to protect intestinal mucosa.

Others—Secondary

- Atomodine.
- Apple pectin.
- Chlorophyll.
- Cod-liver oil.
- Garlic (with care): used in cases where infection or bacterial overgrowth is suspected.
- Raw adrenal or lymph tablets: 2 tablets 2-3 times daily.
- Raw thymus tablets.

Botanicals—Primary

Bayberry: specific, circulatory stimulant
Slippery elm: excellent for healing mucous membranes. Steep $^1/_4$-$^1/_2$ tsp of powder in cup of hot water; cool and drink 1 cup 4-6 times daily.
Goldenseal.
Marshmallow root: an excellent demulcent, tincture, or use powder, 10-30 grains, 3-4 times daily.
Wild yam: anti-inflammatory, antispasmodic
Aloe: 2 fl oz (60 mL) juice 3 times daily
Chamomile: nervine sedative, carminative and anti-inflammatory.
Peppermint oil: 2-6 drops with meals.

Botanicals—Secondary

Comfrey tea.
Cramp bark: antispasmodic.
Spotted cranesbill: especially astringent with bloody stools.
Wild ginger.

Therapeutic Suggestions

Due to the extreme irritability of the bowels and prolonged malabsorption syndrome most vitamins, minerals, and essential fatty acids are usually deficient. In early stages use vitamin injections to bypass the bowels and ensure introduction into the system. Liquid or liquefied supplements are better absorbed than intact pills, which may be used later in therapy. Micellized fat-soluble vitamins are better handled in these cases than oil forms.

CONSTIPATION

DEFINITION

Difficult and/or infrequent bowel movements.

SYMPTOMS

Infrequent and/or difficult bowel movements, headaches, coated tongue, tiredness, bad breath, mental depression, and mental dullness.

ETIOLOGICAL CONSIDERATIONS—PRIMARY

- Diet
  Fiber deficiency; refined foods; excess meat; raw vegetable deficiency; excess milk; fried foods; coffee, tea, alcohol; acid-forming foods; overeating; deficiency of bitter foods
- Inactivity
  Lack of exercise; sedentary existence; bedridden
- Long-term laxative use
- Liver dysfunction
  Gallbladder disease; fried foods
- Stress
  Overwork; anxiety
- Spinal
  Lesions; poor mechanics; visceroptosis, prolapsed colon
- Avoiding call of nature

ETIOLOGICAL CONSIDERATIONS— SECONDARY

Appendectomy; spastic colitis; food allergy; pregnancy; hypothyroidism (associated with hypochlorhydria and constipation); B12 anemia; partial intestinal obstruction (adhesions, scars, cancer); Hirschsprung's disease (absence of normal nerve plexus and ganglia on the wall of the colon); dehydration; hydrochloric acid deficiency; drug use

DISCUSSION

Constipation is more than a troublesome condition. It is an insidious drain on the health of millions of people. As bowel transit time is increased, the stool becomes hardened and difficult to pass due to dehydration. The body slowly reabsorbs the fluid content in the feces and along with it many soluble toxins. This autointoxication is the reason people suffering from constipation have coated tongues, foul breath, lack of energy, and difficulty in thinking. These poisons affect every area of the body.

Fiber deficiency and constipation are associated with diverticulitis, appendicitis, and colon cancer. The small, hardened feces are very difficult for the normal intestinal peristaltic actions to deal with effectively. With the lack of bulk added by fiber in the diet, the intestine resembles a tube of toothpaste that is almost empty. The same difficulty you have in getting out that last bit of toothpaste is exactly the problem your intestine has. The peristaltic contractions are more forceful but less effective and tend to create small outpockets or diverticuli in the intestinal walls (see Diverticulitis).

Associated with both diverticulosis and constipation is a change in the normal bacterial flora. As a result, bile acids normally found in the feces and excreted are altered by prolonged exposure to these abnormal bacteria, and become carcinogenic. Thus we see the cause-and-effect relationship behind low-fiber diets and colon cancer.

Most people habitually use laxatives to regulate bowel movements when constipation is a chronic problem. In many cases this causes a strong intestinal action due to the irritant qualities of the laxative. The unfortunate after-effect, however, is that the bowel reacts to this unusual stimulation by becoming less active just after its use. The result is that in 2–3 days when no further bowel movement has occurred, a second dose of laxative is used—and on and on for years, even decades!

Enemas will also have a similar effect. Laxatives that contain mineral oil not only cause the bowels to become overstimulated and weakened, but also rob the body of fat-soluble vitamins.

Constipation can have its beginnings very early. The normal breast-fed child will have a bowel movement approximately 20 minutes after the start of a feed. This is quickly learned by mothers who breast-feed their infants without first making sure they have diapers on! This bowel action is a true physiological reflex.

Over time, as solid foods are introduced,

this reflex becomes less sensitive and can be affected by the type of foods consumed. Mothers soon become aware of these effects and use foods such as bananas to harden the stool and slow transit time, or prunes and papayas to soften them and encourage a bowel movement. Later, as the child is weaned and cow's milk is introduced, bowel movements become less regular and more difficult to regulate. Once the child is toilet trained, less attention is placed on regularity in some cases, and constipation may take hold. Unless the child is weaned to proper foods such as whole grains, fruit, and raw vegetables, the early years can set up a life-long constipation problem.

In the early years, and also with adults on hectic schedules, the call of nature may be habitually ignored or postponed. This causes the body to discontinue sending these messages to the brain until it has no further choice, due to bowel overload, but to obey.

Regularity has become a meaningless expression in describing or diagnosing constipation. In the past we routinely asked patients if they were regular until we realized that to some people once a week was "normal". It is far more useful to know the consistency of the bowel movement and how often a bowel movement occurs. If the bowels move once or twice daily and the stool is hard or difficult to pass, the patient is constipated, no matter how regular he or she is. This can occur with what we call "loaded bowel syndrome", where nearly the entire transverse and descending colon are filled with hard feces.

Another useful index is bowel transit time, or the time it takes for food to pass through the body. In diets composed of unrefined cereals, fruits, and plenty of raw vegetables the transit time is usually 12 hours or so. On a refined diet this may extend to 24, 48, or 72 hours or longer, as in our example of the once-a-weeker.

Certainly, factors other than diet play a role in many cases of constipation. Lack of exercise removes the mechanical action of the muscles on the intestinal contents, thus slowing bowel action. This also reduces normal circulation throughout the digestive tract. The presence of spinal lesions in any of the segments from the midthoracic region through the lumbar plexus is another major factor.

Eating while under any stressful emotion basically paralyzes all digestive functions, including peristaltic action. Still, all these factors mentioned and those listed under Etiological Considerations account for a very small proportion of cases of constipation. Diet and diet alone stands most prominent as both cause and cure of this disorder.

TREATMENT

Obviously, if the main cause of constipation is a fiber-deficient diet, then both prevention and cure must lie in an unrefined high-fiber diet. If constipation is habitual and of long duration, the weakened bowels must first be strengthened and re-educated, even before a high-fiber diet will stimulate regularity. Often, specific short cleansing fasts or mono diets with herbal aids, hydropathic applications, and spinal manipulations are required to retonify intestinal actions. In the case of long-standing constipation, it is usually beneficial to begin the regimen with a 3-day fruit juice fast with nightly enemas. This is done even where the habitual use of laxatives or enemas is a main contributing factor in causing intestinal weakness. This may or may not be accompanied by colonic irrigation, depending on the case. Following this fast is a 3-day apple mono diet. This consists of 4–5 meals of raw apples with apple juice between meals. On the evening of the third day, the patient takes 2 tbsp of raw, unrefined olive oil. No enemas or laxatives are taken during this mono diet or after in the full anti-constipation diet which follows below.

During the apple mono diet the patient should begin taking 25 drops of cascara sagrada tincture diluted in water four times daily. When taken regularly in low doses cascara acts as a bowel tonic, not a laxative. In the right doses it helps strengthen bowel action, not weaken it. This is continued for 2-3 weeks, then reduced to three times daily for another 2 weeks. If the bowel movements are now regular, the dose is reduced to twice daily for 2 weeks, once daily for 2 weeks, and then stopped entirely.

Follow this fast with the diet below.

On Rising
Fig, prune, and raisin tea (see recipe below).

Breakfast
Choose from the following:
1. Soaked or simmered dried fruit (do not use water in which soaking takes place) with 2-3 tsp of wheat germ and a little soymilk, nutcream, or fruit juice.
2. "Mummy food" (see recipe below)
3. Granola with yoghurt and wheat germ (not on first day following fast).
4. Soak overnight to soften if desired. Chew well.
5. Prunes or figs (stewed or simmered) with yoghurt and wheat germ.
6. Milled nuts may be added.
   Fresh fruit and any whole meal cereal.

Midmorning
Fig, prune, and raisin tea or fruit-bran tea (see recipe below).

Lunch
A large raw salad with milled nuts (no peanuts) or cottage cheese and a slice of 100% whole wheat bread (brown bread is not sufficient) or two crispbreads with tofu, miso, cottage cheese, or nut spread. Stewed apple or soaked or simmered raisins for dessert with wheat germ or bran topping.

Midafternoon
Herb tea, fig, prune, and raisin tea, apple or prune juice.

Supper
Choose from the following:
- Any vegetarian savory meal with baked potato (eat the skin also) and two other vegetables. Any fresh fruit or fruit dessert such as prune whip, stewed fruit

with nutcream and wheat germ, etc.
- Lean meat, fish, or fowl with 2-3 vegetables other than potatoes and brown rice. Fruit-bran tea (see recipe).
- Salad, same as lunch.

On Retiring
Fig, prune, and raisin tea (see recipe below), or herb tea.

Items in diet of special usefulness:
Raw fruit and vegetables, especially apples and celery; unrefined grains; bran (psyllium powder is the best); 1-2 tbsp with water at mealtimes; prunes, raisins, and figs; molasses; olive oil; fluids: 4-8 glasses daily.

Recipes

Fig, prune, and raisin tea
Cut up about 10-12 figs and place in a saucepan together with 10-12 chopped prunes and about 2 tbsp raisins. Cover with 2 pints (1 liter) of water and simmer for about 30 minutes. A little more or less water may be used according to taste, but do not make the juice too weak. If desired, lemon juice may be added to vary the flavor.

Fruit-bran tea
Put 2 heaped tbsp of cleaned bran and 4 oz (120 g) of chopped figs or prunes or raisins in a jug. Pour on 1 pint (500 mL) of boiling water, cover the jug and allow to stand all night. In the morning, strain the essence and take either hot or cold. A stronger drink may be made by simmering the ingredients for 1 hour and then straining and drinking the essence.

"Mummy food"
This is excellent to increase and regulate bowel function and increase eliminations. Take 1 cup (240 g) black or Assyrian figs chopped fine, 1 cup (240 g) dates chopped fine, ½ cup (120 g) coarse yellow corn meal and cook to mush in 2-3 cups (500-750 mL) water. Eat slowly and in moderation.

1–2 tbsp may be taken with any meal or separately as a meal in itself.

Physiotherapy and Hydrotherapy

- General tonic
  Sitz baths—alternate hot and cold; castor oil abdominal packs (see Appendix I).
- Spastic colon
  Hot enemas of chamomile tea; hot compress to abdomen; hot sitz baths.
- Exercises
  General exercise of any nature; abdominal exercises; slant board exercises.
- Spinal manipulation
  General thoracic and lumbar once per week for 4–8 weeks.
- Habits
  Don't eat under stress; don't drink with meals; drink 4–8 glasses fluids daily
  Visit toilet 20 minutes after each meal to establish habit reflex.
- Avoid until bowels are normal
  Refined foods; spicy foods; coffee; sugar; tea; alcohol.

Therapeutic Agents

Vitamins and Minerals—Primary
- Vitamin C: 1000 mg hourly to bowel tolerance, then reduce to 3 times daily.

Vitamins and Minerals— Secondary
- Vitamin B complex.
- Vitamin E.
- Vitamin A.

Others—Primary
- Psyllium seeds or husks: a bulk laxative and lubricant.
- Flaxseed meal, and flaxseed oil: (2 tbsp daily)

- Probiotics: 1 tsp 3 times daily. To help establish normal intestinal flora.
- Bran: 1 tbsp with 1–2 glasses water before or with meals. Bulk fiber source.
- Apple pectin: 500 mg daily not with other supplements. Fiber source.
- Slippery elm: bulking laxative

Others—Secondary
- Brewer's yeast.
- Cod liver oil: 3 capsules twice daily.
- Garlic.
- Hydrochloric acid.
- Chlorophyll liquid: 1 tbsp once or twice daily to eliminate toxins and help prevent bad breath.
- Flaxseed power or oil: 1 tbsp twice daily to aid digestion and as an intestinal lubricant.

Botanicals—Primary
Bitter herbs: will stimulate peristalsis (by stimulating bile flow), e.g. gentian, wormwood, and dandelion.

Cascara: in tonic doses, not laxative doses. For chronic cases addicted to laxatives take 25 drops of tincture 4 times daily for one week, then reduce to 15 drops 3 times daily for one week, then reduce to twice daily for two weeks, then to 10 drops twice daily for two weeks, then 10 drops once daily for one week, then stop. Must be done with proper diet changes.

Senna pods: a stronger, stimulant laxative. Not to be used regularly. Will aggravate chronic constipation.

Botanicals—Secondary
Agar agar.

Aloe: a bitter, and bulk laxative. 2 fl oz (60 mL) of juice 3 times daily.

Chamomile.

Goldenseal.

Guar gum: bulk laxative: 2–4 tbsp daily.

CRADLE CAP
(Seborrheic Dermatitis)

DEFINITION AND SYMPTOMS

Seborrheic dermatitis, common to the newborn and in infancy but can occur at any age, characterized by thick, yellow, crusted lesions appearing on the scalp, and sometimes the face and behind the ears.

ETIOLOGICAL CONSIDERATIONS

- Nutritional deficiency
  Biotin; vitamin A; essential fatty acids
- Yeast overgrowth (*Pityrosporum ovale*)
- Antibiotic use
- Food allergy
- Dairy sensitivity
- Poor hygiene
- Stress
- Obesity

DISCUSSION

Cradle cap is an extremely common childhood problem due to overproduction of sebum, a waxy, oily substance that may plug the sebaceous glands, leading to inflammation and acne formation. The entire scalp may become covered by a thick accumulation of sebum and dead skin cells. The problem often relates to diet and nutrition. Sometimes the infant is sensitive to dairy products either in their own diet or, if breast fed, in the diet of their mother. Nutritional deficiency is also a factor directly in the diet or secondary to deficiency in the mother's milk. Vitamin A, biotin and essential fatty acid deficiency is most frequent. Overgrowth of the yeast that accumulates in the hair follicles may also be a cause. Similar causes of yeast overgrowth as occurs elsewhere in the body are factors, especially too many sweet foods in the diet and improper weaning. Stress and obesity are factors in adults, as well as immune deficiency. Hygiene and care of infant's hair and scalp are often the only cause and only required treatment.

TREATMENT

Avoid dairy foods, especially cow's milk (If breast-feeding, mother should avoid dairy foods also). Diet of the breast-feeding mother needs to be corrected to supply adequate essential fatty acids, vitamin A, biotin and little or no refined foods and sweets. Have at least one entirely salad meal with protein daily if breast-feeding. Avoid antibiotic use in the infant and mother if at all possible.

Physiotherapy

- Oil applications: most oils will work. Apply oil and follow with a scalp massage for 5-10 minutes; leave oil on for 30-60 minutes. Brush scalp vigorously (take care not to cause inflammation or bleeding) and then shampoo. Olive oil shampoo is gentle and effective. Repeat 1-2 times per week until cleared. Calendula oil is a favorite choice. It is very soothing to the skin.
- Vinegar scalp massage: massage scalp with diluted vinegar (mix 50/50 with warm water).
- Tea tree oil: apply diluted with calendula in cases of yeast overgrowth 4 times daily.

Vitamins, Minerals and Others

- Vitamin A: high doses in adults are well tolerated up to 50,000 IU twice daily for

187

short periods. Give children carrot juice as source.

- Vitamin B complex: dose depends on age. Very effective in adult cases or to infant via breast milk at 50 mg doses twice daily. Infants and children under 6 require very small doses, no more than one quarter of an adult dose. Use liquid from non-yeast source.
- Vitamin B6: 5–10 mg daily; topical vitamin B6 salve may be useful. See Dandruff.
- Zinc: 25–50 mg twice daily for adults. 10 mg dissolved in juice for infants.
- Biotin: 50 mg twice daily for adults or breast-feeding mothers.
- Essential fatty acids: evening primrose oil or flaxseed oil. As per label. Usually 1 tbsp once or twice daily.
- Probiotics: if antibiotic use is suspected as cause take as supplement or food.

CYSTITIS AND URETHRITIS
(Urinary Tract Infection)

DEFINITION

Inflammation of bladder and/or urethra; infection of either structures.

SYMPTOMS

Frequency and burning on urination; pain and tenderness over bladder area; intense desire to pass urine even after bladder has been emptied; strong-odored urine, which may be cloudy.

ETIOLOGICAL CONSIDERATIONS—PRIMARY

- Poor hygiene
  Thirty times more common in females— the short female urethra and close proximity of urethra to anus are predisposing factors. E. coli (*Escherichia coli*) infections most commonly found in bacteria; this is a normal inhabitant of the intestine. Poor toilet technique in young females is a major cause of transfer to the vagina.
- Antibiotic and contraceptive pill use
  Repeated use of antibiotics and contraceptive pills disturbs the normal flora

ecology and protective balance in the body.
- Improper diet
  Sweets; refined carbohydrates; carbonated beverages; coffee; chocolate; fresh vegetable deficiency; fresh water deficiency
- Irritants
  Emotions (anger, fear, stress, worry); alcohol; drugs; chemicals; spermicides; preservatives
- Urine stasis
  Inadequate fluids, or improper fluids
- Spinal
  T6 to coccyx lesions may cause reflex irritation, congestion, poor circulation, and tissue degradation, leading to infection.

ETIOLOGICAL CONSIDERATIONS— SECONDARY

- Reiter's disease: urethritis, arthritis, and conjunctivitis as a triad is diagnostic.
- Sexual activity: "Honeymoon" cystitis is common due to local irritation.
- Lack of lubrication in elderly may be a cause.
- Obstruction: an enlarged prostate will block urethra, causing reduced urine

flow and congestion. Stricture (narrowing of urethra) may act similarly.

- Venereal disease.
- Poor eliminations: poor bowel functions cause toxins to be retained and recirculate into the blood, to be handled by the kidneys.
- Liver congestion: poor liver function causes excess kidney function as accumulated toxins pass to the kidneys.
- Following childbirth: the bladder position may favor urine retention if postnatal exercises are not performed.
- A prolapsed transverse colon due to poor abdominal tone, multiple births, or poor spinal mechanics may put pressure on the pelvic organs, causing poor local circulation, congestion, and tissue degradation.
- Allergy.

DISCUSSION

Confusion exists as to the real cause of cystitis. The most common assumption is that bacterial pathogens enter the urethra and ascend into the bladder where they grow and multiply, causing a clinical infection. While we don't wish to deny that bacteria may be isolated from the bladder or urethra in a case of urinary tract infection or that proper hygiene is important, the primary cause of these complaints usually lies elsewhere. The mere presence of bacteria will not cause an infection. If this were so, then everyone would have thousands of infections, both inside the body and out. Bacteria are an ever-present part of life.

The bacteria found in urinary tract infections are the *result* of disease, not its cause. Under normal circumstances, with a healthy body or tissue, bacteria can have no harmful effect. The body's resistance or vitality is so strong that bacteria are immediately dealt with and destroyed, or at least kept under control so that rapid reproduction is impossible. Only when the environment is more favorable for the bacteria will disease result.

Diet

Much of what has been written about diet and cystitis is either misleading or incorrect. We are told by many authorities that cystitis is caused by a too alkaline diet, which, to correct, we should avoid fruits and vegetables and eat plenty of grains, nuts, fish, cheese, and anything else that will make our urine (and system) strongly acid. The common explanation is that bacteria cannot live in an acid environment. This is true, by the way, and a very useful fact in the treatment of acute genitourinary infections. However, it is not the cause of cystitis. The dietary causes of cystitis go much deeper and are more complex than the acidity/alkalinity question alone implies.

Our greatest concern should be the health and integrity of the tissues of the genitourinary system. To maintain these tissues, a balanced diet composed of an *abundance* of fresh and conservatively cooked vegetables, whole grains, protein (preferably more vegetarian than animal), essential fatty acids (unsaturated oils), and a small amount of fresh fruit should be eaten. The fluids consumed should be abundant and as natural as possible. Choose from water, fruit juice, vegetable juice, and mild mint teas. (Pure fresh water is the only really natural drink.) This diet should, if at all possible, be based on organically grown foods. On such a diet, and possibly with the addition of a general vitamin and mineral supplement regimens all the essential nutrients should be available for absorption by the body to nourish these vital organs.

Rather than an acid-reacting diet being healthy for the genitourinary system, this average acid diet so prevalent today along with lack of raw vegetables is what causes many nutritional problems, including the predisposition to cystitis. Once tissues are downgraded by improper nutrition, short-term dietary regimens may be necessary for healing.

Digestion and Eliminations

Too little emphasis is placed on the role of assimilation and eliminations in causing cystitis. If the digestion is weak, even the best of foods cannot provide real nourishment. What good are the best vitamins and minerals if they are never absorbed? Eliminations, too, are very important. Constipation and liver congestion both cause toxins to be recirculated and cause the kidneys excess work. Once the kidneys are overworked, the rest of the genitourinary system becomes irritated. Stress also profoundly affects digestion and elimination, and should always be considered a factor in disease causation.

Spinal Imbalances

One of the most ignored factors in internal complaints, especially those thought to be caused by infection, are spinal lesions. Any injury that causes a lesion in the area from the midback (T6) all the way down to the tailbone (coccyx) can set up what is called a somaticovisceral reflex. This is mediated by nervous and hormonal pathways and may cause reflex irritation, poor circulation, congestion, and tissue degradation in the kidneys, bladder, urethra, uterus, ovaries, prostate, or any other internal structures. This may then cause these structures to become more susceptible to infection by lowering their tissue vitality. Antibiotics and the contraceptive pill are also important factors in upsetting the body's ecology, producing a predisposition to cystitis.

These factors, and to a lesser extent the rest of the etiologic considerations, should all be weighed carefully in each case of genitourinary disease, to diagnose the real cause of the complaint and not just relieve the immediate symptoms with antibiotics or other artificial measures.

TREATMENT

Diet

Purify kidneys, bladder, and urethra.

Stage 1
Liquid fast (5-7 days) on the following fluids:
- Cranberry juice: slightly acidifies urine, increases urine flow, and reduces the adherence of bacteria to the mucous membrane walls; drink 4 glasses daily.
- Watermelon seed tea: purifies.
- Potassium broth: heals and nourishes (see Appendix I).
- Parsley tea: diuretic action.
- Apple cider vinegar, water, and honey (1 cup 3 times daily).

Stage 2
(7-10 days), until condition clears:
- Non-citrus fruits and juice; watermelon and watermelon juice; cranberry juice.
- Salads and vegetable juices; asparagus; apple cider vinegar plus honey.
- Vegetarian meals (no eggs or dairy products); whole grains; baked potatoes.
- Kidney beans; garlic; parsnips; carrots and carrot juice; fluids: 8 or more glasses daily.

Hydrotherapy and Physiotherapy

- Hot sitz bath (pain relief); hot compress; trunk packs; hot glycothymoline packs over pubic area with 50% water, 50% glycothymoline; short-wave over bladder for 15-20 minutes; eliminate toxic elements by encouraging good bowel function (see Constipation).
- Enemas with liquid fast; laxative foods with Stage 2; acidophilus douche—1 tbsp in 2 pints (1 liter) warm water.

Therapeutic Agents

Vitamins and Minerals—Primary

- Vitamin C with bioflavinoids: 500–1000 mg 3–6 times daily, or to bowel tolerance. Acidifies urine and has antibacterial effect. Stimulates immune function.
- Vitamin A: 25,000 IU 2–6 times daily, for short periods. (See warning under Vitamin Toxicity, page 56.) Essential for mucous membrane health.
- Beta-carotene: 10,000 IU twice daily provitamin A.
- Vitamin E: 400 IU 1–2 times daily; healing factor.

Vitamins and Minerals—Secondary

- Folic acid: 40–80 mg daily.
- Pantothenic acid: 100 mg twice daily (with a B complex).
- Niacin: 100 mg twice daily (with a B complex).
- Zinc: 25 mg twice daily. To help with tissue repair and immune response.

Other

- Probiotics (acidophilus): usually 2 capsules 3 times daily. Needed to restore better internal ecology. Use especially when antibiotics have been a cause of condition developing in the first place. Also used as a douche.
- Colloidal silver: acts as a natural antibiotic.
- Chlorophyll: antibiotic and internal cleanser.
- Garlic: 2 capsules 3–4 times daily. Antibiotic.

Botanicals—Primary

Buchu: diuretic, urinary tonic, antiseptic. 10–15 drops tincture 3–4 times daily.
Bearberry: diuretic and gastrointestinal antiseptic. 20–30 drops tincture 4–6 times daily.

Botanicals—Secondary

Comfrey.
Cornsilk: urinary tract demulcent, and diuretic.
Couch grass: demulcent, diuretic. 5–20 drops tincture 3–4 times daily.
Goldenseal: tea 3 times daily.
Juniper berries: diuretic.
Marshmallow root: excellent demulcent, diuretic. Use powder in warm water, 10–30 grains, 3–4 times daily.
Parsley root and seed: use as tea or tincture, 5–15 drops 3–4 times daily.

DANDRUFF

DEFINITION

A chronic scaling inflammation of the skin occurring on the scalp and eyebrows.

SYMPTOMS

Diffuse scaling of the scalp; variable itching.

ETIOLOGICAL CONSIDERATIONS—PRIMARY

- Seborrheic dermatitis
  Dysfunction of the sebaceous glands with increased oil production.
- Diet
  Excess carbohydrates; deficiency of green vegetables; sugar; excess alcohol

191

Excess citrus; salt; excess saturated fats and fried foods; essential fatty acid deficiency

- Vitamin and mineral deficiency
- Vitamin A; vitamin E; vitamin B complex; vitamin B6; zinc; selenium
- Allergy
- Wheat; dairy products; citrus

ETIOLOGICAL CONSIDERATIONS— SECONDARY

Stress; hormonal; acidity; poor eliminations; fungus; strong irritant shampoos or hair treatments; digestive enzyme deficiency

DISCUSSION

Most people consider dandruff of cosmetic importance only. The usual mode of treatment is to attack the offending white scales with various shampoos and other topical agents. This is rarely successful in permanently removing the problem and demonstrates that symptomatic treatments are useless.

Dandruff is a symptom that may be caused by many different factors. Although this condition is commonly considered the result of what is called seborrhea, or an excess secretion of oil by the sebaceous glands, this tells us very little. Many patients with dandruff have excess sebaceous gland activity. This oil in fact is what binds the dead skin cells together to form visible plaques. The excess oil itself must have some unusual irritant quality not normally present if this is the major cause. In some cases this can be found from dietary errors such as excess acidity, allergy, improper fat consumption, or other irritants such as salt, sugar, or alcohol. This will cause irritant elements to be excreted in the body's oily secretions and may cause the body to react with an irritation and rash.

Another possibility is that nutritional deficiency may cause improper function of the sebaceous glands and scalp. Evidence of various forms of dermatitis is readily available in most severe B complex deficiencies as well as in essential fatty acid and zinc deficiency.

Scalp irritation and rash may also develop from the use of strong acid or alkaline shampoos, very hot hair dryers, or unnatural and strong hair treatments or dyes. Hormonal factors also may play a part.

TREATMENT

Diet

A common finding in cases of dandruff is improper diet. This many times is an excess consumption of citrus. As a first step in treatment we forbid the consumption of any but the blandest of fruits and allow only papaya, avocado, and a very few bananas. Later we add other fruits but exclude the entire citrus family until complete cure has been attained. Since most cases show a diet high in carbohydrates and animal fats and low in green vegetables, we restrict or entirely eliminate carbohydrates and saturated fats for a time, and advise a diet primarily of raw and cooked vegetables and vegetarian proteins. These include sunflower seeds, pumpkin seeds, a few nuts, beans, and tofu.

It is best to begin this regimen with 1–3 days of vegetable juice fasting and enemas. This is followed for 1–2 weeks by a diet made up of a small amount of bland fruits and a great quantity of both raw and conservatively cooked vegetables, plus raw vegetable juices. For a further 2 weeks it is useful to continue to restrict the diet to a purely vegetarian cuisine. This may then be followed by a diet similar to that found under Acne, a condition to which dandruff is closely associated. This diet severely restricts saturated fats.

Physiotherapy

- Scalp massage: to 4 fl oz (120 mL) pure distilled water add 20 drops of 85% grain alcohol and 2-6 drops of oil of pine. Massage into scalp and then follow this by massaging a small amount of white vaseline into the scalp. You may alternate this with peanut oil and lemon juice mixture. Use 2 fl oz (60 mL) of peanut oil mixed with the juice of half a lemon. Rub in scalp and leave in for 10-20 minutes before shampoo. See Cradle Cap for scalp treatments.

- Shampoo: use pine tar shampoo or alternate with olive oil shampoo.
- Crude oil scalp massage: 2 times per week (see Baldness)
- Vinegar and water scalp rub: use 20% vinegar to 80% water. Leave on 20 minutes before shampoo.
- Vitamin B6 cream application: apply small amount to scalp twice daily after shampoo.

Therapeutic Agents

Vitamins and Minerals—Primary

- Vitamin A: 25,000 IU 1-2 times daily. Needed in all dry skin conditions to speed healing.
- Beta-carotene: 10,000 IU daily. Antioxidant and needed as a precursor to vitamin A. Less toxic for long-term use than vitamin A.
- Vitamin B complex: 50 mg 2-3 times daily. (If yeast allergy exists, use non-yeast source). B complex deficiency linked to dandruff. Needed for healthy skin and hair.
- Vitamin B6: 100 mg twice daily. Needed for healthy skin and hair.
- Vitamin B12: 1 mg intramuscularly per week.
- Selenium: 200 mcg daily. Helps with dry scale conditions.
- Zinc: 25-30 mg 3 times daily. Helps heal dermatological conditions.

Vitamins and Minerals—Primary

- Vitamin E: 400 IU daily; folic acid: 2 mg daily; vitamin C with bioflavinoids: 1000 mg 3 times daily.
- Biotin: essential for scalp and hair health.

Others—Primary

- Flaxseed meal, and flaxseed oil: (2 tbsp daily).
- Evening primrose oil: 1-2 capsules 2-3 times daily.
- Lecithin: as much as possible. 4 capsules 3 times daily and/or as granules in food.
- Atomodine (or other iodine source).
- Cod-liver oil: 2-4 capsules twice daily.
- Eicosapentaenoic acid: 2-4 capsules 3 times daily.
- Urine therapy: collect first morning urine from mid-stream, bathe scalp and allow to soak for several minutes before rinsing out with pure water.

Others—Secondary

- Kelp: 1000 mg daily. Iodine is useful for hair growth and to heal the scalp. Trace mineral source.
- Hydrochloric acid: if HCL deficiency is the cause of poor absorption.
- Raw thymus: immunological support.
- L-cystein: 500 mg daily. For healthy skin and hair.
- Lecithin: 1000 mg 2-3 times daily. For healthy skin, hair and scalp.

Therapeutic Suggestions

Although saturated fats in the diet are avoided, essential fatty acids are encouraged. EFA, EPA, GLA, and evening primrose oil may show very good responses along with the rest of the suggested supplements. The scalp treatments outlined in detail under the section on Baldness are an essential part of therapy.

DEHYDRATION

DEFINITION AND SYMPTOMS

Excessive loss of body fluid through the bladder, skin (perspiration), lungs (exhaled air contains water droplets), bowels.

Acute symptoms: range from thirst, dry mouth, dry tongue, dry nasal mucosa, skin turgor (loss of elasticity) and headache, to disorientation and coma.

Chronic symptoms: often subclinical in presentation, consequently commonly left undiagnosed by the physician.

ETIOLOGICAL CONSIDERATIONS

- Failure to drink sufficient water (lack of natural thirst).
- Dietary lack of water-containing fresh fruit and vegetables.
- Failure to consume or absorb minerals.
- Excessive exercise, causing perspiration and droplet loss from lungs.
- Intake of caffeine (tea, coffee, etc.), alcohol, soft drinks.
- Airconditioning.
- Pharmaceutical drugs (especially those with diuretic side-effects).
- Poor absorption, or lack, of dietary proteins.

DISCUSSION

Water is by far the largest single component of the body, making up (ideally) about 80% of the total body weight. Water is a biochemical solvent, it participates in the tens of thousands of chemical reactions occurring within our bodies at any one time, it helps maintain electrical balance and acid–alkali balance, it helps regulate our body heat and serves as a lubricant, it makes up the bulk of the lymphatic and blood systems, as well as does many other things.

There is no part of our anatomy or physiology which is not water-dependent.

Dehydration is a state in which excessive fluid has been lost from the body; it can be acute or chronic, sub-clinical or clinical to the point of "drying out". Even just living indoors the average adult needs a minimum of $1\frac{1}{2}$ liters a day, depending on other lifestyle practices; time spent outdoors requires much more, given that we perspire, and lose water merely by breathing. We get water from fluid intake and from food which contains water such as fruit.

Dehydration is caused partly by poor fluid intake; we don't drink enough water, and we eat foods with low water content. But compounding the problem is our intake of diuretic substances such as coffee, tea, soft drinks, alcohol, and powerful prescription drugs which cause the body to excrete excessive amounts of fluid and electrolytes (minerals which help maintain fluid balance within the body).

Another important factor in proper hydration of blood is protein digestion. Protein structures are important in helping to retain plasma concentrations (viscosity). Poor digestion of proteins (e.g. poor levels of gastric acid) will further compromise hydration levels.

Today, many if not most people suffer with some level of dehydration. Clinically, we notice that especially elderly people suffer from it. In fact, aging might prove to be defined as "the process of drying out". Because it seems so simple, it is almost always completely overlooked as a factor in disease causation. Instead, water balance problems are treated at the symptom level, with powerful drugs.

Some common examples are as follows:

An individual with fluid retention is almost always dehydrated. You would think that when the ankles swell up with water, you could not possibly be dehydrated.

However, the lack of water and improper balance of electrolytes transported by serum (water-based) can produce the initial changes that lead to fluid retention. Instead of attempting to correct this water and electrolyte imbalance with safe natural means, we instead force even more water from the body using powerful diuretics. This leads to more dehydration problems, exacerbating the condition.

Another example involves allergies or histamine reactions. When you become dehydrated your body naturally begins to increase production of histamine. A function of histamine is to retain water. Histamine irritates the body's tissues and immune system, and so you suffer the consequences of allergies, immune problems or worse. What do many doctors do? Give you antihistamines. After all, a prescription for water or some form of electrolyte-rich water would seem too ridiculously simple. Yet that is exactly what your body is crying out for.

The Sodium Pump

Most of the fluid balance in your body is maintained by what is called the sodium pump. This is where two minerals, sodium and potassium, are exchanged in and out of body cells, designed partly to ensure proper cellular metabolism.

If you are permanently hampered by powerful prescription drugs that force the body to drain or dehydrate, you have little or no chance of ever achieving homeostasis in the fluid balance area, and you face a lifetime of drugs to try to maintain symptom control.

And as with all powerful drugs, you are prone to all their side effects. In the case of diuretics, these can be dangerous or even life-threatening. Diuretics cause unnatural fluid and electrolyte loss, and in the case of heart disease, you are losing the priceless trace minerals that are needed to heal and maintain the health of your heart and circulatory system.

Dehydration Causes Disease

When you do not have enough water in your body, several things can occur: your kidneys overwork, your digestion is hampered, your heart cannot function properly, your lungs and breathing mechanisms are impaired, your joints suffer, your entire lymphatic system (waste elimination) becomes sluggish and your immune system including the mucous membranes diminish in effectiveness. And at the cellular level, normal cellular functioning becomes impaired, including the capacity to produce energy and remove wastes.

So when it comes to diseases of the heart and blood vessels, kidney or stomach, allergies, arthritis, skin diseases, asthma, and in fatigue states, hydration may be the single most important factor in the cause of the condition, your recovery from it and even your survival.

DIGESTION

Without enough water, your stomach cannot "churn" food properly. Without this churning action, food is not exposed to enough acids and enzymes to be digested. The water for this is supplied from within, rather than by drinking with meals. Excess fluids with a meal reduce the effectiveness of the digestive juices by diluting them. Strong acid is needed in the stomach at all times. A small drink of water or a glass of wine with a meal is OK. Excess fluids with a meal will reduce the effectiveness of the digestive juices by diluting them.

The next stage of digestion in the small intestine will be hampered also. When food leaves your stomach, it is extremely acidic. It must then be handled in the small intestine, which is a more alkaline environment. Your pancreas gets involved here, secreting bicarbonate and alkaline enzymes (all mixed in water) into the small intestine to neutralise the acid food from the stomach. Without adequate water this function is severely hampered.

In fact, when your body knows that an extremely acid food mass is about to pass into the small intestine without adequate buffering, a reflux is usually started. This reflux will cause muscle spasm at the junction between the stomach and the small intestine in a effort to delay the passage of this acid food. This muscle spasm is extremely painful and mimics the pain from ulcers.

In chronic dehydration states, movement of waste product through the gut becomes sluggish, given that bile (a prime mover of peristalsis) is a water-based substance. This can result in states of constipation, which in turn can cause a whole host of disease states, including autoimmune diseases, irritable bowel syndrome, diverticulitis and even cancer.

What is usually done to treat these problems? Drugs are dispensed to treat the symptoms, masking the underlying cause of the problem and ensuring usually permanent indigestion and disease.

A more rational approach would be to drink a glass of pure water a half hour before each meal. In addition, digestive enzymes could be utilized until your system begins to normalize itself.

Lung Problems, Allergies and Asthma

All tissues involved in breathing are dependent on pure water; the trace minerals and elements are water-soluble. Without adequate water, breathing will become labored. Your body will produce histamine in order to retain water. This excess histamine will irritate the mucous membranes of your lungs and respiratory tree, and damage your immune system. Tissues will become sensitized and allergies develop.

As time goes on, the tissues and muscles that make up your breathing mechanism can go into spasm, resulting in severe breathing problems and asthma. Again, antihistamines and chemical dilators are employed with very little effort directed towards getting at the root cause of the problem.

How much better instead to use plenty of water and trace elements. In fact, for those with severe breathing problems, *at least* 4 pints (2 liters) are needed daily. And that means water, not soft drinks, tea, coffee or alcohol. Over time, breathing problems will begin to disappear as rehydration and then tissue rejuvenation will occur. With this type of therapy, the only side-effect is having to urinate frequently.

HEART AND BLOOD PRESSURE PROBLEMS

These may be two of the most misunderstood problems facing medicine. With cardiovascular problems, the body retains fluid. However, earlier on, dehydration can weaken the heart. And no matter what, increased water intake is necessary to regain proper heart and blood vessel function.

For example, when an individual is at risk of thrombosis, stroke, angina or heart attack, it is perceived by the doctor that "the blood is too thick" (and a blood-thinning drug is usually prescribed, such as aspirin or warfarin). But why is the blood "too thick"? Mostly because it is dehydrated. All the system needs is to be properly hydrated, by more water in the blood.

KIDNEY PROBLEMS

Heart and kidney diseases go hand in hand. When fluid balance is disturbed (as in heart disease) the kidneys overwork and as they overwork blood pressure usually rises. And for the most part there is usually insufficient water in the body to help maintain proper kidney function.

One sure sign of dehydration is concentrated urine. If your urine is always concentrated, watch out! That can mean it is full of concentrated inorganic minerals, which your body cannot use, there being too little water in the blood and lymph. This can lead to kidney stones and other problems. Concentrated urine is a strong signal to increase intake of pure water.

ARTHRITIS

Did you ever wonder why people go to hot springs for arthritis relief? Well, part of it is the warm water, which increases circulation. But another factor is transdermal absorption of trace elements (like sulfur) from the water. It is these trace elements that are needed for proper joint function. And it is plenty of water and proper nutrients (including trace elements found especially in fresh fruit and vegetables) that are prerequisite for healing of arthritic joints.

Plenty of water serves as a lubricant needed for proper joint maintenance and health.

LYMPHATIC SYSTEM

The lymphatic system is a water-based system, and its importance deserves special consideration. The vital role of the lymphatic system to the health of the body has largely been overlooked by western medicine. Unless you have a swollen lymph node, inflamed tonsils or appendicitis, doctors rarely say anything about the lymphatic system. When was the last time your doctor said "Looks like your lymphatic system is sluggish?" One can only suspect that doctors either do not understand its importance, do not recognize when it is sluggish, or do not know what do about it. Yet its role is central to so many aspects of health, and improved lymphatic functioning is vital to recovery from many disease processes.

Roles of the (Healthy) Lymphatic System

- Lymph fluid removes wastes from tissue. These are carried in interstitial fluid which bathes body cells. Lymph fluid and intestinal fluid are one and the same, the difference being location; when the fluid is in lymphatic tissues it is called lymph fluid. Some wastes accumulate in tissue as normal by-products of cellular metabolism. Other wastes are absorbed into the bloodstream from food, water, medications, etc. via the intestinal mucosa, e.g. "leaky gut"; also from polluted air via the lungs, skin, etc.

- Lymph fluid is drawn from blood plasma via venous capillaries (by osmosis, diffusion and filtration). It supplies nutrients to various avascular areas of the body such as cartilage in joint spaces.

- Some blood plasma proteins escape from the blood; the lymphatic capillaries pick up these leaked proteins and return them to the blood. Failure to do this results in edema (fluid build-up).

- The spleen is a major lymphatic organ. One of its jobs is to filter and destroy bacteria and worn-out or damaged red blood cells and platelets from the blood. It also recycles the iron for reuse in hemoglobin molecules in red blood cells, which carry oxygen, and carbon dioxide to and from the tissues.

- The lymphatic system plays a major role in immune system functioning. In lymphatic tissue there are dense concentrations of immune system cells (e.g. T-cells, macrophages, B-cells and plasma cells). The thymus is a lymph gland that matures T-cells. The spleen also transforms B-cells into lymphocytes, white blood cells important in specific immune defenses, as (together with T-cells) they produce antibodies that defend against bacterial invasion.

- The lymphatic system also carries dietary fats (lipids) such as cholesterols, and fat-soluble vitamins such as vitamins A, D, E and K.

- The lymphatic system empties lymph into the bloodstream, from where the contents are detoxified in the liver, packaged in bile and transported to the small intestine, and then to the bowel for elimination.

How Does the Lymphatic Flow Become Impaired?

Proper lymph flow depends on proper hydration, and a number of dietary and lifestyle factors such as regular exercise and proper breathing (breathing creates a type of vacuum effect on the lymphatic trunks). Although as wide spread throughout the body as blood, lymph does not have its own "pump"; it depends largely on the exercise of skeletal muscles, and the action of minerals (in this context called electrolytes).

Lymph flow can be impeded when the body is not obtaining adequate net amounts of water, when breathing and exercise is inadequate, when lymphatic fluid, capillaries, ducts and nodes become congested by mucus and fatty deposits (e.g. diets high in saturated fats and proteins), sclerosing (thickening) of lymphatic tissue, or when body fluid (interstitial fluid) becomes too "thick" (in the same way blood is said to be "thick") such as occurs in even subclinical dehydration with lack of water and electrolyte imbalances, or where there are abnormal and excessive interstitial protein concentrations.

Implications of Congested Lymphatic Flow

There are many and varied impacts on the health of a person with a sluggish lymphatic system. In almost every chronic disease state (e.g. chronic susceptibility to infection, arthritis, cancer and dementia) poor lymphatic function at the very least will contribute to the cause processes of these diseases, and any treatment which fails to address lymphatic functioning will prove to be inadequate in progressing cure.

For example, in osteoarthritis, cartilage has lost its integrity, and there is a build-up of wastes around the joint. Why has the cartilage become impaired? One common reason is that it was not receiving adequate nourishment from the lymphatic fluids which provide the bulk of nutrients to the cartilage in the first place. Maybe the diet was deficient in the nutrients, but maybe also the lymph was not flowing adequately in the area.

Lymph carries wastes, including cells which naturally break off from cancer tissue, for example skin cancer) to the blood, and then to the liver for elimination. If the lymph is sluggish, these cancerous cells are much more likely to become lodged somewhere within the body, or within the lymphatic system itself (e.g. in lymph nodes), thus allowing secondary tumors to develop, and preventing the body from what it may be trying to do, that is, to get rid of the primary tumor via metastasis.

What about fluid retention? What about acute infections? And chronic infections? What about in states of fatigue after infection (as in chronic fatigue)? These may be fairly obvious connections to make with the condition of the lymphatic system, lymph flow, etc. in the light of what has been mentioned above.

Naturopathic philosophy says that when the body receives all the right nutrients in the right amounts, when congestions are relieved and wastes eliminated, and when we refrain from further polluting the internal body environment, the body's homeostatic mechanisms, the "mind-body" will act to reverse the disease processes. In our clinical experience, when proper attention is given to stimulating the lymphatic circulation, healing comes more rapidly and surely for any chronic disease.

THE SIMPLE CURE

Pure water, together with proper nutrition and nutritional supplements are needed to correct as well as to maintain health. Water is a powerful broad spectrum tonic for those suffering from chronic degenerative disease, especially the aged.

How to Ensure Adequate Hydration

Dehydration usually results from the unconscious, and the poor habit; changing habits must be an exercise in consciousness, carefully getting into a new habit pattern of good hydration living.

- In order for the body to actually *retain* some of the water you now start to drink, rather than just urinate it out all the time, you need to have mineral salt intake. We recommend Celtic salt, a totally unrefined, natural product which will help restore proper hydration levels. This is to be used instead of other salt. It contains 84 minerals, and can be simply added to cooking, sprinkled on food, put in salad dressing, etc. to taste.

- Cut down on your diuretic intake. This means coffee, tea, alcohol, and pharmaceutical diuretics. Each of these robs the body of hydration status.

- Drink more hydrating fluids. Such fluids can include water, fruit and vegetable juices, herbal teas, miso, even "sports drinks" (avoid aspartame and sorbitol sweetening agents). You can actually prepare your own sports drink by mixing a little Celtic salt and glucose with pure water (e.g. spring water), to taste.

- It is important to drink fairly regularly throughout the day. Half a glass of water with a meal is good for the digestion, but of course, do not drink too much with meals as you do not want your gastric acid levels impaired. Start the day with a drink of water with a squeeze of lemon in it. Do not drink too much after dinner, as it can cause unnecessary waking to go to the loo. Sleep with a glass of water beside the bed.

- If you perspire easily, or spend a lot of time in the sun, you must be doubly sure to ensure best hydration practice.

- The length of time you have been dehydrated (some people have been dehydrated the bulk of their lives!) will largely determine how long it will take you to achieve optimal hydration. It sometimes takes 6–12 months to rehydrate properly, and fully enjoy the many health benefits of proper hydration.

DEMENTIA
Age-Related Memory Impairment, Cognitive Dysfunctioning, Senility, Alzheimer's

DEFINITION

Memory dysfunction due to organic brain disease that is characterized by the premature death of large numbers of brain cells.

SYMPTOMS

Early symptoms include memory loss, cognitive dysfunction, inability to do everyday things, inability for abstract thought, impaired judgment. Later symptoms can include gross memory loss, a loss of personality, and ineffective movement.

Some indicators may be present up to 60 years beforehand, but more typically symptoms onset within 20 years of death. Note that in mid-life memory impairment can simply be age-related (see Memory Loss), and is *not* a definite predictor of senility.

There are recognized stages of mental dysfunction characteristic of dementia, and these are measured via the "global deterioration scale" as follows:

1. No memory decline.
2. Forgetting names of acquaintances, placement of familiar objects, mental fatigue, poor concentration, etc. (age-associated memory impairment).
3. Decreased retention of written material, decline in concentration, with anxiety (this is a mild neurocognitive disorder—can last 7 years)
4. Decreased knowledge of current events; decreased ability to handle travel, finances, complex tasks, and lack of emotion (mild Alzheimer's—can last 2 years).
5. Inability to recall a major event in current life; moderate time disorientation, forgetting family members names (moderate, or early Alzheimer's—can last 18 months).
6. Forgetting name of spouse, birth date, most recent life events; requiring assistance with daily living; delusional and paranoid behavior; anxiety and agitation; urinary and fecal incontinence (moderately severe Alzheimer's—can last 2–3 years).
7. Loss of (in chronological order) speech, ability to walk, to sit up, to smile (severe Alzheimer's can last 7–10 years).

ETIOLOGICAL CONSIDERATIONS

- Genetics
- Metal poisoning by aluminum, copper, iron
- Lente virus
- Toxins (environmental, pharmaceutical)
- Autoimmune factors
- Chronic vitamin deficiency (e.g. B12, folic acid)
- Brain injury/trauma
- Cholinergic nerve destruction due to excitatory amino acids (glutamate, aspartate)
- Gluten/gliadin sensitivity or allergy to wheat
- Hypothyroidism
- Elevated homocysteine levels
- Excess cortisol (from adrenals, a stress hormone) destroys optimal brain functioning

DISCUSSION

We tend to favor the model developed and successfully practiced by Dr Dharma Singh Khalsa. Dr Khalsa has developed the hypothesis that chronically excessive levels of serum cortisol leads to gross deficiency of acetylcholine (ACh), a primary brain neurotransmitter. *"A deficit of acetylcholine is probably the single most common cause of age-related cognitive dysfunctioning."* (Khalsa, *Brain Longevity*, p. 209).

Excessive cortisol levels have particular effects on human biochemistry:

- Inhibit the utilization of blood sugar in brain, affecting the hippocampus, the primary memory center, because they stimulate excessive adrenalin which in turn causes excessive insulin secretion.
- Interfere with neurotransmitters in the brain, especially acetylcholine, which is the primary memory neurotransmitter.
- Kill brain cells; excessive cortisol disrupts normal brain cell metabolism, causing an excess of calcium to enter brain cells, which generates free radicals that destroy cells.

Cortisol (hydrocortisone) is a steroid hormone naturally synthesized in and secreted by the adrenal cortex. It is important for normal carbohydrate metabolism and energy production, and for the normal response to stress. When one is constantly under emotional or psychological stress, the hypothalamus releases corticotrophin-releasing hormone (CRH), which stimulates the pituitary gland to produce ACTH. This stimulates the production of large amounts of cortisol which circulates throughout the body as well as in the brain.

Having developed a hypothesis, Khalsa

has implemented a program that has been running for nearly a decade and is demonstrating significant clinical success, not merely in halting the progress of the disease, but in even reversing it. This program works, where most others have very limited success with treatment of dementia.

TREATMENT

Khalsa has developed basically a 4-part treatment program, the aim of which is to improve brain function. Each part of the program is integrated with each other part, and involves the following:
1. Dietary/nutritional (Stage 1 for 2 weeks, then Stage 2 until symptoms have gone).
2. Stress management.
3. Exercise and lifestyle changes.
4. Medication/supplements.

Dietary Principles

- Low fat intake. Reduce/eliminate saturated fats from everyday meals, but ensure adequate essential fatty acids, especially the omega-3s.
- Eat nutrient-dense foods, that is unrefined or minimally refined, and preferably organic, fresh foods.
- Avoid hypoglycemia. Avoid low blood sugar states; soy is excellent; grazing with good foods minimizes risk of hypoglycemia (see Hypoglycemia).
- Low-calorie program is best (1500–2000 is best level).
- Select your diet from a broad cross-section of foods—fruits, vegetables including legumes, nuts and seeds, and whole grains (e.g. brown rice, soy beans, oats, millet, buckwheat).
- Feed your neurotransmitters. Acetylcholine is synthesized in part from choline, abundant in such foods as soy, chlorophyll-rich foods especially, also in whole grains, egg yolk, lecithin, beans and liver.

- As a rule, have a good amount of protein for breakfast (e.g. soy smoothie which can include lecithin, flaxseed oil); have a high-protein lunch (e.g. salad and tuna or salmon) to provide mental acuity; and have a high-carbohydrate dinner (to relax).

Foods to Avoid
- Eliminate dairy milk from the diet.
- Eliminate red meats and processed meats, in favor of cold-water fish such as salmon or tuna.
- Eliminate fast foods and fried foods altogether. They contain too many free-radical-forming agents.
- Reduce alcohol. French studies show that light alcohol consumption (1–2 wines per day) and maybe even moderate consumption (2–4 wines per day) is prophylactic when compared to non-drinkers, which probably highlights the legitimate role of alcohol in stress management, as well as the noted antioxidant activity of oligomeric proanthocyanidins of red wine.
- Eliminate any foods containing aspartame/Nutrasweet/Equal or saccharine.
- Eliminate all aluminum from intake (e.g. use a reverse-osmosis filter) and drink 4 pints (2 liters) of water daily.
- Avoid antacids (esp. if they contain aluminum)
- Avoid citrates.
- Check heavy metal status.
- Check food sensitivity, especially to milk and wheat.
- Eliminate licorice (it potentiates cortisol, and compromises potassium intake which can lead to hypokalemia).

Note: Ensure there is no pain in the body, as pain is a significant stressor which generates neurotransmitter abnormalities.

Stress Management

"The normal (i.e. healthy) state of mind is *not* uptight. It is really relaxed, creative, intuitive, vibrant and intelligent. It's almost

201

magical; I call the fully relaxed mind the 'magical mind'." (Dr Herbert Benson, pioneer of stress management). A calm mind promotes a calm body, and vice versa.

We know from the pioneering work of Hans Selye into stress (Hans Selye, *1956 General Adaptation Syndrome*) that stress disrupts normal hormone levels, and one effect is the release of excessive amounts of adrenalin and cortisol into the bloodstream.

If stress is not properly managed, this can become a chronic situation, and the end result will be organ failure, in this case, the brain.

See also Stress.

Exercise and Lifestyle Changes

Many of the body's eliminative functions require exercise for optimal results. The lymphatic system is a rubbish removal system which works at a cellular level, removing toxins produced in the normal course of cellular metabolism, as well as those which come from outside the body. Lymphatic health requires, among other things, regular exercise which assists flow in this fluid-based system. Bowels work much better, as do the other organs of rubbish removal such as the lungs, skin and kidneys, when adequate exercise is undertaken. Any program that wants to address dementia must involve exercise as well as other lifestyle changes consistent with general good health.

Medicinal and Nutrient Supplementation

Vitamins and Minerals
- Vitamin A: micellized, up to 100,000 IU daily. (See warning under Vitamin Toxicity, page 56.)
- Vitamin B: studies show that deficiency of each B vitamin (B1, B3, B6, folate and B12) has been linked with dementia.
- Vitamin C: (up to 10 g daily, or to bowel tolerance).
- Vitamin E: (800–2000 IU daily).
- Antioxidant minerals: e.g. magnesium, zinc, selenium.

Others—Primary
- Amino acids: phenylalanine, glutamine, methionine, arginine, tryptophan.
- Lecithin: phosphatidylcholine, precursor to ACh. Preventative 1500 mg daily; therapeutic, 10,000 mg daily.
- Phosphatidyl serine: (capsule form) a fat naturally occurring in every body cell, concentrated in brain (cell membranes of neurons). Lowers stress hormones, increases alpha-waves 15–20%, relieves depression. Stimulates memory of faces and facts. Dosage 100–300 mg daily.
- ALC (acetyl L-carnitine): improves mitochondrial efficiency of brain cells. Improves intercerebral communication (as does piracetum). Up to 1500 mg daily.

Others—Secondary
- Green juices: high in chlorophyll; e.g. Spirulina, wheat grass, chlorella; contain peptides, which are precursors of neuropeptides; also rich in the nine essential amino acids.
- Green tea: rich in flavonoids, polyphenols (including catechins and quercetin) which are potent antioxidants; 1–2 servings or more daily
- Coenzyme Q10: 100 mg daily.
- Probiotics.

Botanicals
Ginkgo biloba: anti-platelet. Has been demonstrated to be effective especially where there is impaired cognition, and can elicit a rapid response (1 hour after 600 mg dose). 2 mL 2 times daily.

Panax ginseng: adaptogenic, adrenal tonic. Curtails release of cortisol by reducing demand for it

Nettles and horsetail: contain silica which leaches aluminum; prevents aluminum absorption from the gut.

Garlic: especially for age-related memory loss.

DIABETES

DEFINITION

A disease characterized by carbohydrate intolerance of varying degrees, due to inadequate production of insulin by the beta cells of the islets of Langerhans, or insulin insensitivity of the body cells, but also involving other glandular organs and body tissues.

SYMPTOMS

Sugar in urine, raised blood sugar, excessive thirst, polyuria (excess urination) and frequency of urination, excess hunger, muscle wasting, weight loss, weakness, electrolyte loss, dry skin, itching, rashes, paresthesia, numbness, tingling of hands and feet, neuropathy with severe pains, vascular degeneration, atherosclerosis, retinopathy, loss of sight, kidney disease, gangrene in dependent limbs due to poor circulation leading to amputation, ketosis, acidosis, coma, and premature death.

ETIOLOGICAL CONSIDERATIONS—PRIMARY

- Diet
  Excess refined carbohydrates and sugar consumption, syndrome X; dairy; excess saturated fat consumption; nutritional deficiency
- Pancreatic insufficiency
  Refined foods; coffee; alcohol; smoking; stress; nervous exhaustion
- Viral infection
- Allergy (e.g. dairy products)
- Obesity
- Spinal: T6 to T10 lesions causing imbalance of function of liver, pancreas, spleen, adrenals, and other organs with congestion and sluggishness
- Heredity

- Pregnancy and severe infection: latent diabetes appears, due to increased insulin requirements at this time
- Autoimmune disease

ETIOLOGICAL CONSIDERATIONS— SECONDARY

- Emotional: longing for what might have been, deep sorrow
- Sudden severe shock (causing constriction of blood flow to vital organs causing damage); lack of exercise; adrenal exhaustion; sedentary existence; hyperthyroid; toxemia
- Hyperadrenocorticism; liver damage, toxicity, or congestion; pancreatitis or other pancreas damage due to trauma, tumor, or infection; poor eliminations

DISCUSSION

Diabetes affects up to 5% of the people in the United States, with many more undiagnosed. The most obvious physiological abnormality recognized in the past is a deficiency of secretion of insulin by the beta cells of the pancreas. Elevated insulin levels also may occur where the body has developed a decreased sensitivity to insulin. In general, high-insulin diabetics tend to be overweight, while insulin-deficient patients become thin and emaciated. The high-insulin diabetic may simply be at an earlier stage of the disease, later to become insulin-deficient with sudden weight loss.

Insulin's role in the body is to facilitate uptake of glucose from the bloodstream by the body's cells for energy utilization. In diabetes the pancreas either does not produce enough insulin, or the body has become less sensitive to it, causing a wide range of metabolic results.

The normal level of glucose in the blood is kept within the narrow range of 80–120 mg %. If, due to insulin deficiency or insensitivity, this rises to 170–180 mg %, sugar spills over into the urine, carrying with it vast amounts of water, water-soluble vitamins, and minerals. This causes a severe electrolyte imbalance and dehydration, stimulating excessive thirst. Since the body's glucose fuel cannot make its way into the cells where it is needed, the body begins to convert fats and protein into sugar as an emergency measure. This results in wasting of the body with weight loss and dehydration. As excess fats are broken down ketone bodies accumulate, resulting in ketosis, dizziness, nausea, vomiting, hyperventilation, and eventually coma. Excess protein breakdown also leads to a general acid condition of the body's fluids.

Characteristic changes occur within the cardiovascular system, leading to atherosclerotic changes that reduce blood flow to the feet, causing slow healing, tendency to infection, ulceration, and finally gangrene, leading to amputation of the toes or feet. Small vessels in the eyes are weakened, leading to rupture and blindness.

Not all cells of the body require insulin for glucose uptake. Certain cells called "insulin insensitive", found in the eye, kidney, myelinated nerves, and red blood cells, take up glucose passively along concentration gradients. Therefore, as glucose increases in the blood, these cells take up large amounts of glucose. Since this amount absorbed is far in excess of the energy needs of these cells, the body must convert it to fructose and then sorbitol to get it out of the way. These two sugars are relatively insoluble and soon exceed their solubility, tending to crystallize out within the cell. In the eye this results in the typical cataract formation found in diabetes. In the kidney it reduces glomerular filtration, causing kidney damage. It damages the nerves, leading to diabetic neuropathy, and reduces the oxygen-carrying capacity of the red blood cells.

The pancreas not only produces insulin, but also secretes digestive enzymes and bicarbonate essential for the breakdown of the basic food groups. When the pancreas is functioning at a low ebb due to overstimulation, it not only may have a reduced insulin output, but will also secrete less digestive enzymes. This sets up a vicious cycle when it comes to protein metabolism. Due to insufficient proteolytic enzymes, protein is not efficiently broken down into its amino acid components.

Since digestive enzymes and hormones (e.g. insulin, cortisol, adrenalin) are composed of amino acids, this maldigestion may eventually lead to further digestive enzyme deficiency and reduced hormone output, resulting in an aggravation of the diabetic syndrome.

In addition to this undigested protein, molecules may pass into the bloodstream, initiating allergy or allergy-like hypersensitivity reactions. (See Allergies and Food Intolerances for more discussion on results of this protein maldigestion.)

The deficiency of fat-digesting capability is also a problem that may be directly related to the complications of arteriosclerosis and other cardiovascular problems associated with diabetes, by altering the relative lipid ratios.

In short, diabetes is a terrible disease, responsible for one in every eight deaths in the United States, and one in every three cases of blindness. The saddest part of this disease is that it is almost entirely preventable.

Diabetes is clearly a disease of civilization. Studies of various populations show that as the consumption of sugar and refined carbohydrates such as white bread and white rice increases, so does the incidence of diabetes. In groups where no refined sugars are consumed and the diet includes unrefined whole grains, little or no diabetes can be found.

Studies done in Finland, Italy and America within the last 10 years have shown there is an cause-and-effect relationship between milk consumption and juvenile diabetes. There are more than 20 different protein components in milk that are implicated in a number of possible immunologically mediated reactions. For example, it is now suggested that juvenile diabetes starts with an allergy to whey protein in cow's milk. Undigested whey gets into the bloodstream, and the immune system produces antibodies to this foreign protein. Pancreatic beta cells (which produce insulin) closely resemble the antibody-initiating the immune response called "stretch" in the whey protein, that is, they are chemically similar, and so these antibodies may attack and destroy the body's own cells because their recognition has been impaired.

Scandinavians are among the world's heaviest milk drinkers and they have the highest rates of diabetes. Studies show feeding an infant a cow's milk formula in the first 3 months of life significantly increases the risk of diabetes.

Diabetes is closely associated with obesity. At least 80% of all diabetics are or were obese. The consumption of refined carbohydrates seems to be the major contributing factor in this obesity. It is possible to consume a large amount of refined carbohydrates in the form of sugar or refined grains such as white bread, macaroni, or white rice in a short time, since the bulky fiber has been removed. If, however, carbohydrates were taken in their natural, unrefined state, it would be impossible to consume even one-fifth of this amount. For example, if a person drinks only one soda drink in 5 minutes (which may contain up to 7 tsp of sugar), it would have taken him or her hours to eat the equivalent carbohydrate value found in apples, carrots, or whole grain bread. Refined carbohydrates, especially in their disaccharide form (i.e. sucrose, which is composed of one molecule of fructose and one molecule of glucose), are especially a problem since they stimulate triglyceride formation associated with the cardiovascular complications of diabetes.

Adult-onset diabetes normally has an incubation period of about 20 years before it becomes manifest. As our children are exposed earlier and earlier to a vast amount of refined cereals, sweets, and soda, we are now finding what would be considered "adult"-onset diabetes in younger age groups.

Although deficiencies of many nutrients have been found to induce diabetes in experimental situations, no single nutrient deficiency is the real cause; nor will there be a real cure. Diabetes is not simply a disorder of the pancreas, but affects the entire body, especially the liver, nervous system, circulatory system, thyroid, spleen, kidney, hypothalamus, pituitary, and adrenal glands. It is not just a disorder of carbohydrate metabolism, but also affects utilization of both fats and proteins. The entire metabolism is upset, as well as all the hormones that normally control it.

Although consumption of refined carbohydrates is one of the major causes of diabetes by causing the pancreas to secrete excess insulin, or the body to become insensitive to insulin, and overworking the pancreas and eventually weakening it, other factors play their part. Stress and adrenal exhaustion are factors in many cases of diabetes. Although the pancreas, with its production of glucagon, which causes an increase in blood glucose levels, is the major antagonist to insulin in the control of blood sugar levels, the adrenal glands are also involved. Normally food is consumed and converted into glucose, raising the blood sugar level. The pancreas secretes insulin to remove the glucose from the blood. If the sugar level falls too low (as in hypoglycemia) the adrenal glands secrete hormones that trigger the conversion of stored sugar in the liver and muscles in the form of glycogen back to sugar for use. These glands, the pancreas, liver, and adrenals, are all under stress with either *hypo*glycemia or *hyper*glycemia. Stress is interpreted in the body as an emergency situation and the adrenal glands respond by secreting adrenalin to derive energy to deal with the supposed threat. If this is too often repeated, or too prolonged, as in chronic nervous tension, the pancreas, adrenal glands and liver become severely depleted and fail to respond properly and hypoglycemia or diabetes may result.

Vitamin deficiencies such as B complex and vitamin C may be the result of this situation since the adrenal glands need large amounts of these nutrients to function.

Refined carbohydrates, stress, coffee, nicotine, and alcohol or recreational drugs all cause the adrenal glands to work in excess, and as we have already seen, overstimulation eventually will lead to inhibition of function. Thus we see that the civilized way of life is the largest factor in the causation of pancreatic and adrenal malfunction leading to diabetes.

Another recent and very interesting clinical observation is that blood sugar levels react differently for different people in response to the same food. Although consumption of refined carbohydrates is considered a primary factor, many seemingly safe foods can cause similar reactions depending upon individual sensitivity. The same endocrine reactions of high or low blood sugar levels, along with pancreatic and adrenal gland depletion, can occur following ingestion of literally any food or food group, including protein, fats, and even unrefined carbohydrates, as well as chemicals or tobacco. These reactions can be considered as an allergy, or probably more appropriately, may be labeled hypersensitivities. In such cases, where standard high complex carbohydrate regimens fail to control the blood sugar level adequately, the individual must have his or her blood sugar reactions tested for all commonly ingested foods, or undertake a rotation diet where individual foods are not eaten more frequently than every 4 days.

Other glands and organs are related to diabetes as well. The liver, where sugar is stored in the form of glycogen as an energy reserve, is found to suffer fatty degeneration in diabetes. Liver disease may be either the result or one of the causes of diabetes. Liver damage, toxicity, or congestion all seem to be associated with the onset of diabetes.

Spinal lesions in the midthoracic region are a common finding in diabetics. These may cause imbalances of function between the liver, pancreas, spleen, adrenal glands, and other organs, causing congestion and sluggish function or hyperactivity.

Insulin, discovered in the early 1920s, has been used in various forms to treat diabetes and has been clearly lifesaving in the short term and does help control the blood sugar level in diabetes.

The insidious cardiovascular changes characteristic of this disease may be more difficult to deal with. These changes in the arteries can cause loss of sight and limb, and may result in early death.

The problem with insulin use is that it is very difficult to prescribe it so that it mimics exactly the body's own production of insulin. In the past, insulin was given in rather large doses, 1–2 times daily. This causes elevated levels of insulin in the bloodstream for longer than usual. Normally the body secretes insulin in response to food, causing an elevation of blood sugar, and feedback controls moderate its level. With injected insulin, the problem is even more complex. Normally, insulin secreted from the pancreas goes first to the liver, where over half of it is used up, the rest then going into the general circulation. With insulin injections, however, all the insulin courses through the bloodstream before reaching the liver. The result is a temporary hyperinsulinism.

The problem with too much insulin in the blood is that excessive insulin levels stimulate the synthesis of cholesterol in the blood vessel wall, and may be a factor in arteriosclerosis. (This fact also provides a partial explanation of how a diet high in refined carbohydrate, which sensitizes the pancreas to produce excess insulin and is the main cause of hyperinsulinism-related hypoglycemia, favors the development of cardiovascular disease.)

Newer methods of insulin administration are currently being introduced which may correct this serious problem, and many physicians are now attempting to prescribe insulin along more physiological lines. There certainly is no question, however, that if diet can control glucose levels, it is a far safer and more desirable form of therapy than is insulin.

TREATMENT

Diabetes is a chronic degenerative disease. As such, by definition, vital organs and tissues have begun to be destroyed. The possibility of cure by natural means depends on the severity of the case and the length of insulin dependency. While some forms of diabetes, such as congenital or juvenile-onset diabetes, can never be corrected through diet alone and will always require insulin, even in these cases diet does help moderate the problem.

Certainly, mild cases of adult-onset diabetes are usually easy to correct. Even once insulin has been taken, if not for too prolonged a period, cure is fairly simple. Prolonged cases, however, require much more effort and total cure may not be possible if the pancreas has been so damaged over years of improper diet and drug suppression that it has literally ceased to function. Exogenous insulin certainly does not cause diabetes; however, the body can become dependent on it and reduce its own insulin production. Sometimes the best that can be done in these cases is to reduce the insulin need through proper diet and the consumption of insulin-like substances found naturally in some foods.

Diet

Until very recently diabetics were routinely counseled to reduce carbohydrates. No distinction was made between refined or unrefined, except that sugar and products with sugar were reduced. The typical diabetic then reduced carbohydrate consumption but continued to eat all manner of devitalized foods. To derive needed energy, which normally would have come from carbohydrates, most ate far more animal fats and proteins. These saturated fats only aggravated the dangerous cardiovascular disease from which most diabetics suffer (see Heart Disease). The type of diet prescribed by most naturopathic physicians for adult-onset diabetes for years has recently found favor.

Rather than a low-carbohydrate diet being the best approach, a diet high in unrefined carbohydrates is the most beneficial.

In one study 70% of the diet was composed of high-fiber unrefined carbohydrates and the average insulin requirement fell drastically during this regimen. Even more surprising was the fact that nearly all the overweight patients *lost* weight while those at a normal weight remained stationary. Many of the patients were able to discontinue insulin therapy altogether.

A good diabetic dietary regimen excludes any and all refined foods such as sugar, sweets, pastry, white flour products, and white rice, and replaces them with natural, high-fiber carbohydrates that take longer to be digested. The key is to supply the body with slow-burning fuel that will not cause a sudden increase in sugar in the blood and therefore require excess insulin. Most of the fats eaten should be vegetarian or unsaturated in nature. No red meats are allowed, and even chicken and fish are restricted to several times per week. The best proteins are vegetarian, with special emphasis on soy proteins due to their high concentration of lecithin, which is a fat emulsifier and contains large amounts of choline, found useful in preventing and treating neurological complications of diabetes. Acid and subacid fruits are allowed in moderation in some cases if eaten with some protein to slow digestion. Many diabetics, however, must strictly avoid all fruit and fruit juice, at least initially. All sweet fruits and dried fruits are forbidden. Meals should always be kept small and taken six times daily. As much as 75% of the diet should be composed of raw foods.

Some foods have an insulin-like action in the body, or other specific usefulness, and should be included in the diet regularly. These include:

- Jerusalem artichokes; fiber (e.g. wheat bran, oat bran, flaxmeal and guar gum); brussels sprouts.
- Cucumbers; oatmeal or oat flour products; green beans; soybeans and tofu; garlic.

- Avocado; Spirulina; wheat germ; brewer's yeast; buckwheat; raw green vegetables.

The following is a sample diet that has been very useful in diabetes:

On Rising
1 tsp Spirulina in warm water.

Breakfast
Choice of one of the following:
1. Whole grain cereal (e.g. oatmeal, whole wheat cereal, etc.).
2. Fruit, yoghurt, and nuts (not peanuts) and wheat germ.*
3. Yoghurt, nuts and wheat germ.
4. Once or twice per week, poached eggs on whole wheat toast.
5. ½ grapefruit or other citrus with some protein.*

Midmorning
Whole grain snack (e.g. bread, crackers, biscuits)
1 tsp Spirulina in warm water.

Lunch
Always include a raw salad composed primarily of green vegetables such as lettuce, cucumber, celery, watercress, parsley, spinach, broccoli, brussels sprouts, garlic, avocado, cabbage, sprouted alfalfa, beet tops, onions, cauliflower. Carrots may be included in small amounts only in the early stages of the diet, with larger portions later in the diet regimen. Also, any of the following:
- Cottage cheese.
- Crisp breads, 100% whole grain bread or other unrefined starch.
- Nuts (e.g. almonds, walnuts, brazil nuts, hazelnuts).
- Beans or tofu, fish, fowl, or lean meat.

Midafternoon
Same as midmorning

Supper
1. Same selection as lunch, or

2. A selection from the following conservatively cooked vegetables: green beans, onions, spinach, brussels sprouts, green peppers, zucchini, kale, artichokes, cabbage, broccoli, okra, beet tops, or other vegetables, especially those that grow above the ground.
3. Soybeans in any form (beans, tofu, etc.).
4. Whole grain (especially buckwheat or oats).
5. Fish.
6. Fowl or lean meat.
7. A small Jerusalem artichoke (hen's egg size) five times per week, cooked in its own juices in patapar paper (Cayce product).
8. Low-fat dairy protein

Evening
Same as midmorning and midafternoon.
Take 1 tsp brewer's yeast and 1 tsp raw bran three times daily.
A large portion of each meal should include a slow-burning carbohydrate.

Potassium Broth Recipe
See Appendix I (may be taken at any time).

Physiotherapy

- Spinal manipulation to midthoracic area and any other specific lesions once per week for 6-8 weeks; rest 2-3 weeks and repeat 1-2 times.
- Alternate hot and cold compresses over pancreas.
- Castor oil packs (see Appendix I) over entire abdomen from lower ribs to pubis.
- Increased exercise is essential, along with normalization of ideal weight to lean body mass.
- Daily "salt glow": mix 1-2 lb (500 g-1 kg). of salt with water until soupy. Stand in shower and rub the mixture vigorously all over the body. Rinse with cold water and dry briskly with a rough towel.

---

*On doctor's approval.

- Alternate hot and cold showers to increase circulation.
- Alternate hot and cold leg baths to increase local circulation.

Therapeutic Agents

Vitamins and Minerals—Primary
- Vitamin A: 25,000-50,000 IU daily.
- Vitamin B complex: balanced 50 mg 2-3 times daily; essential for proper carbohydrate metabolism and adrenal function. Needed with stress. Lowers need for insulin.
- Vitamin C and bioflavonoids: 3000-12,000 mg daily. Strengthens capillary walls, essential for adrenal function, needed in excess in stress. Potentiates action of insulin, therefore reduces insulin need. Bioflavonoids (1000 mg daily) help prevent and help stop progression of diabetic cataracts. Quercetin, for example, is an aldose reductase inhibitor (aldose reductase converts glucose to sorbitol, which then accumulates in lens tissue; the enzyme is present in retinal cells, the cornea, Schwann cells, nerve tissue and kidney cells, correlating with various diabetic complications).
- Chromium: a good source is glucose tolerance factor (GTF) yeast tablets: 2 mg 1-2 times daily. Recently chromium has been combined with picolinate, which aids the absorption and usage. Dose for chromium picolinate is 400-600 mcg daily. You may also use brewer's yeast with added chromium. Needed in small amounts as catalyst for insulin, to act in the uptake of glucose.
- Vitamin E: 400 IU 2-3 times daily. Beneficial in heart disease, essential for healing, lowers insulin need, improves ability of muscles to take up glucose and store as glycogen. Also is antioxidant, and has anti-platelet activity.
- Essential fatty acids: 2 capsules 3 times daily; use EPA, GLA, or evening primrose oil.

- Vitamin B6: 250 mg twice daily, especially useful in pregnancy-onset diabetes and to prevent complications of arteriosclerosis. Vitamin B6 also helps to restore beta cell function. Vitamin B6 is specifically useful to help diabetic neuropathy. A daily intramuscular dose of 50-100 mg vitamin B6 along with 1 mg of vitamin B12 and 500 mcg folic acid is used until pain reduces in intensity; then the dose and frequency is gradually reduced.
- Vitamin B 12: IM injections to prevent diabetic neuropathy or sublingual form at 2000 mcg daily if IM injections are not available.
- Manganese: 5 mg twice daily. This helps heal the pancreas and acts as a co-factor for essential enzymes involved in glucose metabolism. Deficiency is very common in diabetes.
- Zinc: 15-30 mg twice daily. Essential for insulin secretion.
- Coenzyme Q10: 80 mg daily. Helps stabilize blood sugar levels and improves circulation.
- Quercetin: 100 mg 3 times daily. Protects the lens of the eye from damage. See Vitamin C above.

Vitamins and Minerals— Secondary
- Inositol: 500-1000 mg 3 times daily. Helps prevent and treat diabetic neuropathy.
- Magnesium: 500 mg to 750 mg daily Prevention of heart attacks
- Calcium: 1000-1000 mg daily

Others—Primary
- Brewer's yeast (glucose tolerance factor—GTF): necessary for proper production and utilization of insulin. Animals on GTF-deficient diet soon get diabetes. 1 tsp 3 times daily.
- L-carnitine: 500 mg twice daily, on an empty stomach. Helps to mobilize fat.
- L-glutamine: 500 mg twice daily, on an empty stomach. To reduce sugar cravings.

- Taurine: 500 mg twice daily, on an empty stomach. Helps in the release of insulin.
- Phosphatidylcholine (concentrated): 2-4 capsules 3 times daily, or 1 tbsp liquid 3 times daily.
- EPA (eicosapentaenoic acid): 1 capsule 2-3 times daily.
- Lecithin: 2 tbsp granules (or more).

Others—Secondary

- Garlic: 2 capsules 3 times daily.
- Kelp: 3-4 tablets 2-3 times daily.
- Spirulina: lowers insulin need. 1 tsp 3 times daily.
- Bran: 1 tsp 3 times daily.

With doctor's prescription:

- Raw adrenal tablets.
- Pancreatic enzymes: 1-3 tablets with, or just following, meals. The exocrine function of the pancreas (the secretion of digestive enzymes and bicarbonate) is often even more inhibited in pancreatic exhaustion and insufficiency than is its endocrine function of insulin secretion.
- Atomodine: (do not take with other iodine-containing foods such as kelp).

1 drop twice daily, increasing 1 drop daily until 3-5 drops twice daily are taken; then decrease 1 drop daily until back to original dose. Rest 1-2 weeks and repeat, only with doctor's prescription.

Botanicals

Jambul.
Bilberry: hypoglycemic, and rich in bioflavonoids
Goat's rue: hypoglycemic (inhibits gluconeogenesis), and potentiates the effects of insulin.
Gymnema: a favorite hypoglycemic agent.
Fenugreek.

Note: Diabetes is a serious disorder and should always be monitored by a physician. Sudden change of diet, especially the introduction of brewer's yeast and other factors that tend to reduce insulin need, can cause an unexpectedly low blood sugar unless insulin needs are frequently monitored. No diabetic should ever reduce or stop his or her insulin without being under the care of a physician well aware of the consequences of uncontrolled diabetes.

DIAPER RASH
Ammoniacal Dermatitis, Napkin Rash, Irritant Contact Dermatitis

DEFINITION

A common dermatitis of infants affecting the diaper region with or without secondary infection with bacteria or fungus.

SYMPTOMS

Redness, tenderness, edema, inflammation, thickening of skin, raw, oozing skin; second-

ary yeast infection appears bright red with well-defined borders, and often has distinct red papules.

ETIOLOGICAL CONSIDERATIONS

- Irritant chemicals
  Ammonia and urea from urine; fecal enzymes from stool; detergents

- Moist heat and abrasion
  Plastic diaper covers or plastic diapers
- Allergy
  Citrus; cow's milk; fruit; wheat; other
- Antibiotics
  Allergic reaction; secondary yeast infection (e.g. *Candida albicans*)
- Vitamin B complex deficiency
- Essential fatty acid deficiency
- Saturated fat excess
- Cow's milk; formula

DISCUSSION

Diaper rash affects most babies to some degree periodically throughout infancy. The most common cause is prolonged contact with irritants such as urine, stools, or detergents in the moist, warm environment created by not changing the diaper frequently enough. A local irritation or contact dermatitis develops, confined to the diaper region and thighs, which may be complicated by fungal or bacterial infection.

Although prolonged contact with irritants does play a part in the average case of diaper rash, these rashes frequently are the most obvious symptom or manifestation of a primarily dietary problem. Certainly, direct irritation of the baby's delicate skin by diapers washed with strong detergents and not rinsed well will cause a rash. This type of diaper rash, however, is fairly uncommon. If a mother leaves her baby for prolonged periods in a wet or dirty diaper, a rash will also develop, due to the continual maceration of the skin and the normal urine and fecal irritations. This type of rash is perhaps more common than a detergent-caused rash, but still it is uncommon to find a mother so busy or unconcerned about her baby's comfort as to leave the child too long in such an unpleasant condition.

The real problems causing diaper rash are not usually local hygiene, but dietary. Breast-fed infants may respond with a diaper rash to something the breast-feeding mother eats or drinks, or to any new food

or drink added in her diet. Unless the mother becomes aware of this relationship, a slight rash can develop into a chronic one, which is impossible to remove by normal external measures. The offending food in the mother's diet may be literally anything, but citrus or acid foods are the most common. Nearly every infant will develop a diaper rash if the mother eats an excess of vitamin C, pineapples, or oranges. Later, as weaning begins, a diaper rash usually indicates a food sensitivity. This may be due to adding a food too rapidly to the diet, or in too concentrated a form. It may, however, be a true allergic reaction. In either case, this reaction must be carefully watched for and the offending food totally eliminated for 4-6 weeks or longer, and then slowly reintroduced. Often no reaction will occur the second time, but if it does, discontinue the food and introduce it much later in the weaning process.

Cow's milk is another common offender and may represent a true allergy or a reaction to excess saturated fat. In general we suggest discontinuing cow's milk permanently. Goat's milk seems to be much better tolerated and may be used as a dairy source by most infants and children.

Wheat or gluten grains are always suspect with diaper rashes. We usually advise that these grains, especially any yeasted preparations, be added as one of the last foods in the weaning process, some time after the first birthday.

Formula-fed infants who develop a rash may have a specific allergic reaction to the type of formula, or may be suffering from exposure to excess saturated fat, vitamin B complex deficiency, or essential fatty acid deficiency.

Many diaper rashes that follow the use of antibiotics for any reason have the possibility of being an antibiotic reaction, or a secondary fungal infection. These occur fairly commonly since antibiotics destroy many friendly bacteria that act to prevent normal and ever-present bacteria and fungi from gaining too strong a foothold.

TREATMENT

Obviously, cure will come only when the cause is removed. No amount of exterior medication will be of lasting benefit if the conditions favorable for the rash development are not removed. We often see unfortunate infants who have received a barrage of corticosteroid creams, nystatin (for *Candida albicans* infection), and even oral antibiotics. Often the distressed parents have taken the child to nearly every pediatrician in town, receiving conflicting diagnoses of anything from simple diaper rash to ringworm complicated with yeast infection and staph. These cases are very upsetting, especially since the rash is usually of internal dietary origin and could have been treated easily and rapidly in its early stages. Once the local skin has been severely inflamed and thickened, a chronic condition settles in, which can take months of proper therapy to remove. From our experience, the use of corticosteroid creams should be forbidden for the treatment of diaper rash. All that it does is calm the inflammation down for a short period, and once its use is discontinued, the rash flares up again with a vengeance.

Diet

Once a rash has been allowed to develop for any extended period of time, great difficulties arise in finding which particular aspect of the mother's (if breast-feeding) or baby's diet is at fault. Sometimes the infant must be totally reweaned, a very painful process for baby and mother alike. Before this is resorted to, it is often sufficient to analyze both mother's and infant's diet to first attempt to exclude the probable offender. This is usually easier than it sounds. The mother is placed on a highly nutritious, mostly vegetarian diet, excluding citrus fruit, citrus juices, tomatoes, strong spices, alcohol, coffee, and any junk foods. Fruit and fruit juice, even non-citrus juice, is either excluded or drastically reduced. Raw salads

are encouraged at least twice daily. 1–2 glasses of carrot juice should be taken daily. All supplements are discontinued except for vitamin A, vitamin B complex, vitamin E, essential fatty acids, and zinc. The infant's diet must be analyzed individually, depending on age and progression in the weaning process. The most commonly offending foods are fruits and fruit juices, especially citrus; also tomatoes, and wheat or other gluten grain, although literally any food may be a factor. The above foods are totally excluded from the diet. Little or no fruits are allowed. The bulk of the diet should be vegetables and brown rice, if grains have already been introduced. Carrot juice is also encouraged, 1–2 times daily. Formula-fed infants are converted to goat's milk. The infant supplements are the same as for the breast-feeding mother, except in much smaller doses.

Physiotherapy

Although the most common cause of the problem is internal and dietetic, attention must still be given to local therapy.

- Diapers. The best diaper for an infant with a rash is no diaper at all. Keep the child bare and exposed to air and sunlight as much as the climate will permit. When diapers must be worn, make sure that the diaper is antiseptically cleaned and well rinsed or, use disposable diapers. Change the diaper frequently. Wash the area with cool water and gently dab dry using a soft cotton diaper. Apply prescribed powder, oil, or cream as discussed below, depending on the type of rash. Make sure the area is completely dry before applying cream or oil medication, to prevent water from being trapped below this layer.
- Ultraviolet light or sunlight. Expose the infant to small daily doses of sunlight or ultraviolet light. Be careful not to burn the baby's very thin and sensitive skin. No ocean swimming is allowed until the rash is gone. Fresh pool water, especially

rainwater, is fine. If the climate is agreeable, let the child play for hours in the pool, under supervision, of course. It is best if the water is very cold. This should only be done on a warm and sunny day to prevent the onset of hypothermia. Vinegar added to the pool water is useful.

Therapeutic Agents

Vitamins and Minerals

- Essential fatty acids: 4 capsules 3–4 times daily for the mother; contents of 1–2 capsules 2–3 times daily for the infant. GLA (gamma-linoleic acid) is a good source.
- Zinc: 30 mg 2–3 times daily for the mother; a quarter to a half of a 15 mg tablet twice daily for the infant; or 2 drops of liquid zinc, 2 times daily.
- Vitamin A: 25,000 IU 3 times daily for the mother; 2000–5000 IU 3 times daily for the infant. (See warning under Vitamin Toxicity, page 56.)
- Vitamin B complex: 50 mg 3 times daily for the mother; 10–25 mg 2–3 times daily for the infant. Use yeast-free sources in cases of yeast infections.
- Vitamin E: 400 IU twice daily for the mother; 25–40 IU twice daily for the infant.
- Evening primrose oil: 1 capsule twice daily for the infant.

Local Applications

Different combinations of local therapies are effective in individual cases. Sometimes trial and error is the only way to determine which will be most effective. Naturopathic physicians tailor each medication to the individual, using a little more or less of a particular ingredient, depending on the case history and how the rash presents itself. The following applications or combinations of these are effective:

- Powders: calendula powder; clay; slippery elm powder; comfrey powder; Peruvian balsam powder; zinc stearate powder; goldenseal powder; lycopodium powder.

- Ointments and oils: calendula cream; tea tree oil (antibiotic, antifungal); vitamins A and D ointment; liquid lecithin; lanolin; gentian violet (for yeast infection). Apply twice daily. Combine: 3 parts castor oil, 1 part tea tree oil, $\frac{1}{2}$ part Peruvian balsam tincture. Apply every 2 hours after a mild green soap wash.
- Another approach is to powder by day and oil at night. A useful combination of powders includes: clay, 4 parts; zinc stearate, $\frac{1}{2}$ part; Peruvian balsam powder, $\frac{1}{2}$ part; slippery elm powder, $\frac{1}{2}$ part; comfrey powder, $\frac{1}{2}$ part; calendula powder, $\frac{1}{2}$ part. Powder after each diaper change, at least every 2 hours. At night apply the above oil or calendula cream, liquid lecithin, or other water-repellent medicinal ointment.
- A further useful approach is to apply liquid lecithin day and night every 2–4 hours.
- A useful preventative (and part of many treatment regimens) is to wash the diaper region with dilute vinegar—1 to 2 tbsp per 2 pints (1 liter) of water. Repeat with each diaper change. Often this is the only treatment needed.
- Others: aloe; cod-liver oil; vitamin E; poke root ointment (for ringworm); evening primrose oil; tincture of green soap.

Botanicals (External)

Aloe.
Calendula.
Comfrey.
Peruvian bark: combined with castor oil for ringworm.
Poke root (highly toxic, see page 60).
Slippery elm.
Tea tree oil.

Therapeutic Suggestions

If the rash has a definite bacterial infection, begin therapy with a mild tincture of green soap wash, hydrogen peroxide rinse, and tea tree oil applications repeated every 2-3 hours for about 7-14 days. This is an effective procedure for use in bacterial and fungal rashes.

Mild, uncomplicated diaper rash usually responds to changes in mother's diet, or possibly a change of diaper type. (Some diaper service diapers are good to prevent rashes, while others cause diaper rashes; and some infants do better with cloth diapers, others with disposable diapers.) We rarely use therapeutic supplements for infants with mild rashes; more prolonged or severe rashes may need them. Vitamin A, B complex, zinc, and essential fatty acids are often useful. The most useful powder and cream is calendula for mild rashes. A cod-liver oil and zinc oxide ointment such as desitin is also useful. *Be sure to change diapers frequently.*

DIARRHEA

DEFINITION AND SYMPTOMS

Frequent loose and watery stools with or without gas or abdominal discomfort.

ETIOLOGICAL CONSIDERATIONS

Infant

- Overfeeding
- Allergy
- Mother's diet
- Bottle feeding (rare in breast-fed infants)
- Teething Infection (viral or bacterial)
- Or other causes, as for adults.

Adult

- Food allergy (milk—lactose intolerance); wheat (celiac disease, others); gastritis; colitis
- Food poisoning; infection (viral or bacterial); water supply; overeating; intestinal parasites; digestive enzyme deficiency; heavy metal poisoning; toxicity; stress, fear, emotional upset; pancreas, adrenal malfunction; anemia; excess vitamin C; antibiotic use

DISCUSSION

It is important to remember that diarrhea is a symptom and not a disease. Nearly every person will suffer an occasional bout of diarrhea. This may be due to gastric flu, mild food poisoning, or simply injudicious eating. These acute episodes are usually of short duration and are the result of the body's attempts at internal cleansing and purging. As such they should not be suppressed, but encouraged. If, however, a loose bowel condition becomes chronic, a serious problem exists. With each passing day of chronic diarrhea nutrients are lost in the stool, lowering general vitality and creating a vicious cycle of downgraded health.

It is extremely important to resolve acute diarrhea of infants as soon as possible, to prevent severe dehydration with catastrophic results. Episodes of infantile diarrhea occur much more frequently among bottle-fed babies, with gastroenteritis being a serious threat to the bottle-fed child under 6 months of age. Most children at some time will suffer periods of diarrhea with colds, gastric flu, or even teething. Many food sensitivities, intolerances, or allergies first manifest themselves with bouts of diarrhea which may later become chronic, or paradoxically, disappear altogether if the condition is not attended to. In this case the more superficial reaction of loose bowels has been replaced by progressively deeper symptoms.

Breast-fed infants may respond with diarrhea to foods in the mother's diet. Severe dehydration from violent or prolonged diarrhea (six or more watery stools daily in the absence of oral fluid intake) may occur rapidly in infancy or childhood. *These cases require hospitalization for intravenous replacement of fluids. Never attempt to treat severe diarrhea at home without medical supervision.*

Diarrhea occurring later in life may have many possible causes. Food allergy is one of the commonest factors, with gluten (see Celiac Disease) or lactose (milk sugar) intolerances being fairly common. Other foods may cause similar reactions. Gastritis and colitis are also a cause of loose bowels. Improper diet and stress are the usual factors involved in these cases. A digestive enzyme deficiency will cause food to pass undigested into the lower bowel, causing fermentation and diarrhea. This may be congenital or acquired, due to overeating, stress, glandular imbalance, or old age. Severe B complex deficiencies and anemia will also result in diarrhea. On the other hand, excess supplementation with vitamin C and sometimes zinc will cause intestinal irritation and diarrhea. Many cases of chronic bowel irritability can be traced to parasitic infection and is corrected once these are removed. Acute and chronic diarrhea is also frequently found to be caused by the water supply, especially in areas on water catchment systems. A history of previous antibiotic therapy just prior to the onset of diarrhea pinpoints this as a cause of altered internal ecology, a frequent cause of loose bowels.

TREATMENT

Obviously, the treatment chosen will depend on the type of diarrhea, acute or chronic, and its cause.

Acute diarrhea is an action by the body to re-establish internal equilibrium. This purging action is a self-defense mechanism to rid the body of unwanted and possibly dangerous material as rapidly as possible. This acute internal cleansing should never be suppressed. One of the oldest and most effective therapies for acute diarrhea is to fast and encourage further elimination with a purge and an enema. By fasting, the irritated digestive system is given a chance to rest and heal. Occasionally an enema may help flush the system rapidly. This should not be done if colitis is suspected. Diarrhea of infancy can be extremely dangerous. Any diarrhea in infants that does not clear in 24 hours should be seen by a physician.

Be sure enough fluids are taken to prevent dehydration. This is extremely important. Several foods and drinks have been found useful to control acute diarrhea after the initial fasting period of 1–3 days. These include the following:

- Green apples (no skin); bananas (remove central vein of banana); carob powder (rich in pectin) and amaranth powder; barley water; carrot and cabbage juice; carrot soup.
- Yoghurt; white toasted bread (this is an old treatment from the original works of Hippocrates). We have found it quite useful. Eat only well-toasted 100% refined white bread for 1–2 days. This is just about the only use we have ever found for white bread.
- Slippery elm tea; blackberry leaf tea or juice; sauerkraut and tomato juice: 1 tbsp of each every hour.

Acute diarrhea should not last longer than 2–3 days. If it is not getting better with only clear fluids at this time, it may be considered *chronic diarrhea,* which may be much more difficult to treat. The source of the loose bowel condition must be traced and eliminated. Refer to Colitis, Digestive Disturbances, Celiac Disease, or other related topics in this book. The following dietary suggestions may be useful in individual cases:

- Green apple mono diet (no skin).
- Bananas plus carob powder; yoghurt.

- Yoghurt plus carob powder (equal portions).
- Brown rice mono diet.
- Blackberry juice and gelatin.

Therapeutic Agents

Vitamins and Minerals—Primary

- Liquid B complex: 25-50 mg twice daily, plus B complex and B12 intramuscular injection 1-3 times per week.
- Potassium: 100 mg daily. Needed to replace the potassium lost in loose stools.

Vitamins and Minerals—Primary

- Vitamin B3: if long-term or pellagra-type syndrome exists.
- Vitamin A (micellized): 10,000-25,000 IU 1-4 times daily. (See warning under Vitamin Toxicity, page 56.)
- Folic acid, glutamine, and zinc: to reverse damage to intestinal villi.
- Magnesium supplementation may be in order if there is any cramping pain.

Others—Primary

- Non-wheat bran (psyllium): can be very beneficial in some chronic cases.
- Probiotics: 1 tsp powder 3-4 times daily. Useful in correcting proper bowel ecology.
- Pectin: a bulking agent, useful in most cases. The apple mono diet is high in pectin, and is the basis for its use.
- Psyllium powder: (2 heaped tsp in a small amount of pure apple juice).

Others—Secondary

- Pancreatic enzymes: when chronic, due to digestive enzyme deficiency.
- Chlorophyll: to heal mucosa.
- Charcoal tablets.
- Garlic capsules for infective causes.

Drinks—Primary

- Raspberry juice: 3-4 cups daily, astringent.

- Peppermint tea.
- Distilled water: water is always the best for short duration cases where fluid loss has not been too severe, resulting in extreme electrolyte loss.

Drinks—Secondary

- Carrot juice and cabbage juice.
- Meadowsweet tea.
- Chamomile tea; slippery elm tea.
- Blackberry juice or tea.
- Raspberry leaf tea and cinnamon (or oak if severe); ½ tsp 4-6 times daily for patient under 1 year.
- Barley water.

Botanicals—Primary

Blackberry tea: 3-4 cups daily. Astringent; especially good for children.
Cranesbill: astringent.
Marshmallow: soothing.

Botanicals—Secondary

Amaranth: astringent.
Cinnamon: astringent, hemostatic. Use strong tea, 4-6 times daily, or 10-30 drops tincture in warm water.
Goldenseal: especially if chronic, helps to restore structure and function of the bowel wall
Oak bark tea: astringent.
Peppermint essence: 3-15 drops every 2-3 hours.
Spotted cranesbill: used especially with blood loss. *Note:* blood loss could be an indication of a serious problem and anyone with this symptom should always be seen by a doctor.
Tormentil.
Wild yam: antispasmodic, where there is pain with spasm.
Witch hazel: astringent. Used as dilute retention enema.

Therapeutic Suggestions

Be careful not to give too many medications and thus further irritate the condition. Keep therapy simple whenever possible. Use all supplements with caution in this and other irritable bowel complaints. The best therapy is a water fast for 1–3 days for both acute and chronic cases. Chronic cases require intramuscular vitamin injections and the use of botanicals. Diarrhea due to parasites may be best treated with ortho-dox measures.

DIGESTIVE DISORDERS
(Gastritis, Heartburn, Indigestion)

DEFINITION AND SYMPTOMS

Acute or chronic abdominal discomfort, pain, irritation, bloating or gas, often accompanied by general malaise, headache, nausea, and sometimes vomiting.

ETIOLOGICAL CONSIDERATIONS—PRIMARY

- Improper diet
- Refined carbohydrates and sugar; poor food combinations; overeating; insufficient chewing of foods; hurried meals; too-frequent meals (snacking); strong spices; salt; coffee, tea, alcohol, carbonated beverages; drinking with meals; acid-forming foods
- Excessively hot or cold foods; food additives, preservatives, colorings; food allergy or digestive incompatibility (milk, wheat, etc.)
- Stress
- Digestive enzyme deficiency
- Hydrochloric acid deficiency common in older age groups

ETIOLOGICAL CONSIDERATIONS—SECONDARY

- Constipation; smoking; *Candida albicans* overgrowth; bacterial overgrowth; drugs (aspirin and others); spinal lesions; psychological; heavy metals; aluminum cookware
- Water catchment systems; obesity; pregnancy; hiatal hernia; gallbladder disease
- Hypothyroidism (hydrochloric acid deficiency associated); liver disease; ulcer; lack of exercise

DISCUSSION

Indigestion, heartburn, and gastritis are not really diseases in themselves, but are symptoms of abnormal digestion. The usual treatment for these common problems is the prescription of antacid medications aimed at removing the unpleasant symptoms without attempting in any way to treat the cause. Sodium bicarbonate preparations are the most frequently used antacids. This rapidly neutralizes gastric acid and will relieve heartburn caused by excess acid. Used on a regular basis, however, it disturbs the body's acid/alkaline balance, creating a condition of alkalosis. Sustained alkalosis with a substantial intake of calcium in the form of milk or calcium-containing antacids creates milk–alkali syndrome, causing irreversible kidney damage. Clearly this "cure" is not as benign as the commercials would have us believe.

The real causes of these digestive disorders are usually very simple to diagnose and treat. The largest number of factors, obviously, center around diet. We are constantly amazed at the incredible combinations some people cram into their mouths. We begin the treatment of all digestive complaints by asking the patient to compile a list of everything he or she eats, solid or

217

liquid, for a 3-day period. The results are usually quite revealing.

Following is a summary of the most common dietary mistakes.

Consumption of refined carbohydrates (especially sugar): Refined carbohydrates cause a rapid secretion of gastric acid. This acid is normally buffered by the protein content of a food substance. In this case the bran and fiber have been removed through the refining process, with the end result being excess gastric acidity. Sugar is the worst offender in this class since it is devoid of any real substances whatsoever for the acid stimulated to work upon. (For more detail see Peptic Ulcer.)

Poor food combinations: The average person pays absolutely no attention to proper food combinations. Often a meal will consist of raw fruit, cooked fruit, raw vegetables, cooked vegetables, soups, several types of protein, starch, coffee, alcohol, and sweets. Indigestion, here we come! Always keep meals simple and never combine:

• Fruit with vegetables.
• Fruit (especially citrus) with starches Liquids with solids.

Some nutritional advisers warn against eating starches with proteins due to their different requirements for digestion. This, however, does not seem logically possible since many foods are composed of a large percentage of starch and protein. With specific reference to concentrated starches and concentrated protein, Airola suggests in *How To Get Well* and *Everywoman's Book* to eat proteins first. This allows for their normal exposure to the stomach's hydrochloric acid, which is essential in protein digestion, but not that of carbohydrate. The person with an average healthy stomach, however, can ignore this rule.)

Excessively large meals: When the stomach is overloaded the amount needed to be digested can exceed the body's supply of digestive enzymes. Food then passes into the lower small intestine, is only partly broken down, and causes fermentation, indigestion, and gas. Never eat until completely full.

Too-frequent meals: If food is eaten too soon after a previous meal its normal digestive process is disturbed. It is usually best to allow at least $1\frac{1}{2}$ hours after a fruit meal, 2-$2\frac{1}{2}$ hours after a vegetable meal, and $3\frac{1}{4}$-4 hours after a combined meal with proteins, carbohydrates, and fat. Be especially careful to allow complete digestion of a starchy meal before having any fruit, especially citrus.

Insufficient chewing of foods: The digestive enzyme salivary amylase (ptyalin) initiates carbohydrate digestion of starch in the mouth and continues to act for 20-30 minutes in the stomach before it is inactivated by gastric acid production. Chewing stimulates salivary amylase secretions, breaks food down into smaller particles for more complete exposure for enzymatic digestion, and also stimulates secretion of digestive enzymes in the stomach, pancreas, and small intestine for further digestion. Chewing is especially essential to break down the indigestible walls of cellulose found in all vegetables, to expose their inner food substances to digestive juices. The habit of bolting down food in hurried meals is a major cause of indigestion.

Drinking with meals: Any liquids taken with solid meals dilute the action of digestive juices, making complete digestion more difficult. This applies to any drinks, even soup. These should be taken at least 15 minutes before other foods are eaten and not sooner than $\frac{1}{2}$ hour afterwards.

The use of strong spices or other gastric irritants: Salt is the most common irritant to the stomach. It causes extreme acidity and irritates the delicate mucous membranes. Other irritants include sugar, pepper, curries, coffee, soda, and alcohol.

Excess acid-forming foods: Overconsumption of refined carbohydrates, sugar, and other acid-forming foods is a common finding. Green vegetables are the best alkaline elements for proper pH balancing.

Excessively hot or cold foods: These irritate the delicate stomach linings which cannot cry out with pain since they have little sensation of temperature. This is why food that burns your mouth or esophagus no longer hurts once it reaches the stomach. If done repeatedly the stomach becomes deranged and poor digestion results.

Eating under stress: When food is eaten under stressful conditions, or when anxiety, anger, or other similar emotions are present, digestion is severely disturbed. The emotions cause the parasympathetic branch of the nervous system, responsible for normal digestive enzyme secretion and gastric motility, to cease functioning so that the sympathetic branch of the nervous system may prepare for what it interprets as an emergency situation. Always spend 10-15 minutes in some quiet, soothing activity before meals. Prayer or a few minutes of meditation before meals is also advisable.

Eating when sick: All animals fast during an illness. This is nature's law and should be followed.

Fried foods: Deep frying makes any food difficult to digest and may be a factor in the high incidence of stomach cancer in civilized nations.

Although disregard of the above rules of eating are the major causes of indigestion, other factors may exist.

Food allergy: This is a fairly common cause of digestive upset. Milk and wheat are the two most frequent offenders, but any food may be at fault. This disturbance may be caused by a true allergy or simply a food intolerance due to a specific digestive enzyme deficiency such as the lactase deficiency of milk intolerance.

Other digestive enzyme deficiencies: These can cause gastric disturbances in the digestion of carbohydrates, proteins, or fat. These may be associated with a disorder of the pancreas, liver, or gallbladder.

Hydrochloric acid (stomach acid) deficiency: This is a common problem (especially in the over-50 age group) causing gas, bloating, poor protein digestion, and chronic malabsorption of most minerals and some vitamins. Although we frequently associate hyperacidity with heartburn symptoms, in fact hyperacidity is a very rare

condition. Hypoacidity is the much more common cause of this condition.

This point deserves more attention. So often, antacid medications are sought (by the patient, over the counter) or prescribed (and this is negligence if it is done, as is so often the case, without proper testing and diagnosis), the thinking being that there is too much acid in the stomach, causing heartburn. In fact, too little acid is most likely to be the cause; when there is some stress going on, or when you're rushing, or the food is rich, or there is too much protein present, the stomach will not be secreting enough hydrochloric acid or digestive juices, so it will signal with a little reflux to tell you it doesn't want the contents in the stomach. What little acid that might be there will enter the lower esophagus and cause the sensation of "burning", another of Nature's warning wonderful messages not to do it again. The problem is, we either do not heed the message, or we misinterpret the message and so "treat" the messenger (the pain) instead of listening to and heeding the message. The long-term consequences of antacid usage is that you will not be digesting foods (especially proteins) very well, and you will be at risk of nutrient deficiency, which places you at risk for the diseases of older age, including cancer.

Hydrochloric acid deficiency is also associated with many other digestive complaints, as well as with hypothyroidism, asthma, allergies, rheumatoid arthritis, osteoporosis, lupus, pernicious anemia, diabetes, systemic candidiasis, chronic hepatitis, intestinal parasites, eczema, vitiligo, and others. Milk consumption is a common cause or aggravating factor in many cases, since it takes so much hydrochloric acid to acidify milk, leaving little or no reserve for other protein in the meal. The result is incomplete breakdown of protein, causing gas, bloating, and other more systemic problems such as allergy.

Emotional causes: Stress and other destructive emotions upset the normal digestive cycle, making even the best of food indigestible. Prolonged stress, anger, or worry also create an acidic condition of the entire body.

Spinal lesions in the thoracic region: These can alter the nerve and blood supply to the stomach or other organs of digestion, making normal function impossible. This area should always be treated in cases of chronic indigestion.

Heavy metal poisoning: This may be a factor in some cases. Certainly the use of aluminum cookware is to be avoided, especially if indigestion is a problem. Many other heavy metals may produce the same effects (see Heavy Metal Poisoning).

Some indigestion during pregnancy is normal. This may be minimized by proper diet with plenty of alkaline foods such as vegetables and proper exercise. Avoid large meals if this is a problem, in preference to 4–6 smaller ones.

TREATMENT

Diet

For acute or chronic indigestion the first course of action is always to fast. Any of the following fasts are used with this complaint:

- Water with a twist of lemon; dilute apple juice; carrot juice; carrot and cabbage juice.
- Slippery elm tea.

These may be followed by a mono diet regimen such as:

- Apple mono diet; carrot mono diet; brown rice diet.

In severe cases strict regimens similar to those found under Colitis or Peptic Ulcer are needed.

In cases where *Candida albicans* overgrowth is suspected from the case history and symptomatology (gas, bloating, rectal itching, ear itching, vaginitis, constipation, diarrhea, nail bed fungus, infantile colic, depression, fatigue, skin rashes, allergies, psoriasis, autoimmune diseases, antibiotic use, and contraceptive pill use) the dietary regimen and supplement plan are a bit different. The emphasis still is to avoid refined

carbohydrates and excess fruit or fruit juice, since yeast grows best in a highly refined carbohydrate diet. A yeast-free diet is also recommended, even though the yeast in foods is a different type of yeast from Candida. A significant proportion of patients report aggravation of a yeast infection upon consumption of yeasted foods. Yeast-free vitamin supplements are to be used as well. The main portion of the diet should be vegetables and proteins. Non-glutinous grains (such as rice, millet, spelt or corn) seem to be better tolerated during the regimen. Garlic is useful, in the diet and in supplement form. Acidophilus in the form of yoghurt or in supplement form (probiotics) is beneficial when taken several times each day. Used to inhibit yeast growth are biotin, garlic, caprillic acid, aloe vera juice, olive oil, and the anti-yeast herb taheebo. Many cases require nystatin for 2–6 months. However, with a change of bowel ecology from proper diet, and possibly hydrochloric acid supplementation (yeast grows poorly with adequate hydrochloric acid secretions), this may sometimes be avoided, but the treatment program is prolonged, and the diet must be adhered to rigidly.

Therapeutic Agents

Vitamins and Minerals
- Vitamin A: 10,000–25,000 IU 1–2 times daily.
- Vitamin B complex (liquid): 25–50 mg 1–2 times daily.
- Vitamin B12 (may require intramuscular injection if hypoacidity is a problem).
- Folic acid.
- Vitamin C: sodium ascorbate if hyperacid; ascorbic acid if hypoacid.
- Vitamin E: 400 IU twice daily.

Other—Primary
- Hydrochloric acid: if hypoacid. Capsules work best when 20–40 grains are taken before meals as the adult dose, 10–20 grains for children. If this causes discomfort, begin with a 5–10 grain

dose and increase after 3-5 days. Some cases need very slow acid increase and may require the gradual introduction of lemon juice and water—1-8 fl oz (30-250 mL), gradually increasing to a 50/50 mixture, to accustom the stomach to acid before hydrochloric acid capsule supplementation.

- Pancreatic digestive enzymes.
- Probiotics: to normalize bowel ecology.

Other—Secondary

- Bromelain enzyme.
- Charcoal tablets: 1 tablet every 1-2 hours in acute cases.
- Aloe vera juice: 2 fl oz (60 mL) 3 times daily.
- Fiber: e.g. psyllium powder.
- Kelp.
- Lemon juice.
- Papaya enzyme.
- Pepsin.
- Sodium alginate.
- Soured milk or yoghurt.

Botanicals

The choice of a particular botanical formulation will depend precisely on just what the problems are, but the following herbs are commonly used in various gastric upset type conditions

Angelica.

Anise.

Chamomile: anti-inflammatory and sedative.

Comfrey.

Dandelion.

Fennel.

Ginger root: anti-nausea and anti-inflammatory.

Goldenseal: especially if chronic.

Meadowsweet: helps normalize stomach acid.

Peppermint.

Slippery elm.

Therapeutic Suggestions

Begin therapy with fast and diet changes. Only use supplements and botanicals later if still required. Often, they are not.

DIVERTICULITIS AND DIVERTICULOSIS

DEFINITION

Diverticula: spherical pouches protruding from the lumen of the intestine through the bowel wall. Most commonly found in the sigmoid colon.

Diverticulosis: uncomplicated diverticula.

Diverticulitis: diverticula with inflammation present.

SYMPTOMS

Diverticulosis often causes no symptoms or may cause irritable colon symptoms (may be coincident).

Diverticulitis: Symptoms of "left-sided appendicitis"

- Pain in lower left quadrant.
- Nausea, vomiting, abdominal distention, colic.
- Constipation and/or diarrhea (may alternate).
- Tenderness, fever if infection is present.
- Fiber deficiency.
- Refined diet; white bread; white rice.
- Constipation.

ETIOLOGICAL CONSIDERATIONS— SECONDARY

Nutritional deficiency: muscular weakness in intestinal wall; obesity; visceroptosis (poor abdominal tone, prolapse, poor spinal mechanics); spinal (poor abdominal circulation of blood and lymph); stress (reduced peristalsis); poor bowel habits; thyroid deficiency; adhesions due to previous appendectomy; spastic colon; allergy (especially to dairy products)

DISCUSSION

Diverticulitis is another of the "civilized diseases". While 30% of Americans over 45 suffer the discomfort of diverticular disease, it is extremely rare in undeveloped nations living on a diet of unrefined foods. It has become increasingly obvious that our low-fiber diet of highly refined foods is the major cause of diverticulitis and colon cancer.

Diverticulitis occurs when the neck of the diverticulum becomes blocked by swelling or feces. This causes a condition of stasis which favors bacterial invasion. An abscess may form and spasm may result in intestinal destruction. This in itself may require surgery. Perforation of the abscess may also occur, leading to peritonitis, a severe surgical emergency. Healing of any of these complications may result in fibrosis and narrowing of the colon. This in turn may later require surgery. As you can see, prevention in this case is much better than cure.

Diverticula become filled with bacteria in many cases and these consume a large amount of B vitamins. Occult blood loss also may occur, explaining the commonly associated condition of anemia found so often in diverticular patients.

Clearly, since a lack of fiber is the major cause, the commonly employed low-fiber diet is not the best treatment. Lack of fiber in the diet causes chronic poor eliminations and constipation. This constipation in turn causes an increase in the gas pressure against the colon walls. To make the situation even more conducive to diverticula formation, the low-residue, low-fiber diet takes 2–3 times as long to pass through the colon. This encourages excessive water absorption and leaves a very concentrated small stool, which is very difficult to expel and demands more forceful peristaltic contraction to move it along its course. The excess work puts increased pressure on the colon walls, helping to produce outpouchings of diverticula.

A high-fiber diet composed of unrefined grains and raw fruits and vegetables helps prevent diverticular disease and favors proper intestinal action in several ways. On such a diet the stools are 2–3 times as bulky as those formed on a low-fiber diet. The fiber absorbs water, making a softer stool that is passed easily with less forceful peristaltic contractions. Transit time is also reduced, with an average of 12–24 hours as compared to 36 hours (or significantly longer) on a low-residue diet.

Contrary to the situation with a low-fiber diet where the excess abnormal bacteria produce harmful carcinogenic substances from normal bile acids, cellulose actually encourages friendly bacterial development, which in turn produces several of the B complex vitamins for use by the body. In addition, while a low-fiber diet with its sticky feces tends to cake the intestinal membrane, fiber will help clean these walls and stimulate local circulation.

TREATMENT

While a low-fiber diet is the major cause of diverticular disease, often the initial stages of treatment actually require adherence to a low-fiber diet. This, however, is of short duration, lasting only as long as it is necessary to be able to reduce local irritation. Once the inflammatory stage of diverticulitis is under control, the gradual introduction of high-fiber foods is essential to reach maximum results.

Diet—Acute

Choose from any of the following, consuming only one type of liquid at any single meal:

- Water (best fast, but most difficult); carrot juice; carrot and lettuce juice.
- Celery and lettuce juice; beetroot juice; watercress juice; grape juice.
- Apple juice; slippery elm tea; comfrey tea
- Marshmallow tea; chlorophyll liquid; Spirulina liquid drinks.

This liquid diet (fast) should be continued until all painful symptoms have subsided. At this point semisolids may be added slowly and carefully, watching for any adverse reaction. Add papaya, mashed banana, steamed carrots, baked yams, or sweet potatoes.

Once it becomes apparent that these foods are well tolerated, other cooked and pureéd foods of higher fiber content may be added. Some people at this stage can handle grated raw foods. Begin with raw grated apple and raw grated carrot. It still will be necessary to avoid fruit skins and fruit, and fruit and vegetables with small hard seeds such as tomatoes, cucumbers, figs, strawberries, raspberries, guavas, etc.

The next stage includes addition of grains and proteins. Brown rice well cooked and well masticated is a good initial choice of grains. Tofu and steamed fish are good proteins. Once these are well tolerated the diet can rapidly be expanded to include all natural unrefined food. Thorough mastication is absolutely essential in the initial stages of this diet.

Most patients can be weaned to a high-fiber diet fully in 6–8 weeks. This diet will then help heal the intestinal walls and prevent further severe attacks of diverticulitis. In long-standing cases the diverticula may remain, as shown by x-ray, for years. Others simply never go away. Most cases, however, remain symptom-free irrespective of the presence of old diverticula as long as the high-fiber diet is adhered to and bowel eliminations remain regular.

Physiotherapy—Acute

- Castor oil packs (see Appendix I).
- Alternate hot and cold sitz baths: very beneficial for long-term cure.
- Cold trunk packs: tonic effects.
- Hot moist compress: pain relief.
- Hot sitz bath: pain relief.

Spinal Manipulation

Twice per week for 3–4 weeks; 2 weeks off, then repeat three times or as required.

Therapeutic Agents

Vitamins and Minerals— Primary

- Vitamin C with bioflavonoids: 250–1000 mg 2–6 times daily.
- Zinc: 25–50 mg, 2–3 times daily.

Vitamins and Minerals— Secondary

- Vitamin A: 10,000–25,000 IU 2–6 times daily in acute cases; for maintenance 1–2 times daily. (See warning under Vitamin Toxicity, page 56.)
- Vitamin B complex: 25–50 mg 1–3 times daily. Liquid B complex may be best in these conditions.
- Vitamin E: 400–800 IU daily.

Other—Primary

- Atomodine: at doctor's prescription: 1 drop for 7 days; 5 days off 2 drops for 7 days; 5 days off 3 drops for 7 days; 5 days off (repeat 2–3 times).
- Psyllium powder/husks 3 times daily: (3–5 tsp daily). Helps normalize bowel function and establish more normal bowel ecology.
- Probiotics: especially *Bifidobacterium bifidis* and *Lactobacillus bulgaricus*. 2 capsules 3 times daily. Helps correct bowel ecology.
- Raw, unprocessed, finely milled oat bran and soaked prunes.

Other—Secondary

- Pancreatic enzymes: with meals where digestive enzyme deficiency exists.
- Garlic.
- Hydrochloric acid: if hypoacid.
- Liquid chlorophyll.
- Molasses: helps correct bowel function. Also molasses, mashed banana, and low-fat yoghurt.

Botanicals

Slippery elm: $^1/_2$ tsp in warm water 3-4 times daily. Demulcent; soothes mucous membranes.

Comfrey: with slippery elm as a warm tea, 3-4 times daily.

Ginger root: anti-inflammatory.

Goldenseal: cholagogue, antimicrobial, mucous trophorestorative.

Marshmallow: to soothe inflamed tissue.

Picrorrhiza kurroa: to stimulate the immune system.

Wild yam root: for colic.

Therapeutic Suggestions

In general, the diet change is 90% of the solution. Bran helps add fiber and speeds up normal bowel function. Stick to the high-fiber approach even with 7-10 days of gas or discomfort. Your body is readjusting. Add supplements later in the regimen. Mild botanicals such as slippery elm may be taken early on without aggravation. The daily consumption of 6-8 large glasses of water is a very useful aid to proper bowel function, especially in conjunction with the bran.

EARACHE
(Otitis Externa and Otitis Media)

DEFINITION

Otitis externa: inflammation and infection of external ear.

Otitis media: inflammation, infection, or serous congestion of middle ear.

SYMPTOMS

Infective: pain, fever, throbbing, discharge

Serous: feeling of fullness, loss of hearing acuity, little or no pain, ringing in ears

ETIOLOGICAL CONSIDERATIONS

- Diet
  Excess mucus-forming foods; allergy (cow's milk, wheat, other); green vegetable deficiency; refined diet; excess sugar
- Lowered immunity
  Diet; stress
- Preceding infection
  Colds; measles; mumps; pneumonia; tonsillitis; enlarged adenoids (common before puberty); localized boil, external
- Improper treatment of acute disease
- Repeated antibiotic use
- Bacterial infected swimming water
- Excess earwax
- EFA deficiency
- Impacted wax
- "Q-tip syndrome"
- Forceful clearing of nose
- Breast-feeding while lying down

DISCUSSION

Ear infections affect most people at some time in their lives, usually following an upper respiratory infection. They are often the result of blocked Eustachian tubes.

Eustachian tubes allow air to be behind the ear drum, to allow the "drum" to resonate. For whatever the reason, when this narrow tube becomes clogged up with mucus, the accumulated mucus within the ear acts as a medium for bacterial proliferation. Infants are particularly susceptible to this problem and may develop an ear infection with nearly any viral or bacterial upper respiratory infection. Other less commonly related agents are allergies, nursing while lying down, and second-hand smoke. Many chronic or recurrent middle ear infections have a nutritional basis, in which excessive amounts of mucus are released in the Eustachian tubes causing congestion, and inviting infection.

The average case presents with a diet high in refined mucus-forming foods and a deficiency of raw green vegetables. This is certainly true with children. Allergy often is related—not the type most doctors blame (dust, molds, grasses, etc.) but food allergies. Dairy and wheat allergies or excess are often a factor with ear problems.

Chronically enlarged adenoids may cause blockage of the Eustachian tubes, leading to congestion and fluid exudation into the middle ear, creating serous otitis media, which may remain uninfected, or act as an ideal medium for bacterial proliferation. Although the adenoids are an immediate and obvious cause of Eustachian tube blockage and therefore ear congestion, the enlarged adenoids, which you cannot see without special equipment, are in reality only symptoms of a deeper disorder. Tonsils or adenoids do not enlarge without a cause, and it is in correcting the conditions that led to their enlargement that a true cure may be found (see Tonsillitis).

Another aspect of improper diet directly related to recurrent infections is decreased immunity. If the diet does not supply essential nutrients for the immunological system, or if stress depletes the body's vital reserves, resistance to infection is reduced. The body is then very susceptible to colds, flu, tonsillitis, and other acute diseases, which may eventually affect the ears. Once a weakness is established in the ears due to damage from an infection, it makes recurrent infections more likely.

External ear infections are generally less obviously related to diet and nutrition, and more readily influenced by changes in the local environment of the external ear. "Swimmer's ear" is a common disorder caused by repeatedly wetting and softening the earwax, which then becomes an ideal medium for bacterial development. This is very common where the swimming water is stagnant or polluted.

The people most often affected by external ear infections are heavy wax producers. This seems to be at least partly related to diet and it is the proportion of saturated versus unsaturated fats that are implicated. To reverse the tendency to produce excess wax we advise restricting saturated fats and taking daily doses of essential fatty acids in capsule or liquid form.

It is crucial to begin treatment for all ear infections at the very first sign of a problem. If you are attentive to the early signs or sensations that indicate infection (fullness in the ear, loss of hearing, pressure or mild pain, or the inability to clear your ears), it is possible to treat many of these problems with natural means. Once the infection has progressed to acute pain, antibiotics may be required. Whenever you have an upper respiratory infection, it is essential to begin a mucus-cleansing diet immediately, and to make certain that your ears can be cleared frequently, especially after blowing your nose.

TREATMENT

Diet

Minor ear congestion or infection may benefit by the mucus-cleansing diet (see Asthma). Recurrent cases of infective or serous otitis media require a diet very high in raw vegetables, with little or no starch or dairy products. This should be combined with intermittent periods of 3 days on the mucus-cleansing diet. Similar regimens to those found under Asthma and Tonsillitis will be useful.

Physiotherapy

Local applications

- Mullein essence: We advise parents of young children to have some mullein essence on hand at all times, because this is the most effective application for all ear infections. Apply 6-10 drops in affected ear 3-4 times daily and insert cotton. It will relieve pain almost instantly and is anti-infective. Mullein oil preparations are better when fungus is a factor.
- Garlic oil and propolis ear drops.
- Garlic foot compress (see Appendix I): very useful for children who refuse or cannot adhere to a mucus-cleansing diet.
- Probe palatal end of Eustachian tube with index finger. Apply Hydrastis (goldenseal) tincture or olbas oil to this area with tip of finger.
- Onion poultice (raw or cooked), plus heat. Apply to ear.
- Chamomile, hops, and lobelia fomentation, plus heat (for pain).
- Botanical ear oil: 1 part lobelia, 1 part myrrh, 1 part mullein, ½ part sassafras, ½ part hemlock, 4 parts olive oil. 4 drops in ear 3 times daily.
- Hydrogen peroxide plus oils, then ear lavage, for excess wax.
- 70% isopropyl alcohol: 1 drop in ear following swim, to prevent infection.
- Hot compresses for acute pain.
- Alternate hot and cold compresses for chronic pain.

Therapeutic Agents

Vitamins and Minerals

- Vitamin A: 10,000-25,000 IU 3-4 times daily for acute cases; twice daily for chronic cases. (See warning under Vitamin Toxicity, page 56.)
- Vitamin C: 500-1000 mg up to every hour.
- Zinc: 15-30 mg twice daily.
- Vitamin B complex: 25-50 mg twice daily.
- EFA and EPA: for chronically hardened earwax.

Others

- Garlic: 2 capsules 3 times daily.
- Thymus: 1-2 per hour in acute; 2, 3 times daily in chronic.
- Sour apples: serous otitis.

Botanicals

Mullein: antibacterial. 4-6 drops in ear 4 times daily.

Eyebright.

Golden rod: anti-catarrhal.

Echinacea.

Angelica.

Therapeutic Suggestion

Most acute earaches are immediately helped by mullein essence, 4-6 drops four times daily in the affected ear. This will give nearly *instant* pain relief, and is effective against both external and middle ear infections. If you do not have mullein handy, a few drops of onion juice in warm flaxseed oil, is decongestive and anti-inflammatory. Apply to both ears (works within minutes).

This should always be accompanied by the mucus-cleansing diet (onions) and plenty of carrot juice, raw green apples, garlic, vitamins A and C, zinc, and thymus.

Chronic ear infections may be very obstinate. A trial of nutritional therapy is suggested prior to allowing tubes to be placed in the ears. This is a last resort.

EDEMA

DEFINITION

Excess fluid retention locally or systemically.

SYMPTOMS

Swelling of hands, ankles, feet, face, abdomen, or other areas of the body. Premenstrual syndrome, headaches, leg ulcers.

ETIOLOGICAL CONSIDERATIONS

- Allergy; congestive heart failure; kidney disease; poor circulation.
- Severe protein deficiency; anemia; adrenal malfunction; liver disease.
- Hypothyroidism; premenstrual; pregnancy; physiological; toxemia.
- Excess salt, meats, dried fish; potassium deficiency; varicose veins.
- Vitamin B complex deficiency; vitamin B1 or B3 deficiency; oral contraceptives.
- Vitamin B6 (premenstrual fluid retention); drugs (steroids); sprain; obesity.
- Constipation; lack of exercise.

DISCUSSION

Edema may be a symptom of an extremely severe internal disorder. At the first onset of unusual fluid retention, a complete physical examination is suggested. Once serious problems such as congestive heart disease, kidney disease, or liver disease are ruled out, more subtle causes may be safely dealt with.

Severe anemia and protein deficiency are rarely a cause of edema, except under extreme conditions. The only such case we have seen was a young lady of 22 who followed a strict fruit and raw vegetable diet for 14 months. She consulted us not for her lack of energy, cardiac irregularity, emacia-tion (69 lb), or hair loss, but because she was now having difficulty in getting her shoes on over her extremely swollen feet. We were shocked to find how ill-informed she was regarding general nutrition. She was surprised that her various symptoms were due directly to her no-protein diet. It was explained to her that she was 2–3 months from death due to liver, kidney, and heart failure, and she was placed on a new diet including protein. Within 4 weeks her edema was almost completely gone. We emphasize this case since it clearly demonstrates the lack of knowledge that some people show in relation to their health. She had read somewhere that protein was harmful to the body, causing all kinds of poisons to accumulate and lead to disease. She had further read of people living for long periods on all fruit or all fruit and vegetable diets to cleanse themselves and increase their vitality. It is our hope her case makes clear that these diets are for *short-term use* only, and are not intended for people to live on indefinitely.

Other more common causes of edema are related to the menstrual cycle. Premenstrual edema is extremely common and is dealt with in detail under Premenstrual Syndrome. The use of contraceptive pills has also been found to cause fluid retention. The contraceptive pill severely depletes many of the B complex group, especially vitamin B6, which is given with great success as therapy for many cases of edema. Fluid retention during pregnancy also occurs in many women. This can be due to an increase by 50% of the blood volume during pregnancy, pressure exerted by the fetus which restricts venous return from the legs, or constipation, which also may restrict blood flow. Obesity during pregnancy exaggerates these effects. Toxemia of pregnancy is also characterized by edema.

Diet may also play a role in fluid retention. The habitual consumption of excess salt as a condiment or salt-containing foods such as dried meats, fish, and pickles, and canned and restaurant foods (especially Chinese) upsets the body's fluid equilibrium, favoring fluid retention. Potassium deficiency will act in the same manner. This can really be a problem with older people who consume vast amounts of salt (salt taste dulls over a period of years, requiring more and more to be used). These people also tend to eat less potassium-containing vegetables due to denture problems, get much less exercise, and sit for prolonged periods of time. Each of these factors plays a part, along with the general tendency towards reduced heart and kidney function, to produce the common edema of old age.

It is important to remember that edema may be the body's response to internal toxins which it attempts to dilute.

TREATMENT

The common treatment for edema is the use of powerful diuretic drugs that help get rid of accumulated fluids. This only treats the symptom without attempting to find or correct the cause. Not only is fluid excreted, but many vitamins and minerals are lost, causing generalized weakness, mental dullness, and reduced vitality. The only cure for edema is finding and removing the cause. For edema of heart, kidney, or liver origin, consult those topics for detailed treatments. The therapy given below is fairly generalized to help as many with edema as possible. Many cases of edema are serious and are best treated in conjunction with a sympathetic physician.

Diet

Nearly any fluid retention problem can be benefited by a vegetable and fruit juice fast emphasizing vegetables, as carrot or carrot and beet juice, This may be continued anywhere from 3-21 days with supervision.

Another useful regimen is the all-watermelon diet for 2-3 days.

Follow this regimen with an all-raw-foods diet with plenty of raw green vegetables. A good lacto-vegetarian diet should then be followed until complete cure is established. Absolutely no animal proteins other than fermented dairy products (yoghurt, kefir) are allowed. (*Note:* This diet does not apply to edema due to anemia. See Anemia if this is the main cause.)

Physiotherapy

- Alternate hot and cold sitz baths.
- Slowly increase general exercise.
- Hourly leg and calf exercise.
- Alternate hot and cold leg sprays.
- Alternate hot and cold hip sprays.
- Alternate hot and cold showers.
- Sauna (if no contraindication) to induce perspiration.

Therapeutic Agents

Vitamins and Minerals— Primary

Edema is a symptom of disease, not a disease of itself. Specific supplementation will depend on the primary cause. Refer to treatment sections elsewhere in this text once a specific diagnosis is established.

- Vitamin B6: diuretic. 50-250 mg 1-2 times daily. Of special use with fluid retention related to menstrual cycle.
- Bioflavonoids: reduce capillary permeability.
- Vitamin C: 500-1000 mg 3-6 times daily.

Vitamins and Minerals— Secondary

- Vitamin A: 25,000 IU 1-2 times daily.
- Vitamin B3: 50-400 mg 1-2 times daily.
- Vitamin B complex: 25-50 mg 1-3 times daily.
- Vitamin E: 400 IU 1-2 times daily.
- Potassium: 100 mg daily.

Botanicals

Apis: homeopathic dose; for edema due to stings or swelling.

Herbal treatment should be aimed at causative processes, and diuretics selected accordingly. The following have diuretic action should it be necessary to mobilize fluids rapidly to reduce pressure on sensitive systems temporarily during systemic treatment:

Aphanes: edema of kidney or liver origin.

Bladderwrack: as a tincture, or in tablets has diuretic function.

Broom tops: with weakened heart.

Buchu: diuretic.

Cactus: edema of heart origin.

Cleavers: diuretic.

Cola syrup (Cayce product): kidney origin.

Dogbane: edema of heart origin.

Hawthorn berries: edema of heart origin.
10-20 drops tincture 3-4 times daily.

Juniper berries: diuretic.

Lily-of-the-valley: edema of heart origin.

Pareira root: edema of kidney origin.

Parsley: diuretic.

Pipsissewa and poplar bark

Wahoo: edema from convalescence.

Watermelon seeds: diuretic. Use infusion of dried seeds.

EMPHYSEMA

DEFINITION

A degenerative disease of the lungs characterized by enlargement, distention, and destruction of the alveolar spaces.

SYMPTOMS

Wheezing, chronic non-productive cough, expectoration, shortness of breath, foul breath, cyanosis, and difficulty in exhalation.

ETIOLOGICAL CONSIDERATIONS—PRIMARY

- Smoking
- Pollution
  Smog; radioactivity (nuclear)
- Occupational
- Glassblower's lung; metal worker's lung; miner's lung; others
- Cadmium exposure
- Industrial; auto exhaust; smoking; galvanized pipes

ETIOLOGICAL CONSIDERATIONS— SECONDARY

- Diet (excess refined carbohydrates; excess dairy products; deficiency; allergy)
- Poor body mechanics; spinal; lack of exercise; poor circulation; obesity
- Toxicity; poor eliminations

DISCUSSION

Emphysema literally means "inflation", which accurately describes the condition of the small air exchange sacs (alveoli) in the lungs which become over-distended, filled with mucus, and inelastic. This destruction of the alveoli reduces the effective oxygen exchange surface of the lung, so that the victim is in a state of slow suffocation. This general lack of oxygen and consequent increase in carbon dioxide within the system causes the patient to breathe more rapidly. Due to loss of tissue elasticity in the lungs, air is difficult to expel, leaving the patient with expanded chest and great difficulty in exhaling. As the air sacs break down, mucus accumulates, which further reduces the active oxygen exchange surface. The cough reflex is stimulated but is not efficient enough to remove mucus from the lower parts of the lung. The small cilia, whose job it usually is to waft mucus towards the throat to be expelled (the muco-ciliary escalator), are also destroyed, in most cases by smoking, and so do not function. The result is extremely difficult breathing, chronic cough, and inability to perform even mild tasks. Over time this progressive degeneration may lead to lung infection, high blood pressure, enlargement of the heart, and heart failure.

Emphysema is commonly associated with bronchial asthma and chronic bronchitis, and often follows a history of either. In general, the same factors are responsible for all these conditions, with special importance being placed on one or another aspect, depending on the condition.

Cigarette smoking is more related to chronic bronchitis and emphysema than it is to asthma, which often has more of an allergic or psychological basis. Certainly, cigarette smoking is central to most cases of emphysema, unless other inhalants are a factor. Smoking dries and irritates the delicate mucous membranes, destroys available sources of vitamin C, increases the need for vitamin B complex and vitamin A, and destroys the delicate cilia essential for cleansing the lungs of unwanted foreign matter. Apart from these well-known effects, cigarettes have been found to contain a large amount of the toxic element cadmium, which has been found to cause emphysema in laboratory animals. It is also found in high concentrations in the lungs of humans with emphysema. Other sources of cadmium are air pollution, auto exhaust, and galvanized water pipes

Air pollution and radioactive fallout have both been implicated in the rapid rise in emphysema. Any irritant inhalant from industrial pollution can be a factor, as well as any occupation that exposes the lungs to irritants. Well-known occupational emphysemas are miner's lung, glassblower's lung, and metal worker's lung.

With emphysema, diet plays a role similar to that in chronic bronchitis and asthma. A common fault is an excess of refined carbohydrates and a general lack of raw green vegetables. This mucus-forming diet predisposes to minor lung ailments which, if too often repeated or improperly treated, may become asthma or bronchitis and later emphysema.

Poor body mechanics can affect the respiratory excursion, reducing oxygen exchange by the lungs as well as local circulation and nutrition. Kyphosis, a forward bending in the midback, or scoliosis, a side-bending deformity in the midback, both may reduce the space allowed for the lungs to expand. Lack of demanding exercise and habitual shallow breathing allow the ribs to become less mobile, reducing the vital capacity or lung excursion, predisposing to lung disease.

Spinal lesions in the upper and midback can also severely upset local nerve, blood, and lymph supply to the lungs, resulting in downgraded tissue vitality.

TREATMENT

Emphysema is a degenerative disease. It comes at the end of years of abuse and results in tissue breakdown and scar formation. Even early cases of emphysema already have permanent lung damage that can never be totally corrected.

Prevention is obviously the best way of avoiding lung damage, but even advanced cases may be improved significantly with proper care. In a case of emphysema so severe that the patient can barely walk without complete breathlessness and prostration, sometimes improvement to the point of being quite active can be achieved.

Diet

Similar dietary regimens to those found under Asthma and Bronchitis are very useful with emphysema. In advanced cases vitality is usually very low and therapy must be moderated accordingly. Mucus solvents such as onions and garlic should always be included in the diet, as well as citrus fruits with their pulp, these being high in vitamin C and bioflavonoids. Foods high in vitamin A are essential for lung health and should be included regularly. The bulk of the diet should be raw vegetables. Dairy products, wheat, and excess starches are to be avoided. Alternate the diet with periods of citrus or vegetable juice fast (especially carrot juice and watercress). Also, 3-4 days on the mucus-cleansing diet (see Appendix I) strictly or modified to include carrots as well as raw salads, is beneficial. Results will be slow but steady, and perseverance is essential.

Physiotherapy

- Postural drainage with percussion: hang from the waist over the edge of a bed with a bowl placed at the head for easy expectoration. Apply a hot, moist compress to the back repeatedly for 5-10 minutes and then have a friend pound vigorously on the back with open palms. As mucus is loosened it should be expectorated. Repeat 1-3 times daily.
- Alternate hot and cold chest packs: to stimulate circulation, respiration, and mucus elimination.
- Alternate hot and cold showers: as above, and also to improve general skin function.
- Exercise: progressively increase the amount and speed of whatever exercise you are capable of. Exercise is best done in a warm, moist environment, not outdoors on a cold day, which would cause drying of the mucous membranes. Stationary bicycling has been used in various studies to great benefit, although any exercise that requires progressively more exertion will do.
- Inhalation therapy: inhalations of various herbal steam mixtures are beneficial to help heal the lungs and aid expectoration. These include:

Mixture 1: eucalyptus oil, fir balsam, tolu, benzoin.
Mixture 2: sage, thyme, rosemary, cloves
Other: olbas inhalation and chest compress
- Diaphragmatic breathing: (See Asthma).
- Breathing exercises (See Asthma).
- Spinal manipulation: weekly manipulations to entire thoracic region, including ribs and intercostal deep muscle massage.

Therapeutic Agents

Vitamins and Minerals
- Vitamin A: 25,000-100,000 IU daily. (See warning under Vitamin Toxicity, page 56.) Essential for health of mucous membranes.
- Beta-carotene: 10,000 IU twice daily. Helps repair and protect lung tissue.
- Vitamin B complex: 50 mg 2-3 times daily.
- Vitamin C and bioflavonoids: 3000-12,000 mg of vitamin C daily.
- Vitamin E: 800-1200 IU daily; reduces oxygen needs; antioxidant; healing agent.

Others
- N,N-dimethylglycine (DMG): 100-250 mg 3 times daily. Increases endurance.
- Carrot juice: 1 glass 1-2 times daily.
- Coenzyme Q10: 60 mg daily. Eases breathing by increasing oxygen utilization.
- L-cysteine and L-methionine: 500 mg of each twice daily on an empty stomach. To help protect and repair lung tissue.
- Adrenal tablets: 1 or 2 tablets 2-3 times daily. To help restore the adrenal glands which become overworked do to the constant stress and fear this disease places on the individual.
- Garlic: 2 capsules 3 times daily.
- Honey/onion syrup (see Appendix I): 1 tsp 3-6 times daily.
- Raw thymus tablets: immunological support.

- Protein supplements.
- Free form amino acids: to aid in lung repair.
- Cayce expectorant (number 49).
- Chlorophyll.
- Lecithin.

Botanicals

Quebracho blanco: respiratory stimulant. 5-25 drops tincture 3 times daily.
Grindelia: antispasmodic, and expectorant.
Hawthorn: circulatory stimulant, to improve blood flow to the lungs.
Pleurisy root: reflex stimulating and diaphoretic.

Boneset.
Comfrey.
Passion flower: nervine sedative.
See also Bronchitis.

Therapeutic Suggestion

Emphysema responds slowly due to its degenerative nature. Mucus solvents (garlic, onion syrup) are very useful. Very high doses of vitamin A are needed, along with B complex, C, and especially E. The patient must stop smoking and avoid exposure to occupational inhalants.

EPILEPSY

DEFINITION

Epileptic seizure: a brief disorder of cerebral function usually associated with a disturbance of consciousness and accompanied by excessive neuronal discharge.

SYMPTOMS

Grand Mal

Prodromal phase: a warning phase lasting hours or days with a mood change.
Aura: an apprehension of brief duration that a seizure is about to occur.
Loss of consciousness: a sudden fall occurs.
Tonic stage: loss of consciousness with muscular contraction, including contraction of the respiratory muscles, which creates a "cry" as the air is forced out through a partially closed glottis. This stage lasts 20-30 seconds.
Chronic stage: tonic spasm is replaced by interrupted powerful jerks or spasms of face, mouth, jaw, body, and limbs. Foaming of the mouth may occur, along with inconti-

nence of urine and biting of the tongue. This stage lasts 20-30 seconds.
Relaxation stage: the person lies flaccid and falls into a deep sleep lasting a few minutes to 1 hour or more. After regaining consciousness the person is often confused and may have a headache.

Petit Mal

A transient loss of consciousness with blank stare lasting 10-15 seconds. Some myoclonic jerks of the extremities may occur at this time. In rare cases this is also accompanied by total loss of consciousness, falling to the ground, and immediate recovery of consciousness.

Partial or Focal Epilepsy

The commonest site of dysfunction is the temporal lobe. This form is manifested by hallucinations of smell, taste, sight, or hearing and "deja-vu" feelings. There also may be experienced a dream-like quality which may be accompanied with well-coordinated, seemingly purposeful motor actions of which no memory will be retained.

Jacksonian

Disturbance of function in one part of the body spreads to involve adjacent areas. An example is an involuntary twitch of a hand that spreads to the entire arm or whole side of the body. Consciousness may or may not be lost.

ETIOLOGICAL CONSIDERATIONS—PRIMARY

- Lymphatic lesion (Peyer's patches).
- Digestive disturbances.
- Over-distended stomach due to excess intake of food; poor eliminations.
- Spinal lesion.
- Incoordination of cerebrospinal and autonomic nervous systems.
- Head injuries.

ETIOLOGICAL CONSIDERATIONS—SECONDARY

- Nutritional or toxic causes.
- Aluminum toxicity; copper toxicity; lead toxicity; mercury toxicity; chemical toxicity; pesticides; food additives; calcium deficiency; magnesium deficiency.
- Manganese deficiency; selenium deficiency; trace element deficiency; zinc deficiency.
- vitamin A deficiency; vitamin B6 deficiency; vitamin D deficiency; taurine deficiency.
- Allergy.
- Metabolic abnormalities (increased B6 need)
- Anoxia (heart block, anemia, vasoconstriction due to reflex from upper cervical vertebrae lesions).
- Sensory triggers (flickering light, TV-induced epilepsy, sounds).

- Emotional triggers.
- Heredity.
- Glandular imbalances, adrenals (hypoglycemia), pancreas (hypoglycemia), gonads, pineal, pituitary, liver).
- Cerebral tumors.
- Cerebrovascular disease.
- Uremia.
- Hypoglycemia (insulin-secreting adenoma).
- Sudden alcohol or drug withdrawal.

DISCUSSION

The usual medical approach to epileptic seizures of unknown cause is the use of sedatives and anti-convulsants, with Dilantin the most frequently prescribed drug. Dilantin does not cure epilepsy, but does help control the frequency and intensity of seizures. Many cases are completely controlled. Most anti-convulsant drugs, however, tend to deplete the body's folic acid, thus creating folic acid deficiency. Hyperplasia of the gums can also occur.

Other side effects of anti-convulsant drugs include rashes, irreversibly enlarged lymph nodes, osteomalacia (rarefaction of bone), slurred speech, mental confusion, dizziness, insomnia, blood abnormalities, hyperglycemia, and possible liver damage. Obviously, no physician would prescribe such a strong drug unless he or she carefully monitored the patient for side effects, and unless it was essential. Unfortunately, we have observed some cases where its prescription has been seemingly more cavalier. One patient in particular who experienced one seizure and was placed on Dilantin "for the rest of his life". Upon investigating his case it was discovered that he had been spraying with pesticides for 3 days prior to his seizure. Unfortunately, none of this ever came out in his initial case history, and Dilantin was prescribed. Certainly such cases are in the minority, but it does emphasize the importance of a complete case history prior to the administration of any drug medication.

The problem thus far in treating epilepsy through natural means has been an incomplete understanding of the multiple causes of the disorder. A clear picture of its causation has been sadly lacking. The more individualized holistic approach that naturopathic physicians employ has been successful in some cases in bringing about remarkable improvements.

The work of Edgar Cayce[27] has helped to present a fresh model to explain the complexity of this disorder. With his special sensitivity and ability to see hidden causes, some new insight into epilepsy has been presented. Cayce found the most frequent causative factor was an incoordination between the cerebrospinal and autonomic nervous system. This is caused by a lesion in what Cayce calls the "lacteal ducts", which coincide loosely with Peyer's patches, lymphatic structures in the small intestine. This area, according to Cayce, but not yet substantiated by current medical knowledge, is a crucial center where both the cerebrospinal and autonomic nervous systems meet. A lesion, or a twisting of these meeting places, causes reflex lesions in the spine and brain, resulting in excessive abnormal neurological impulses. These reflex changes may also involve the endocrine system, causing disturbances.

Another common factor Cayce found was a digestive incoordination. Poor elimination can overload the lymphatic regions just past the duodenum and produce toxic substances which may affect the whole body and also contribute to the lacteal lesion as described above. Spinal lesions were also cited as a factor in many of the Cayce readings. Evidence from other sources sheds further light on this perplexing disorder.[28]

Some research points to vitamin B6 deficiency as a possible factor in some cases of epilepsy. One study revealed a B6 deficiency in certain baby formulas causing infantile epilepsy which was reversed by supplying vitamin B6. Some infants have also been found to have an increased need for B, as the result of a metabolic abnormality.[29]

Deficiencies of vitamin A, vitamin D, folic acid, zinc, and taurine (an amino acid) have also been linked with epilepsy in some patients. Other studies found that magnesium deficiency was a common cause with supplemental magnesium being curative. This was especially true in infants with excess calcium intake resulting in magnesium loss.[30]

It has been known for a long time that magnesium deficiency may cause muscle tremors and convulsive seizures. In 1976 magnesium was shown to be at lower levels in epileptics than in normal subjects. A magnesium supplement of 450 mg daily has successfully controlled seizures in a trial of 30 epileptic patients, restoring a proper physiological balance.[31]

Calcium deficiency also must be considered a possible cause. As far back as 1983 the *International Clinical Nutrition Review* reported cases of epilepsy successfully treated by restoring normal calcium levels.[32]

Toxic metals such as lead, copper, mercury, and aluminum have long been known to cause seizures. These toxicities are increasingly common in our modern society with aluminum cookware, auto exhaust, industrial pollution, and copper water pipes. Several other correlations have been found, pointing to nutritionally related causes of epilepsy.

Hypoglycemia has long been associated with convulsions. Serum glucose levels have been shown to fall just prior to seizures. It is estimated that between 50-90% of all epileptics have either constant or periodic episodes of low blood sugar, and 70% show abnormal glucose tolerance levels of the hypoglycemic type.

Allergy is another fairly well documented cause of epilepsy in some patients. Many case studies exist where exposure to chemicals, pesticides, food additives, or common foods such as peanuts or tea has been the sole cause of seizures for individual patients. In these cases drug therapy is not only clearly inappropriate, it is often detrimental.

Certainly, not all patients with epilepsy can be helped with natural therapies, but a careful investigation into each case may reveal possible avenues of therapy that may eventually help the patient reduce or in some cases even entirely eliminate the need for drug therapy.

TREATMENT

Diet

The diet should include low-fat (no fried foods, meat, or milk), low-carbohydrate foods, and no alcohol, salt, or sugar. This will promote regularity. The principles of a hypoglycemic diet regimen should then be followed for long-term care. Avoid MSG, chemical exposure, and stimulants such as caffeine.

Physiotherapy

- Castor oil packs: should be used in series—3 days on, 1 day off, for at least 6 months. This is to help heal the intestinal lesions present in the majority of epileptic patients, according to Cayce. Use 3–4 thicknesses of undyed wool. Saturate this with hot castor oil and wring out lightly. (This is heated in a special pot used for this purpose only. You may reuse the same cloth 20–40 times. just store it in the pot and add more castor oil with each use.) This cloth is applied as hot as the body can comfortably bear, to the area on the right side of the abdomen, from the lower rib border to the iliac crest covering the liver to cecum and umbilicus. The pack is covered with oiled cloth or plastic and kept warm by a heating pad. If necessary, the bed may also be protected with plastic. The pack should stay on 1–3 hours. After finishing, wash the area with a weak solution of bicarbonate—1 tsp to 2 pints (1 liter) warm water. These packs should be done at the same time of day, in the evening. Take 2 tbsp unrefined olive oil the evening of the third day of packs.
- Massage: after the castor oil pack, a deep abdominal massage to help break up any adhesions is useful. Use a combination of peanut oil, olive oil, and tincture of myrrh.
- Spinal manipulation: on the fourth day, after 3 days of castor oil packs, obtain a spinal treatment of C1, 2, 3, T9, 10, and sacrococcygeal areas, plus any specific lesions. These treatments are to be done about twice per week for 3 weeks, with 1 week of rest. Repeat the cycle over a 6-month period, minimum.
- Exercise; walking; swimming; calisthenics; keep active.

Therapeutic Agents

Vitamins and Minerals—Primary
- Vitamin B complex: 50 mg 3 times daily; essential to proper central nervous system function.
- Intramuscular B complex: B12 plus folic acid: 1–2 times per week.
- Vitamin B6: 100 mg twice daily; anticonvulsant.
- Vitamin C: to bowel tolerance.
- Vitamin E: 400 IU twice daily. This alone can reduce seizures by 50%.
- Calcium: 800–1000 mg daily; sedative.
- Magnesium: 400–2000 mg daily. Anticonvulsant; increases cellular uptake of taurine; antihomocystein.
- Folic acid: 1 mg twice daily.

Vitamins and Minerals—Primary
- Vitamin A: 25,000 IU 1–2 times daily.
- Trace minerals.
- Zinc: 25 mg 2–3 times daily.
- Selenium: increases glutathione peroxidase, a free radical scavenger enzyme.

Others—Primary
- Adenosine: sublingually. Especially indicated where CNS trauma is the main cause of the seizures.
- Melatonin: MAO inhibitor; anticonvulsant

- Coenzyme Q10: 30 mg daily. Improves oxygenation of the brain.
- Taurine: 1–3 g daily. Modulates neuromuscular excitation and calcium flux
- L-tyrosine: 500 mg 3 times daily. Needed for proper brain function.
- Atomodine: 1 drop daily.
- Melatonin: 2–5 mg daily. Anti-convulsive, acting as an MAO inhibitor

Others—Secondary

- Pancreatic enzymes
- Tryptophan (a precursor to seratonin and melatonin)
- EFA (essential fatty acids): 4 capsules 3 times daily.
- Fletcher's castoria as needed.
- Lecithin: 4 capsules 3 times daily, or in granular form in drinks or on food.
- Octacosanol (wheat germ oil concentrate): 2500–5000 mcg daily.

See also Hypoglycemia, Allergies and Food Intolerances.

Botanicals—Primary

Passion flower: whole plant extract plus elixir of wild ginseng (Cayce product).

Sedative, antispasmodic. 1 tsp 4 times daily and $1/2$ hour before retiring. Decrease other medication slowly over 3–6 weeks with doctor's permission.

Bacopa monniera, skullcap, and kava: anti-convulsives.

Valerian root tea.

Lobelia: emetic doses at first signs.

Botanicals—Secondary

Chamomile.

Catnip.

Gotu kola.

Rehmannia and Siberian ginseng: adrenal tonics.

Hyssop: petit mal.

Peony root.

Useful Prescriptions

- Antispasmodic tea: black cohosh, lady's slipper, skullcap, valerian. dose: 2–3 cups at first sign of attack.
- Kloss antispasmodic: tincture of cayenne, $1/2$ part, cohosh, 1 part, lobelia seed, 1 part, skullcap, 1 part, skunk cabbage, 1 part. 8–15 drops, up to 1 tsp on tongue at first sign of attack.

FATIGUE
(Including Chronic Fatigue)

DEFINITION AND SYMPTOMS

Abnormal tiredness and lack of energy. Weakness, mental and physical; lethargy; depression; inability to perform ordinary daily duties.

ETIOLOGICAL CONSIDERATIONS—PRIMARY

- Hypoglycemia (adrenal exhaustion and other results)
- Stress (nutritional and glandular reactions)
- Anemia
  Iron; vitamin B12; folic acid; copper; vitamin C and others
- Viral
  Cytomegalovirus (CMV); Epstein-Barr virus (EBV); others
- Leaky gut (implying bowel toxemia—Candida, parasites, protozoa, destruction of intestinal flora or chronic antibiotic use.)
- Toxicity

Diet; pesticides; additives; drugs; polio vaccines (reactions to); smog; smoking
- Allergy
- Glandular imbalances
  Hypothyroidism; pituitary; adrenals; pancreas
- Poor eliminations or assimilation
  Constipation; enzyme deficiency, poor digestion and absorption of essential nutrients
- Poor skin function; liver, gallbladder disease
- Cardiovascular causes
  Low blood pressure; high blood pressure; arteriosclerosis and atherosclerosis
- Improper diet
  Excess saturated fats; excess refined carbohydrates; junk foods, vitamin and mineral deficiency; excess cow's milk (early infancy anemia); overeating; skipped breakfast; coffee, alcohol, soda, sugar; excess animal protein; protein deficiency
- Degenerative disease
  Cancer; arthritis; most others
- Lack of demanding exercise

ETIOLOGICAL CONSIDERATIONS— SECONDARY

- Excess sex or excess masturbation
- Contraceptive pill; overweight
- Overwork
- Lack of sleep
- Sedentary occupation
- Psychological, e.g. depression
- Heavy metal poisoning
- Old-age nutrition syndrome (lack of teeth, resulting in little fresh vegetable intake)
- Shallow breathing

DISCUSSION

Probably the most common complaint of people today is fatigue. This is not a disease per se, but is a major symptom of many disturbances. Often, however, it must be dealt with generally as the single most obvious presenting disorder, without much else to aid in diagnosis. As you may understand from the long but still very incomplete list of possible causes, such a seemingly simple complaint can be very complex in its proper diagnosis and treatment.

A complete case history and good physical examination will usually reveal other clues to the origin of the fatigue. Although many etiologic factors are listed, in reality most of these in turn have a nutritional basis. Hypoglycemia, or low blood sugar, is one of the most frequent causes of a type of fatigue that is more obvious in the mid-morning and afternoon in its early stages, becoming more continuous as the system becomes less able to cope with its repeated stress. The adrenal glands and pancreas become overburdened and eventually fail to function properly. The type of diet usually responsible for hypoglycemia, high in refined carbohydrates, is also deficient in the very vitamins and minerals essential for the health and well-being of these and others of the body's glands and organs.

Stress is also a common factor in fatigue. It may cause a form of hypoglycemia by depleting the adrenal glands which respond to any fear, anxiety, worry, or similar emotion, as if they were emergency conditions. A wide range of physiological actions are evoked to provide sufficient energy to meet this "danger". Eventually the adrenal glands become exhausted and, as vital energy reserves become overtaxed, fatigue results. Unlike true nutritional hypoglycemia, this type of fatigue does not necessarily occur between meals, but may be more related to an incident of intense stress or emotion. If this stress fatigue is coincident with a refined diet and especially if coffee or other caffeine-containing drinks such as black tea or cola are routinely consumed, the hypoglycemic state may take on a totally unpredictable character.

Caffeine is in reality a drug; a socially accepted drug, but a drug just the same. Unlike sugar, which at least draws part of its energy surge from its caloric nature, caffeine and caffeine-containing drinks such as unsweetened coffee or tea have no intrinsic energy value whatsoever. They do not give energy, but cause an endocrine emergency action to extract energy from the body's vital reserves in the liver and muscles. Caffeine causes glycogen stored in these tissues to be mobilized and converted to the body's fuel, glucose. Ultimately this extraction of energy leaves the energy reserves severely depleted, just as an unwise spender soon finds his or her pockets empty. The result is profound weakness and chronic fatigue. Caffeine drinks are probably the greatest curse to the body, after refined sugar. Habitual coffee or tea drinkers become literally addicted to their brew. So often we hear of people who just can't get going without their morning coffee, or who get a morning headache unless they drink coffee. What could be a clearer sign of dependency than this? Absolutely no progress will be made with chronic fatigue as long as coffee is a part of the diet.

Diet may influence the energy reserves in ways other than by the upsetting effects of low blood sugar. Many vitamin and mineral deficiencies are related to a lack of energy. The most widely accepted of these relate to the production of anemia. Deficiency of iron, B12, folic acid, B complex, vitamin C, vitamin E, copper, and others may be involved. Relative magnesium deficiency can cause fatigue when there is excess calcium in the diet. These deficiencies are fairly common as a result of devitalized food consumption; or may be related to conditions of blood loss such as profuse menstrual periods or bleeding ulcers.

Protein deficiency may be a cause of fatigue in some cases, while excess proteins may also be a factor. The habit of skipping breakfast or just having a sweet roll and coffee is associated with both low blood sugar and morning fatigue. Often, a change to a substantial high-protein breakfast will completely remove the morning "blahs". Excess protein, especially saturated animal fat proteins, cause a host of problems, including cardiovascular disease, liver and gallbladder disease and toxicity, all with symptoms of fatigue. Even excess vegetarian proteins may become a problem for a sedentary person. In general, the more demanding exercise a person does, the more protein he or she can eat and deal with effectively. Any excess clogs the system, causes toxicity, and lowers the body's vitality as it attempts to deal with the excessive amounts of unneeded and often toxic waste products of protein metabolism.

Another form of toxicity results from poor eliminations. Slow bowel transit time (loaded bowel syndrome, constipation) causes toxic residues in the colon to be reabsorbed, causing lethargy, depression, coated tongue, fatigue, and other signs of ill health. A high-fiber diet corrects this situation quite easily. One of the primary roles of the liver is detoxifying harmful or unwanted elements in the body. If the liver is overworked, general toxicity results. A congested liver due to excess toxins such as pesticides, food colorings, preservatives, etc., from foods, excess fatty foods, excess protein, chemical exposure, or drugs also will leave the person in a sluggish, toxic state.

Lack of demanding exercise and poor skin function cause poor circulation of blood and lymph. This results in stagnation and ultimately toxicity in various organ groups, causing lowered vitality and fatigue. It is paradoxical that exercise, which initially requires energy, produces such an abundance of vitality and more energy. Occupations that require little physical exertion are much more fatiguing than good, hard physical work. Exercise stimulates blood and lymph circulation, aids in tissue nutrition, stimulates the endocrine system, tones and cleanses the cardiovascular system, and generally acts to "grease" our entire body machine. Exercise also helps keep our energies directed and concentrated, preventing many emotional and mental disorders.

Food allergy is a frequently ignored cause of poor vitality, depression, listlessness, fatigue, and other similar symptoms. This may be caused by any food and may cause sudden acute symptoms almost to the point of prostration, or the more subtle chronic fatigue if the allergen is consumed on a regular basis.

Cardiovascular disease, arteriosclerosis, and atherosclerosis can reduce the efficiency of the blood circulation. If the blood flow to the brain is reduced due to narrowing of the vessels of blood supply, mental fatigue and lethargy may result. A similar effect occurs due to cervical arthritis, where the bony changes encroach on the vessels which pass through them and supply blood to the brain.

Other degenerative diseases such as cancer usually are first noticed by vague feelings of tiredness and lack of energy or vitality. All the other factors listed under Etiological Considerations not previously mentioned may be involved in individual cases. As you can see, "simple fatigue" can be fairly complex and nothing to ignore.

Chronic Fatigue Syndrome (CFS)

CFS, a so-called "new" disease, it is the chronic form of myalgic encephalomyelitis (ME), and also used to be called "post-viral fatigue syndrome". Just because one might have been feeling "tired for months" doesn't fit the definition of CFS. Fatigue of uncertain etiology, of minimum 6 months duration, associated with EBV antibodies, and with other symptoms has been the generally accepted definition of CFS. Women, especially between the ages of 20–40 seem to be more prone to CFS than males (2:1).

CFS appears to be characterized by a chronically disturbed or compromised immune system, with a demonstrated history of immune system hyperactivity, often with suppressive therapies leading to exhaustion. Being a syndrome means that while fatigue is the primary presenting symptom, other symptoms are variously associated with the fatigue, generally involving the immune system such as recurrent fevers, muscular pain and weakness, shifting pains, joint pains, sore throats, depression, anxiety, headaches, emotional lability, intestinal discomfort, lymph node swelling, disordered sleep, swollen glands, and general flu-like symptoms.

Despite much research, and although there are several theories, the etiology remains uncertain. EBV is a herpes virus, the infectious agent implicit in glandular fever, and is a suspected causative agent. EBV targets primarily the B-lymphocytes, liver, and brain. EBV in the brain can cause more severe symptoms such as mental confusion, fatigue, poor concentration, insomnia. EBV grows within throat epithelial tissue, and is transmitted by saliva.

The thing to note here is that simply having been exposed to EBV in the past, with or without the overt symptoms of glandular fever does not mean one is going to get CFS. Glandular fever is said to be caused by EBV, is a very contagious infectious disease, and has been called the "kissing disease", and the "yuppie flu". Most people probably have antibodies to this virus, which, like its other herpes cousins remains latent within a host for life, as an envelope virus, and tends to become active only if the host is "run down", or overloaded with toxins. Any suppression of the immune system, for example pharmaceutical medications, emotional upsets, illness, stress, and allergy will provide opportunity for EBV to multiply.

It is not clear at all if EBV is the primary cause, or even a cause at all, of CFS. After all, EBV infection has been described as "inevitable". Most people have it, and it is associated with a whole range of diseases. Whether EBV is simply an innocent bystander is still to be determined; simply because antibody titres are high in *some* CFS sufferers, begs the question. Which gets back to the fundamental question again, as to what causes what. We suspect that EBV and other herpes viruses, CMV, Hepatitis, even HIV, while commonly present in huge proportions of the populace, can and will only become players when the immune system is otherwise under stress.

Some researchers think that CFS represents a type of autoimmune disease caused by endotoxins produced by EBVs which hide in various immune cells. This view will adopt protocols of treatment which aim to restore the integrity of the bowel wall (see Leaky Gut).

Some have pointed out that during times of viral stress, chemicals stored in adipose tissue can be mobilized into systemic lymphatic and blood circulation, which can result in symptoms consistent with those of chronic fatigue. This "synergy" between virus and chemicals points out the need for liver detoxification as well.

TREATMENT

An attempt must be made to discover the basic cause of the fatigue and then treat specifically.

Diet

The hypoglycemic regimen using the blood-building foods found under Anemia is usually a safe choice. Some cases may benefit with periodic fruit or vegetable juice fasting and periods on a raw foods diet. No refined foods, coffee, or drugs are allowed. If this simple dietary approach does not prove effective, food allergy tests and a hair analysis may prove useful. If constipation is a problem, make sure the diet supplies adequate fiber. Always assume the lymphatic system needs rehydrating and decongesting, so avoid allergy foods, drink copious water, ensure Celtic salt intake, and gently exercise within one's capacity.

Physiotherapy

- Meditation: 20 minutes, twice daily; deep breathing exercises; aerobics.
- Outdoor exercise daily (ought to induce perspiration); ice-cold foot baths; massage.
- Daily morning wet grass walks; alternate hot and cold showers; alternate hot and cold head baths or sprays (for brain fatigue); "salt glow" skin rub (see Appendix I); dry body brush (see Appendix I); saunas; general spinal therapy; head stands, inversion therapy.

Therapeutic Agents

Vitamins and Minerals
(Choice depends on the cause)
- Vitamin B complex: 50 mg 2–3 times daily. Deficiency of this group can cause fatigue.
- Vitamin B3: active in mitochondrial energy production.
- Vitamin B12: oral, sublingual 250 mcg daily, plus 1 mg intramuscularly per week.
- Vitamin C and bioflavonoids: 2000 mg 3 times daily, or more.
- Multivitamin, multimineral preparations: use where multiple vitamin and mineral deficiencies are suspected.
- Vitamin A: 25,000 IU once daily.
- Pantothenic acid.
- Folic acid.
- Vitamin E: 400 IU 1–3 times daily.
- Chromium: with hypoglycemia.
- Iron: Due to iron deficiency anemia, 25–50 mg daily.
- Calcium: 800–1000 mg daily.
- Magnesium: due to relative calcium excess, stress, etc. 500–2000 mg daily.

Others
- Probiotics: take daily.
- Brewer's yeast: with hypoglycemia.
- Coenzyme Q10: (up to 300 mg daily).
- Dimethylglycine: increases oxygenation of the tissues and boost energy levels.
- L-acetyl-carnitine.
- Bee pollen.
- Desiccated liver tablets.
- Desiccated thyroid: with prescription.
- Kelp.
- Lipoic acid: detoxifies nitric acid.
- Methionine.

- Pancreatic enzymes.
- Raw adrenal tablets.
- Raw pituitary tablets.
- Raw thyroid tablets.

Botanicals
- Ginseng: general.
- Oats: mental.

Note: There are many herbal medicines that can really help the body's energy systems recover homeostasis. Causative factors must be taken into account, and if you suffer from prolonged fatigue you should consult a trained herbalist, or a naturopath trained in the use of botanical medicine as part of your therapy.

Stress Management

Stress management is an important element of any treatment which attempts to rebuild the immune system, consequent to and regardless of what may have led to, or caused the dysfunction along the way. In CFS, this aspect must indeed be central.

FEVER

DEFINITION

Elevation of the body temperature above normal. 98.6°F (36.8°C) is considered average but this will vary from person to person and with time of day.

SYMPTOMS

Skin is hot, dry or wet; the person suffers from malaise, general lassitude.

ETIOLOGICAL CONSIDERATIONS

- Toxicity:
  Impurities in blood and lymphatic system
- Infection:
  Bacterial; viral; parasitic

DISCUSSION

Body heat is normally generated at about 98.6°F (36.8°C). This temperature is produced by the body's internal work being performed day and night in its multitude of various tasks. The heart pumps, blood moves, muscles contract, air is expelled, food digested, hormones produced, etc.

Fever, or excessive body heat, is also produced by internal work performed by the body. In response to toxicity or infection the body institutes special defense mechanisms to help re-establish normality. These include an increase in the number of white blood cells and their transport to the area of need; antibody production; increased respiration to provide more oxygen; increased heart rate to pump blood, white blood cells, oxygen, and antibodies throughout the body; and formation of new blood vessels in areas of infection to allow closer and more effective contact of white blood cells, antibodies, and oxygen with foreign elements. These, along with many more activities, are all designed for defense. The best definition for fever is not a morbid or pathological disease state, but rather a state of hyperfunctional repair.

From this short explanation it becomes clear that fever is not the problem to be cured, but the *result* of the problem and *part* of the cure. Hippocrates once said, "Give me fever and I will cure all disease." This gives us insight into the true nature of fever.

241

Fever aids in eliminating toxins and helps destroy pathogenic bacteria. These bacteria usually have a very narrow optimum temperature range. Being pathogenic they live comfortably within the normal range of human temperature and can then actively reproduce. As the body's temperature rises to the upper limits of the bacteria's viable range, the generation time increases so that reproduction becomes slower and the body's defenses can combat them more effectively. At a critical point in the fever process, the body's defenses will engulf and destroy the bacteria faster than they can reproduce, resulting in a cure.

Recent research supports these views of fever. In a series of experiments on fever with fish, amphibians, birds, reptiles, and mammals, fever has been found to confer a clear advantage to the organism against any invading pathogens. Each of these groups of animals was found to respond in similar ways to fever. When the onset of fever is first noticed the animals seek a warmer part of their environment. A fish will swim to a warm-water niche in its local habitat; a reptile will migrate to a sun-drenched sandhill, and a tree frog will climb to the uppermost branches to maximize its exposure to the warmth of the sun. Once a warm, comfortable location has been found, the animals become very inactive and cease to feed. Animals deprived of the ability to migrate towards warmth or kept active were slowed in their recovery and had a higher death rate.

Fever response in humans follows a similar course. The onset of fever is usually announced by an abrupt chill that occurs after the temperature has begun to rise, This is fever's most dramatic paradox. This chilly sensation usually causes the patient to seek warmth in bed, covered by several blankets, and even with a hot water bottle at the feet. Fever is also associated with a desire to rest and reduce all normal activities. As the fever progresses, general weakness and muscular aches encourage this withdrawal and inactivity. Body movements become minimal. External stimuli become aggravating and the personality begins to disintegrate. The mind becomes dull and speech less articulate. The entire concentration is focused on the febrile condition. The appetite is characteristically depressed and even the most favorite dish is unappealing. As the temperature peaks and sweating begins, the second paradox of the febrile state is observed. In spite of the elevated fever, the aches and chills cease with the onset of sweating and a state of relative comfort supersedes.

This entire process of what is called *adaptive withdrawal* has been proven to be a definite survival advantage. When human subjects are given medication to lower their fever and eliminate the chills and muscular discomfort, discouraging the desire for warmth, rest, and abstinence from food, it has been found that their illness is lengthened and the prognosis diminished. In other words, subjects allowed to follow their normal instincts produced by the febrile state got better sooner and suffered less complications than those given fever-reducing medications.

Another study has conclusively found that antibiotics work far more effectively when the fever is not suppressed by aspirin. Once again, fever is a self defense mechanism and is both a healing and cleansing process. Fever, *if properly managed* with natural means, does not cause brain damage. In fact, a real danger in fever is when it is artificially suppressed. Death can then result as toxins accumulate and attack susceptible organ groups.

The presence of fever by itself is not very informative. A normal high fever may be anywhere from around 104–105°F (40°C) and does not indicate how severe a disease really is. Children, however, develop notoriously high fevers in a very short time due to some fairly harmless bacteria and viruses, and if the fever is allowed to reach 106°F (42°C), brain damage can occur. In some isolated cases, however, severe complications or death have occurred after even relatively low fevers, depending on the cause. Obviously, a doctor should be consulted for all severe or prolonged fevers.

As important a consideration as how *high* the temperature, is how long it has lasted, how the patient is coping, and whether the patient is *sweating*. A normal fever will run anywhere from 1–4 days. If it is prolonged it can indicate trouble. The patient's defense mechanisms may be weak and not up to the task on their own. If the fever is allowed to last too long, the body's energy reserves may be depleted, leaving it defenseless against the invader. If the patient is suspected of extremely low vitality, a more active approach to the problem is advisable. If the patient is not coping well with a very high fever, this also may be an indication for external intervention. And lastly, if the patient has a fever and is not sweating this *always* demands external intervention. Fever and sweating are two partners that should never be separated. Sweating is needed to help expel toxins and keep the temperature regulated.

One very important footnote to the discussion on fever is that fevers in the newborn and infant should never be allowed to rise too high and never without medical supervision. The temperature control mechanisms in the newborn are still immature, and with a high fever will sometimes become uncontrollable. Infants' fevers climb very rapidly. If allowed to reach 106°F (42°F), brain damage can occur. There have been rare cases of brain damage and death reported as low as 103–104°F (39.4–40°F). All moderate to high fevers in infants should be medically monitored.

For older children and adults we normally allow a fever to reach 104°–105°F (40°–40.5°C) before advising simple hydrotherapeutic procedures to be used. Obviously, this will depend on the cause. Some fevers should be kept under control at a lower temperature. This certainly varies from case to case, and with children it depends very much on the condition of the child. We usually don't allow the fever to be lowered to less than 102°F (38.5°C) in most circumstances.

Once an investigation is made so that you are sure that the cause of the fever is not serious and life-threatening, the following treatments may prove useful.

TREATMENT

Diet

All animals will fast when ill. Infants will refuse food and often even breast milk when they have a fever. Therefore we have before us the best example of the laws of nature at work. When you have a fever the best diet is the *liquid fast*. The old saying "feed a cold, starve a fever", although misunderstood, is at least correct when it comes to fever. The following liquids may be of benefit: water; diluted fruit juices; hot water and lemon juice; hot teas (to sweat).

It is important not to allow infants to become dehydrated. If the infant refuses fluids, he or she must receive intravenous fluid and electrolyte replacement.

Physiotherapy

When advised:
- Cold compresses.
- Tepid—body heat 98.6°F (36.8°F), 30-minute bath.
- Baths followed by brisk towel rubs to increase skin function where patient's vitality is high.
- Trunk packs: these are advisable in most fevers. They work with the healing process and lower the body temperature by relieving internal congestion, increasing skin function with sweating, and increasing elimination. In this case a cold trunk pack draws blood from the congested interior to the surface, and then induces sweating as the pack heats up.
- Hot blanket baths, hot compresses, etc. (if goose skin). Use in conjunction with sweating teas.
- Hot Epsom salts bath (see Appendix I) followed by sweating in bed under many blankets.

Therapeutic Agents

Vitamins and Minerals

- Vitamin C: 250–1000 mg per hour or as instant powder to drinks. Helps reduce fever.
- Vitamin A: 5000–25,000 IU 2–6 times daily. (See warning under Vitamin Toxicity, page 56.) Enhances immune function to help defend against infection.

Others

- Garlic: 2 capsules 3–4 times daily. Acts as an antibiotic and immunostimulant.
- Propolis: 10–15 drops tincture 3–4 times daily. Antibiotic.
- Thymus: 2 tablets every 1–2 hours. Immunostimulant.

Botanicals

Catnip tea.
Coneflower: blood purifier.
Elderflower tea.
Pleurisy root: to induce sweating.
Boneset.
European vervain.
Garlic.
Lemon balm.
Peppermint.
Yarrow.

Therapeutic Suggestions

The key to the proper treatment of fevers in general (please refer to comments on fever of infancy) is to allow the fever a wide range of action up to 104–105°F (40°C). Sweating must be encouraged and stimulated. The diet should be liquid only. The general situation and what symptoms accompany the fever (e.g. cough, body aches, excess mucus) influence if and what other medications are prescribed.

FIBROCYSTIC BREAST DISEASE
(Cystic Mastitis)

DEFINITION AND SYMPTOMS

Breast tenderness and cystic development, which may recur with each menstrual cycle or become continuous. The breast becomes nodular, with freely movable cysts near the surface of the breast. Deeper cysts can occur.

ETIOLOGICAL CONSIDERATIONS

- Methylxanthines (e.g. coffee, tea, cola, chocolate)
- Hormonal imbalance Estrogen excess; thyroid
- Allergies
- Vitamin deficiency (especially vitamin E)
- Constipation/toxemia: studies showing women with 3 or less bowel evacuations a week have 4.5 times the risk of developing cystic breasts

DISCUSSION

Although the cysts of cystic mastitis are benign there is a three- to seven-fold increase in the chance of cancer for those women with chronic fibrocystic disease. The condition usually progresses until menopause, when it is unlikely for new cysts to develop. There is an obvious correlation with the menstrual cycle. Approximately 20–50% of women are affected. Overstimulation of the breast by the female hormone estrogen is implicated. Until recently, little was known about the causes of this disorder. Within the past few years it has been observed that food and drinks containing methylxanthines, including coffee, tea, cola, and chocolate, are capable of aggravating this condition. Removing these substances from the diet is the most effective form of treatment for most women. Vitamin E supplementation has also been found to be very effective, in conjunction with these dietary changes.

TREATMENT

Although only foods containing methylxanthines have been implicated in this disorder, we usually suggest removing all negative health factors, to get the most complete cure. This includes eliminating not only coffee, tea, cola, and chocolate, but also smoking and alcohol, if possible. The diet should be composed of as many raw foods as possible, with emphasis on a more vegetarian protein-base diet, to avoid the hormones found in commercially raised meats, especially chicken and lot fed pig and beef. Changing to a diet high in soy foods will also reduce the estrogenization of the female reproductive organs and tissues, and will help prevent estrogen-dependent cancers.

Vitamins and Minerals—Primary
- Vitamin A: 25,000 IU twice daily. Needed to maintain the health of the ductal system of the breast.
- Vitamin B6: 200 mg 2-3 times daily. Use especially if PMS symptoms coexist.

- Vitamin C: 1-3 g 2-3 times daily. Essential for proper adrenal hormone balance.
- Vitamin E: 400-800 IU daily. As an antioxidant this vitamin protects breast tissue from cellular damage.
- Coenzyme Q10: 100 mg daily. Acts as a powerful antioxidant to protect breast tissue.
- Methionine: 500 mg daily on an empty stomach. Detoxifies estrogen (methylation) thus reducing excess.
- Evening primrose oil: 6-8 capsules daily.
- Flaxseed oil: 1-1½ tbsp daily.
- Probiotics.

Vitamins and Minerals—Secondary
- Zinc: 50 mg daily. To enhance immune function and repair tissue.
- Vitamin B1: 100 mg twice daily.
- Vitamin B complex: 50 mg 1-2 times daily.
- Calcium: 1000 mg daily.
- Arginine: 500 mg daily.
- Kelp or other iodine source.
- Bromelain: 1-2 tablets daily taken on an empty stomach. Anti-inflammatory.

Botanicals
Poke root: a lymphatic decongestant; specific. May also be used as an external poultice to relieve breast tissue inflammation (highly toxic, see page 60).
See Hypothyroidism, as conditions often are linked.

FLAT FEET
Pes Planus, Fallen Arches

DEFINITION

Collapse of the internal longitudinal and transverse arches of the foot. Eversion of the foot is associated in many cases.

SYMPTOMS

A sensation of weakness and strain on the medial (inner) side of the foot. Pain and aching at night, which is increased on weight-bearing. The pain usually centers on the inner border, or at the metatarsal heads. Referred pain to the calf, knee, hip, or low back is common. Loss of "spring" in step, with awkwardness. Feet tire easily, numbness, cramping.

ETIOLOGICAL CONSIDERATIONS

- Excess weight-bearing (carrying heavy weights, obesity, pregnancy); weak muscles
- Prolonged standing; improper foot wear; previous strain, sprain, or fracture; knock-knees
- Poor body mechanics: weight-bearing center incorrect; external rotation of leg; heredity
- Congenital (abnormal talus bone); shortening of achilles tendon; improper walking habits (walking with foot everted; claw toe walking)
- Arthritis, rickets, or calcium deficiency
- Muscle paralysis or weakness—due to disease such as polio or muscular dystrophy; spinal lesions

DISCUSSION

The foot is a very complicated functional unit, composed of 26 articulating bones. It is supported by an internal longitudinal ligament (spring ligament), external longitudinal ligament, and anterior and posterior transverse ligaments. It is not the function of the ligaments, however, to withstand prolonged weight-bearing. It is the muscles that provide the foot with its real support.

In the weight-bearing position there is a natural tendency of the foot to evert (turn outward), which is counteracted by the muscles of the feet. If these muscles weaken and eversion becomes chronic, the weight distribution on the foot becomes severely altered. Instead of a balanced distribution of weight through all the ligaments of the foot, the whole weight is thrown onto the internal spring ligament, which is not designed to handle such stress.

In the normal foot, weight is first carried by the heel (calcaneus), passed down the outer border of the foot to the five metatarsal bones in the front of the foot, with a final push-off from the big toe. If the muscles become weak, the ligaments are overburdened and they begin to stretch. This leads to bone displacement and, finally, permanent bone changes. In specific medical terms, what occurs is a movement of the talus bone forward and medially (towards the midline). This can then be found displaced towards the inner side of the foot. The navicular bone is depressed and the heel (calcaneus) rotates posteriorly downward and everts, so that walking is done more on the inner border. With these actions, the entire foot can be seen to evert in the typical flat-footed position, The foot then widens as the transverse arch collapses and the forefoot abducts or moves away from the midline.

These foot changes may further affect muscular balance in the calf, leg, hip, and low back, causing tiredness, pain, rotation of the fibulae, and sacroiliac or lumbar spinal lesions.

The most detrimental influences causing flat feet are a combination of excess weight-bearing, weak muscles, calcium deficiency, and poor body mechanics.

The most obvious cause of excess weight-bearing is obesity. Occupations that require repeated or prolonged lifting also may be a factor, Muscles may become weakened by lack of general muscular tone, excess burden, nutritional deficiency (especially calcium deficiency), spinal lesions upsetting nutritional and nervous supply to muscles, trauma or previous strain, or poor spinal mechanics causing muscle imbalances and weakness.

Poor spinal mechanics may also be a factor in several ways. Habitual walking with the foot everted places the weight burden on the weaker inner spring ligament, straining the arch and overburdening the muscles, which then weaken, allowing the ligaments to stretch. The big toe is then forced to push off in a position of adduction, creating the complication of hallux valgus, where the toe rotates and then crosses over its neighbor. The increased lumbar curve caused by wearing high heels throws the weight center forward onto the front part of the foot. The same situation occurs with the condition called visceroptosis, where the abdomen sags due to weak abdominal muscles, obesity, or spinal lesions, causing the center of gravity to alter, affecting the feet. The muscles between the toes (lumbricals and interossei) then weaken, due to the excess burden. The toes may also begin to "claw", favoring a collapse of the anterior transverse arch which is associated with the condition called metatarsalgia.

TREATMENT

Normally the arches only begin to form when the child has been walking for a year or so. This means that it is normal for a toddler to show some degree of flat feet and no cause for alarm. In some cases, however, arches do not form due to congenital causes and special shoes are required. Three degrees of flat feet are recognized:

- First-degree flat foot: is a postural deformity with alteration in the muscles and ligaments but only minor displacement of bone or pain. Complete correction is possible with proper treatment.
- Second-degree flat foot: shows slight bone change and muscle damage. Complete correction is no longer possible, but stabilization and strengthening will relieve the symptoms of pain and weakness to a large degree.
- Third-degree flat foot: shows permanent bone changes with some arthritis and rigidity. No cure is possible.

As you can see, it is very important to treat flat feet in the earliest stages to prevent permanent joint deformity.

Diet

It is essential that the diet contain a large amount of readily absorbable minerals, especially calcium. Contrary to popular belief, dairy products are not the most desirable source of calcium. A far better source is raw green vegetables taken with a slightly acidic salad dressing containing apple cider vinegar or lemon juice. Salads or cooked vegetables should be eaten in large quantities with both lunch and supper. Dairy products, in most cases, should be reduced if a large portion of the diet has been concentrated on this source in the past. Less red meats and more fish or vegetarian proteins are also suggested. Soy milk contains more bio-available calcium than dairy milk by nearly 2.5 times.

Physiotherapy

The main part of therapy lies in physical therapies. These must be done daily for any real results.

Exercises—Standing

- Spring up: stand on hard floor, rise gently onto toes and then "spring up". This should be done in the morning before shoes go on, and repeated 15–30 times. Repeat again in evening.
- Rise and sink: stand on forefoot with hands over head and slowly rise onto toes. Lower arms in front of body and gradually sink down to the flat foot and heel. Repeat 10–20 times twice daily.
- Heel-to-toe rock: stand on the flat feet and rock heel to toe for 2–3 minutes twice daily.
- Scrunch: with shoes on scrunch the toes up against the bottom of the shoe so that the foot arches. Do this 6–10 times and repeat up to 10 times daily.
- Pick up: pick up a ping pong ball or a large marble with the toes. Make this into a game.
- Bean bag game: make 3 inch (8 cm) square or round bean bags. Pick up bags

with toes and then toss them into a target such as a small wastebasket or hat.

- Ostrich step: walk in a straight line with weight on the outer borders of the foot and toes curled downward and inward. Raise each foot so that it is opposite the other knee before placing it down to the ground.
- Incline board walk: nail two 9 ft (3 m) × 10 inch (25 cm) wide boards together at their long edges to make an equilateral triangle with the ground. Walk along the boards with one foot on each board. Repeat 10-20 times twice daily.
- Hip rotation: stand with feet 2-3 inches (5-8 cm) apart. Contract gluteal muscles (seat) and rotate the hips outward while keeping the toes, outer foot, and heels firmly on the ground.
- Push out: stand with the feet 2 inches (5 cm) apart and attempt to force them apart, thus putting weight and stress on the outer portions of the foot, but do not move the feet. Slowly relax and repeat 10-20 times.
- Toe rise: rise onto the toes and slowly tilt the weight onto the outer borders of the foot. Repeat 10-20 times twice daily.
- Outer foot stand: knees are held parallel and then slowly rolled outward so that the weight is placed on the outer borders of the foot.
- Outer border walk: walk on outer borders of foot.

Exercises—Sitting
- Heel raising and lowering.
- Sit with feet crossed resting on outer borders.
- Sit cross-legged.
- Press toes against ground but do not raise any part of foot off ground.
- Place thin book under toes and flex forefoot, keeping toes straight. This is a very important exercise.

Local Therapy
- Postural and muscular re-education and exercises, with special work on Achilles tendon, calves, quadriceps, gluteals, paravertebral lumbar muscles, and abdominals.
- Deep muscle massage to plantar fascia, entire foot and lower limbs with: peanut oil: ½ pint (250 mL), witch hazel: 2 fl oz (60 mL), rubbing alcohol: 4 fl oz (125 mL), oil of sassafras: 3-10 drops; tincture of capsicum: 2 drops mix well and repeat massage twice daily.
- Tannic acid foot and lower leg baths: made by boiling old coffee grounds and water for 10 minutes. Apply hot and massage feet and lower legs while soaking. Time: 20 minutes daily.
- Alternate hot and cold foot baths.
- Spinal therapy (to specific lesions).
- Local manipulation: general joint mobilization. Treat talus which has rotated anteriorly and medially, navicular which is depressed, and calcaneus which is everted.
- Footwear: the front of the shoe should not compress toes and should have a straight inner border from heel to big toe. Soft, resilient arch supports are useful. In later stages of the disorder an inner wedge heel lift of ¼ inch (6 mm) may be needed. This raises the inner border of the heel to counteract its tendency to evert.

Therapeutic Agents

Vitamins and Minerals
- Calcium: 400-800 mg daily.
- Vitamin C: 500-3000 mg daily or more,
- Vitamin A: 4000-25,000 IU twice daily.
- Vitamin B: 25-50 mg twice daily.
- Multiminerals: e.g. Celtic salt.
- Magnesium: 200-400 mg daily.
- Silica.

Botanicals
Horsetail.

Therapeutic Suggestions

Exercise, Exercise, Exercise!

FLATULENCE
(Adult and Infant Colic)

DEFINITION

Flatulence: abnormal amounts of gas passing upward or downward, with or without intestinal discomfort.

Infant colic: abdominal pain, distension, insomnia, extreme fretfulness, and hysteria.

SYMPTOMS

Excess gas, abdominal distention, abdominal discomfort.

ETIOLOGICAL CONSIDERATIONS—PRIMARY

- Improper diet
  Excess acidity; poor food combinations; beans; hurried meals; frequent meals; allergies; food intolerances (e.g. dairy or wheat/gluten); liquids with meals
- Digestive enzyme deficiency
- Inadequate mastication
- Weakened digestion, poor eliminations
- Gallbladder/liver disorder
- Poor absorption
- Abnormal intestinal flora (yeast overgrowth)

ETIOLOGICAL CONSIDERATIONS— SECONDARY

Spinal (midthoracic); visceroptosis: poor spinal mechanics; diverticulitis; anemia; parasites; improper weaning

DISCUSSION

Flatulence is not only uncomfortable and embarrassing, it is also a sign that some aspect of the digestive system is not functioning properly. What flatulence means, irrespective of its cause, is that food is not being completely digested, or is digested inadequately, for the particular part of the digestive system it is currently passing through to deal with it effectively. Digestive enzymes are essential in the digestive process to break down complex proteins, fats, and carbohydrates into small molecules for proper absorption. The result of food that is too complex passing out of the stomach and upper small intestine into the rest of the intestinal tract is fermentation, gas, and abdominal pain.

Diet is the most important consideration in all cases of chronic, excess gas formation. Certain foods such as beans are well-known gas producers. They contain oligosaccharides (raffinose and stachyose) which have digestive enzyme resistant chemical bonds between their sugar molecules causing food to be incompletely broken down and passed into the small intestine where fermentation and gas result. Many other foods will affect particular individuals in a similar way. These are usually easily determined and avoided. If this is the only cause, the problem is quickly solved.

More often, however, the problem is deeply ingrained. Food allergies or intolerances are a common cause of severe intestinal disorders with gas. Any food may cause a reaction, but the most frequent offenders are dairy products and gluten grains (see Celiac Disease). Generally unwise food combinations also may cause gas. The usual citrus/starch combination for breakfast is definitely a problem. These two require entirely different acid/alkaline levels for proper digestion and the two in the stomach at the same time simply become indigestible. Fruit and vegetables at the same meal or melons with anything else will have a similar effect. If these foods then pass into the intestine undigested, gas results.

The habit of drinking, especially milk, with meals is another bad nutritional habit. The liquids dilute digestive juices and hinder proper digestion. Excessively large meals also upset digestion by depleting the body's digestive enzyme capacity. Some food is then undigested or only partly digested, leading once again to fermentation and gas

Meals taken at too-frequent intervals tend to upset the digestion of the meal taken previously, and also may cause enzyme depletion as above.

Hurried meals with inadequate chewing do not allow sufficient breaking down of vegetable cell walls. Cellulose, the main component of vegetable cell walls, is normally indigestible and unless food matter is thoroughly masticated, it may lead to gas formation and irritation in some people. Salivary digestive enzymes in the mouth, although of little use in partial breakdown of starches, have been overemphasized as a major digestive source. However, the process of chewing and tasting foods, along with the passage of sufficient salivary enzymes into the stomach, signals the secretion of other digestive enzymes absolutely essential to the digestive process.

Eating while under stress results in very poor digestion. Stress stimulates the sympathetic nervous system which governs danger responses and turns off the parasympathetic nervous system responsible for the secretion of digestive enzymes and intestinal motility.

Disorders of the liver and in particular the gallbladder upset fat digestion. Gallbladder disease is commonly associated with indigestion and gas.

Under normal circumstances the intestines are inhabited by friendly bacterial flora, absolutely essential for proper digestion. If the diet is high in vegetable matter and fiber, these bacteria do not cause any problems. If the diet is composed of sweets, refined carbohydrates, excess meat, and is low in fiber content, the amount and type of bacterial flora change, becoming less favorable to proper digestion and vitamin synthesis, and more favorable for gas production. Antibiotic use can totally upset this internal ecology, as can repeated enemas.

Poor eliminations and constipation may also be a cause of flatulence directly, or indirectly by causing diverticulitis with abnormal pain and gas.

Spinal lesions in the mid-thoracic region T4 to T10, or the condition of visceroptosis with poor abdominal tone, may cause abnormal secretion of digestive enzymes, reduced stomach or intestinal activity, or pressure on the intestinal tract, resulting in abnormal function.

Parasitic infections should always be considered as a possibility with any abnormal intestinal conditions. Some cases of infant colic are the result of Candida infections. This may be suspected in an infant whose mother had a yeast infection during her pregnancy, or if the infant has received antibiotic therapy for any reason. It is essential to re-establish normal bowel ecology as soon as possible. A preparation of Lactobifidus powder added to the milk may be useful to correct this condition. If the infant is being breast-fed, express a small amount and add the Lactobifidus powder ($1/8$–$1/4$ tsp) to the milk, 2–3 times daily. Other stronger medications should be avoided if possible.

Infant colic is included within this section on flatulence since some of the considerations apply. The most common cause of colic in the totally breast-fed infant is the mother's diet. Literally any food may cause the baby to suffer infant colic, gas, or diarrhea, but cabbage, onions, garlic, wheat, yeast, brussels sprouts, and broccoli are common offenders. Outside of the single irritating foods that may affect the infant at one time or another, the problem is usually a totally inappropriate diet of fried foods, junk food, and refined food in all manner of chaotic combinations. An example of this in our practice was one couple that came in red-eyed and extremely distressed since their 8-month-old daughter kept them up day and night with nearly constant screaming. Once the mother was placed on a "normal" diet the infant settled down within 2 weeks into a sweet, well-tempered child

Colic that develops in a formula-fed infant obviously implicates the food given. The infant may be allergic to the milk, wheat, soy, or sugar in the formula. If breast milk is absolutely not available to the child, vitamin- and mineral-enriched goat's milk is a better alternative to formula. Usually, however, the mother can breast-feed, or at least can with some effort, but has either been improperly educated about what is best for her child, or has some psychological hang-up about breast-feeding. Even if the mother did not begin breast-feeding she can, with perseverance, develop a milk supply for her infant literally any time after birth and sometimes even years later by frequent attempts at breast-feeding over several months. If the infant does have colic and the mother could breast-feed, it is the best course of action in these formula-intolerance cases.

If colic has developed after weaning has begun, the obvious cause of the problem is one or several of the foods added to the diet. We are constantly amazed at what little understanding some parents have regarding the weaning process. One couple came to us about their 3-month-old infant's colic. When asked what the child ate, the proud answer was that he ate *everything* they ate! This was even more horrifying when you understand that their diet included fried eggs, bacon, pork, pastry, spaghetti, pizza, hamburgers, french fries, Coca-Cola, and so on.

When each new food is not slowly added and the infant carefully monitored for reactions such as colic, rashes, or any other unusual symptom, it can become very difficult to determine which food is the offender without totally reweaning the child. This is a difficult process for both parents and child, but is the only way to proceed if the diet has already become fairly complicated without care in weaning.

The two food groups, wheat and dairy products, are especially suspect and should be eliminated as a first step in all cases. Food allergies or intolerances to these two food groups are very common. In general, wheat and other grains are introduced far too early in the average infant's diet. Digestive capacity for concentrated starches only begins around 5–6 months in most infants. We usually advise grain to be introduced as one of the last foods and yeast bread added well after the first year of life. Fresh boiled goat's milk is usually less of a problem than cow's milk and this should be the choice if at all possible, to be introduced just before weaning is to commence. If these two simple rules were applied, there would be far fewer people with allergies in the world.

TREATMENT

Diet

General Rules

An old proverb states that nine-tenths of what we eat goes for our health, while the other one-tenth goes to the health of our doctor. In the case of indigestion and flatulence, this is clearly so.

Never eat to the stage that you feel full. Meals must be unhurried. It is wise to spend 10–15 minutes before each meal in quiet activity, and have a minute or two of silence before eating, to allow the nervous system to relax. Never eat when hurried or under stress, since the food will only cause you harm.

Each bite of food must be chewed thoroughly. A person with a healthy stomach may gulp food with no obvious ill effect. The person with weak digestion must carefully chew each bite until almost liquid, to make the food more accessible to enzyme digestion.

Do not eat between meals. Some people may benefit by eating between meals for conditions such as hypoglycemia, but usually it is better to allow complete digestion of each meal before eating again. We know some people who eat only one meal each day; however, it begins upon waking and continues until late at night. This will

251

overburden the digestive system, leading to disease.

Do not drink with meals. The dry feeding regimen is often sufficient in itself to correct many digestive complaints.

Never eat fried foods, hydrogenated fats, sugar, refined carbohydrates, or other junk food.

Be careful in combining foods.

The actual dietary regimen employed varies from patient to patient. With some it is enough to remove any allergic or irritating foods and follow the simple dietary rules above. Others need to be treated by treating the major causes affecting their case, such as constipation, gallbladder disease, etc. The following regimens are useful, depending on the patient:

- 3–14-day fruit juice or vegetable juice fast.
- 10-day brown rice diet.
- Apple diet (no skin).
- Raw foods diet.
- Constipation diet.
- Liver-cleansing diet and gallbladder flush.

Physiotherapy

- Hot sitz bath (acute).
- Hot compresses (acute).
- Alternate hot and cold sitz bath (chronic).
- Enemas (acute and with cleansing diet regimens).
- Spinal manipulation.
- Abdominal exercises.

Therapeutic Agents

Vitamins and Minerals

Dependent upon major cause, or none required. It is usually best to discontinue all pill supplements except those specifically recommended below for the flatulent condition, until full recovery has been attained.

Others

- Bran: adds fiber and regulates bowel; not to be used in wheat sensitivity. May aggravate condition for first 7–10 days. 1 tsp with water before meals.
- Charcoal tablets: 1–2 per hour in acute flatulence.
- Pancreatic enzyme tablets: 1–2 with meals.
- Garlic: some cases find this very effective; may aggravate others.
- Glutamic acid hydrochloride.
- Hydrochloric acid: if hypoacid condition has been verified by test.
- Probiotics: not to be used if dairy sensitivity exists. 2 capsules 3 times daily.
- Lemon juice and hot water.

Botanicals—Primary

Gentian: digestive bitter.

Fennel: carminative.

Chamomile: if of nervous system origins.

Wild yam root: works rapidly in acute adult or infant colic. Adult dose: 15 to 25 drops of tincture in water every $\frac{1}{2}$ hour for 1–2 hours; then every 4–6 hours. Child dose: $\frac{1}{4}$ to $\frac{1}{2}$ adult dose.

American saffron: infusion. Adult: 1 cup 2–3 times daily.

Infant colic: 1 tsp three times daily on empty stomach.

Botanicals—Secondary

Anise: tea.

Caraway.

Cinnamon.

Cloves.

Comfrey.

Coriander.

Cumin.

Dill.

Flaxseed.

Ginger.

Goldenseal: 25 drops in water 3 times daily as a bowel tonic.

Parsley.

Peppermint.

Peppermint oil: 1–4 drops in hot water for flatulent colic.

Slippery elm: 1 cup tea 3–6 times daily.

Thyme.

GALLBLADDER DISEASE
(Gallstones and Cholecystitis)

DEFINITION

Gallstones (cholelithiasis): concretions in the gallbladder.
Cholecystitis: inflammation of the gallbladder.

SYMPTOMS

- Right upper quadrant abdominal discomfort (may be symptom-free for years); biliary colic (knife-like pain)
- Dyspepsia (fatty foods cause gas, fullness, nausea, bloating, and/or belching)
- Chronic constipation, headaches, irritation, quick temper, nervousness, pain between shoulder blades on right referred to right shoulder, possible fever and chills with positive Murphy's sign (acute)

Note: In chronic cases the gallbladder is shrunken and scarred. Long-term complications of gallbladder disease include cancer.

ETIOLOGICAL CONSIDERATIONS—PRIMARY

- Diet
  Fiber deficiency; fried foods; saturated fats; excess dairy products; excess sugar and refined carbohydrates; overeating
- Bile stasis: Dietary fats must empty the gallbladder frequently and forcibly. Bile stasis allows the bile to become too concentrated. Incomplete emptying is a major cause of gallbladder disease plus stone formation.
- Bile blockage: 95% of all cholecystitis is caused by a stone in the neck of the gallbladder, in the cystic duct, or is due to inspissated bile (thickened bile). The gallbladder distends, becomes edematous, and inflamed. Secondary infection may then occur.
- Obesity: overburdened gallbladder; sluggishness
- Liver sluggishness and toxicity
- Contraceptive pill: doubles chances of gallstones
- Lack of exercise: decreased bile secretion
- Stress

ETIOLOGICAL CONSIDERATIONS— SECONDARY

Food allergy; non-steroidal anti-inflammatory drugs; constipation; pregnancy, many children: (associated with gall bladder disease)

DISCUSSION

Gall bladder disease and gallstones in particular are most common in the developed nations and are fairly rare in undeveloped nations. This places gallstones in the unique class of diseases called diseases of civilization. With this understanding it becomes clear that much unnecessary surgery can be prevented by simple changes in cultural, dietary, and social habits.

The surgical removal of the gallbladder (rarely necessary) robs the body of a useful organ and does nothing to correct the cause of gallstones or disease. To understand fully the real causes and treatment of these disorders, a little physiological background is useful.

Bile is secreted by the liver at the rate of about 4 pints (2 liters) a day. It is then stored in the gallbladder in a concentrated form (10×). Bile contains 90% water, mucus, bile

253

pigments (bilirubin from hemoglobin breakdown—red blood cell pigment), cholesterol, bile salts (help emulsify fats), lecithin, and inorganic salts. Bile aids digestion and absorption of fat by increasing the solubility of fatty acids and emulsifying fats to make them more easily accessible to lipase, a fat-breaking enzyme from the pancreas. Bile salts are necessary for the absorption of fat-soluble vitamins. They help promote peristalsis and are mildly laxative. Bile is reabsorbed in the intestine, returns to the liver, and stimulates more bile secretion. Bile is initially secreted from the gallbladder due to the hormone cholecystokinin from the intestinal mucosa which is liberated when fatty foods enter the small intestine. This hormone causes the cystic duct and gallbladder to forcibly contract and expel its bile contents. With these few facts, you can see that the gallbladder is essential for proper digestion of fat and fat-soluble vitamins, and aids in keeping the bowels regular.

Cholecystitis is almost always secondary to gallstones or thickened bile. Gallstones form due to a combination of factors, the most prominent being faulty diet and bile stasis. The typical American diet of high cholesterol and saturated fatty foods such as fried eggs, bacon, white toast, butter and coffee with sugar and cream is a fine example of a diet carefully designed to cause gallstones, as well as other serious diseases. Saturated fats, such as excess eggs, milk, cheese, butter, meats, and hydrogenated margarine are all a major factor in causing gallstones. Ninety percent of gallstones are primarily cholesterol in composition. The problem with gallstone formation is not only excess cholesterol, but also a deficiency of many foods that normally keep cholesterol under control

Refined carbohydrates and sugar upset cholesterol metabolism, and increase blood cholesterol levels. They also decrease bile flow. This effect is enhanced on a high-protein diet. When whole grains are refined, bran is stripped away. Bran has been found to therapeutically lower cholesterol levels. It influences the amount of chenodeoxycholic acid, a natural bile acid which lowers cholesterol and dissolves stones.

Vitamin E, also lost in carbohydrate refining, has been found to both prevent and dissolve gallstones. Vitamin E is commonly deficient in women on the contraceptive pill and during pregnancy. Lecithin, an element deficient in most modern diets, is a well-known fat emulsifier, and helps keep cholesterol in solution. Vitamin A helps keep the mucosal walls healthy and prevents excess dead cells from entering the gallbladder and bile. A diet rich in vitamin B complex helps empty the gallbladder more efficiently. Vitamin C helps convert cholesterol into bile acids and renders it harmless.

Unsaturated oils help stimulate the gallbladder to contract vigorously and thus cleanse itself on a regular basis. Raw, unrefined olive oil is the most efficient of all oils. This is the reason that Italians, who consume large amounts of olive oil in their diet, have a low incidence of gallstones. Olive oil has been used for therapy in gallbladder disease as far back as the Roman empire. (Note: A no-fat diet or very low-fat diet will actually cause gallstones by decreasing bile flow and allowing the bile to become concentrated

Most gallstone patients are hearty eaters and high livers. While not all patients are "fat, flatulent, female, and over forty", certainly the majority are. Excess food puts an unnecessary burden on the digestive organs. Once the ingested food reaches a point of exceeding the body's enzymatic capacity, the rest remains undigested, or partially digested, causing bowel toxemia, gas, discomfort, and constipation (or diarrhea). A headache may soon follow. Smaller, more frequent meals increase bile flow, stimulate the gallbladder, and keep bile from getting too concentrated.

Exercise stimulates bile secretion by the liver. Too little exercise, therefore too little bile, causes a deficiency of bile digestion, especially if the foods eaten are of the wrong type.

Anger, fear, excitement, worry, and hate all cause bile to cease flowing, and therefore encourage stone formation.

TREATMENT

Therapy for gallstones and gallbladder disease is aimed at first flushing the gallbladder of its stones by use of specific time-tested dietary regimens and herbs. Many variations exist as to the type of foods and liquids consumed, and the relative proportions of the flushing agents. Several different examples will be given. Nearly all these regimens are based on the therapeutic effects of olive oil. Prior to attempting these methods, an x-ray of the gallbladder is advised, to determine the size of the stones. If they are too large to be successfully passed and become lodged in the ducts, severe pain and possible surgery may be the result. For very large stones special methods are required to dissolve the stone so that it may be safely passed. We strongly recommend that if this therapy is undertaken, it should be closely supervised by a naturopath experienced in this regimen.

Diet

Liver and Gallbladder Diet

Stage 1: Begin treatment with a 3-to-5-to-7-day grapefruit mono diet

Breakfast
Fresh grapefruit.

Midmorning
Fresh grapefruit juice.

Lunch
Fresh grapefruit.

Midafternoon
Fresh grapefruit juice.

Supper
Fresh grapefruit.

Evening
Fresh grapefruit juice.

Stage 2

Breakfast
Fresh grapefruit.

Midmorning
Fresh grapefruit juice, black cherry juice, parley tea, carrot and watercress juice, raw beet juice, apple juice, or dandelion root tea.

Lunch
A large, varied raw salad with nuts (other than peanuts) or soy-based protein with 1–2 whole wheat crisp breads. Olive oil plus lemon, garlic, and honey as salad dressing.

Midafternoon
Same as midmorning.

Supper
1. Same as lunch; or
2. Any vegetarian meal (excluding the use of dairy products or eggs), with baked potato and two other green or root vegetables; or
3. Steamed vegetables and brown rice or other whole grain.

Dessert
Any fresh, baked or stewed fruit.

Evening
Grapefruit juice.

Olive Oil Therapy

Olive Oil Flush 1

8.00 a.m.
½ pint (250 mL) raw unrefined olive oil plus juice of 2 lemons.

9.00 a.m.
Repeat.

10.00 a.m.
Repeat.

1.00 p.m.
2 tsp Epsom salts in a glass of warm water.

Olive Oil Flush 2

On empty stomach, drink 4 fl oz (125 mL) raw unrefined olive oil mixed with 4 fl oz

(125 mL) lemon juice. Lie on right side with hips elevated for 2 hours.

Olive Oil Flush 3:
1 pint pure olive oil
8–9 lemons (juiced)
Drink plenty of apple juice or grapefruit juice for 24–72 hours before starting diet. Begin at 7 p.m.: 4 tbsp olive oil with 1 tsp lemon juice, separately or mixed. Repeat every 15 minutes until all the oil is gone.

Gallbladder and Liver Flush 4:
Follow Stage 1 of the liver diet for 3–5 to 7 days, then continue Stage 2 for 7–14 days. Five days preceding the day of the olive oil therapy, take as much apple juice as can be consumed, in addition to your normally pre-scribed Stage 2 diet. On each of these 5 days also take 90 drops of orthophosphoric acid diluted in water. (After flush take 10 drops daily unless otherwise directed.) Three hours after lunch take 1 tbsp Epsom salts in approx-imately 1 fl oz (30 mL) water (chase with citrus juice to avoid the bitter taste). Instead of supper, have citrus juice (grapefruit). At approximately 7 p.m. take a strong coffee enema in which 2 tbsp Epsom salts are dis-solved. Then do either of the following:

Straight Flush
Just before bed, take ½ cup of unrefined olive oil and ½ cup citrus juice. They may be blended or taken separately.

Royal Flush
Eight 2 fl oz (60 mL) doses of olive oil taken over 2–4-hour period, approximately every 15 minutes. Citrus juice may be blended with it. (*Note:* Some people find olive oil difficult to get down. Sometimes sipping it through a straw so that the oil does not come in contact with the lips helps considerably.)

Therapeutic Agents

Acute Cases
- Apple juice; beet extract tablets; beetroot tops, beet juice; beet tops, carrot, and lemon juice.
- Chamomile tea: to dissolve; dandelion tea and dandelion greens: clears obstruction.
- Grapefruit juice; olive oil plus lemon; pear juice; peppermint tea; pineapple juice.
- Potassium broth, radish, watercress, nasturtium.

Chronic Cases—Supplements
- Vitamin C: 500–2000 mg 3–6 times daily.
- Vitamin A (micellized): 10,000–25,000 IU twice daily. Use emulsified form.
- Vitamin B complex: 25–50 mg 2–3 times daily.
- Vitamin B6: 50–100 mg 1–2 times daily.
- Vitamin E (micellized): 400 IU 1–3 times daily.

Other—Primary
- EPA (eicosapentaenoic acid): 5–10 g daily.
- L-glycine: 500 mg daily. Needed for bile acid synthesis.
- Olive oil: include in diet daily.
- Choline, inositol, and methionine: useful lipotrophics and bile stimulants.
- Black radish plus olive oil (to dissolve): 2 tbsp grated radish with 1–2 tbsp olive oil, mixed.
- Eat ½ hour before breakfast for 40 days.
- Peppermint oil: 2 capsules 3 times daily. To cleanse the gallbladder.
- Bran: 1 tsp with water 2–3 times daily.
- Lecithin (as concentrated phosphatidylcholine): take 1–2 capsules 3–4 times daily.

Other—Secondary
Alkaline foods; beet tablets; brewer's yeast; corn oil; laxative foods; orthophosphoric acid; smaller meals; taurine—thins bile (for prevention).

Botanicals
Black root: to reduce gall bladder inflammation.
Boldo: helps dissolve gallstones; cholagogue.

Wild yam root: for colic.

Fringe tree: increases bile flow.

Globe artichoke.

Barberry: positively affects the quality of bile salts.

Celandine: reduces inflammation of bile ducts.

Chamomile.

Dandelion.

Oregon grape root: stimulates bile.

Yellow dock: stimulates bile.

Note: Be sure to drink 6–8 glasses of water daily to help prevent gallstone formation.

GLAUCOMA

DEFINITION

Elevated intraocular pressure with gradual vision loss. No early symptoms; later, colored halos around lights, eye ache, headache, tunnel vision, visual abnormalities, frequent changes of eyeglass prescriptions.

ETIOLOGICAL CONSIDERATIONS—PRIMARY

- Blockage of outflow of aqueous humor or Increased production of aqueous humor
- Prolonged stress (adrenal exhaustion).
- Glandular imbalance (adrenals or thyroid).
- Collagen metabolism abnormalities.
- Spinal lesion (cervical, upper thoracic and cranial)
  Disturbed nervous and blood supply; autonomic system disturbance
- Blood sugar abnormalities (diabetes associated)
- High blood pressure and arteriosclerosis
- Drugs
  Antispasmodics; steroids, including eye-drops; tricyclic antidepressants

ETIOLOGICAL CONSIDERATIONS— SECONDARY

Toxicity; allergy; heredity; coffee, caffeine, nicotine, and alcohol; blood vessel constriction; trauma

DISCUSSION

Glaucoma involves an increase in fluid pressure within the eye which eventually damages the delicate optic nerve at the back of the eye. This nerve is the connecting link between what your eye sees and its interpretation by the brain. Intraocular pressure depends on an equilibrium between inflow of fluid called aqueous humor from an area called the ciliary body and its outflow from the tissues of the iridocorneal angle. If fluid production is too great, or more commonly, if fluid outflow is obstructed, pressure builds, causing tissue (nerve) damage. The higher the pressure above normal, the more serious and rapid is the damage. However, even lower pressure increases over a prolonged period of time may cause nerve damage and thus vision loss.

Once damage has occurred and vision is partly lost, it can never be regained. Since early symptoms are not present, or are not very noticeable in most cases, an early diagnosis depends on routine eye pressure checks. Many optometrists offer this check as part of a normal eye examination.

The actual cause of glaucoma is not entirely clear. Some cases clearly show a hereditary predisposition. Blood sugar abnormalities, specifically diabetes, are also associated with glaucoma. Prolonged stress may precede glaucoma, as may a history of improper eye use such as reading in dim lights, watching excessive amounts of television or movies with poor lighting, or habitual use of sunglasses. Some physicians feel that there is a clear connection between glandular imbalances such as adrenal exhaustion or hypothyroidism. Others point to general toxic causes as a factor.

Whatever the actual cause, it seems likely that the way in which these tissues suffer damage is by reduced nutrition in the form of altered blood lymph, or hormonal or nervous supply. This may be due to hormonal or glandular imbalance, constitutional toxicity, spinal lesions, cranial lesions, habitual use of coffee, tea, alcohol, tobacco, or any other factor such as allergy, which might disturb the body's normal functioning.

TREATMENT

Orthodox treatment for glaucoma consists of eyedrops designed to reduce the fluid production in the eye, or to increase its outflow. Should these fail several types of surgery are now available, including laser procedures.

However, there is hope for a more complete and natural cure of glaucoma for some patients. The best-documented treatment alternative in reducing intraocular pressure is megadoses of vitamin C. In studies where 5–7 g of vitamin C were given up to 7 times daily, remarkable decreases in eye pressure were noted. The higher the initial pressure, the more dramatic the pressure reduction. However, even with mildly elevated pressures, significant reductions occurred.

Another well-recognized substance found in experimental studies to lower intraocular pressure is marijuana. This, at present, is a controlled drug, but available by prescription for this purpose from a sympathetic ophthalmologist.

Other less well-known approaches to glaucoma involve generalized constitutional treatment along with local physiotherapy and spinal manipulations. These therapies base their methods on correcting hormonal imbalances, circulatory and nervous supply deficiencies, and toxic causes.

Diet

The basic dietary changes are aimed at supplying adequate nutrition, encouraging internal cleansing, and establishing equilibrium. Periods on vegetable juice (carrot) and fruit juice fasting are recommended, followed by short, exclusively raw food diets. The interim diet emphasizes carrots, greens (lettuce, celery, sprouts, beet tops, etc.) and plenty of seafoods (fish, oysters, seaweeds, kelp, etc.). Potassium broth should be taken regularly or as a stock base for other soups. Gelatin should be included whenever possible in this regimen. These three stages (fast, raw foods, and interim diet) should be rotated at intervals, the length of each depending on the condition of the patient.

Absolutely no alcohol, coffee, black tea, cola, or smoking is permitted during the diet, since these interfere with the normal blood circulation to the eyes and upset the hormonal stability in the system as a whole.

Physiotherapy

- Spinal manipulation: specific lesions will usually be found in the upper cervical region (especially C1) with others in the general cervical and upper thoracic regions. Cranial lesions may also be found as a result of trauma. The endonasal technique (see Appendix I) may be useful. Precede all spinal therapy with moist heat.
- Atomodine fume baths: put 1 tsp of Atomodine in 1 pint (500 mL) of boiled water. Make an improvised steam tent by placing pot under wooden chair and covering chair and body up to neck with a blanket. This will allow the Atomodine fumes to settle upon the body, helping to correct hormonal imbalances. Repeat twice per month.
- Sweat baths, saunas: 1–2 times per week.
- Massage: follow each spinal therapy, sweat bath, and especially each Atomodine fume bath with massage from the

midthoracic area up to the occiput, along the paravertebral muscles. This should be deep neuromuscular type massage with the following mixture: 2 fl oz (60 mL) olive oil, 2 fl oz (60 mL) peanut oil, ¼ fl oz (7 mL) oil of sassafras, 1 tsp liquefied lanolin.
Follow each massage session with alternate hot and cold showers, including alternate hot and cold head douches.

- Ice-cold baths: fill a large basin with ice-cold water. Immerse both eyes in the container and rapidly blink eyes open and shut 5-10 times. Rest and then repeat 2-3 times, twice daily.
- Alternate hot and cold eye compresses: apply a hot, moist towel or folded washcloth to both eyes for 2-3 minutes; then apply an ice-cold cloth for 2-3 minutes. Repeat 3 times, ending with cold.
- Ice-cold eye compress: apply ice-cold moist towel or folded washcloth for 2-3 minutes; rest 1 minute and reapply 3-4 times. Repeat twice daily.
- Bates eye exercises (Found in *The Art of Seeing,* by Aldous Huxley).
- Neck exercises.

Avoid dark TV viewing, excessive movie attendance, reading in poor light, or wearing sunglasses excessively.

Therapeutic Agents

Vitamins and Minerals— Primary

- Vitamin A with beta-carotene (micellized): 25,000 IU twice daily.
- Niacin.
- Vitamin B1: 100 mg twice daily.
- Vitamin C: 5-7 g 7 times daily; average for 150 lb (68 kg) person 35,000 mg daily (extra B6 and magnesium is

required to prevent increased calcium excretion which is associated with the tendency to form kidney stones). Helps maintain collagen structures.

- Vitamin E: 400-800 IU daily. Antioxidant. Protects tissues of the eye.
- Bioflavonoids. especially quercetin.
- Rutin: 20-30 mg 3 times daily.

Vitamins and Minerals— Secondary

- Vitamin B2.
- Vitamin B6: diuretic.
- Vitamin B12.
- Vitamin B complex: 50 mg twice daily.
- Calcium: 800-1000 mg daily.
- Chromium.
- Magnesium: 400-500 mg daily.

Others

- Lipoic acid: (especially in open-angle glaucoma).
- Kelp or other iodine source (e.g. Atomodine or 636—Cayce products).
- Evening primrose oil: reduces intraocular pressure.
- Probiotics.
- Spirulina: 1 tsp 3 times daily.
- Taurine.

Botanicals

Bilberry, the "vision herb", and Oregon grape: both contain berberine, a potent antioxidant with specificity for the eye.

Note: Non-toxic therapies may help control glaucoma or reduce pressure levels to prevent need for surgery. *In all cases remain under the care and supervision of your ophthalmologist, who can regularly check your intraocular pressure.*

GOUT

DEFINITION

A recurrent form of arthritis affecting the peripheral joints. The metatarsophalangeal joint of the great toe is the most common site affected.

SYMPTOMS

Acute joint pain, warmth, swelling, acute tenderness, and redness. The skin is tense and shiny red or purple. First attacks usually occur at night with pain that is throbbing and excruciating. These first attacks are usually short-lived, but subsequent ones last longer, for weeks or even months. Gradual joint destruction may occur. Chalk-like soft tissue nodules may form in the earlobes, tendons, and cartilage.

ETIOLOGICAL CONSIDERATIONS—PRIMARY

- Diet
  Excess meat consumption; excess refined carbohydrates and sugar (increases uric acid levels); overindulgence in alcoholic beverages; excess coffee; lack of fresh fruit and vegetables; lack of dietary fiber (intestinal toxemia); vitamin E and B5 deficiencies
- Hereditary
  Enzyme deficiency causes excess production of uric acid, resulting in uric acid kidney stones and gout.
- Reduced renal clearance of uric acid
- Excess puride synthesis
- Stress
  Causes increased uric acid levels; executive syndrome, adrenal exhaustion
- Obesity

ETIOLOGICAL CONSIDERATIONS— SECONDARY

Acidosis; hyperlipidemia, hypertriglyceridemia; sedentary existence; previous injury to area; previous oral antibiotics causing friendly intestinal bacteria deficiency; lead poisoning; drug-induced: penicillin, insulin, diuretics; Candida infections. Gout may be associated with psoriasis, thyroid and parathyroid disease, cardiovascular disease, kidney disease, obesity, and hypertension.

DISCUSSION

Gout results from the deposition of sharp crystals of monosodium urate in tendons and joints. It also may be deposited in the intestine and kidney tissues, and may cause kidney disease and death. Hyperuricemia is associated with disease in affluent societies. It has been considered a disease of the wealthy. As such it has often been called "the rich person's disease". Throughout history the sufferer of gout has been depicted as a portly, middle-aged gentleman sitting in a huge leather chair with one foot resting painfully on a soft cushion as he consumes great quantities of meat and wine. This picture has arisen from the fact that many an acute attack of gout follows an evening of wining and dining. Certain nucleic acids (purines) in many foods increase the uric acid content of the blood. This occurs because uric acid is the ultimate oxidation product of the purine bases adenine and guanine. Organ meats and alcoholic beverages are the worst offenders. While meat actually contains purines and so helps raise uric acid levels directly, alcohol inhibits uric acid excretion by the kidneys, thus retaining uric acid in the body.

Other factors also influence the amount of uric acid in the body. A high-fat diet will increase the uric acid level. Also associated with raised uric acid levels is obesity. As weight increases, so does the uric acid level in the blood.

Another form of gout, which can be called "poor person's gout", results from consumption of an excessive amount of refined carbohydrates and sugar.

The dietary explanation of gout has come under some disrepute in recent years. Although it is not denied that a large portion of uric acid comes from dietary sources, it has become clear that this is not the only source. Endogenous uric acid, or uric acid made in the body through the breakdown of purine bases, is also a major source. This discovery has led many physicians to abandon the classic uric acid avoidance diets and employ new drugs that are aimed at lowering the uric acid levels artificially. On such therapy a person is enabled to continue moderate alcohol and meat intake.

The drug-dependence approach is short-sighted. A raised uric acid level and consequent gouty arthritis are valuable danger signals telling us that something is wrong with our manner of living. Once we understand this message we have the opportunity to re-establish proper equilibrium and prevent other diseases also associated with excess meat, fat, and alcohol intake.

TREATMENT

Diet

Non-citrus alkaline fasting is the best method for eliminating uric acid from the system and establishing equilibrium. These fasts need to be very short (3–4 days) in duration and repeated often over a period of at least 6 months, however, since uric acid levels rise sharply as keto acids increase in the blood due to fat breakdown. A highly alkaline urine helps keep uric acid in solution and a high fluid intake helps remove uric acid from the system. For these reasons non-citrus fruit juice, vegetable juice, or potassium broth are excellent liquids to use in the fast.

It is important to understand that gout has taken many years to develop and will also take some time to correct. Naturopathy does not offer quick and easy ways to remove symptoms. What it does offer is the possibility of a total cure. True treatment and cure is possible if the patient both understands and is willing to follow these simple methods. For those who truly wish to rid themselves of the pain and disfigurement gout causes, the road is long but very rewarding.

Liquid Fast (Any or All)
- Non-citrus juice (may make worse at first); vegetable juice (celery as the main base).
- Celery and parsley juice; red cherry juice (neutralizes uric acid); carrot juice.
- Potassium broth.

Diet between fast

Low uric acid, low purine, low fat, and no alcohol. In general, the diet should consist of 75% raw foods, with the greatest portion of these being non-starchy vegetables. Vegetables to include in large quantities are celery, carrots, alfalfa sprouts, kale, cabbage, parsley, and any other green leafy vegetable (other than spinach). As far as fruit is concerned, black cherries, bananas, and strawberries are especially useful.

If possible, this cleansing diet, devoid of any carbohydrates or protein, should be adhered to for 5-day intervals between the first two 3-to-4-day fasts. This will encourage elimination and weight reduction and help detoxify the system. Should this diet become too difficult, the next stage of the treatment should then be started. This consists of the addition of low-purine foods such as raw goat's milk with yoghurt, poached eggs, low-fat cheese, a few nuts, brown rice, millet, and corn bread. The bulk of the diet still remains as above (green vegetables).

The following chart will help give some basic guidelines for the long-term diet

High-Purine Diet (Avoid): Group 1

Anchovies; mussels; meat broth; porridge (oatmeal); meats; roe; heart; sardines; herring; scallops; kidney; sweetbreads; liver; yeast; mackerel; spices; meat extracts; organ meats.

Moderate-Purine Diet: Group 2

Bran; spinach; fish; beans; fowl; lentils; shellfish; mushrooms; asparagus; peas; cauliflower; whole wheat.

Low-Purine Diet: Group 3

Rice; green vegetables; millet; nuts; goat's milk; cornbread; goat's yoghurt; fruit; sea vegetables; low-fat cheese; eggs.

A high fluid intake is essential, as well, to cleanse the system of uric acid. The best therapeutic procedure is to alternate the fast and low-purine diet every 7–14 days, fasting 3–5 days, and then going on the diet for 7–14 days.

Therapeutic Agents

Vitamins and Minerals

- Vitamin C with bioflavinoids: up to 5000 IU daily. Helps to lower serum uric acid levels.
- Vitamin A: 25,000–75,000 IU. (See warning under Vitamin Toxicity, page 56.) Lowers uric acid levels.
- Vitamin E: 400–1200 IU daily. Antioxidant. Deficiency associated with gout.

- Vitamin B complex: 50–100 mg 1–3 times daily. Essential for proper digestive function and all enzyme systems. Anti-stress.
- Folic acid: 25 mg 3 times daily.
- Pantothenic acid: 100–250 mg twice daily. Anti-stress vitamin. Deficiency associated with gout.
- Zinc: 25–50 mg daily. Needed in tissue repair and protein metabolism.

Others

- Lecithin: 2–4 capsules 3 times daily.
- SOD (superoxide dismutase): 2–3 tablets 3–4 times daily. Antioxidant and free radical destroyer.

Botanicals

Burdock root.

Colchicum: 5–15 drops tincture 3 times daily during acute attack only.

Celery: 10–30 drops use tincture of seeds 2–3 times daily. Eat stalk in very large amounts daily.

White bryony: for pain made worse by motion; use as tincture or low-potency homeopathic dilution.

Therapeutic Suggestion

For acute gout, we have found black cherries and juice (from a tin) for an evening dessert over a couple of days to be effective over that period. It is good as a palliative, but causes of gout must be sought and processes reversed See Arthritis for physiotherapy.

HALITOSIS
(Bad Breath)

DEFINITION AND SYMPTOMS

Offensive mouth odor.

ETIOLOGICAL CONSIDERATIONS—PRIMARY

- Digestive disturbances
  Digestive enzyme deficiency; hydrochloric acid deficiency; food intolerance;

improper diet or food combinations.
- Diet
  Overeating (exhaustion of digestive enzymatic capacity); food allergy (milk, wheat, and others); fiber deficiency; excess meat; excess refined carbohydrates; mucus-forming diet
- Gum or tooth disease (poor dental hygiene); improper diet
  Pyorrhea; gingivitis; cavities
- Constipation (poor eliminations)

ETIOLOGICAL CONSIDERATIONS— SECONDARY

Sinusitis; post-nasal drip; tonsillitis; respiratory problems; smoking; anxiety (stomach derangement); heavy metal poisoning (selenium and others); liver disease; diabetes; dehydration; mouth breathing

DISCUSSION

Foul breath is *always* a sign of some internal disorder and should never be treated only with palliative mouthwashes. The first investigation should be of the teeth and gums. A visit to a good dental hygienist or dentist will reveal if tooth or gum disease is the cause. If the mouth is healthy, all other local problems should then be eliminated, including sinusitis, chronic nasal allergic symptoms, post-nasal drip, tonsillitis, and chronic lung conditions. Should these problems be absent, the most probable cause of the offense is a digestive disturbance, usually due to improper diet. The most common problem involves poor eliminations and constipation. As the bowel contents are retained for prolonged periods within the body, toxins are reabsorbed, which cause coating of the tongue and foul breath. (See Constipation for further discussion and treatment.)

Another common factor is digestive enzyme deficiency. In a few cases an actual deficiency of hydrochloric acid or other digestive enzymes may be the primary cause. In most cases the enzymes were of normal character and amount, but have over a period of time become depleted in their production by dietary abuse.

Very large meals or too-frequent meals exceed the body's ability to produce digestive enzymes. This causes large portions of only partly digested foods to enter the small intestine, setting up fermentation that causes both flatulence and halitosis. Improper food combinations also create conditions impossible for proper digestion. Such foods as citrus fruits and complex carbohydrates (e.g. bread), a common combination at breakfast, are a common offender. Mixing fruits and vegetables or melons with just about anything else also will upset digestion.

Fiber deficiency and an excess consumption of refined carbohydrates along with too much milk or meat seems to be the worst dietary regimen as far as breath is concerned. Not only is this diet highly mucus-forming, but it favors tooth and gum disease, digestive weakness, constipation, and a host of other diseases, both related and unrelated to halitosis.

Certain individual foods may be the culprits in isolated cases. Many people simply cannot digest either milk or wheat. Others have special food intolerances or allergies that may upset digestion. These need to be diagnosed and eliminated. Useful tests include the cytotoxic food allergy test, RAST test, pulse test, or food elimination diets.

Stress and anxiety are often the main cause of bad breath. Prolonged stress will make normal digestion impossible by affecting both the nervous and endocrine systems.

Certain heavy metal poisoning may cause halitosis. Selenium has been known to give a garlic-like odor to the breath.

TREATMENT

Dental Hygiene

If dental problems are the cause no treatments will be beneficial until the offending cause is treated. Pyorrhea must be treated with a proper high-fiber diet, herbs, Ipsab (Cayce product), or myrrh, goldenseal and glycothymoline mouth rinse, proper brushing, and dental flossing.

Diet

Proper digestion and elimination may be reestablished by a short 3-day apple mono diet or a longer brown rice mono diet. This is then followed by the constipation regimen, or simply by converting to a high-fiber diet with sufficient raw vegetables and fruit. Meals should be smaller than normal and taken dry, without drinks or soups. Don't drink liquids within the half hour before meals and not until an hour to an hour and a half following meals. This helps prevent digestive juices from becoming diluted and therefore less efficient. Although water is easily acidified by the stomach acid normally, a hydrochloric acid-deficient individual needs all the acid he or she can produce for digestion. Milk is particularly detrimental if taken with meals, since it requires such a great amount of acid to be acidified, leaving little or none left for the meal itself. This may be why kosher laws do not allow dairy products to be consumed with meat at the same meals. Hydrochloric acid is essential for proper protein digestion. Drinking water between meals, however, is very important to help cleanse the body. Cases of bad breath are improved by drinking 6-8 glasses of water daily. In some cases more prolonged liquid fasting with enemas or colonics may be useful. Often the mono diet or fast will need to be repeated several times to gain complete results.

Physiotherapy

Colonics; enemas; outdoor exercise; skin brushing (see Appendix I); "salt glow" skin rubs (see Appendix I).

Therapeutic Agents

Vitamins and Minerals
- Vitamin A: 25,000 IU 1-2 times daily.
- Vitamin B6.
- Vitamin B complex: 250 mg 1-2 times daily.
- Zinc: 15-50 mg 2-3 times daily.

Others
- Liquid chlorophyll: as much as possible.
- Glycothymoline: 6 drops internally daily.
- Fresh vegetables: especially carrots and greens.
- Lactobacillus: normalizes bowel ecology; 2 capsules 3 times daily.
- Bran: 1 tbsp with water before all meals. Helps correct fiber deficiency.
- Ipsab (Cayce product): applied to gums where gum health is cause.
- Charcoal.
- Pancreatic enzymes with meals.
- Fresh fruit, especially apples.
- Laxatives (see Constipation).

Botanicals
Anise seeds.
Cardamom seeds.
Caraway seeds.
Fennel seeds.
Parsley
Whole cloves.
Coneflower.
Goldenseal: for internal causes.
Goldenseal and myrrh: gargle for gum disorders.
Peppermint tea: for digestion.

HEADACHE AND MIGRAINE

DEFINITION

Headache: pain in or around head.
Migraine: recurrent attacks of headaches with visual and gastrointestinal disturbances.

SYMPTOMS

Headache: irregular attacks of pain in various parts of head or in the sinuses in the facial area.
Migraine: recurrent pain with associated nausea, vomiting, and photophobia. The pain is usually confined to one side of head or eye. The patient is irritable and desires seclusion without direct light. Attacks may be preceded by flashes of light due to intracerebral vasoconstriction and followed by head pain due to dilation of extracerebral cranial arteries in the dura and scalp.

ETIOLOGICAL CONSIDERATIONS—PRIMARY

- Spinal
  Atlas (C1); axis (C2); C1 to C7; cervical/thoracic junction (C6 to T2)
- Muscular spasm
  Suboccipital triangle, neck and shoulder tension, toxicity
- Arthritis
  Nerve compression (direct and indirect due to osteophytes or inflammatory disease)
- Stress
  Teeth grinding; anxiety; perfectionist; depression; insomnia
- Digestive problems
  Constipation; indigestion; intestinal toxicity; inflammation of stomach
- Disease of eye, ear, nose, throat, sinuses, teeth
- Toxic

Drugs; infections; kidney disease; liver disease; arthritis; food additives; gas appliances; paint fumes; nicotine excess; vitamin overdose; coffee excess; monosodium glutamate (Chinese restaurant syndrome due to excess MSG for sensitive individuals leading to headache, nausea, vomiting, and diarrhea)

ETIOLOGICAL CONSIDERATIONS— SECONDARY

Coffee (including coffee withdrawal, called the "rebound headache"), junk foods, tea, cocoa, salt, fats, excess carbohydrates and sugars; hypoglycemia; dehydration, whether acute or chronic; allergy; liver disease; head injuries; high blood pressure; circulation; cerebral hypoxia; anemia; water retention; menstruation; premenstrual tension; pregnancy; vitamin B1 deficiency; contraceptive pill; menstrual disorders; after spinal puncture; meningitis; tumor; eye strain (poorly fitting glasses, prolonged concentration, poor vision)

DISCUSSION

Headaches and migraines are frequently confused and the terms have been used by many almost synonymously. However, they are two very distinct entities and should always be accurately diagnosed. The case history usually is sufficient to establish a migraine with its recurrent one-sided nature and the associated visual and gastric disturbances. A migraine diagnosis is important since this condition is deep-seated and therefore may take longer to correct. Specific allergy is commonly found in migraine patients and tyramine-containing foods such as cheese, wine, citrus, and then to a lesser extent, avocados, plums, bananas, raspberries, and alcoholic beverages all have been known to initiate an attack. The exact mechanism by which tyramine, a breakdown product of the amino acid tyrosine, works is not proven. It is suspected that tyramine causes a release of norepinephrine, causing vasoconstriction of the blood vessels in the scalp and brain. This results in a reduced blood supply, which may be the cause of the visual symptoms that so often warn of a migraine. As the norepinephrine supply is exhausted, the blood vessels respond by dilating, according to the law of dual effect where every action has an equal and opposite reaction. The enlarged vessels are the postulated cause of the migraine pain. Other food allergies or sensitivities may be a factor. Chocolate is a common offender, but any food may be the cause. It is estimated that at least 25% of migraine cases are due to food sensitivity. Refer to Allergy for more detail on allergy diagnosis and treatment.

From the lengthy list of possible etiologic considerations, it becomes obvious that to first cure chronic headaches a thorough case history is important to help isolate the major cause. Often, several factors will coexist and all these must be dealt with to obtain permanent relief. The most frequently occurring causes are spinal lesions, intestinal disturbances, liver congestion, poor circulation, hypoglycemia, allergy, menstrual disorders, sinusitis, muscular tension, and arthritis.

Headaches of cervical origin are the most common cause of all headaches. This type of headache is very easy to diagnose and treat. No matter how long the patient may have been suffering from chronic or recurrent headaches, and we have treated many cases where these headaches have been a constant problem for as long as they can remember, they usually respond to osteopathic care in a relatively short period of time. The site of the problem is almost always between the occiput and C1, or between C1 and C2. However, any region of the cervical spine or the muscles in this area can be the cause. Since headaches of cervical origin are by far the single most common cause of all reported headaches, examination and treatment by a qualified practitioner of spinal therapy should be the first choice, not the last.

In regard to stress, muscular tension, and cervical arthritis, these are often progressive. The most common syndrome we see is the middle-aged (usually female) patient with severe headaches due to stress and inability to relax. This slowly restricts cervical movements and circulation. Chronic muscle hypertonicity causes local toxicity (due to accumulated metabolites) and decreased disc space. The result is chronic headaches with or without other referred pains down to the hands. Over the years this lack of circulation and restricted movement becomes recognizable on x-rays as osteophytic lips and spurs, the classic findings in osteoarthritis. This is a perfect example of how improper emotions eventually affect the physical body, causing disease.

An interesting note about migraines and coffee consumption comes from the action of coffee, which constricts blood vessels and therefore helps relieve many headaches of vascular origin (a migraine headache is one type of vascular headache). Many people report chronic morning headaches until the first cup of coffee is consumed. This "coffee cure" has little real curative effect. In fact, due to the law of dual effect which governs all drug activity in the body, any agent which elicits a given action by the body will later cause an equal but opposite reaction. Therefore the vasoconstriction caused by caffeine is followed by vasodilation (the cause of vascular headaches) later on. This is one of the reasons a midmorning and midafternoon headache will recur in heavy coffee consumers.

TREATMENT

Treatment depends on predisposing causes. If liver congestion is a major factor, as it often is, a liver-cleansing fast and liver-cleansing herbs are indicated. Intestinal toxemia also calls for fasting and enemas. Hypoglycemia-related headaches require frequent high-protein meals and specific nutrients related to that disorder (refer to the specific headings that apply). In general, alkaline fasts repeated 3-7 days are usually very therapeutic, with an enema taken on days 1, 2, 3, 5, and 7.

Fasts

- Apple juice (general).
- Fruit juice (general).
- Grapefruit juice (liver congestion).
- Mucus-cleansing diet (see Appendix I): sinusitis.
- Hot water and lemon juice (general, liver).
- Fruit diet (less severe general).

Enemas

Coffee: to relieve acute migraine.

Emetics

The induction of vomiting will usually abort an early migraine and may help relieve a severe headache in many cases. Lobelia is taken in emetic doses.

Hydrotherapy

Ice compress to base of head while lying in darkened room.
Ice to forehead with simultaneous hot foot bath is also effective to abort an attack.

Exercise

Vigorous daily exercise seems to help reduce frequency of attacks.

Therapeutic Agents

Vitamins and Supplements

Selection of appropriate supplements very much depends on the individual case history, and professional guidance ought to be sought. The following would need to be considered:

- Vitamin B complex: 25-200 mg 1-2 times daily.
- Vitamin B12: 10 mg 3 times daily in acute conditions.
- Niacin/niacinamide: 50-200 mg 3 times daily in acute conditions.
- Vitamin B6.
- Vitamin C complex.
- Calcium: 800-1000 mg daily or 200-400 per hour in acute attacks.
- Magnesium: 400-800 mg daily or 100-200 mg per hour in acute attacks.

Others

- Atomodine.
- Garlic.

Botanicals

Betony: with vertigo.
Black cohosh: relaxing nervine, antispasmodic, sedative, especially for headaches of menstrual origin.
Blue flag.
Celandine: liver involvement.
Chamomile: peppermint plus catnip tea for sick headache and nervous stomach.
Culver's root: with liver involvement.
Fringe tree: for bilious headache.
Goldenseal: for bilious headache.
Hops: hypnotic.
Jamaica dogwood
Lady's slipper: headaches of climacteric; hysterical headaches; reflex headaches from ovaries or uterus.
Lavender: apply to forehead.
Lobelia.
Mistletoe: headaches due to increased blood flow to brain, high blood pressure.
Pulsatilla, or pasque flower: nervous and gastric headache, neurotic headache with menstrual disorders.
Passion flower.
Peppermint: headaches of stomach origin.
Salicin willow.
Senna.
Skullcap.
Valerian.

Wintergreen.

Yellow jasmine: drink $\frac{1}{2}$-1 cup infusion every $\frac{1}{2}$-1 hour until headache is relieved.

Useful Prescriptions

- Chamomile, peppermint, rosemary, skullcap, valerian.
- Catnip, chamomile, peppermint.
- Chamomile, senna.

Note: Severe headaches may be due to a serious medical disorder. An example is the headache of glaucoma that may, if left untreated, lead to vision loss or blindness in a very short period of time. Another example is the severe headache with vomiting that results from intracerebral hemorrhage that must be considered a medical emergency.

HEART DISEASE
(Arteriosclerosis, Atherosclerosis, Angina, Coronary Heart Disease)

DEFINITION

Arteriosclerosis: a degenerative change in the arterial walls, affecting first the middle and later the inner layers, and resulting in loss of elasticity and possible calcification. Commonly referred to as hardening of the arteries.

Atherosclerosis: a degenerative change in the arterial walls which principally affects the larger arteries such as the aorta, coronary, and cerebral vessels. Systemic changes in other arteries also occur. The basic lesion is plaque formation on the inner walls of the vessels, causing narrowing and possible embolism when the plaque breaks loose into the circulation, with possibly disastrous results. The plaque is composed primarily of 70–80% tissue, cholesterol and other fats.

Angina: recurrent substernal pain lasting $\frac{1}{2}$-1 minute, which may be precipitated by stress, exertion, a large meal, emotion, extreme cold, or other factors. Pain is characterized by the sensation of a viselike tight band drawn across the chest. Coronary atherosclerosis is the major cause.

SYMPTOMS

Cold extremities, lethargy, dizziness, senility, difficulty thinking, high blood pressure, pain in legs on exertion, angina, blurred vision, enlarged heart, difficulty breathing, palpitations, heart attack, embolism.

ETIOLOGICAL CONSIDERATIONS—PRIMARY

- Diet
  Rancid oils in the diet; antioxidant deficiency; use of unsaturated vegetable oils in cooking; margarine; homogenized dairy products; excess saturated fats; deficiency of fat emulsifiers; excess refined salt; excess refined carbohydrates and sugar (sugar increases triglycerides, platelet adhesiveness, uric acid levels, and blood pressure); vitamin and mineral deficiency; excess vitamin D (3000 mg or more daily is atherogenic)
- Coffee
- Alcohol
- Lack of exercise
- Smoking
- Obesity

ETIOLOGICAL CONSIDERATIONS— SECONDARY

Emotional; heavy metal poisoning; soft water; contraceptive pill; diabetes; hyperinsulinism: may cause atherosclerosis; family history; gout; high blood pressure; elevated triglyceride, and uric acid levels; long-term ox bile supplementation

DISCUSSION

Heart disease is still the number one killer in civilized nations. Evidence clearly shows that the incidence of heart disease is directly related to our abnormal dietary habits, but there are still ambiguities, and diet is only a part of the picture. Wherever people live on a diet high in polyunsaturated vegetable oils, refined carbohydrates and animal fats, high blood pressure, arteriosclerosis, atherosclerosis, angina, and other degenerative heart changes occur most frequently.

A great deal of confusion still exists about the role of animal fats in the causation of heart disease. Until a few years ago it was a commonly accepted assumption that excess consumption of saturated fats found in meat, eggs, and dairy products was the main cause of these disorders. This view, however, never could adequately explain why Inuit or other tribal people who eat a very large amount of animal fats do not show an increased incidence of heart disease, or indeed a host of other anomalies. Still, most doctors stuck to their beliefs and reiterated the meat-heart maxim regularly. It may not be totally correct, but at least it is simple and easy to quote without having to go into too much time-consuming detail.

The problem with much past research has been the traditional tendency to try, whenever possible, to find a single, simple "something" that will explain a particular disease, such as "cholesterol". However, this is rarely possible. Heart disease, and most other degenerative diseases for that matter, is the result of a total lifestyle, holistic causes, and not a simple dietary excess or deficiency.

In analyzing the true causes of degenerative heart disease, it is essential always to bear in mind that people are individuals and as such respond to various causative factors differently. Diet is definitely a major factor in degenerative heart disease. Saturated fats (those commonly found in animal products) are a problem, as has long been suspected, and the situation is getting worse, not better. Certainly the western diet contains a significantly larger amount of animal proteins than many other populations with less heart disease.

The problem, however, is not only how much meat or dairy products we eat, but also what kind. Domesticated animals have a much higher percentage of saturated fat than wild animals, due to a different diet, activity level, and the hormones used by various cattle and poultry industries to fatten their stock artificially. The meat or poultry we eat now is very different from that our grandparents ate, much to our detriment. So one has to be careful in comparing the types of saturated fats the Eskimos eat compared with those we eat today.

Cow's milk, ignoring for the present the fact that this product was not designed by nature for humans, has also changed considerably over the past 100 years. We now break the fat molecules in milk up into easily absorbed particles by homogenization, and feed this food to our infants, resulting in cases of atherosclerosis by the age of five. We also pasteurize milk, a process of high temperature application, and this creates trans-fatty acids, agents known for their capacity to damage arterial walls and initiate sclerosing with subsequent risks of stroke and heart attack. It is no wonder that heart disease, once a disease of middle age, is now being found in people in their late twenties.

Homogenization allows a substance called xanthine oxidase to enter the bloodstream. Kurt Oster, former chief of cardiology at Park City hospital, Bridgeport, Conn., co-author of *The XO Factor* believes that this milk fat enzyme, xanthine oxidase "initiates over 50% of all heart disease". This substance gets into arterial walls and destroys plasmalogen which makes up about a third of the arterial cell membrane, leading to an integration of cholesterol into the cells, creating more rigidity and other pathologic changes to arterial tissue.

The cholesterol story also is far from simple. Over the past few years other extremely interesting research has helped clarify many of our previously unanswerable questions about the cholesterol/heart disease link. One study examined some of the original research data which showed that cholesterol in high amounts fed to experimental animals led to a high percentage of developing coronary heart disease. This study has often been quoted to prove the causative link between cholesterol and coronary heart disease. In recent tests, however, using proven pure cholesterol, no such results were found. However, when cholesterol that was allowed to go *rancid* was used, coronary heart disease did result. The conclusion was that the harmful effects of rancid oil products were the primary factor, not simply cholesterol. This study has particular significance when we compare it with studies showing the usefulness of antioxidants (anti-rancidity factors) in the diet for both prevention and treatment of heart disease.

The Other Side of the Cholesterol Story

Firstly, let's point out that cholesterol is not bad in and of itself. The body needs cholesterol to ensure proper cell membrane function. From cholesterol the liver makes up bile acids, vital in digestion and absorption of fats, oils and fat-soluble vitamins. Very important hormones (e.g. sex hormones, adrenal corticosteroids such as aldosterone and cortisol) and vitamin D are made from cholesterol, and the skin uses cholesterol to protect us against the wear and tear of sun, wind and water. Cholesterol helps damaged skin to heal, and prevents infections from foreign agents. It also acts as an antioxidant when needed, and protects us from certain cancers. Without cholesterol, we would die, and too little cholesterol is implicated in many disease states.

The liver makes enough cholesterol for the needs of the entire body from 2-carbon acetates it derives from the breakdown of fruit sugars and protein, as well as from essential fatty acids. Cholesterol is not "essential", that is we do not need to take any cholesterol as such into our bodies through food, because body cells synthesize it, when and as required.

The body's cells make the cholesterols it needs in response to daily needs. For instance, when we drink alcohol, it dissolves in and fluidizes cellular membranes. In response cells build more cholesterol into the membrane bringing it back to a normal (less fluid) state. As the alcohol wears off, the membrane hardens, so some membrane cholesterol is removed to re-establish normal (greater) membrane fluidity, the excess cholesterol is hooked up to an essential fatty acid (EFA), for example omega-3, shipped via blood to the liver to be changed into bile salts for excretion (given the presence of necessary vitamins, minerals and enzymes in the liver). Bile salts are dumped into the intestines where they are picked up by bowel fibre, and provided the bowel is sufficiently active, they are eliminated before they can be reabsorbed and recycled (see Leaky Gut).

The Medical Cholesterol Dogma: "Cholesterol Causes Heart and Vascular Disease"

The most commonly accepted theory of cardiovascular disease (CVD) states that when too much cholesterol builds up in the body, it is deposited in the arterial walls causing atherosclerosis, a narrowing of the arteries and vessels. Excess cholesterol and saturated fatty acids can make blood platelets "sticky" increasing the risk of a clot thus increasing the risk of angina and heart disease, heart attack, stroke, gangrene, as well as blindness, deafness, edema and kidney failure.

This unproved theory that time has honoured has now become dogma. For all the cholesterol lowering of the past 40 years, CVD is still on the increase. All the recent evidence suggests that we have been barking up the wrong tree. In fact it is worse than this. There is no other substance as widely publicized by the medical profession. "The cholesterol lowering enterprise threatens to turn a large percentage of the healthy population into patients ..."[33]

The cholesterol scare is big business for doctors, laboratories and drug companies. The new-generation cholesterol-lowering drugs like simvastatin and pravastatin are very expensive, but offer a risk reduction of heart attack of only 2% (if that).

There is no such thing as "good and bad" cholesterol; it is all good. LDLs (so-called "bad cholesterol") is just as important and good as HDLs (so-called "good cholesterol"). LDLs carry cholesterol, triglycerides and fat-soluble vitamins to cells where they are needed, HDLs take them back to the liver as required. The confusion exists because a high LDL reading simply means that our system is being overloaded by cholesterol either from food, from abnormally high synthesis, and/or from too slow a removal. It does not mean we are at a greater risk of heart disease or stroke. Consider the following:

- Cholesterol consumption has remained constant over the past 100 years, while CVD has skyrocketed.
- The US Framington Heart Study found that there is "no discernible association between the amount of cholesterol in the diet and the level of cholesterol in the blood ..."
- People in many other cultures consume far more cholesterol than we do, and have far less heart disease. For example, the Masai consume mostly meat, blood and milk, up to 2000 mg of cholesterol daily, yet maintain a 3.5 mmol/L serum cholesterol and have a low incidence of heart disease.

- *The Lancet* said in June 1931 that heart attack was almost unknown before 1926, before margarine, when butter, lard, tallow and other saturated fats were eaten without fear.
- The BMJ reported in 1989 the results of the Renfrew and Paisley survey which showed that serum cholesterol levels (high or low) made no difference when it came to fatal heart attacks.
- The Roseta study showed that American Italians with high serum cholesterol actually had less than 50% of deaths from heart attack than the rest of the USA. Several other more recent studies also show the benefits of the "Mediterranean diet", which confirm less death from heart attack *and* cancer.
- CVD (coronary vascular disease) risk factors which are at least as important, if not more so than serum cholesterol, include the consumption of refined sugar, animal fats, food additives, and especially *trans*-fatty acids, e.g. margarine.
- Drugs that lower cholesterol do not (statistically) reduce heart attacks or deaths from atherosclerosis.
- Lp(a) and its adhesive protein apo(a), which looks like LDL, is a strong risk factor for CVD. Measurements on which cholesterol dogma is based have erroneously lumped LDL and Lp(a) together. Disassociated from Lp(a), LDL appears to be only a weak risk factor. This means LDL has been wrongly blamed for damage done by Lp(a). Lp(a) often increases when serum vitamin C levels are low, and decreases when vitamin C is high.
- Increased intake of vitamin C (to several grams daily) and other antioxidants can keep Lp(a) levels down, build strong, thin artery walls with strong connective tissue, and reverse and cure cardiovascular disease.

One must look to the advent of polyunsaturated vegetable fats (e.g. margarine) and oils to explain the paradox. "MI [heart attack] deaths have increased in direct ratio

271

to the consumption of polyunsaturated fats as oils and margarines". When you heat natural, unsaturated vegetable oils (as in refined, heat-treated, and partly hydrogenated oils), the oils undergo a transformation from the chemical *cis* form to the more stable but abnormal *trans* form. The *trans* form, not normally found in these oils if cold pressed or unheated, is more reactive with oxidants, producing rancidity by-products that cause an elevation in the circulation of possible mutagenic substances which may initiate damage to the arterial walls. This may be a significant factor in the production of atherosclerotic plaque build-up, plaque being the local lesion found associated with coronary heart disease.

Margarine may also be a factor. Originally many people converted from butter to margarine to reduce their total dietary cholesterol intake, thinking they were making a healthy choice. This seemed logical in light of the cholesterol–heart attack hypothesis; however, it turns out that the use of partly hydrogenated oils not only does not decrease blood cholesterol levels, it increases them. Hydrogenated oils are high in *trans* forms of fatty acids. This form inhibits a liver enzyme responsible for converting cholesterol into bile acids. Bile acids transport cholesterol out of the body. If cholesterol is not converted to bile, it accumulates in the blood, the exact opposite of the desired result.

Recent research warns against low levels of serum cholesterol. Indiscriminate lowering of cholesterol actually increases the risk of cancer, as LDLs transport the fat-soluble antioxidant vitamins E, A, and carotene. Studies have shown that elderly females with cholesterol *over* 7 mmol/L survive *longer* than those with cholesterol of 4.5 mmol/L or lower. Mortality was 5 times higher in the lower group than in the 7 mmol/L group! Low cholesterol levels also reduce the numbers of serotonin brain receptors thus increasing anxiety, depression and psychoses, attempted suicides, and possibly predisposing to dementia. Low cholesterol levels also affect the capacity of the endocrine system to manufacture the hormones, and will create imbalances there as well, which affect libido, menstrual cycle (e.g. amenorrhoea), among other things.

There is no doubt whatsoever that low levels of serum cholesterol do not prevent heart attacks. But worse, low cholesterol levels may be associated with the causes of cancer. Cancer patients seem almost invariably to have low serum cholesterol levels. Cholesterol may be, in fact, part of our defense system against cancer. Cholesterol for one thing acts as antioxidant against lipid peroxydation.

We know a lot more about cholesterol today than we did in 1956 when the cholesterol–CVD theory was spawned. The majority of studies show that there is no truth in the theory, but for whatever reasons the dogma remains. It is important to realize that the damage caused by polyunsaturated oils and margarines is at least partly to blame for the increased incidence of CVD and sudden heart attack, and probably lung and other cancers as well, in affluent countries.

Abnormally elevated serum cholesterol is more a sign of nutrient deficiency than a problem in its own right. The best solution is to ensure adequate nutrient intake and waste elimination, and trust to Nature. Rather than merely reducing cholesterol levels, we must heed the signs, and take all the appropriate lifestyle and dietary steps to avoid atherosclerosis and heart disease, not "shoot the messenger"

Saturated fats, although a central factor in heart disease, do not work in isolation in the diet. Refined carbohydrates and specifically sugar are also known to increase fat levels in the blood. The combination of sugar or refined carbohydrates taken with saturated fats seems to cause the highest of all increases of cholesterol and triglycerides in the blood. This combination of foods is extremely common in the modern diet from early childhood on. Take, for example, the typical milkshake (sugar and milk) or a hamburger and Coke (meat, refined white flour bun, and sugar). While saturated fat consumption has increased only 10% in the past

100 years, the increase in refined carbohydrates and sugar has gone up to an incredible 700%. This increase in consumption of refined carbohydrates, especially sugar, is the single most important factor effecting a rise in blood triglycerides. There is a definite link between societies with an extremely high sucrose consumption and coronary heart disease.

A second major cause of heart disease is lack of demanding exercise. Lifestyles have changed drastically over the past 100 years, and as general physical activity levels have decreased, heart disease has increased. Demanding physical exercise really gets the blood flowing, helps clear the arteries of any early deposits, and prevents atherosclerosis and high blood pressure. In general, a very active person will develop heart disease later than his or her sedentary peer, or not at all. Activity alone, however, is no real protection. To be effective, the heart rate as well as the respiration must escalate to the point of breathlessness for at least 5 minutes each day.

Stress, coffee, smoking, alcohol, and obesity are all contributing factors to be considered in individual cases. Stress causes an increase in cholesterol, glucose levels, and triglycerides. It also causes an elevation of blood pressure. There is a well-known association between stress and coronary heart disease.

Caffeine potentiates the action of adrenalin by blocking its breakdown. This results in the same physiological responses as does stress. Heavy caffeine consumption results in a twofold greater risk of coronary heart disease. Cigarette smoking is now a well-documented risk factor in heart disease. Stress, coffee, and smoking all cause a vasoconstriction or narrowing of the arteries which is especially important in cases of angina where atherosclerosis is present

A lot of work is being done at the level of psychoneuroimmunology, and by many other mind–body physicians such as cardiologist Dean Ornish, who are studying the psycho-emotional factors impacting on diseases such as heart attacks and strokes. They say that one's feelings about certain things have direct physiological bearing on stroke and heart attack.

Although all the answers to the heart disease question are not in, it is clear now, as it has been for quite some time, that the only true prevention and cure is to be found in a *total* lifestyle change. For those who are waiting for a simple answer, or one that comes in a little package or easy-to-swallow pill, we offer no hope.

TREATMENT

Coronary bypass operations have become commonplace as the "cure" for coronary atherosclerosis and severe angina. A segment of vein from the leg is grafted to bypass the narrowed artery segments in one or all three of the coronary arteries. Dramatic as this therapy is in relieving the immediate threat of imminent death due to heart failure, it neglects the fact that the disease is systemic in the first place, and affects the entire circulatory system, not just the heart. It also does nothing to prevent further degeneration of even the new transplanted arteries. At best it is an emergency repair job which does not in any way remove the cause, and often serves to provide a patient with a false sense of security. All of this would be acceptable if the cause were not known, or the cure impossible, both of which are not true. Even the most advanced cases, short of a terminally fatal heart attack or severe infarction, can be benefited by natural treatment.

The common practice of prescribing aspirin "to thin the blood" and therefore prevent angina or a stroke, is without scientific basis. No study has demonstrated that aspirin can prevent a heart attack or stroke, and the thinning the blood approach fails to take account of the cause of the disease processes and lulls one into what is a false sense of security. The much-touted Physicians Heart Study failed to demonstrate the myth, because it was a flawed study; they used aspirin which contained magnesium in it. It is unfortunate that they didn't actually test the usefulness of magnesium on its own which has now been shown to help prevent heart attack. Aspirin usage has some very negative side effects, including nausea and vomiting, gastric ulcers, liver damage, gastrointestinal bleeding, allergic reactions, deficiencies in iron, and other minerals and vitamins cause cerebral hemorrhages which cause bleeding strokes.

Magnesium will do what aspirin fails to do; it reduces abnormal platelet adhesiveness, it is a potent vasodilator and anticoagulant; it is a natural calcium channel blocker, and it has no side effects within recommended dosage guidelines.

Diet

The basic diet regimen should be similar to that found under Hypertension. Periods of vegetable juice fasting are interspersed with a high-fiber, unrefined carbohydrate, mostly vegetarian protein diet, emphasizing plenty of fruits, vegetables, vegetarian proteins, and high-fiber whole grains. Perseverance and rigid adherence to the diet are essential to obtain permanent results. Weight reduction is a primary aim for the obese. It is important to remember that degenerative heart disease usually takes 20 or more years of wrong living for the effects to become noticeable, and cannot logically be totally reversed overnight. Natural therapies are generally slow, but sure.

Diet for a Healthy Heart
The following diet may be of some use as a guideline.
Choose from the following:

Breakfast
1. Whole-grain cereal. Use soy milk or buttermilk if desired. A little honey or sweetener is allowed, but not necessarily suggested.
2. Low-fat yoghurt, fresh wheat germ, brewer's yeast, and a little fruit, especially green apples.

3. Two poached eggs plus whole grain bread (2–3 times per week only).
4. Fresh fruit salad plus nuts and/or yoghurt.

Midmorning
1. Whole grain snack (e.g. crackers, muffins, bread).
2. Cereal-grain coffee, or herb tea.
3. Vegetable juice.
4. Spirulina in water.
5. Miso soup.
6. Yoghurt.
7. Mixed nuts (unsalted).

Lunch
1. Always have a fresh, raw, mixed salad including seed sprouts, plus any of the following:
2. 100% whole grain (e.g. brown rice, wheat, oats, etc.).
3. Vegetarian protein (e.g. tofu, soybeans, beans, nuts, seeds, or low-fat fermented dairy products).
4. Cold water fish (e.g. cod, salmon); other fish less frequently.
5. Chicken or turkey without skin.

Midafternoon
As midmorning.

Supper
1. Cooked vegetables.
2. Vegetarian protein.
3. Whole grain.
4. Cold water fish (cod, salmon, etc.); other fish less frequently.
5. Chicken or turkey without skin.

Physiotherapy

• Aerobic Exercise: obviously all exercise programs must be instituted slowly, with care, and under the supervision of a doctor in the case of heart disease. No surer way exists, however, to correct the problem. Whatever exercise you are initially able to do, it must be increased gradually over a period of time until true aerobic conditioning is possible, involving continuous vigorous exercise for 15-20 minutes or more each day. If you can now walk only 50 yards slowly before becoming tired or breathless or suffering angina pain, gradually increase the distance and the pace, with the aim of soon being able to jog and then run. The same procedure is applied to any other activity: bicycling, rowing, swimming— anything as long as it is steady and continuous, once again with a doctor's supervision.

- Alternate hot/cold showers: these are excellent at stimulating the circulation, but must be done gradually, to prevent sudden shock that the heart cannot yet stand. Begin by taking alternate hot then lukewarm showers, alternating the hot/warm every 2-3 minutes. Slowly, over the next 2-6 months, depending on the severity of the initial condition and your general improvement in health through diet, exercises, and the rest of your new health program, increase the difference between the water temperatures to hot/cool and then to hot/ice-cold.
- Skin brush and "salt glow": stimulates circulation, encourages proper skin function, and aids in elimination.
- Chelation therapy for arteriosclerosis.
- Daily meditation or prayer.
- Spinal manipulation: lower cervical/upper thoracic, 1-2 times per week, especially where spinal lesions may be aggravating or causing angina due to imbalance in the deep versus superficial circulation.
- Massage.
- Colonics or enema series, where bowel loading is affecting angina. General toxemia may be a factor in all degenerative heart disorders.
- Liver flush: often the liver is found to be congested in these conditions. See Gallbladder Disease for details of liver flush.
- Hot compress: in acute angina apply hot moist compress to chest or midback,

then massage the muscles deeply along the spine and follow with spinal manipulation.

Therapeutic Agents

Vitamins and Minerals— Primary

- Vitamin E: 100-400 IU 2-3 times daily. Vitamin E is stripped away with the germ of grains and lost in the refining of oils. It is essential or a healthy heart. It helps dissolve blood clots, inhibits platelet aggregation, dilates blood vessels, and conserves oxygen so that the heart needs work less. As an antioxidant it prevents fatty acids from becoming toxic within the body. It takes time to build up optimal levels of vitamin E, (so simply taking vitamin E at times of stress is not the best way). Gradually increases dose of natural mixed tocopherols from 100-400 IU 2-3 times daily. Higher doses of up to 2400 IU have been used. We generally recommend 400 IU daily, as the best possible preventative measure you can take against any form of heart or vascular disease.
- Vitamin C with bioflavonoids: 500-2000 mg 3 times daily Helps keep plaque from forming, lowers triglycerides, strengthens capillaries and increases HDL.
- Vitamin B3: 400-500 mg of mixed niacin and niacinamide 2-4 times daily. Especially useful for angina.
- Magnesium chelate, citrate or orotate: 300 mg to 2 g daily. More may be useful in some cases up to a ratio of 1:1 with calcium. Especially useful in ischemic heart disease after a myocardial infarction, or for those on diuretic therapy. Magnesium is a natural calcium blocker (calcium blockers are used in angina and cardiovascular disease). An anti-stress mineral.
- Selenium: 100-200 mcg daily. Helps improve vitamin E efficiency. Low selenium levels are a risk factor in heart disease.

Vitamins and Minerals—Primary

- Vitamin A: 10,000–25,000 IU daily.
- Vitamin B complex: 25–50 mg 1–3 times daily.
- Vitamin B6: helps in production of EFA, antithrombic agent, anti-aggregation of platelets.
- Inositol.
- Choline: 1 tsp 3 times daily. High-potency phosphatidylcholine as lecithin.
- Folic acid: 75 mg daily in some cases. Vasodilator.

Others—Primary

- Bromelain: 2 tablets 3 times daily on an empty stomach. Acts as fibrinolytic agent to aid in dissolution of thrombi. Anti-inflammatory.
- Essential fatty acids as found in salmon, cod, and other cold-water fish oils rich in omega-3 EFA decrease platelet adhesion, increase bleeding time, and reduce risk of heart disease. This is the key preventive factor in the traditional Inuit diet. Flaxseed oil, 2 tbsp daily, for the omega-3s
- EPA (eicosapentaenoic acid): 5 g daily as preventative, 5–20 g daily as therapy.
- Garlic: 2 capsules 3 times daily. Decreases blood viscosity.
- Lecithin: contains choline of the vitamin B complex group and is essential for the proper use of fat and cholesterol in the body.
- Probiotics: Lactobacillus lowers cholesterol levels by normalizing bowel ecology, preventing excessive endogenous cholesterol production.
- L-carnitine: 1500–3000 mg daily. Increases HDLs, promotes transport of fatty acids into mitochondria, reduces triglycerides; useful in angina.
- Coenzyme Q 10: 50–100 mg daily. Increases oxygenation to the tissues of the heart and useful to prevent recurrences of heart attack.

Others—Secondary

- Atomodine: with angina take 1 drop twice daily for 5 days; stop 5 days and repeat 5 times.
- Bran: 1 tbsp 3 times daily.
- Brewer's yeast: high in vitamin B complex, selenium, and chromium. Causes regression of atherosclerotic plaque.
- Citric acid: a nutritional chelating (binding) agent.
- Desiccated thyroid: in hypothyroid-related heart disease.
- Chlorophyll.
- Cod-liver oil: 1 tsp 3 times daily
- Citrus fruits.
- Grape juice.
- Phosphatidylcholine: the most concentrated form of lecithin.
- Low-fat fermented milk products: yoghurt, buttermilk, and kefir.
- Evening primrose oil: decreases platelet aggregation.
- Wheat germ oil.

Botanicals

There are many botanical medicines used in cardiovascular therapy, depending on particular requirements, and we advise the services of a competent herbalist. Here are some of those more commonly used.

Cardioprotective: hawthorn; *Inula racemosa*, sage, Panax ginseng.

Cardiotonic (to improve pumping action): hawthorn, coleus, astragalus.

Systemic vasodilators: hawthorn, yarrow, coleus, lime flowers.

Hypotensive vasodilators: mistletoe, garlic, olive, *Scuttelaria baicalensis*, astragalus, valerian.

Portal hypotensives: fringe tree, globe artichoke

Anti-hemorrhagic: rehmannia, yarrow, horsetail, cranesbill.

Anti-platelet aggregation: coleus, ginger, *Salvia miltiorrhiza*, dong quai, garlic.

Hypertensives: licorice, prickly ash, cayenne

Anti-anemia: most bitter herbs, withania, dong quai, yellow dock, nettle, alfalfa.

Other useful herbs include: angelica; black cohosh plus yellow jasmine for angina; cactus for angina with irregular heartbeat.

HEAVY METAL POISONING

DEFINITION

Excess exposure and absorption of heavy metals in toxic clinical or subclinical doses.

SYMPTOMS

These are dependent upon the type of metal and degree of exposure.

Lead

Cumulative doses may cause:
Constipation; nausea; vomiting; diarrhea; learning difficulties; difficulty in concentration; mental retardation; confusion; emotional instability; restlessness; vertigo; hyperactivity; insomnia; muscle aches; gout; arthritis; fatigue; kidney damage; pituitary damage; birth defects; impotence, sterility; ataxia; tremors; muscle weakness; seizures; degeneration of motor neurons; loss of appetite, anorexia; schizophrenic-like behavior; growth problems in long bones; cirrhosis of liver (jaundice); cataracts; metallic taste; headaches; thyroid dysfunction; impotence, sterility; lead colic (painter's colic); anemia; lead line on gum margin; peripheral neuritis: (e.g. painter's wrist drop); lead encephatopathy

Cadmium

Cumulative doses may cause:
Emphysema; kidney damage, nephritis; hypertension; arteriosclerosis; abdominal cramps, colic; nausea, vomiting; diarrhea; liver disease; acne, slow healing (zinc deficiency); anemia.

Mercury

Cumulative doses may cause:

Tremors; chromosome damage; birth defects; insanity; kidney damage; abdominal pain; nausea; vomiting; loss of hearing or vision; mental retardation; sore gums, gingivitis; tooth loss; vertigo; headaches; nervousness; skin eruptions; fatigue.

Aluminum

Cumulative doses may cause:
Digestive disorders; seizures; colic, gas; motor and behavioral dysfunction; gastritis; skin rash; brain degeneration; headache; senile dementia; Alzheimer's disease.

Copper

Cumulative doses may cause:
Mental disorders; schizophrenia; anemia; copper deposits in kidney, liver, brain, eyes; arthritis; hypertension; insomnia; nausea, vomiting; autism; hyperactivity; stuttering; rheumatoid arthritis (high copper levels); myocardial infarction; toxemia of pregnancy; post-partum psychosis; Wilson's disease; inflammation and enlargement of liver; cystic fibrosis.

ETIOLOGICAL CONSIDERATIONS

Lead

Auto exhaust; industry (smelters, paint factories); water; lead pipes (soft water is the worst); industrial pollution; pesticides runoff; water catchment: lead-headed nails; especially severe if acid rain occurs (industrial or volcanic origin); paint ("painter's colic"); roof paint (water catchment systems); children eating lead-based wall paint or paint on cribs due to lead's sweet taste (sugar of lead); cigarettes (lead arsenate used on tobacco as insecticide); Insecticides/fungicides; newspaper ink (burning newspaper increases lead in air); soldered cans; gardens near main roads; children playing near main roads jogging on main roads; commercial baby milk; industrial materials: nails; solder; plating; plaster; putty; lead; shellfish, oysters; gasoline: lead tetraethyl forms lead oxide in engine exhaust; bullets; lead weights: melting down and casting without proper ventilation, including soldering; auto body workers; organ meats; dolomite; cosmetics; paper clips; cooking utensils; enamel and cloisonne work; lead paint on goblets, lead crystal; hair colorings; wines; ceramic glasses: improperly fired lead-glazed ceramics when used with acidic foods such as citrus, tomatoes, etc.; old pewter; machine shops.

Cadmium

Cigarettes; fertilizers; water pipes (impure galvanized pipes); soft drink dispensers coal burning; zinc deficiency; zinc smelters; low melting point alloys; refined foods (low zinc/cadmium ratio); "silver solder" gives off cadmium when overheated; catchment from galvanized roofs; hardware; cadmium-plated nuts, bolts, and wood screws have dangerous potential when heated above 626°F or if sanded or power buffed. Gives off onion/garlic odor.

Mercury

Dental fillings; large fish; pesticides/fungicides; coal burning; pollution; cosmetics; canned tuna/salmon; water-based paints; adhesives; chemical fertilizers; fabric softeners; calomel laxatives; drugs

Aluminum

deodorants; antacids; cookware; foil; emulsifier in cheese processing; salt (anti-caking ingredients); baking powder; beer and soda cans; construction materials; catchment water.

Copper

Copper water pipes and copper water heaters (especially where water is acidic); meats (copper sulfate given as growth enhancer); soybeans (high copper); frozen greens, canned greens (copper added to produce ultra-green color) zinc deficiency; alcoholic beverages from copper brewery equipment; instant gas hot water heaters; hormone pills; soft water; pesticides, insecticides, fungicides; copper jewelry; copper cooking pots, especially if acid foods are cooked.

DISCUSSION

From the above list of possible harmful effects of heavy metal toxicity, it is obvious that these substances can pose a serious health risk. Knowledge of these dangers has come slowly and with much suffering. The entire Roman Empire routinely dosed itself with toxic lead by drinking out of lead goblets, lining its aqueducts with lead, or even adding it to wine in the form of lead acetate, called "sugar of lead", to enhance its flavor and sweet taste. In the seventeenth century the serious condition of "painter's colic" was recognized as being lead-related. Later, laws were enacted to prevent rum from being made in lead containing pots. In the eighteenth and nineteenth centuries lead poisoning was epidemic in the upper classes, who habitually drank an excess of lead-containing port wine.

Exposure of workers to toxic metals has been the major source of knowledge about their harmful effects. Industrial toxicology now recognizes that toxic exposure to lead, cadmium, mercury, aluminum, copper, and other less common metals may cause serious disease and even be fatal. With this awareness came the establishment of permissible levels or threshold limit values to monitor workers and their environments. Blood and urine tests have been used primarily to diagnose a suspected toxicity, but for the most part estimation of probable heavy metal levels is the major preventive measure. Even among the orthodoxy there is dissatisfaction with these inexact methods and the heavy reliance on threshold limit values which do not take into consideration individual differences between heavy metal susceptibility (biochemical individuality), other sources of contamination off the job, the effect of a closed environment, or the fact that some heavy metals (e.g. lead) are *cumulative* in their effects.

The real question, however, has been at which point do these toxic substances cause even a slight deviation from health? The assumption is usually that some toxic metal absorption is harmless; however, many now feel that even *slight* amounts may cause abnormal physical and mental responses. Threshold limits are clearly designed to protect the *majority* of workers from *clinical disease*. It is the subclinical symptoms of heavy metal poisoning, however, that may be the greatest threat to the health and well-being of the industrial worker.

With the rise of industrialization, heavy metal pollution of the air, water, and the food chain became an increasing problem. Now environmental exposure is clearly unavoidable. Studies of snow layers in Greenland, far from industrialization, clearly show this increase, which progresses yearly. By the 1950s routine tests of "symptomless" US children showed hundreds of thousands with toxic lead levels.

In reviewing the sources of metal pollution, the variety of ways in which we poison ourselves will become obvious. Cigarettes, auto exhaust, newspapers, canned foods, frozen foods, aluminum cookware, insecticides, fungicides, food additives, water piping, cosmetics, hair dyes, antacids, and even deodorants!

PREVENTION AND TREATMENT

In this day and age prevention of heavy metal poisoning is not easy, but it is absolutely essential to health and well-being. The most obvious preventive measure is to avoid consuming food or water likely to be contaminated. All canned food or frozen green foods are suspect. Lead-containing solder is often used in canned foods and copper sulfate is used frequently in treating canned or frozen green vegetables to help give an ultra-green color to enhance marketing. Any food exposed to insecticides, pesticides, or fungicides may have high levels of lead, cadmium, mercury, copper, or other toxic chemicals and should be strictly avoided. The safest vegetables are organically grown. Make sure, however, never to grow food within 25–50 ft (7.5–15 m) of a major road, to avoid lead toxicity. The further the better!

Cooking utensils with copper or aluminum cooking surfaces should be discarded. Use only tempered glass, stainless steel, or non-lead-glazed earthenware. Since heavy metals tend to concentrate within the ocean food chain, passing from bacteria to algae, then to small fish and later big fish, it is important to avoid frequent consumption of large fish such as tuna, marlin, and swordfish. In many areas swordfish is not allowed to be sold due to high heavy metal levels.

The source of fish, especially clams and other shellfish, is equally important. Avoid any shellfish caught near industrial towns. The best fish are freshwater lake or river fish from unpolluted waters, and small ocean reef fish.

Commercial meats are generally unfit for regular human consumption for many reasons, including heavy metal poisoning. Wild game may also have excessive amounts of heavy metals unless far from civilized areas.

Water supplies are difficult to change for most people. Those living in very old houses should check the plumbing to ensure that lead is no longer used anywhere in the system. The most potent dose of heavy metals from water comes in the morning after the water has been in the pipes for prolonged periods. The best prevention is to allow the water to run 1–2 minutes to drain away the pipes' reserve before you use it. Water filters also may be used.

Although it is considered the duty of the employer to prevent occupational heavy metal poisoning, many seem truly unaware of any health risk. We conducted informal spot checks on local auto body repair shops and did not find a single shop that required workers to wear air filter masks while on the job. Day after day, year after year, these workers are exposed to an incredible amount of heavy metals in the grinding, sanding, and painting process, completely oblivious to the dangers to which they are being subjected. Other occupations are equally exposed and just as unprotected. Any worker involved in such an industry should make the problem known to his or her employer or union. A routine yearly hair analysis should be provided for in all industrial contracts, as a preventive measure.

The human fetal brain concentrates heavy metals very rapidly. It is essential that pregnant mothers especially make all efforts to avoid these poisons. Children also are very susceptible. Playgrounds near major roads are possible sources of lead poisoning. Even soft drinks from beverage dispensers may cause toxic metal poisoning. Any child with behavior disorders or learning difficulties should be given a hair analysis to exclude toxic metals before being subjected to other treatments, This applies to adults as well.

Detoxification

Once heavy metal toxicity is diagnosed or suspect, the following regimen and nutritional supplements will help slowly reverse the process, provided the cause has been eliminated. It is important that the elimination take place in a controlled and gentle manner, since toxins will be released from body stores in muscles, organs, and bones, creating elevated blood levels for a short period of time. This can be extremely serious if the elimination process is too pronounced, causing exaggeration of the patient's symptoms, or even stimulating uncontrolled psychotic behavior.

Diet

Short periods of citrus fruit or apple mono diets are useful in the elimination process. Each case will determine the length of the initial mono diet. The more severe the toxicity, the shorter will be this first elimination. The usual period for the first mono diet is 3–7 days. This fairly rapid detoxification is followed with a mostly raw foods regimen with the exception of cooked beans as protein. A typical diet outline is as follows:

On Rising
Hot water and lemon juice.

Breakfast
Fresh grapefruit or just-ripe green apples.

Midmorning
Carrot juice.

Lunch
Raw green salad with cooked beans.

Midafternoon
Carrot juice

Supper
As lunch, or cooked vegetarian meal with plenty of ultra-green vegetables, seaweeds, and beans.

Evening
Raw apple or carrot juice.
1 tbsp raw bran is to be taken with all meals. Spirulina should be added whenever possible. All water should be distilled. No alcohol or smoking is allowed, and all foods should be organically grown, if at all possible.

This diet may last 1–2 weeks and then alternated with the mono diets previously mentioned. The second mono diet series may be much longer than the first, since we now need to extract deeper stores of heavy metals. Some cases may benefit from a prolonged citrus fruit juice fast at this time.

Another 1-2 weeks on the mostly raw foods diet with cooked beans is then followed by a further fast or mono diet. By this time all symptoms will have disappeared and the patient must be educated on how to avoid all toxic heavy metals and placed on a mostly vegetarian diet, allowing fish three times per week, if desired. No other meat is allowed for at least 3 months or longer. Periodic fast, mono diets, or mostly raw food diets should be undertaken for at least 3 days twice per month.

Therapeutic Detoxifying Supplements

Vitamins and Minerals—Primary

- Vitamin C plus bioflavonoids: 1000 mg 6 times daily, or more in acute toxicity, to bowel tolerance. High dose of C plus calcium. Vitamin C is a detoxifier and chelator (binding agent) of toxic metals. Given intravenously in high dose (30 g) for acute toxicity.
- Vitamin B6: 50-100 mg daily. This helps protect against kidney stone formation on a high C supplement regimen.
- Calcium orotate, calcium lactate, or bone meal: 600-1500 mg daily. Calcium decreases gastrointestinal absorption of some heavy metals and aids in their elimination. Milk as a calcium source is associated with increased lead levels and is not advised.
- Selenium: 200 mg twice daily. As an antioxidant it helps to detoxify heavy metals.

Vitamins and Minerals—Primary

- Vitamin A: 25,000 IU twice daily for 1 month, then once daily.
- Vitamin D: 400 IU twice daily.
- Vitamin E: 400 IU 2-3 times daily.
- Vitamin B complex: 50 mg twice daily.
- Zinc: 1 5-30 mg 2-3 times daily.
- Magnesium orotate: 300 mg.
- Potassium iodide: 1000 mcg daily for 1-2 months.

Others

- Pectin: found in just-ripe apples and white inner lining of citrus peels. It absorbs heavy metals and prevents absorption from gastrointestinal tract. It is a chelating (binding) agent.
- Sodium alginate: 250 mg 4-8 times daily; helps chelate and eliminate toxic metals. Algin is found in sea vegetables such as kelp.
- Sulfhydryl amino acids (L-lysine, L-cysteine, dimethionine): as found in legumes and as supplement form in many detoxification tablets.
- Kelp: 2 tablets 3 times daily.
- Chlorophyll: use as a supplement and in deep green vegetables. Helps to detoxify heavy metals
- Bran: 1 tbsp 3 times daily. Fiber in diet helps carry heavy metals through the system.
- Citric acid.
- Distilled water.
- Garlic.
- Lecithin: 4 capsules 3 times daily or 1-2 tbsp granules.

Note: Once heavy metal poisoning has reached the stage of severe confusion, seizures, and disorientation (all signs of encephalopathy), the condition is a medical emergency and is best treated in hospital with chelating agents. Due to the chance of brain damage these severe symptoms should not be treated at home.

HEMORRHOIDS
(Piles)

DEFINITION

Varicose veins of the hemorrhoidal plexus, external or internal.

SYMPTOMS

Burning, itching, and pain with bowel movement; blood loss with bowel movement; dilated, painful, enlarged, and often protruding swellings in the anal region.

ETIOLOGICAL CONSIDERATIONS

* Diet
* Refined foods (fiber deficiency); over-eating
* Constipation (straining at stool)
* Laxative habit
* Poor abdominal tone (visceroptosis)
* Lack of exercise/sedentary existence
* B6 deficiency
* Pregnancy
* Improper heavy lifting (without breathing, increasing intra-abdominal pressure)
* Toxicity

DISCUSSION

Hemorrhoids are extremely rare in countries where whole unrefined cereal grains are a major part of the diet. This places hemorrhoids in the class of "diseases of civilization". The western diet, with its refined carbohydrates such as white bread, white rice, and macaroni, is one of drastically reduced total fiber intake. Associated with this low-fiber diet is chronic constipation, and addiction to the habitual use of laxatives.

The major mechanical cause of hemorrhoids is increased intra-abdominal pressure. This can occur during heavy lifting when the breath is held. More common, however, is the increased intra-abdominal pressure created by straining to pass hard fecal matter during a bowel movement. With a lack of fiber in the diet, the stool becomes dehydrated, hard, and extremely difficult to pass. Laxatives are then resorted to, which act in several ways to ease bowel movements. Some act as irritants, while others are lubricants, softeners, or fiber additives. Of these only the fiber additives could be considered relatively harmless, as this approach is designed to *add* fiber removed from the diet by consumption of refined food. Most other laxatives, however, set up a vicious cycle of bowel movement followed by constipation, needing further laxatives. The powerful bowel movements so created leave the bowel in a flaccid state, further weakening future peristaltic action. We have seen patients literally addicted to both laxatives and enemas which, when used habitually, also cause bowel weakness and reduce peristaltic action (see Constipation).

Obesity with visceroptosis (sagging abdominal region) caused by weak abdominal muscles and lack of exercise will also predispose to hemorrhoids. This usually coincides with improper dietary habits.

TREATMENT

The prevention of hemorrhoids is much easier than their cure. Once the small blood vessels have been grossly dilated and fibrotic scar tissue has formed, it can be very difficult to totally remove the local damage. Surgical removal of hemorrhoids only gets rid of the immediate symptom and does nothing to prevent a recurrence. Surgery also creates more scar tissue. In spite of this, some hemorrhoids will need to be removed surgically if natural therapies fail to eliminate them. After this, prevention of further hemorrhoids should be the main priority.

The obvious dietary solution is to add fiber to the diet naturally through unrefined whole grains, fruit, raw and conservatively cooked vegetables, and nuts. While the addition of fiber alone in the form of bran will help most people have shorter transit times, larger stools, and will reduce constipation, this approach is not advised as the sole dietary change. Rather than eating refined foods and adding fiber later, it is much better to eat unrefined foods with all their protein, vitamins, minerals, and fiber intact. It is true, however, that bran is very useful in many stubborn cases of constipation and hemorrhoids. The dietary therapy for hemorrhoids is the same as for constipation.

Exercises

- Slant board exercises.
- Abdominal strengthening exercises.
- Hemorrhoid-specific exercise: stand with hands at side at attention. While inhaling, raise the hands over the head and rise on the toes. Stretch as far as possible, then breathe normally and lean as far forward as possible without falling. Retain this position for 3–5 minutes. Repeat twice daily.

Hydrotherapy

- Heat for pain relief.
  Hot compress; hot sitz bath.
- Alternate hot and cold, to cure:
  Alternate hot and cold sitz baths; alternate hot and cold compresses; alternate hot and cold perianal sprays
- Ice-cold: in acute cases; also to help replace prolapsed internal hemorrhoids. Cold compresses; cold sprays; cold sitz baths
- Ice: in acute cases:

Ice compresses. icicle suppository (may be made by placing a small copper tube in a halved potato—to act as a stand and prevent water draining away, filling with water and freezing). Insert in the rectum for 30 seconds at first, later increasing to 1–2 minutes; repeat 1–2 times daily.

Compresses and poultices

- Witch hazel: continuous day and night. Recommended in all cases.
- Lemon juice compress, or inject juice of lemon and 1/2 pint (250 mL) cold water into rectum and retain 10 minutes, followed by cold sitz bath.

Therapeutic Agents

Vitamins and Minerals

- Vitamin C: 1000–2000 mg 2–3 times daily. Tonifies bowel wall tissue.
- Bioflavonoids.
- Vitamin E: 400 IU 3 times daily.
- Vitamin A: 25,000 IU twice daily.
- Vitamin B complex: 25–50 mg 1–3 times daily.
- Vitamin B6: 25 mg 3 times daily.

Others

- Blackstrap molasses.
- Bran: 1–2 tbsp with meals.
- Increase fluids.
- Lemon.
- Olive oil: 1 tbsp prior to meals.
- Raw carrot cure.

Botanicals

Stone root: 2 capsules 3 times daily.

Psyllium seeds.

Aloe plus goldenseal: topical.

Bloodroot tea.

Calendula lotion: topical use.

Goldenseal

May-apple or American mandrake: for complete prolapse (highly toxic; see p. 60).

Mullein tea.

Peony root: 1 cup infusion twice daily.

Rhatany.
Wintergreen: for painful hemorrhoids.
Suppositories:
Goldenseal: insert one nightly.
Stone root.

Stramonium: for extremely painful
hemorrhoids.
Witch hazel, stone root, and Peruvian
balsam.

HEPATITIS

DEFINITION

Inflammation of the liver due to infection or toxic substances. Infectious agents include viruses, bacteria, and parasites. Toxic agents include antibiotics, drugs, industrial solvents, anesthetics, carbon tetrachloride, and others.

SYMPTOMS

Begins similar to influenza with weakness, lassitude, drowsiness, nausea, fever, and headache. Jaundice may or may not develop, with or without dark urine, gray stools, and skin irritation. The liver is tender and enlarged. Appetite is poor. Possible depression. Liver may develop necrosis or cirrhosis. Severe cases may be fatal.

ETIOLOGICAL CONSIDERATIONS

*   Infection: (viruses, bacteria, parasites) Hepatitis symptoms may be simulated by parasitic amebiasis, abscess of liver.
*   Infectious hepatitis 2–4-week incubation period. May be prevented by immune serum globulin injections. Contracted via blood, feces, contaminated food, water, and shellfish.
*   Serum hepatitis (Australian antigen) 4–23-week incubation period. Parenteral transmission.
*   Toxic hepatitis (via inhalation, ingestion, skin absorption).
*   Drugs (a large number).
    Chemicals (carbon tetrachloride); insec-

ticides; solvents; metallic compounds and others.
*   Improper diet
    Downgraded liver function; reduced vitality
*   Bile obstruction: alcohol

DISCUSSION

As a general rule, disease occurs only when resistance is low. Certainly, with hepatitis, contamination by the infective agent is a major consideration. In both infectious and serum hepatitis, feces and blood are considered infectious. Both types may be spread by the fecal and oral route, with poor sanitation a factor. However, a healthy system will resist such invasions more efficiently than would otherwise be the case in downgraded health. Improper diet will leave the liver more susceptible to infection by clogging it with unnecessary chemicals or toxins which must be detoxified, and by supplying it with deficient nutrients. Gallbladder malfunction and liver toxemia are also major causes of degraded liver vitality.

TREATMENT

The treatment of acute hepatitis and chronic hepatitis is somewhat different than in other liver diseases. Although short liver-cleansing diets may be useful in isolated cases, a high-protein diet rich in nutrients favors recovery. The type of protein foods used are important and should be primarily lacto-vegetarian. Yeast, wheat germ, egg yolks, low-fat yoghurt, acidophilus low-fat milk, tofu, soybeans, and Spirulina are good sources. The diet should also contain high-chlorophyll foods such as raw and cooked green vegetables. Of special importance in treating acute hepatitis are vitamin C injections (25–50 g of sodium ascorbate intravenously daily) with calcium gluconate (1 g per 10 g of vitamin C). Also useful are vitamin B complex and B12 injections intramuscularly in addition to multiple oral nutritional supports. Lecithin is of special significance and should be consumed as food and as a food supplement.

Diet

High protein, lacto-vegetarian, low-fat: wheat germ, yeast, lecithin, egg yolks, low-fat goat's milk, eggnogs, and lecithin; low-fat acidophilus milk and curds; low-fat yoghurt; hot water and lemon; tofu, soy products; beets plus beet tops; greens, Spirulina; papaya; plenty of fluids

This diet may cause ammonia build-up if liver damage is severe. This must be monitored. Lactobacillus helps prevent this build-up from becoming aggravated by excess protein consumption.

Note: Absolutely no saturated fats or alcohol can be consumed.

Physiotherapy, Hydrotherapy, and Spinal Manipulation

- Trunk packs (abdominal): leave on for 1–3 hours or overnight.
- Coffee enema: 1–2 times daily (see Appendix I).
- Alternate hot and cold compresses over liver area.
- Rest and sunlight baths.
- Spinal manipulation: thoracic and lumbar.

Therapeutic Agents

Vitamins and Minerals
- Vitamin C: 1000 mg per hour in acute cases, 25–50 g sodium ascorbate intravenously (with 1 g calcium gluconate to 10 g vitamin C daily). Antiviral.
- Vitamin A: 10,000–25,000 IU emulsified, 2–6 times daily. (See warning under Vitamin Toxicity, page 56) Promotes healing.
- Vitamin E: 400–1200 IU daily. Prevents hemorrhaging and scar formation. Improves circulation. Antioxidant.
- Folic acid: 5 mg 3 times daily.
- Vitamin B complex, oral: 50 mg 3 times daily, plus intramuscularly.
- Vitamin B12: 1 mg intramuscularly 1–3 times per week.

Others
- L-carnitine: 500 mg twice daily on an empty stomach. Transports fatty acids into mitochondria for hepatic repair.
- Glutathione: 500 mg twice daily on an empty stomach. Helps protect the liver.
- L-cysteine and L-methionine: 500 mg twice daily taken on an empty stomach. Detoxifies liver toxins and works with glutathione.
- Free form amino acids: take as per label. Supplies necessary protein for healing and to rest liver.
- Crude liver: intramuscular injections daily.
- Coenzyme Q10: 60 mg daily. Enhances tissue oxygenation.
- Essential fatty acids.
- Chlorophyll.
- Pancreatic enzymes.
- Disodium phosphate.
- Garlic.
- Radish tablets.
- Raw liver tablets.
- Raw spleen tablets.
- Raw thymus tablets.
- Spirulina: 1 tsp 3–4 times daily.

Botanicals—Primary
Hepatic anti-inflammatories: *Scutellaria baicalensis*, licorice, bupleurum, *Salvia miltiorrhiza*.
Hepatic antivirals: phyllanthus.
Immune stimulants: picrorrhiza, astragalus.

Hepatoprotective and trophorestoratives (able to restore liver structure): St Mary's thistle, globe artichoke, bupleurum, astragalus.

Schisandra chinensis lignans: protective against viral liver damage, stimulates cytochrome P450 detoxification pathway.

Botanicals—Secondary

Celandine: cholagogue. 1–10 drops tincture 3–4 times daily.

Fringe tree: 5–30 drops tincture 3–4 times daily.

Blue flag.

Culver's root: 10–60 drops tincture 3–4 times daily.

Dandelion: cholagogue.

Goldenseal.

Licorice: antiviral.

Oregon grape root: excellent antioxidant.

HERPES GENITALIS AND COLD SORES

DEFINITION

Cold sores, canker sores, fever blisters: a recurrent, contagious viral infection caused primarily by herpes Type 1 virus. *Herpes genitalis, venereal herpes, genital herpes:* a recurrent, contagious viral infection usually caused by herpes Type 2 virus.

SYMPTOMS

Recurrent fluid-filled blisters that rupture, leaving red, inflamed, painful lesions. These are preceded by a slightly irritating tingling. Once the lesion appears, pain is pronounced. Lesions may affect the lips, tongue, nose, face, genitals, thighs, or elsewhere. The first attack is most severe. Lesions tend to dry and crust over in 10–14 days. Repeated attacks in same area may cause scarring.

ETIOLOGICAL CONSIDERATIONS—PRIMARY

- Herpes virus Type 1 and Type 2
- Sexual contact
- Stress (physical or emotional)
- Overwork
- Acid diet
- L-arginine excess

ETIOLOGICAL CONSIDERATIONS— SECONDARY

Fevers; vitamin deficiency; citrus; some drugs; sunburn; menstruation; friction

DISCUSSION

Genital herpes infections now affect over 35% of the population in the US, with over half a million new cases reported each year. Of these victims, 80% are 20–39 years of age, with most of the reported cases being Caucasian. Traditionally, the distinction between herpes Type 1 and Type 2 was that Type 1 infections occurred primarily on the upper half of the body (cold sores) and Type 2 on the lower half (genital herpes). This distinction is no longer considered very valuable, as either type may infect any part of the body. Many consider herpes a worse disorder than gonorrhea or syphilis. At least with these other venereal infections cure is possible. The orthodox medical field, however, can offer little hope presently for the herpes patient.

Although the herpes infection itself is moderately painful, the real concern is not with the lesions themselves. The most painfully difficult aspect of having genital herpes is the fear of giving the disease to someone else. Severe depression, self-reproach, hate, and anger often follow the initial attack, which may deepen into a major psychological problem in some cases. Great difficulties arise for the single herpes sufferer on whether, or when, to tell a prospective bed partner about the infection.

Herpes tends to cause recurrent attacks with intervals without symptoms. The virus is thought to live in the dorsal root ganglia of the dermatome affected and migrate to the lesion site under certain conditions. Gradually, most victims learn which factors lead to an outbreak for them. Commonly observed factors are physical or emotional stress, overwork, anxiety, fevers, friction, or menstruation. Although most herpes infections, either cold sores or genital, are passed from person to person by the intimate contact of a kiss or sexual activity, there is some evidence that herpes can live outside the body long enough for indirect infection to occur. Tests have shown that herpes can live up to 4 hours on toilet seats

Outside of the lesion itself and psychological trauma, herpes has been implicated as a cause or factor in cervical cancer in women, and in severe infections of the newborn. If the mother has an active lesion during delivery, this represents a serious risk to the newborn since the infant's immune system is still too weak to prevent a systemic spread of herpes, which may cause blindness, nerve damage, and may even be fatal. In these cases many obstetricians recommend cesarean section as a preventative.

TREATMENT

To our knowledge, no natural therapy has been successful in eliminating herpes completely. What we have seen in our practice, however, are patients who once had frequent attacks, even lasting 3 weeks out of every 4, who now have only rare incidents, short-lived and fairly mild.

Diet

The nutritional approach to herpes is based partly on the observation that an amino acid, L-arginine, must be supplied in the environment for herpes to grow. L-lysine, another amino acid, has been found to decrease absorption of L-arginine and to increase the speed of its metabolic breakdown in the body. The key then is to decrease L-arginine-containing foods, increase L-lysine foods, or to simply take an excess of L-lysine as a nutritional supplement. High L-arginine foods are peanuts, peanut butter, cashews, pecans, almonds, seeds and chocolate, with peas and untoasted cereal grains being moderate sources. Foods with a better arginine-lysine relationship are brewer's yeast, dairy products, potatoes, meat, and eggs. In clinical practice we encourage these minor changes in diet, but advise L-lysine as a supplement, with the patient taking 500 mg each day when symptom-free, and 500 mg 3-4 times daily when a lesion is present. When L-lysine is taken it reduces the pain of an acute lesion, shortens its duration, lengthens the remission state, and decreases frequency of occurrence.

In general, the diet must be alkaline in reaction, avoiding sweets, refined carbohydrates, alcohol, and, for some people, citrus. All food must be unrefined and in as natural a state as possible. Fermented foods such as plain yoghurt, kefir, or acidophilus milk should be taken daily, along with 1-2 glasses of potassium broth. Foods such as brewer's yeast also should be eaten daily in food as well as in supplement form.

Physiotherapy

- Ultrasound: direct to lesion when acute, or to spinal area related to dermatome affected. Repeat daily for 2 weeks, then 3-4 times per week for 2-3 weeks.
- Meditation: learning to deal with stress is essential to prevent outbreaks.
- Acupuncture.
- Ice applications: topically.

Therapeutic Agents

Vitamins and Minerals

- Vitamin C with bioflavonoids complex: 1000–6000 mg daily (or to bowel tolerance). Increases natural interferon production.
- Vitamin B complex: 50 mg 3 times daily.
- Zinc: 30 mg 2–3 times daily.
- Vitamin E: 400 IU 1–2 times daily; also as topical application to cold sore or genital herpes.
- Vitamin A: 25,000–50,000 IU daily; also topical.
- Vitamin B1: 100 mg plus vitamin B12 (1000 mcg intramuscularly) 1–3 times per week initially, then 1–2 times per month.
- Vitamin B1: 200–300 mg daily.
- Vitamin B6.
- Vitamin B12: 25 mcg twice daily.
- Folic acid.
- N,N-dimethylglycine.
- Pantothenic acid.

Other

- Probiotics *Lactobacillus acidophilus*, and *L. bulgaricus*: 4 capsules 4–6 times daily in acute cases; 2 capsules 3 times daily for maintenance. This must be fresh and refrigerated to be effective. Demonstrates potent antiviral activity.
- L-lysine: 500 mg daily for prevention. 500 mg 3 times daily during an attack.
- Atomodine: apply locally followed by glycothymoline.
- Thymus tablets: 2 tablets 3–6 times daily.

Botanicals

St John's wort: specific for enveloped viruses such as herpes.
Astragalus: antiviral.
Butternut: local application, use decoction of root.
Comfrey: root powder; local.
Goldenseal: powder; local.
Lemon balm topically for 3–4 days.
Green kukul nut: apply sap to lesion 3–4 times daily.
Oregon grape root: 1 oz herb to 1 pint (500 mL) water; 1 cup 2–3 times daily.
Thuja.

HIATAL HERNIA

DEFINITION

Protrusion of the stomach above the diaphragm through the esophageal hiatus, leading to a reflux regurgitation of acid pepsin through the incompetent gastroesophageal sphincter.

SYMPTOMS

Heartburn, pain, difficulty with swallowing, inflammation, ulceration, gastrointestinal bleeding, pain from reflux on reclining, fibrositis, and possible stricture of esophagus.

ETIOLOGICAL CONSIDERATIONS

- Increased intra-abdominal pressure
  Constipation; obesity; pregnancy; heavy lifting; tight, restricting abdominal clothing (girdles, belts, jeans, etc.)
- Diet
  Overeating; fiber deficiency (slow stomach transit time); refined carbohydrates; spicy foods, acid foods, coffee
- Cigarette smoking (nicotine relaxes sphincter)
- Digestive enzyme deficiency
- Poor abdominal tone
- Weak diaphragm (especially in older age groups)

- Poor spinal mechanics "dowager's hump" (kyphosis)

DISCUSSION

Hiatal hernia is one of our "civilized diseases", being uncommon in underdeveloped nations. Looking at the etiologic considerations, it is easy to see why.

The most widely accepted causative factor is increased intra-abdominal pressure. Western diets, with an abundance of low-fiber refined foods, favor constipation. The result is straining at stool with an increased intra-abdominal pressure, literally forcing the stomach through the diaphragm.

Obesity, so common in developed nations, is another major factor associated with hiatal hernia. Restricting abdominal clothing such as girdles, tight belts, and skin-tight jeans is another factor fairly unique to "civilized" nations.

Of all the factors influencing formation of hiatal hernia, it is diet that has the most central effect. As previously mentioned, the western low-fiber diet will favor constipation. However, this is not diet's only role. Refined carbohydrates, stripped of their protective protein and fiber coverings, act to stimulate gastric acid production, without the ability to buffer that acid (see Peptic Ulcer). This causes an excess of acid in the stomach and sets up conditions necessary for gastric reflux into the esophagus, leading to heartburn. In fact, several authorities feel gastric reflux is the primary condition with a hiatal hernia, following *secondarily* from injury to the tissues by the acid.

Another aspect of refined carbohydrates is that due to the lack of fiber an overabundance of carbohydrates may be consumed, leading to obesity. Overeating is a major causative factor in hiatal hernias. Excessively large meals tend to slow stomach transit time. As the food sits for prolonged periods in the stomach, the esophageal sphincter relaxes and allows gastric acids to enter the esophagus.

Another factor slowing stomach transit time is meals containing large amounts of fats and fried foods. This may be the reason hiatal hernias are so often associated with gallstones. Consumption of foods that increase gastric acidity such as sweets, coffee, tea, alcohol, and spicy foods all predispose to hiatal hernias.

TREATMENT

Obviously, the treatment must first reverse the causes.

Diet

If constipation is present, the treatment for habitual constipation should be followed. The diet is changed to a high-fiber one of smaller meals. The bulk of the diet should be composed of raw fruits; raw and conservatively cooked vegetables; whole grains such as brown rice, millet, bulgar, barley, oats, rye, and wheat; nuts; beans; sprouts; and some animal proteins if desired, but little or no red meat. Periods of fasting or the apple mono diet should be alternated with this general high-fiber diet. Bran should be taken with all meals.

Weight loss is a major aim with obese patients. All sweets, coffee, tea, alcohol, fried foods, and spices are forbidden. Patients are told not to drink with meals and to eat only when hungry.

Physiotherapy

- Spinal manipulation: improper spinal mechanics are corrected with spinal manipulation and back exercises to correct thoracic kyphosis.
- Abdominal exercises: good abdominal tone is essential for proper bowel eliminations and diaphragm function. These must be done vigorously daily. Without proper abdominal tone, healing will not be possible with this condition.

Therapeutic Agents

Vitamins and Minerals

- Vitamin A: 10,000–25,000 IU 1–3 times daily. (See warning under Vitamin Toxicity, page 56.) Helps reduce excess acids and enhances immune function.
- Vitamin C plus bioflavinoids: may require buffered forms. Dose depends on how well it is tolerated.
- Vitamin E: 200–400 IU 3 times daily. Helps in healing of irritated tissues.
- Zinc: 25 mg twice daily For healing and repair of tissues.
- Vitamin B: 250–500 mg daily.
- Vitamin B complex: 25–50 mg 2–3 times daily, if well tolerated.
- Pantothenic acid: 250–500 mg daily.
- Manganese: 50 mg daily.
- Choline: 1–2 g daily.

Others

- Proteolytic enzymes with pancreatin: as per label. To improve digestion.
- Bromelain: 2 tablets after meals. Proteolytic enzyme.
- Papaya enzyme: 2 tablets 3–4 times daily or as needed. Aids digestion and healing.
- Bran: 1 tbsp with water before all meals.
- Aloe vera juice: twice daily. Heals and soothes.
- Kelp or other iodine source.
- Lecithin.
- Sodium alginate.

Botanicals

Comfrey.
Goldenseal.
Marshmallow.
Slippery elm: demulcent.

Therapeutic Suggestion

The return to a high-fiber diet is the major therapy. Supplements may aggravate condition in early stages; use intramuscularly or liquid form where possible. Bran may aggravate condition at first, but a non-wheat bran (e.g. psyllium powder) is essential. Slippery elm will help soothe the mucosa and is useful even in early stages.

HICCUP

DEFINITION AND SYMPTOMS

Repeated involuntary, spasmodic contractions of the diaphragm, which are then followed by a sudden closure of the glottis.

DISCUSSION

This usually self-limiting condition is the result of irritation of the afferent or efferent nerves or the medullary centers controlling the muscles of respiration. Most episodes last only short periods of time; however, we occasionally hear of hiccups lasting for several days. Cases lasting for years have even been reported. You can imagine how irritating a prolonged case of hiccups would be. Unfortunately, simple techniques for stopping such a prolonged case do not work since the cause in these situations is usually pathologic. This may include such serious conditions as a tumor in the medulla oblongata, disorders of the stomach or esophagus, pancreatitis, hepatitis, or hepatic metastases. Fortunately, common cases of hiccups are not of this serious nature and are easily relieved. Most cases are caused by overeating or overdrinking, which will distend the stomach and irritate the diaphragm.

TREATMENT

A high blood carbon dioxide level is known to inhibit hiccups. Breath holding and/or rebreathing into a paper bag are the most commonly used techniques. Should these fail it is not difficult to gather tried and true pet techniques from literally anyone you care to ask. The following list reflects years of unscientific, untested, and unproven clinical trial methods, which we are sure will, if not cure the condition, at least entertain you.

A female patient of ours swears that this technique is 100% successful. She recommends taking 10 (not 9 or 11) sips of water in rapid succession. Others are:

- Lie on left side for 10–15 minutes.
- Chew and swallow ice for 10–15 minutes.
- Drink a glass of water from the opposite side of the glass.
- Apply pressure with the flat hand just below the breastbone.
- Hold breath while extending head as far back as possible.
- Eat some sugar.
- Apply ice to neck.
- Take a hot bath.
- Stand on your head.
- Take a roller-coaster ride.
- Induce vomiting.
- Have your stomach pumped.
- Have someone apply traction to your tongue!
- Apply strong digital pressure over the phrenic nerves behind the sternoclavicular joints (We use this one).
- C5 mobilization, percussion, and manipulation (We also use this one).
- Good (hic) luck!

HIVES
(Urticaria)

DEFINITION

Local wheals and erythema of the dermis.

SYMPTOMS

Pruritus (itching), elevated wheals, swollen eyes, possible general and occasionally fatal anaphylactic response (edema of airways causes respiratory distress similar to severe asthma); self-limiting, 1–7 days, except in cases of severe hypersensitivity when death may result.

ETIOLOGICAL CONSIDERATIONS—PRIMARY

- Imbalance between deep and superficial circulation.
- Disordered stomach and bowels; skin: improper eliminations.
- Toxemia, including autotoxemia of leaky gut
- Food allergy: shellfish, milk, eggs, wheat, pork, onions, some fruits.
- Drug allergy (drug sensitivity may be hidden, such as penicillin in milk).
- Food additive (food dyes, preservatives).
- Spinal lesion.
- Insect stings.
- Lymph stasis/poor circulation.

ETIOLOGICAL CONSIDERATIONS— SECONDARY

Chlorine in drinking water (destroys intestinal flora); stress (histamine release); adrenal exhaustion; liver congestion; hydrochloric acid deficiency; acid condition; chronic infection; coffee, alcohol, tobacco may cause or aggravate condition.

291

DISCUSSION

We believe the most common cause of hives is an imbalance between the deep and superficial circulations, accompanied or caused by poor eliminations. Toxins are then thrown into the superficial circulation and cause a typical histamine "wheal" response. Although allergy is the accepted exciting factor, we believe that instead of looking externally for the cause, it usually may be found within, in the intestinal tract (see Leaky Gut). It is also possible to get hives from sensitivity to various foods or various external agents. We then must deal with the reasons for the hypersensitivity such as adrenal exhaustion, stress, diet deficiency, improper weaning, food additives, or pesticides. Many cases follow the use of a particular drug.

Lymph stasis and poor circulation may be caused by lack of exercise, poor skin function, poor eliminations, toxemia, general atony or even spinal lesions. Several interesting cases come to mind where all treatments failed to give relief until spinal manipulation was successfully tried.

With severe anaphylactic reactions causing respiratory distress, immediate hospital care is required.

TREATMENT

Prolonged fasting is the best method to eliminate recurrent hives. This will allow the intestine to heal, eliminate toxins, and re-establish proper eliminations. The following fluids are useful: distilled water; carrot and green vegetable juice; burdock seed tea.

This diet should be continued as long as possible, or repeated at frequent intervals until the hives do not return. Enemas or other eliminants should be used during the fast. If constipation is a problem, follow the regimen under Constipation.

The diet between fasts should reduce sugars, fruits, and carbohydrates to a minimum. Eat an abundance of green vegetables, avoid saturated fats, or fried foods. Organically grown food is advised.

Physiotherapy

- Oatmeal or bran bath to relieve itching: 2 lb of either placed in muslin bag and set in hot bath—104-106°F (40-42°C).
- Cream of tartar and water paste applied to hives. Trunk packs to induce sweating.
- Sodium bicarbonate bath for itching. Ultraviolet light.

Therapeutic Agents

Vitamins and Minerals
- Vitamin C: essential for adrenal function; anti-inflammatory. 1000 IU 3-4 times daily or more. Ascorbates are best.
- Vitamin B complex: 50 mg 2-3 times daily. Helps prevent production of histamine from the amino acid histidine needed for adrenal function and natural cortisone production.
- Vitamin A: 25,000 IU 2-3 times daily for 2 months. (See warning under Vitamin Toxicity, page 56.)
- Vitamin B6: 50-100 mg twice daily.
- Vitamin B12: 1 mg intramuscularly daily in acute stage.
- Calcium: 2000-3000 mg daily in acute, and 1000 mg intravenous with 5 g vitamin C.

Others
- Raw adrenal tablets: helps normalize cortisone production which is an anti-inflammatory and antihistamine.
- Hydrochloric acid: 5-60 grains with meals.
- Wheat germ oil: rub on hives.
- Marshmallow soap.

Botanicals—Primary
Nettles.
Albizzia: anti-allergy.
Alfalfa: blood tonic and cleanser.
Chamomile.
Feverfew.
Sarsaparilla.
Scutellaria baicalensis.

Aloe vera: topically.
Apis mellifera: tincture.
Oatmeal: tincture.

Botanicals—Secondary

Burdock seed: tea.
Catnip: tea.

Cat's claw.
Chickweed: ointment.
Dandelion.
Echinacea.
Elder leaf: ointment.
Rehmannia.
Sassafras: tea.

HYPERACTIVITY (Hyperkinesis, Hyperkinetic Impulse Disorder, Minimal Brain Damage, ADD/ADHD

DEFINITION AND SYMPTOMS

A behavioral disorder of children and sometimes adults, manifested by impulsive activity, low stress tolerance, emotional instability, anger, anxiety, aggressiveness, destructive behavior, hyperresponsive actions, slow learning, short attention span, and sometimes a lack of coordination.

ETIOLOGICAL CONSIDERATIONS—PRIMARY

- Food allergy
- Essential fatty acid deficiency
- Vitamin and mineral deficiencies and dependencies
- Food additives, flavorings, colors, preservatives, salicylates
- Caffeine foods and drinks soda; tea; coffee; chocolate
- Refined and canned foods, junk foods

ETIOLOGICAL CONSIDERATIONS— SECONDARY

- Phosphate-containing foods such as red meat and carbonated drinks; pesticides, insecticides, fungicides; celiac disease; salicylate sensitivity (Feingold concept); heavy metal toxicity; hypoglycemia; fluorescent lights (lack of full-spectrum lighting); history of birth trauma, prenatal hemorrhage, toxemia, low birth weight, prematurity, difficult labor, or lack of oxygen at birth; monosodium glutamate (MSG); environmental; parasitic infestation; glandular imbalance; psychological causes; drugs

DISCUSSION

Hyperactivity of a child can totally destroy the hopes of a reasonably normal life for every member of the affected family. Each time such a child is brought into our office, we find the mother's physical and psychological condition even more upsetting than the child's. These parents suffer incredible tension, profound helplessness, frustration, and guilt, trying to deal with their own pent-up emotions that arise in response to their child's behavior. It is a rare mother indeed who does not break down into tears during the initial consultation. Hyperactivity transforms what was hoped to be the beautiful experience of parenthood into an endless nightmare.

293

Orthodox treatments have included drugs to sedate and tranquilize the child. This may remove some of the more obvious symptoms temporarily, but does nothing to deal with the cause. The mother frequently is told that nothing more can be done, and given the hope that, at least for some hyperactive children, the problem seems to resolve itself by the midteens.

The cause of hyperactivity is unknown. Abnormal conditions of pregnancy, labor, or the immediate post-partum period may account for some cases. This, however, accounts for only a small number of cases where the condition of minimal brain damage may in fact be the sole cause.

The Feingold diet has become popularized, blending the age-old arguments of naturopaths and organic food enthusiasts against the use of refined, devitalized foods poisoned by additives, food colorings, preservatives, flavorings and pesticides; and the more original discovery by Dr Ben F. Feingold that a significant number of hyperactive children have a salicylate sensitivity. Salicylates are not only found in aspirin, but also in many common foods such as almonds, apples, apricots, cherries, cranberries, cucumbers, grapes, nectarines, oranges, tangerines, peaches, peppers, plums, prunes, raisins, and tomatoes.

Further useful research has come out of the orthomolecular psychiatry approach. Many physicians have found that a significant number of hyperactive individuals suffer from vitamin dependencies. In such a situation, the patient may require more of an individual nutrient than an otherwise normal person. This research is very similar to that done with schizophrenia (see Schizophrenia).

Both of these approaches have done a real service in presenting at least a part of the nutritional concept to the public attention. Unfortunately, they are both incomplete, failing to present the entire range of possible causative factors in any given case. It is of course no new discovery that diet and nutrition are the single most influential factors in the cause of hyperactivity. Naturopaths have been successfully treating hyperactivity with simple diet changes. The fact that some children are hypersensitive to the blatantly poisonous substances used in the agriculture or food processing industries should be accepted as common sense. Even if every child does not show the ill effects of such poisons in the form of hyperactivity, other manifestations may result. This is one of the great human mysteries, that each is unique.

Going one step beyond this, it is not too surprising that some people would respond unfavorably to a group of foods containing a naturally occurring substance such as the salicylates. There certainly is evidence that other food groups can cause or aggravate specific conditions, such as the nightshade group (potatoes, tomatoes) in its relation to some cases of arthritis.

Hypoglycemia is another factor commonly found associated with behavioral disorders, including hyperactivity. Low blood sugar is an increasingly common problem as a result of the objectively bizarre diet most people now consume. From bottled baby food onwards we are literally bombarded with highly refined, devitalized foods and incredible amounts of sugar. Even a casual observer must surely be appalled at the typical junk food diet—or perhaps common sense has left us. Not only does the hypoglycemic state itself create glandular and behavior disorders, but some individuals develop such a severe sugar sensitivity that even minute amounts cause allergy-like reactions sometimes manifested as emotional instability or hyperactivity.

Food allergy or sensitivity is another dietary factor often related to hyperactivity. Milk and wheat are the two most common factors, along with sugar, as mentioned above. Any food, however, may be suspect. Celiac disease has been a recognized problem in many cases of behavioral disorders.

Heavy metal toxicity is now becoming more recognized as a cause of behavioral disorders. In children this often accompanies a typical devitalized diet, high in canned and frozen foods. Sometimes the cause may be found in the water supply or some other chronic exposure (see Heavy Metal Poisoning for sources of contaminants).

More subtle factors such as environmental lighting may be important with some individuals. Once again, just because some people might be able to live in a dark, smoggy city in a small box with artificial light does not mean that all could do so unharmed. A wonderful book on the effects of natural and artificial light on humans and other living things is *Health and Light* by John N. Ott.

Diagnosis

Diagnosis of hyperactivity, aggression and/or learning disorders may involve dyslexia, dyspraxia, and ADD/ADHD (hyperactivity). As children naturally grow, learn and develop, aspects of any of these disorders may be seen. For example nearly all children can be hyperactive, inattentive and aggressive at times. But a disorder is diagnosed when the behavior becomes characteristic, extreme, socially disruptive and difficult to manage.

It is also important to note that many children (and adults) with various other neurological disturbances such as epilepsy, autism, Down's, schizophrenia, bipolar and many other conditions sometimes have hyperactivity and/or frustration/aggression as characteristic features of their behavior and will benefit from the treatment protocols proposed here.

ADD/ADHD

Signs and Symptoms

The signs and symptoms of this disorder are many and varied. The American Psychiatric Association's DSM (diagnostic and statistical manual) Rating Scale is used in diagnosis, and different diagnoses can be attributed usually depending on what specific signs are present. Signs and symptoms include:

- Hyperactivity, perceptual motor impairment, coordination deficit.
- Short-term attention span, failure to finish a task
- Poor concentration, inattentiveness and easy distraction, impulsiveness.
- Poor organizing ability, memory and thinking disorders.
- Specific learning disorders, speech hearing and EEG irregularities.
- Irritability, frustration, aggression, destructibility, socially disruptive, depression.

Onset of the disorder typically is evident before 4 years of age. Early warning signs can occur in infancy and include difficulty feeding, constant thirst, frequent tantrums, head banging, and rocking the cot.

Pathophysiology

While causes (in strictly scientific terms) remain uncertain, abnormalities in neurological function especially the neurotransmitters, are characteristic diagnostic findings. Thyroid dysfunction can also cause signs and symptoms.

ADD sufferers demonstrate abnormal glucose metabolism in many parts of the brain, especially the premotor cortex and superior prefrontal cortex, areas responsible for the preparation and execution of motor activity, inhibition of inappropriate social responses, and attentiveness.

The sympathetic nervous system (the one which governs the "fear, fight and flight" response) becomes impaired given the abnormal response of the adrenal glands to glucose.

However, models are emerging which clearly implicate nutritional considerations, which include allergies and sensitivities, and nutrient deficiencies.

Medical Approach

The medical approach, like so many medical approaches to illness, does not attempt to deal with the causes but with the symptoms. The classic approach remains the use of stimulants (to increase attention span) and/or antidepressants if needed. Also some adjunctive intervention therapies such as assistance with schooling, cognitive/behavior modification, and personality and relationship counseling.

Methylphenidate (Ritalin) is the drug of choice for ADD/ADHD. It is a psychostimulant, an amphetamine and the MIMS Annual (1996; 20:268–269) states:

"Its mechanism of action is not completely understood, but Ritalin presumably exerts its stimulant effects by acting on the brain stem arousal system and cortex. There is neither specific evidence to clearly establish the mechanism whereby Ritalin produces its mental and behavioral effects in children, nor conclusive evidence as to how these effects relate to the condition of the central nervous system."

The use of Ritalin has increased by up to 500% in the past 5 years. The drug is not effective in all cases. In a third of cases there is no benefit, and it aggravates some others.

We express concern that many doctors are prescribing Ritalin as a diagnostic tool ("If it calms the child, then the child is considered to have the condition"—the point being that a positive response to a psychotropic drug is not uncommon and in no way demonstrates ADD as a diagnosis). One study suggested that up to 40% of pediatricians in the US were using Ritalin as just such a "litmus" test for ADHD.

The use of stimulant drugs does show at least some short-term benefits, such as improvement in attention span, social and family function, self-esteem and cognition. But there is no indication of long-term benefits from drugs. Long-term side effects are unknown (for example, the effect on the important adrenal glands, and the brain itself, in later life), so the use of these drugs including Ritalin is highly experimental.

Biochemical Considerations

We follow what is becoming known as the biochemical hypothesis. This model suggests that the cause, in most cases and very commonly, has to do specifically with nutrient deficiencies in association with food sensitivities, intolerances and allergies. Practitioners are achieving significant therapeutic effects in following the treatment protocols explicit in this model.

The mind and body are continuous. A happy body generally means a happy mind, and a happy mind means a happy body. What happens when the body becomes unhappy for some reason? The mind becomes unhappy.

With hyperactivity, one is observing a mind which is preoccupied with disturbances within the body including the brain, such as severe disturbances of the gastrointestinal, immune and nervous systems, that there is a condition of "no peace" in the brain. When the body is not happy, the brain is not happy, and learning anything becomes too hard.

We follow this hypothesis because of recent papers over the past decade implicating certain food groups in this biochemical hypothesis, and because when the model is followed, patients get better. In other words it works and it is a practical way to address the problem.

Culprit Food Groups

There are three major food groups that can cause brain allergies and brain chemical imbalances. These are:

- Dairy foods, including milk, cream, butter and margarine, ice-cream and other foods containing dairy products.
- Wheat and other similar protein.
- Refined sugar (sucrose) and foods containing same.

There are some other problem foods such as corn, chocolate, oranges, peanuts, eggs, cocoa and occasionally some others as well. Certainly foods and drinks containing certain artificial food colors (e.g. red—tartrazine), flavors and preservatives can also be a problem, but the main culprits are the three categories mentioned above.

If an immune system is bombarded with particular food groups over a period of time, there is the likelihood of allergy, especially if the immune system is subject to stress, and nutrient deficiency.

Nutrient Deficiencies

Nutritional research reveals that the average Australian and American child is nutrient deficient, as testified by the growing number of cases of asthma, eczema, obesity, emotional disorders and disturbances in immune function including leukemia. Given the popularity of convenience shopping today, in which most food is highly processed, and there is very little consumption of raw foods causing a broad-based deficiency of minerals, vitamins and enzymes, one has to expect that things are going to get a whole lot worse.

Apart from being overwhelmed with so much saturated fat, the average child (and adult) is deficient in the essential fatty acid omega-3 (EFA). Typical western diets provide an omega-3 to omega-6 ratio that is far too high. This is a classic case in which the relative excess of one nutrient creates a relative deficiency of another, because many nutrients need to be in proportional balance. This is the situation with so many different nutrients, and the consequences of such imbalances we are seeing more and more. An optimal ratio is 4 (omega-6) to 1 (omega-3). Currently We see a 14:1 average and even higher in some children. Major studies are demonstrating that supplementing omega-3 fatty acids (e.g. flaxseed oil) ought to be the first line of therapy in these conditions. Omega-3s are specific for the ADD/ADHD condition, and are therapeutic.

Zinc is an essential mineral specific for this condition. Low zinc levels in developing animals and humans produce a broad range of defects, including immunological, neurological, endocrine and behavioral disorders including hyperactivity. Given the enormous levels of stress experienced in today's society, we are seeing more and more cases of relative zinc deficiency. Zinc in a combi-

nation of vitamin B6 and magnesium is specific for these conditions.

In reference to studies into thyroid function and ADD/ADHD, certain specific nutrients are required to activate the thyroid, including iodine, tyrosine, zinc, vitamins B2 and B3, copper, chromium, potassium and selenium.

Current studies in the US are also finding that hyperactive children may not get good quality sleep. Snoring is one factor of deprivation, but there are many others as well (see Insomnia).

Restoring the Balance (Homeostasis)

Instead of prescribing Ritalin and other amphetamines to literally speed the adrenal glands to exhaustion (a very *un*natural therapy and experimental in its long-term effect), we must focus on causes; deal with those, so that one can get on with having a long, happy and healthy life. Merely treating the symptoms is not curative, as any long-term sufferer will tell you.

Based on the individual child, an individualized treatment plan which is reasonable, flexible, which addresses dietary factors, with supporting therapeutic supplementation of particular nutrients, along with botanical (herbal) and specific medicines to assist in bringing the body and mind back into harmony and health, can be devised by a competent naturopathic physician.

The treatment protocols we offer here aim to restore vitality to the immune system, calming and balancing the nervous and gastro-intestinal systems. Restoring the required nutrients to the body will result in restoring balance and affecting what can sometimes seem like a miraculous cure.

TREATMENT

Diet

The most obvious, and for many the most difficult change in diet must be the conversion to 100% organically grown, unrefined foods, with absolutely no additives, colorings, preservatives, pesticides, or any other chemical adulterations. This includes avoiding sugar, salt, most soy sauce, yeast, canned foods, frozen foods, most commercially baked goods, most restaurant foods, etc. You must be absolutely sure of the contents of every item consumed. This rarely is an easy process unless you happen to live in an area where organic foods are readily available, or can have your own garden. Unlike other conditions where organic foods are highly recommended, they are an absolute necessity in hyperactivity. Even a small amount of the offending chemicals can trigger an attack of behavioral problems lasting up to 5 days. If you only allow one minor slip every 5 days, and it happens to be the primary irritant, the child will experience a continuous reaction. In other words, no improvement will be seen.

Specific allergy tests may be very revealing. Unfortunately, no food or chemical allergy test is perfect and none has as yet been devised that tests for all types of allergic reactions. Still, the RAST, cytotoxic, and pulse tests should be used to find any specific factors that may be present. Don't be confused if one test shows a specific allergy and others do not confirm this. Each tests for a specific type of reaction and they often do not overlap.

The basic diet is similar to the hypoglycemia regimen with the exclusion of wheat, gluten grains (see Celiac Disease), dairy products, and yeast. These foods are so commonly dietary problems that they are eliminated routinely until all symptoms are gone. They may be carefully reintroduced later to see if a recurrence takes place. Use rice and oat cereal and breads. The first to be reintroduced is dairy foods in the form of goat's yoghurt. Next comes organically grown wheat in any unyeasted preparation. Last of all, yeast is tried.

It is important to reduce dietary intake of phosphate-containing foods such as meat and carbonated drinks, sodas, soft drinks, etc., as high phosphate levels when combined with low magnesium levels can precipitate hyperactivity.

A most important inclusion in the diet is flaxseed oil (See Appendix for recipe for AJ's Salad Dressing, or in a soy milk smoothie).

A hair analysis is performed to determine any excess heavy metal toxicities and to trace the source. A general heavy metal detoxification program is then instituted if significant levels are found (see Heavy Metal Poisoning).

Once the body has been normalized by proper diet and the child has returned to normal, it is essential to maintain the program for at least 6 months. At this time it is often possible to become more flexible with the diet, but any return to the old habits will certainly result in a return of the old behavioral patterns.

Physiotherapy

- Saunas: 1–2 times per week.
- Daily exercise: whatever the activity, it must induce sweating.
- Throw out your TV.
- Spinal manipulation: once per week.
- Massage: 1–2 times per week. Massage along spine with cocoa butter.

Therapeutic Agents

Vitamins and Minerals—Primary

- Zinc: 15–30 mg 2–3 times daily.
- Vitamin E: 400 IU daily, antioxidant (protective of possible GLA toxicity effects, where GLA is more than 20% of caloric intake).
- Vitamin B complex: 25–50 mg 2–3 times daily, plus intramuscular injection.
- Vitamin B3 (nicotinamide): from 300–1000 mg daily, or higher, until flushing occurs.
- Vitamin C and bioflavonoids (esp. quercetin): 1–6 g daily. Antistress, adaptogenic.
- Magnesium: to 2000 mg daily; calming,

- relaxing.
- Chromium: 200 mcg daily for glucose intolerance.
- Selenium: 200 mcg daily.

Vitamins and Minerals— Secondary
- Vitamin A: 10,000–25,000 IU 1–2 times daily.
- Vitamin B6: 100–400 mg daily.
- Pantothenic acid (B5): 200–500 mg daily.
- Vitamin B12.
- Calcium: 800–1500 mg daily.
- Folic acid.
- Trace minerals: e.g. Celtic salt.

Others—Primary
- Essential fatty acids: especially omega-3 (GLA—gamma-linoleic acid), specific in high doses, flaxseed oil (1 level tsp, 3 times daily); especially if excessive thirst.
- Adenosine: decreases brain damage.
- Atomidene: source of iodine (Cayce product).
- GABA (gamma-aminobutyric acid): 600 mg daily; tranquilizing.
- Histidine hydrochloride: promotes alpha wave activity, antistress; heavy metal chelator.

- Kelp: source of iodine.
- DL-phenylalanine: increases brain enkephalin, endorphin; improves gastric acid secretion.

Others—Secondary
Taurine, methionine, choline and tyrosine: lipotropes which assist in detoxification pathways in the liver.
Raw brain tablets.
Raw pancreas tablets.
Raw adrenal tablets.
Glutamine.
Evening primrose oil.
N,N-dimethylglycine.
Yeast.
L-cysteine: if heavy metal toxicity.

Botanicals—Primary
Passion flower.
Valerian.

Botanicals—Secondary
Lime flowers, hops, lobelia, skullcap, and zizyphus: nervine sedatives.
Chamomile.
Other herbs include the important adaptogenics, such as Panax and Siberian ginseng, gotu kola, schisandra, and withania.
See also Allergies and Food Intolerances.

HYPERTENSION

DEFINITION

Increased blood pressure that cannot be ascribed to a single cause. Average blood pressure is 120/80 for males and slightly lower for females. The 120 (systolic pressure) is the pressure in the arteries when the heart is in the middle of its contraction; the 80 (diastolic pressure) is the pressure in the arteries when the heart is at rest. A reading of 140/90 is considered suspicious. Higher readings are considered clinical hypertension. The diastolic is usually con-sidered the most important, as this is the pressure the arteries are under when at rest.

SYMPTOMS

Headache, dizziness, nervousness, irritabil-ity, energy loss, fatigue, insomnia, and inter-mittent increase in blood pressure, later becoming permanent. Late symptoms are hypertensive heart disease with enlarged heart and possible left ventricular failure, myocardial infarction, possible senility, cerebral hemorrhage, paralysis, and death.

ETIOLOGICAL CONSIDERATIONS

Although there are several factors that may raise blood pressure, such as increased cardiac output, an increase in the viscosity of the blood, or increased peripheral resistance, in most cases of hypertension we find that increased peripheral resistance is the primary cause, with little or no change in the other two factors. This increased peripheral resistance or narrowing of the blood vessels occurs chiefly in the arterioles (small arteries) and may be anatomical or functional. The initial cause may be vasoconstriction (narrowing), added to by stress or spinal lesions. This sets up a vicious cycle of narrowing and resultant hypertension, which in turn causes further vascular narrowing, etc. The renal arteries may play a key role in the process and seem to be the most sensitive to change due to increased blood pressure.

Another postulated cause of hypertension is narrowing of the blood vessels due to cholesterol and other fatty molecules. Research over the last thirty years implicates saturated fats, such as those found in red meat and butter, with their high cholesterol content. Many authorities, however, seriously question the high blood pressure/ heart disease/high cholesterol hypothesis. We feel the current hysteria over cholesterol is unfounded and misinterpreted, and the true causes of heart disease and high blood pressure has more to do with "unnatural" fats such as margarine and heat-modified oils than to any naturally occurring food fat or oil that has been consumed by our ancestors from the time of creation.

Some studies implicate the consumption of unsaturated oils in the causation of heart disease and high blood pressure. These studies do not, however, differentiate if it is the unsaturated oils themselves or the artificially processed unsaturated oils that may cause this effect. To our knowledge, no research has been done to differentiate the effects of refined unsaturated oils from the effects of unrefined cold pressed unsaturated oils. The refined oils are a questionable health risk since many changes occur in the natural oil as it is processed at high temperatures. Certainly, hydrogenated oils such as margarine are a definite risk factor. The fatty acids found in this preparation have been altered from the *cis* form to the entirely unnatural trans form, which has no known metabolic function. It also interferes with essential fatty acid metabolism. One of the known symptoms of essential fatty acid deficiency, in fact, is high blood pressure.

Cold-pressed unsaturated oils should retain their vitamin E content as well as their normal essential fatty acid content, which keeps them from going rancid. Both of these factors are essential for good health, and have been used therapeutically to help reverse and control high blood pressure. Further research on this is needed.

Drugs given to treat high blood pressure either reduce cardiac output, reduce peripheral resistance, or are diuretic in action to reduce total blood volume. The common approach is to begin with very mild diuretics and mild hypotensive drugs and increase the dose as required, or change to more powerful drugs when the milder ones are no longer effective. An important factor to understand here is that in most cases the progression from mild hypertensive drugs having few side effects to stronger hypotensive drugs having significant side effects is the rule, rather than the exception. In practice, we frequently see the situation where a person has been treated for hypertension with drugs that have lost their effectiveness. These patients have been lulled into a false sense of security, feeling that their blood pressure is under control with diuretics and other drugs, only to find on examination a reading of 160/100 or even 110! On questioning, this was the very figure that had prompted drug therapy in the first place, several years before.

The most revealing and upsetting fact of all is that in our experience over 85% of all cases of high blood pressure are both treatable and preventable *without* drugs and most physicians know it. The problem is that both the prevention and treatment of hypertension require lifestyle changes which are both difficult and time-consuming to accomplish.

The evidence supporting lifestyle causes of hypertension is readily available. Certainly, excess weight is a known factor, as is excess consumption of animal fats (vegetarians have long been known to have both lower blood pressures and less incidence of hypertension, but then vegetarians eat a whole lot more whole grains, seeds and nuts, and vegetables than most meat eaters usually consume), fiber deficiency due to consumption of excess refined carbohydrates, stress, lack of demanding exercise, and excess refined salt intake. The common argument from physicians is that patients are simply unwilling to change. They show as evidence that even if patients are told to cut out salt, increase their exercise, and lose weight, very few ever do more than reduce their salt intake without making other lifestyle changes. We concede that many patients are unwilling or incapable of change; however, from experience We have found a growing number who are ready for change, and most willing to do so if educated properly.

It is true that this education process takes considerable time and effort on the part of both doctor and patient, but rewards are high. The end result is a patient carefully weaned off high blood pressure medication and nearly ecstatic with a feeling of self-control of his or her health; and a physician satisfied that yet another human being has begun to understand the true causes of high blood pressure.

TREATMENT

The first and most important stage of treatment begins by exploring in detail with the patient all the common causes of hypertension, and showing which of these factors relate to the patient's condition.

Diet

In most cases diet remains the single most important factor in the causation of high blood pressure. The ordinary western diet of fried eggs, white toast, bacon, and fried potatoes for breakfast, a meat sandwich for lunch, and meat again for supper (all usually highly salted), not to mention excess dairy products (saturated fats again), coffee, sugar, tobacco, and alcohol, is a prescription for physical disease, especially high blood pressure. (*Note:* There is no one aspect of the western diet that causes high blood pressure, but rather the multitude of improper foods and eating habits.)

We find the best procedure is to have the patient make a list for 3 days of every bit of food, solid or liquid, that enters his or her mouth. We can then gently and carefully analyze the diet in the light of a few clinical facts. The first is that most people who are overweight and have hypertension can usually lower their blood pressure significantly simply by losing weight. The other is that it has been shown over and over that most people with hypertension can lower their blood pressure by eating less meat and more vegetables. In fact, the most effective way to lower blood pressure safely, rapidly, and permanently, is an entirely vegetarian diet.

Obviously, not all people are able or willing to become totally vegetarian. This is where the skill of the physician comes into play. It is the physician's job whenever possible to convince the patient that a regimen of total vegetarianism for from 3-6 months is in his or her best health interests, and that such a diet can and should be not only bearable, but enjoyable. Once blood pressure is under control, moderate meat eating, especially fish and fowl, can once again be resumed, but this is by no means suggested. A diet based on mostly whole grains, with a large proportion of fresh vegetables, can allow some saturated fat in the form of animal products and still maintain a healthy blood pressure, especially with adequate exercise in the regimen. It is just until proper cardiovascular health has been re-established that an all-vegetarian diet is essential, especially in cases of severe or long-standing high blood pressure.

It is essential for the physician to keep firmly in mind the type of diet optimally beneficial, tempering this with what the patient can achieve. It is, however, important not to be so lenient that results are not achieved. We find the best approach is a period of 4–8 weeks of a very strict whole food vegetarian diet, so that both patient and physician can see a true change. This encourages both and makes the long road ahead more achievable.

Below you will find a sample diet regimen for high blood pressure. There is nothing magical about the diet. All that is being stressed is a diet composed of a very large proportion of raw and cooked vegetables, fresh fruits, whole grains, and vegetarian proteins. Refined salt is restricted totally from the diet. This one change alone will help reduce the average blood pressure considerably. Use only an unrefined sea salt such as Celtic salt, as a multimineral. The early stages restrict carbohydrates for weight reduction, if needed; and also protein to achieve a true elimination effect. Brief fasting periods are very useful for rapid blood pressure reductions and then finally eliminating the last of the blood pressure drugs. These diets are alternated as deemed suitable by the physician and are followed by a good general diet, either vegetarian or including light meat-eating (fish or poultry), with plenty of fruit, vegetables, and unrefined whole grains.

High Blood Pressure Diet Regimen

Stage 1:
On Rising
A glass of red grape juice or other fruit juice.

Breakfast Day 1
Any ripe fresh fruit (e.g. apples, grapes, grapefruit, pears, papaya, mango, etc.), excluding bananas.

Breakfast Day 2
Fresh fruit (with or without goat's yoghurt) or stewed fruit or baked apple with a little honey or malt if desired. Wheat germ and soybean lecithin granules are desirable and may be added.

Midmorning
Vegetable juice such as carrot, or carrot and other juices, mixed.

Lunch
A large, varied raw salad with plenty of green vegetables such as lettuce, onions, cabbage, green peppers, parsley, celery, carrots, and a few walnuts or other nuts or nutmeats (excluding peanuts); fresh fruit for dessert if desired.

Midafternoon
As midmorning.

Supper Day 1
Same as lunch.

Supper Day 2
Steamed green leafy vegetables and root vegetables (other than potatoes, including onions, always). Fresh fruit for dessert, if desired.

On Retiring
Same as midmorning.

Drinks
Grape juice, apple juice, spring water, or dandelion coffee between meals when thirsty; drink moderately.

If you are taking any drugs prescribed by a doctor for your condition, you must not on any account stop taking them when you begin this diet. As you progress with the dietetic treatment and your health improves, the dosage may gradually be decreased, but only with the consent of your doctor.

Stage 2:
One of the following:

- Three-day fast on fruit juice (one glass at 4-hour intervals sipped slowly). Grapefruit or apple juice is recommended; however, most fruit juices will do fine. Make sure never to mix juices at any given meal. It is best to restrict oneself to one juice type daily.
- Four-day mono diet of grapes and grape juice. Eat 4–8 oz (125–250 g) of red grapes at 4-hour intervals, with red grape juice to drink when thirsty, between meals.
- Four-day apple mono diet of apples and apple juice.

Stage 3:

On Rising
A glass of red grape juice or other fruit juice.

Breakfast Day 1
Any fresh or stewed fruit with lecithin granules, wheat germ, and a little honey if desired.

Breakfast Day 2
Plain yoghurt (goat's, if possible) with fresh or stewed fruit, lecithin granules, wheat germ, and a little honey if desired.

Midmorning
Vegetable juice.

Lunch
A large, varied raw salad with nuts and 1–2 crispbreads with nut spread, or cottage cheese. Fresh fruit for dessert (especially grapes) if desired.

Supper
Any vegetarian meal (though restricting eggs or cheese to twice per week each. These foods are not encouraged due to their high fat content). Tofu, soybeans, and whole grains or brown rice and buckwheat are especially beneficial. A baked potato may be eaten (including the skin) and two other vegetables. A fresh or stewed apple with soaked and simmered raisins and a little honey for dessert, if desired.

Drinks
Grape juice, apple juice, vegetable juices, dandelion coffee, or herb teas when thirsty, and in moderation.

General Considerations

- No refined salt Use Celtic or another unrefined sea salt sparingly.
- Eat smaller meals than usual and get as much rest from stress as possible.
- No alcohol, coffee, or tea, and no smoking. No licorice.
- Foods especially useful are buckwheat, onions, garlic, brewer's yeast, miso, wheat germ, lecithin granules, soybeans, tofu, the pulp of citrus fruits (inside of skin and outside of fruit), parsley.

Other specialized diets useful in some cases are: brown rice diet; lemon juice fast; vegetable juice fast; fresh juice fast.

In addition to the dietary regimen, certain foods, food supplements, and herbs are useful in speeding up the process.

Exercise

Lack of demanding exercise usually associated with a sedentary occupation is a second major factor in causing hypertension. A person needs a minimum of 12–20 minutes daily of the type of exercise that leaves you breathless. This helps clear artery walls of adhering fatty molecules and prevents narrowing of blood vessels. Obviously, a person who already has hypertension needs careful supervision in increasing his or her daily exercise safely until this minimum has been reached. Any type of exercise is acceptable but it must be done regularly.

Relaxation Exercises or Meditation

Stress is considered a major factor in some cases of hypertension. For patients with tension problems, it is useless to simply say "avoid stress". Usually these people will be overstressed under any circumstances, showing a basic tendency of character

303

rather than a simple reaction to a single life situation. For these people progressive relaxation exercises or meditation will be essential. We usually advise patients to find a class of this type that appeals to them and then practice consistently twice daily. The type of exercise or meditation is of little matter, as long as the result leads to physical relaxation, and hopefully better self-awareness. One very useful relaxation exercise is called the "draining exercise". This was given to us by a very special man who really knew how to relax to the very foundation of his soul.

Sit in a comfortable chair with eyes closed and take a few deep breaths, relaxing as much as possible. Quiet your mind and feelings to the best of your ability and let yourself go, once again to the best of your present ability. Next, imagine that you are filled with tension in a *liquid* form, from the top of your head to the tips of your fingers and toes. Further imagine that your body is like a bathtub filled with this liquid tension, and that all 10 fingertips and toe tips are the plugs where this liquid may be drained away. In your imagination pull these plugs from the fingers and toes and let this fluid tension drain out of your body. First, draw your attention to your scalp and head and visualize and feel this liquid tension lowering out of your scalp into your face and neck. As it passes out of your head feel the muscles of your face relax. At the same time you are aware of a constant draining away of tension out of your fingers and toes. Next, feel the tension lowering into your neck and shoulders and into your upper arms and chest. You will begin to notice your breathing becoming more relaxed and regular as the tension drains through your solar plexus and down into your elbows and lower arms. Next, feel this liquid tension flow into your wrist and hands, as well as your abdomen and lower back. As the liquid drains further into your hands and fingers, feel the tingling as it escapes from your body out of the fingertips.

Continue to allow this tension to flow constantly out of the fingers as it continues to drain into your lower abdomen and pelvic region, deep into your sexual organs, and then down to the thighs. Next, it flows to the knees and calves and on into the ankles. Feel the tingling sensation as this liquid tension drains into the feet and out your toes. Maintain this sensation of feeling the liquid tension now draining out of both your fingers and toes for 3-5 minutes, or longer. Then take 3-4 deep, relaxing, cleansing breaths. The object is that with each of these cleansing breaths, you take in new, pure energy to replace the old tension energy you have just drained away.

At this time, if you are a religious person, be open to prayer and let yourself be filled with that grace that may now flow into your empty, open vessel. If not of such a temperament, many other avenues are open that will help unlock your feelings. One technique is to visualize some real or imagined scene of beauty, trying actually to feel the refreshing air on your face, or smell the sea breeze or flowers. In time you will be able to retreat into this peaceful scene and learn to find rest and relaxation.

If you do this "draining exercise" twice daily, early in the morning and before bed, you will soon find that this peace and relaxation becomes a part of you. At first you may find it difficult to let your mind go, or your feelings. Do not criticize yourself for this but gently redirect your mind to the draining exercise each time it wanders. Your reward for perseverance will be an entirely new approach to life, filled with the freedom and joy of a child's. And more to the point, it will lower your blood pressure.

Physiotherapy

Hot showers or baths are discontinued and replaced by warm showers, alternating with cool showers. These alternating warm and cool showers should be 3 minutes each, repeated 2-3 times. Later, as the cardiovascular system strengthens, the temperatures may be more extreme, with hot and ice-cold water being used. This should be followed by drying with a rough towel to redden the skin, thereby increasing superficial circulation.

Therapeutic Agents

Vitamins and Minerals—Primary

- Vitamin B complex: 50 mg 3 times daily, with niacin/niacinamide (100–400 mg 1–2 times daily). Lowers blood pressure.
- Vitamin B6: 50–100 mg daily. Diuretic.
- Vitamin C complex (with bioflavonoids): 2000 mg 3 times daily.
- Vitamin E: begin with 100 IU twice daily and increase slowly over 1–2 weeks to 400 IU twice daily. In some cases 1200 IU daily is required. A rapid increase in vitamin E intake has been known to raise some blood pressures while a slower increase will lower them.
- Magnesium: 400–2000 mg daily. A vasodilator, and calcium channel regulator. More may be required if on diuretics (diuretics can cause urinary magnesium excretion leading to hypomagnesemia).
- Calcium (orotate, aspartate, citrate): 800–1200 mg (can be up to 3 g) daily.
- Manganese.

Vitamins and Minerals—Secondary

- Selenium: 200 mcg daily. Antioxidant.

Others—Primary

- Garlic: 2 capsules 3 times daily. Lowers blood pressure.
- Coenzyme Q10: 90–240 mg daily. A potent aid in reducing blood pressure.
- Essential fatty acids: GLA (gamma-linoleic acid). Flaxseed oil.
- Tyrosine: works via the CNS to regulate blood pressure amphoterically (up or down depending on needs)
- Taurine: 50–100 mg per kilogram of body weight in three divided doses daily (2 g daily). A hypotensive.
- L-Carnitine, L-glutamine and L-glutamic acid: 500 mg of each; to detoxify ammonia, and transport long chain fatty acids.
- Lipoic acid: antioxidant, hypotensive.
- Japanese 3-mushrooms (maitake, shiitake, reishi): reduces high blood pressure.
- Proteolytic enzymes, bromelain: between meals. Improves protein digestion, cleans circulatory system.

Others—Secondary

- Chlorophyll, barley green, wheat grass, Spirulina: 6–8 glasses daily.
- Lecithin: 1–2 tbsp 3 times daily. Lowers blood pressure, emulsifies fats.
- Rutin: 2 tablets with meals.
- Histidine hydrochloride: 200 mg, 3 times daily. Anti-stress.
- Wheat germ oil: natural source of vitamin E
- Kelp: diuretic.
- Apple pectin: helps reduce blood pressure.

Botanicals—Primary

Systemic vasodilators: hawthorn, yarrow, coleus, lime flowers.

Hypotensive vasodilators: mistletoe, garlic, olive, *Scutellaria baicalensis*, astragalus, valerian

Portal hypotensives: globe artichoke, fringe tree.

Botanicals—Secondary

Cayenne.

Fennel.

Foxglove: for congestive heart failure.

Garlic.

Hawthorn berries: cardiac depressant, hypotensive; helps dissolve deposits on arteries.

Indian snakeroot: hypotensive, contains reserpine. May cause severe depression. Take only under medical supervision.

Lime flowers: for arteriosclerotic hypertension.

Rosemary.

Watercress.

Green hellebore: very poisonous. Take only

under medical supervision. 2–10 drops to lower blood pressure and pulse rate. See also Heart Disease.

Therapeutic Suggestion

Reduction of drug therapy must be done slowly and safely. Medical supervision is recommended. We usually advise 6–12 weeks of strict application of all therapeutic suggestions before reducing drugs. At this point, if we are convinced that the patient has been applying the therapies correctly,

we cut drug medication in half and put the patient on a 3 day strict juice fast of either citrus juices, vegetable juices, or grape juice. This further lowers the blood pressure.

After several more weeks medication may again be cut in half while the patient fasts, then the drugs are taken on alternate days for a week or two before stopping entirely, again during a short fast.

Botanical medication to lower high blood pressure should be used only until the rest of the naturopathic program has had a chance to reverse the cause (refer also to Heart Disease).

HYPOGLYCEMIA AND HYPERINSULINISM

DEFINITION

A defect of carbohydrate metabolism where the blood glucose level (BGL, also referred to as BSL—blood sugar level) reaches levels lower than normal. In some cases, symptoms are better associated with elevated insulin levels.

SYMPTOMS

Nervousness, irritability, emotional problems, fatigue, depression, craving for sweets, inability to concentrate, cold sweating, shakes, palpitations, tingling of skin and scalp, dizziness, trembling, fainting, blurred vision, cold extremities, nausea, midmorning tiredness and mid-to-late-afternoon tiredness, anxiety, indecisiveness, crying spells, allergies, convulsions, hyperactivity. Symptoms are mostly episodic, being related to the time and content of the previous meal, and are usually improved by eating.

ETIOLOGICAL CONSIDERATIONS—PRIMARY

- Refined carbohydrates (e.g. excess sugar, candy, fruit juice, vegetable juice, dried fruit, or refined grains) leading to carbohydrate sensitivity and excess insulin production.
- Adrenal exhaustion: may be primary or secondary due to diet or stress.
- Stress: depletes vitamin B complex, vitamin C, and adrenals.
- Excess coffee and/or nicotine.

ETIOLOGICAL CONSIDERATIONS— SECONDARY

Sucrose sensitivity; systemic candidiasis; immune deficiency; large meals; alcoholism; pregnancy; liver damage; thyroid disorders; pancreatitis, pancreatic tumor; pituitary insufficiency: kidney disease

DISCUSSION

Hypoglycemia is probably one of the most widespread disorders in civilized nations today. It is not a disease as such but a symptom that may result from a wide range of hormonal abnormalities reflecting irregular function of many glands and organs. Unfortunately, it often goes undiagnosed and its multitude of symptoms are frequently labeled as emotional or psychological in origin.

To understand hypoglycemia a little physiological background is essential. The body needs a steady supply of readily available energy to function. It derives this energy from food primarily in the form of carbohydrates which are converted, in the process of digestion, into their simplest common denominator, glucose. Glucose is essential for all bodily activity, and is especially necessary for the function of the nervous system and brain, which responds drastically to abnormal variations of the BGL/BSL.

Normally the BGL/BSL is kept within a very narrow range of variation by various hormones which respond rapidly to even slight changes. Insulin from the pancreas is released when glucose enters the blood from digested food. This lowers the BGL/BSL to the normal range. The sugar is then stored in the liver and muscles in the form of glycogen, or converted to fat for later use. Cortisol and growth hormone counterbalance this insulin action. If any of these hormones are secreted too rapidly or too slowly an imbalance of the BGL/BSL can occur.

If the blood glucose level rises above normal, or if glucose is delivered to the blood too rapidly, as it is following a meal of simple refined carbohydrates, the body deals with this excess in two ways. It initiates a sudden burst of insulin to counteract what the body perceives as a very dangerous imbalance. It also begins to convert the excess glucose in certain "glucose-insensitive cells" found in the eye, kidney, myelinated nerves, and red blood cells, first into fructose and then sorbitol. This is important since both fructose and sorbitol are relatively insoluble within the cell and tend to crystallize out, leading to cataract formation in the eye, basement membrane thickening in the kidney, damage to nerves, and altered oxygen-carrying capacity in red blood cells. This sorbitol pathway is initiated each time the blood glucose levels rise rapidly on the glucose rollercoaster ride that hypoglycemics travel daily.

In some cases of hypoglycemia insulin is often secreted in excess and thus lowers the BGL/BSL too far and too rapidly. This is what is often called hyperinsulinism. In functional hypoglycemia the insulin response may be normal, but the insulin antagonism may be out of balance, once again leading to a low BGL/BSL. The most commonly involved glands are the adrenal glands. Most commonly, both the pancreas and adrenal glands are malfunctioning. The liver is also usually involved in this imbalance. Some cases of hyperinsulinism show normal insulin levels but a reduced sensitivity to insulin. This results in a prediabetes type of glucose metabolism where sugar levels remain elevated for a prolonged period and then fall rapidly below normal.

The causes of the endocrine imbalances of hypoglycemia are usually easy to find in civilized nations. The two most significant factors are diet and stress. The average American diet is literally a prescription for hypoglycemia, with its common foods such as white bread, sugar, soda, and coffee. Sugar and refined carbohydrates are absorbed very rapidly into the bloodstream since they require little digestion due to the stripping of their protein and fiber in the refining process. This rapid increase in the BGL/BSL causes the pancreas to become hypersensitive to sugar. In time the pancreas learns to secrete very large amounts of insulin in response to a rise in BGL/BSL. This causes a rapid lowering of the BGL/BSL, in this case far lower than normal. During this low period the symptoms of hypoglycemia become manifest. This is primarily due to a deficiency of glucose supply to the brain and the resulting adrenal "shock" response.

The adrenal glands recognize the low sugar level as an acute danger and institute an appropriate response. In time the adrenal glands become overstressed by these recurrent emergencies and lose their ability to cope adequately with the situation.

Most people fail to recognize that excess table sugar is not the only "refined carbohydrate" that may cause this disinsulinism leading to hypoglycemia. Excess honey, fruit, fruit juice, dried fruit, or even vegetable juice will cause a rapid rise in blood glucose levels, causing pancreatic hypersensitivity.

Stress also plays a major role via the adrenals since stress also is recognized by the adrenals as an emergency situation and triggers similar responses, thus once again overburdening the adrenals. To further aggravate the complexity of the situation, you should also understand that stress depletes vitamin B complex and vitamin C, both of which are necessary for proper adrenal function, in addition to which vitamin B complex is an essential nutrient in the metabolism of carbohydrates. In turn, the carbohydrates have *already* been stripped of vitamin B complex in the refining process and therefore need extra vitamin B complex for utilization! And we are not off the merry-go-round yet! Coffee stimulates the adrenal glands, which act to mobilize the body's energy reserves in both the liver and muscles. This removes the body's fail-safe mechanism to further keep the BGL/BSL in balance, and further abuses the adrenal glands.

The importance of the diagnosis and proper treatment of hypoglycemia should not be underestimated. In the past, and even to some practitioners presently, hypoglycemia has been considered a non-disease. Some doctors claim that the label "hypoglycemia" is too often used for any emotional problem that enters the practitioner's office. Hypoglycemia can be diagnosed clinically using the 5-hour blood glucose tolerance test. Some cases show normal blood glucose levels but elevated insulin levels, which are associated with hypoglycemic symptoms.

Recent medical research has supported the view that the effects of even mild hypoglycemia may be far-reaching. Hypoglycemia has now been clearly associated with a significant proportion of physical, mental, and emotional disorders including hyperactivity, schizophrenia, antisocial behavior, criminal personalities, drug addiction, impotency, alcoholism, epilepsy, asthma, allergies, ulcers, and arthritis.

As much attention should be placed on preventing and treating hypoglycemia as has been the case with diabetes. These two disorders are often manifestations of a similar endocrine imbalance, due to the same causes.

Back in the 1960s the seriousness of hypoglycemia was often dismissed. Often a physician, upon discovering hypoglycemia, would recommend a candy bar whenever the patient felt weak. This caused a rapid rise in blood sugar which later resulted in an even more precipitous drop. This "candy bar" therapy for hypoglycemia was clearly a case of a short-term solution that ultimately caused the problem it was meant to solve.

The only effective treatment is the removal of the initial causes and the re-establishment of normal hormonal controlling mechanisms. Unfortunately, once the pancreas has been hypersensitive to sugar over a long period of time, complete recovery is not always possible. In experiments with rats that were fed refined carbohydrates until clinical hypoglycemia developed, it was found that the hypoglycemia could be corrected and kept under control with a change in diet, but once the old diet was reverted to, the hypoglycemia returned fairly rapidly.

Obviously, the longer a person has hypoglycemia and the more severe the condition, the less probable is a complete cure. All that can be expected in these cases is that with a change in lifestyle and diet, no hypoglycemic symptoms will be present. These people, however, do remain hypersensitive to sugar and can react with hypoglycemic symptoms should they revert to their old diet and stress patterns.

TREATMENT

Diet

The body is very similar in its proper energy needs to a good wood-burning stove—with a supply of high-fiber fuel, it will burn evenly and at the right consumption rate. If, however, the body is supplied with refined carbohydrates stripped of both fiber and protein, the situation becomes similar to paper burning in the stove at a very high heat for a very short period of time.

The traditional low-carbohydrate diet, or high-protein diet, so often advised for hypoglycemia, is not the answer. What is needed is a high-fiber carbohydrate diet with adequate protein. Instead of three large meals daily, the diet should consist of grazing—having six smaller meals, or three smaller meals and three snacks between meals. The basic concept of the diet is that all foods should be unrefined and slow to digest.

Dried fruit, fruit, fruit juices, and vegetable juice are all considered rapidly absorbable and should be consumed in moderation. When fruit is eaten, it should be taken with some protein such as a handful of nuts, cottage cheese, or yoghurt. Fruit juice, if taken at all, should be diluted 80% with water, taken in small quantities, preferably near the time other food is eaten. The rest of the diet is composed of vegetables, whole grains, and protein.

The following diet is an example of the type used in this condition. Choose from the following suggestions:

Breakfast
1. Granola (unsweetened).
2. Cooked whole grain cereal, especially oatmeal.
3. 1-2 soft-boiled or poached eggs, 1-2 slices whole grain bread. Yoghurt, plus wheat germ and brewer's yeast for dessert, if desired.
4. Yoghurt and wheat germ, kefir, acidophilus milk, buttermilk, or raw unpasteurized cow's or goat's milk. Add brewer's yeast if possible.

5. Fresh fruit with yoghurt and wheat germ (if wheat is tolerated). Sweet fruits are to be eaten only rarely and in moderation. Grapes are too sweet for this diet. Recommended fruits are papaya, apple, grapefruit, orange, bananas or fresh berries. Nuts may be added. $\frac{1}{2}$ tsp honey may be used if desired, but no more.

Midmorning
Choose from:
1. Almond milk: 12 almonds blended with water, a little juice, brewer's yeast, and lecithin.
2. Unsweetened herb tea.
3. $\frac{1}{4}$-$\frac{1}{3}$ handful raw nuts and seeds (almond, brazil, hazel, sunflower, etc.).
4. Whole grain crackers, biscuit, bread, or other source of unrefined carbohydrate.
5. 1 tsp Spirulina in warm water.

Lunch
Fresh raw salad, always as the main part of the meal. Use AJ's Salad Dressing (see Appendix I); or olive oil and lemon and herb dressing, avocado dressing, or yoghurt dressing on salad, or other non-sweetened natural dressing. Then choose from:
- 1 slice 100% wholemeal bread and cottage cheese or other protein.
- $\frac{1}{3}$ avocado plus lemon.
- Whole grain brown rice, millet, or buckwheat.
- A little cheese (white cheese is to be preferred).
- Fish, fowl, or lean meat.
- 100% whole meal sandwich.
- Dessert: if desired, a little yoghurt plus wheat germ and brewer's yeast.

Midafternoon
As midmorning.

Supper
Choose from:
- 2-3 cooked (never boiled or fried) vegetables
- Whole grain (rice, millet, buckwheat, etc.).

- A vegetarian savory meal with cheese, eggs, or vegetarian protein.
- Lean meat or fowl 2-3 times per week only.
- Fish.
- 100% whole meal bread with butter or cottage cheese.
- Baked potato (be sure to eat skin).

Evening
1. Raw goat's milk, cow's milk, or kefir drink, with ½ tbsp brewer's yeast; nuts may be added in a blender.
2. Almond milk.
3. 100% whole grain snacks.

Desserts:
1. Yoghurt and wheat germ plus brewer's yeast if desired
2. Fresh fruit, especially papaya.

If hungry at any time your best choice is a slow-burning fuel food made of 100% carbohydrate sources.

Never Eat
- Sugar (white or brown) or anything that contains sugar. Honey is permitted only in absolute moderation (1 tsp daily) and best avoided altogether when possible.
- White flour and its products.
- Refined grains, rice, macaroni, etc. Use whole grains, whole wheat macaroni, etc., instead.

Very Important to Avoid
- Alcohol.
- Coffee.
- Smoking.
- Dried fruits, dates, figs, plums, grapes. Eat bananas in moderation only.

Foods of Special Usefulness
Whole grains (especially oats and oat flour); nuts; raw milk products (if no sign of allergy exists); soy milk; avocado; brewer's yeast; Jerusalem artichokes

Note: When eating fruit, eat in moderation and slowly. Always eat with some protein. When drinking fruit or vegetable juices, drink no more than 3 fl oz (90 mL) at a time. It may be best to avoid juices altogether. Eat only when relaxed. Avoid stress whenever possible.

Therapeutic Agents

Vitamins and Minerals—Primary
- Vitamin B complex: 50 mg 3 times daily. Aids digestion and absorption.
- Vitamin B3 (niacinamide): very useful for nervous hypoglycemics, stress-induced hypoglycemia, or adrenal exhaustion cases. 500 mg time-release capsules, 2-3 times daily, can be as effective as valium for these patients. If nausea occurs, reduce dose. (Hepatitis has been reported to occur at very high doses of vitamin B3 intake in susceptible subjects. Nausea is an early warning sign and should be heeded).
- Vitamin C: 500-1000 mg 3-4 times daily.
- Vitamin E: 400 IU daily.
- GTF: (glucose tolerance factor composed of chromium, nicotinic acid, and glutamic acid). This is essential for carbohydrate metabolism. GTF is essential for proper insulin function. (GTF is found in yeast or separately in pill form.) 1 tsp brewer's yeast 3 times daily.
- Vitamin B6 helps improve beta cell function.
- Chromium piccolinate: dose depends on type and amount of brewer's yeast (GTF) also being taken. 200 mcg daily is the usual dose, can be up to 600 mcg.
- Zinc: important in all enzyme systems, including insulin production.

Others—Primary
- Digestive enzymes: with meals.
- Probiotics.
- Psyllium powder: 1 tsp 2-3 times daily. Fiber helps regulate absorption of carbohydrate from the intestine.

Others—Secondary
- Spirulina: 1 tsp 3 times daily.

- Lecithin: 1 tsp 3 times daily (a good source of choline).
- Lipoic acid.
- Raw adrenal: 1 tablet 1–3 times daily.
- Raw pancreas: 1–2 tablets 2–3 times daily.

Botanicals—Primary

Gymnema: potentiates insulin response.
Goat's rue: potentiates insulin response.
Bilberry: hypoglycemic herb containing flavonoids
Wild yam.

Botanicals—Secondary

Hypoglycemic agents are found in: jambul, fringe tree, fenugreek, Panax ginseng.
Adrenal adaptogens and tonic herbs: useful in this condition, and include licorice, rehmannia, withania, Siberian ginseng, oats, schisandra.
Hepatics and cholagogues are used to assist liver function as well, such as: fringe tree, St Mary's thistle.

IMMUNE DEFICIENCY

DISCUSSION

The immune defense system is designed to protect against infection. Its actions are mediated by antibodies (immunoglobulins) and the cells of the lymphocytic system (cellular immunity). A deficiency, either genetic or acquired, of either system will increase susceptibility to infections in general and some diseases. Since the discovery of the first immune deficiency disease in the early 1950s, over 20 distinct types have been reported, most of which are hereditary. The immune system, however, is very susceptible to acquired malfunction from a number of directions. One very controversial cause of immune malfunction is the procedure of vaccinations against common childhood and epidemic diseases. The thymus gland seems to be the site most severely affected, altering the function and activity of this all-important kingpin of the immune system.

While severe infectious diseases may be the result of immune deficiencies, they may also be the preceding cause. For example, it is common for allergies, a frequent result of immune malfunction, to follow a severe case of mononucleosis, hepatitis, rheumatic fever, candidiasis, or other acute viral or bacterial disease that may reduce the production by the thymus gland of T-helper cells necessary to moderate the allergic response. Toxic exposure to chemicals or radiation may have similar results.

Another common source of immune deficiencies is single or multiple nutritional deficiencies. The immune system can only be as healthy as its organized cells and tissues. Various nutritional deficiencies have been associated with immune malfunction. Nutritional deficiency may be simply the lack of nutrient intake, or poor digestive and absorption processes.

Stress, pharmaceutical drugs (chemotherapy, including antibiotic usage), undiagnosed or untreated allergy, environmental pollutants, and poor hygiene can all contribute to a weakened immune system.

As the immune system becomes weakened, the body becomes susceptible to any opportunistic virus or bacteria that can take hold with sometimes devastating results. Literally any infectious disease may be considered an immune deficiency. If the immune system is functioning adequately, no such infection could take place. This includes the range of infectious diseases from colds to pneumonia, or diseases of unknown origin such as multiple sclerosis, multiple dystrophy, and AIDS.

AIDS (Acquired Immune Deficiency Syndrome)

AIDS is not a particular disease, but is a term used to describe various possible manifestations of disease that can occur when the human immune system breaks down. Long before the HIV virus was discovered, many different AIDS scenarios were documented, including Kaposi's sarcoma, pneumocystis carinii pneumonia, meningitis, TB; in fact about 27 conditions in all.

The HIV-AIDS theory states that a deadly virus, and a virus alone, called the human immunodeficiency virus (HIV) causes the immune systems of people infected with it to become weak, as the virus somehow kills off particular agents of the immune system (e.g. a particular subset of white blood cells called T4 helper cells, CD4), over a period of time to the point of immune system collapse, and the patient succumbs to rampant infection and usually ends up dying.

From about the time of the development of Robert Gallo's first HIV-AIDS model in 1984, there has been a growing body of dissidents, eminent scientists starting with Professor Peter Duesberg, molecular biologist and retrovirus researcher, to whose voice literally thousands of scientists and AIDS researchers today have been added, which has challenged initial assumptions as well as the evolving HIV-AIDS model as it is today.

From a philosophical viewpoint, the HIV-AIDS model is not holistic enough. It has yet to be proven that any disease can be caused solely by the mere presence of a virus. A seed will only grow and flourish when the environment is right for it—fertile soil, water, sunshine, fresh air, etc. Otherwise it will see out its days quiescent, latent, or the birds of the field will pick it up. It's the same with bugs and viruses. Naturopaths have always recognized this basic fact of health and disease. These so-called "pathogenic" viruses and bacteria are constantly present in the external environment and within our bodies. It is only when our bodies defenses are overloaded or artificially breached that they may gain a foothold to cause "disease". Many healthy, symptom-free people have tested positive to HIV for as long as the virus has been hypothesized.

It may well be that HIV is simply a new virus discovered "opportunistically" at a time that an explanation of AIDS diagnoses were trying to be understood in select groups of gay men. Maybe this newly discovered virus is a two bit player, maybe simply an innocent bystander who gets a little excited at the party, and not a villain after all. Science still cannot tell us. After all, in what way does AIDS-dementia or AIDS-PCP or HIV enteropathy differ from non-AIDS dementia, non-AIDS PCP or non-HIV enteropathy, except for the presence of HIV? A classic case, and there are lots more, of circular reasoning, implicit in the HIV-AIDS model.

Epidemiological studies tend to favor factors other than viral that cause immune suppression as the causes of AIDS. In 1990, Professor Robert Roote-Bernstein stated "AIDS will only be understood when we begin to explore the ways in which anal sex, infections and antibiotics, drugs, blood products, anesthetics and malnutrition interact. All of these agents had been demonstrated to be immunosuppressive prior to the discovery of HIV, and all are highly associated with one or more AIDS risk groups: immunological response to semen following anal intercourse (semen in the blood is a highly toxic substance); the use of recreational drugs such as nitrites ("poppers", "snappers", etc.), chronic antibiotic use (often associated with promiscuity), opiate drugs, multiple transfusions, anesthetics, malnutrition (whether caused by "gay bowel syndrome", drug use, poverty or anorexia), multiple concurrent infections by diverse microbes, and infection by specific viruses such as CMV, EBV, hep-B, all of which are as highly associated with AIDS as is HIV. Several of these agents including CMV, hep-B, opiate drugs and repeated blood transfusions are known to cause the same sort of T-cell abnormalities that are found in AIDS and which are usually attributed perhaps inaccurately to HIV infection".

At the 2000 AIDS world congress in Durban, South Africa the South African president caused a stir at the opening of the conference, by basically standing up alongside these dissidents and saying he doesn't think HIV is the major problem confronting the people of Africa, and there are other primary contributors to the AIDS epidemic such as poverty and crop failures leading to malnutrition, anal sexual practice and personal hygiene, inadequate housing and sanitation, and the effects of war, all are potential factors which create "the milieu", the fertile soil of immune deficiency in so many Africans today. When these factors have been addressed in the west, morbidity and mortality rates from AIDS have started to decline, as indeed these were the factors which have led to the decline in infectious diseases generally.

The cocktail of drugs often prescribed, which can include antibiotics such as bensathine penicillin, themselves quite toxic, contributes to erosion of the bowel flora populations and further predispose to the autointoxication associated with leaky gut, with consequent further immune dysregulation and suppression. Leaky gut may well be a primary etiologic event in the development of AIDS, as well as other immune deficiency conditions.

TREATMENT

Prevention is important, and maintaining a healthy lifestyle is fundamental in any disease prevention strategy. "Safe sex" practices properly understood and practiced help ensure one is not at risk of any sexually transmissible disease.

A basic tenet of naturopathy is, that given the right opportunities, and the right help, the body can heal itself. With any classification of immune system dysfunction, the goal of treatment must be to boost the immune system naturally, and this includes all the lifestyle markers of good immunity, the "Seven Doctors", which are fresh air, sunshine, clean water, clean fresh raw foods, exercise, rest, and a happy heart. One must avoid those things which predispose towards disease, and ensure the body has enough nutrient for self-healing. Dietary and nutritional advice must form the basis of any protocol to regain health. Special assistance can be sought from the more traditional vitamin, mineral and botanical supplements, as well as a whole host of newer ones.

Each case of immune deficiency has to be considered individually. Classic forms of immune deficiency might need to be treated by an immunologist. There are naturopathic physicians specializing in treating AIDS and other severely immuno-compromised patients, and you should seek out those in your area. The treatment protocol must address first things first; for example, any systemic or local infection, especially systemic candidiasis which often underlies chronic infection, must be addressed as a priority, including addressing potential leaky gut syndrome. Then detoxification must be appropriate for the individual person, cellular metabolism at mitochondrial level needs boosting, then the immune system may need rebuilding. So we strongly advise against self-treatment without taking advice from a naturopathic physician familiar with the proper protocols. Other less severe cases may benefit by the following treatment. The tissues affected most will need local therapy, and will give clues to specific nutrients needed.

Diet

Changes must be made to favor a less acidic, less toxic internal environment, and a more alkaline one. Acid-forming foods include animal foods (red meat, dairy) and refined cereal (bread, rice, pasta, etc.). Initially a vegan diet majoring in raw fruit and a "rainbow" salad with herbs, flowers such as nasturtium, steamed vegetables and limited amounts of whole-grain cereal such as oats and brown rice might be appropriate for a period of cleansing, alternating with a few days of juice and broth fasting.

Proteins ought to be those easily digested, to include raw nuts and seeds such as sunflower, pumpkin, sesame seeds, sprouts such as alfalfa and bean, fish such as salmon and sardines, soy foods such as tofu and other soy products like soy milk, cheese, yoghurt, and eggs.

Organic foods are to be preferred, especially and drink lots of pure water to assist with the detoxification of metabolic and exogenous waste products.

Caffeine, alcohol, nicotine, recreational drugs, refined sugar and refined flour are forbidden as they each contribute insult to the immune system, albeit in different ways. The less refined or processed (which includes cooking) the better. Fried foods and vegetable oils and fats (e.g. margarine) are also taboo.

Stress Management

The emotional body as well as the physical one needs nurture and healing, as negative emotions such as worry, anger, fear, anxiety, rejection, hurt, sorrow, depression and insecurity all contribute to immune system depression. Whether you choose massage, yoga, meditation, moderate exercise, a hobby, biofeedback, acupuncture or any other form of stress management, it must become a regular event, and frequently practiced. Ensure you are getting adequate amounts of good quality sleep and rest.

Physiotherapy

- Colonics or enemas.
- Sauna.
- Spinal adjustments.
- Sunbathing.
- Moderate exercise, e.g. daily walking.
- Dry body brushing for the health of superficial lymphatics.
- Cold shower (1 minute all over) following normal warm.
- Support group meetings.

Therapeutic Agents

Following is a list of nutrients found useful in enhancing general immune function. Specific selection and supplementation dosages will depend on individual case history and symptoms.

Vitamins and Minerals—Primary

- Vitamin A and natural carotenes: 50,000–100,000 IU daily. (See warning under Vitamin Toxicity, page 56.) Immune system regulation and antioxidant.
- Vitamin B complex: 50 mg 1–3 times daily. Anti-stress, CNS function, energy
- Vitamin B6: 250–500 mg daily. Needed for protein absorption, enzyme systems.
- Vitamin B12: 1 mg intramuscularly 1–7 times per week.
- Vitamin C: up to bowel tolerance; 30–100 g intravenously may be helpful. Probably the primary immune system vitamin.
- Bioflavonoids: especially quercetin, proanthocyanidins.
- Vitamin E (d-alpha-tocopherol): 400–800 IU daily. Antioxidant; important part of immune functioning. *Note:* Very high doses (over 1200 IU daily) tend to temporarily depress the immune system.
- Zinc: (chelate form is best) 25 mg 3–4 times daily.
- Selenium: 200 mcg daily. Mortality rates from AIDS have been highest where selenium is most absent.

Vitamins and Minerals—Secondary
- Vitamin B5: 150 mg daily.
- Folic acid: 400 mcg to 10 mg daily.
- Pantothenic acid: 250–500 mg daily.
- Iron: dose depending on need and response.
- Magnesium: 400–2000 mg daily.
- Copper: 1–3 mg daily.

Others—Primary
- Mushrooms: (shiitake, reishi, maitake).

- Coenzyme Q10: (up to 240 mg daily): mitochondrial support; improves cellular detoxification and therefore energy levels.
- Protein powder: non-animal sources best, since inadequate protein absorption is immunosuppressive.
- Probiotics: first line of immune system defense, and manufacturers of powerful antiviral chemicals.
- Superoxide dismutase: cellular oxygenation
- Monolaurin: fatty acid from human milk; anti-HIV activity.
- DHEA (dehydroepiandrosterone): antiviral (inhibits replication); thymus protective.
- Cysteine, methionine, lysine: antioxidant, antiviral, hepatoprotective.
- Lipoic acid: has been called the "antioxidant's antioxidant"; helps to detoxify the liver
- Digestive enzymes, pancreatin: taken between meals to destroy circulating antigen–antibody complexes, and as a blood purifier, and virucide; taken with meals to aid digestion especially of proteins.
- DMG (di-methylglycine).
- Essential fatty acids: (GLA, evening primrose oil, EPA, flaxseed oil).
- Carrysin: derived from aloe vera, immunostimulatory, stops night sweats, fever, diarrhea.

Others—Secondary

- Organic germanium Ge-132: (also found in garlic, pearl barley, Siberian ginseng, chlorella).
- Bovine colostrum: contains immunoglobulins and other immune stimulating factors.
- Celtic salt, or some other multimineral tablet or colloidal minerals.
- Green drinks: e.g. Spirulina, barley green, chlorophyll, chlorella.
- Glutathione: antioxidant, detoxifies peroxides, including nitric oxide.
- Raw liver and other glandular preparations: e.g. thymus, adrenals, spleen.
- Bitter melon.
- Royal jelly.
- Glycine.
- Dextran sulfate: improves T-cell counts.

Botanicals—Primary

The following is a short list of herbs that have demonstrated immunostimulant properties; there are many more which might be indicated in specific cases depending on clinical findings and individual biochemical needs, and for this one needs to be consulting a naturopath proficient in the use of botanical medicine.

Echinacea: antibiotic; antiviral; anti-inflammatory; stimulates interferon and activates macrophages; best in combination with goldenseal.

Bupleurum falcatum.

Black bean: reported to inhibit capsid viruses and increase T-cell counts and nutritional status, leading to weight gain.

Picrorrhiza: potent hepatoprotective.

Andrographis.

Globe artichoke.

Rehmannia: hepatoprotective; immunostimulatory; counters side effects of corticosteroid medications.

Panax ginseng.

Astragalus.

Cat's claw.

Pau d'arco.

Tea tree.

Garlic.

St Mary's thistle: potent hepatoprotective.

Pfaffia paniculata: adaptogenic, immunostimulant (not for inflammatory diseases), antiviral, fungicide, vermifuge.

Wild black carrot: antibiotic, antiviral, antifungal, alkalinizing agent (adaptogenic).

Goldenseal.

Aloe vera: antiseptic, anti-inflammatory, antiviral, antibacterial.

Essiac: immunostimulatory, anti-cancer herbal formulation, taken internally.

Ligustrum (nu zhen zi): immunostimulatory; inhibits tumor cell growth.

St John's wort: antiviral.

Licorice root: glycyrrhizin is an antiviral, and immunostimulant.

Botanicals—Secondary

Depuratives, hepatoprotective: e.g. dandelion.

Lymphatic system decongestants, e.g. clivers.

Digestive aids: kelp; meadowsweet gentian.

IMPOTENCE
(Male)

DEFINITION AND SYMPTOMS

Inability to attain or maintain an erection adequate for normal sexual activity

ETIOLOGICAL CONSIDERATIONS—PRIMARY

- Psychological
  Lack of emotional arousal (e.g. marital discord); fear of failure; inhibitions; feelings of inadequacy/ignorance of genital anatomy and function; psychological trauma; stress; depression; feelings of guilt or fear

ETIOLOGICAL CONSIDERATIONS— SECONDARY

Physical abnormalities; endocrine imbalance usually reflecting low testosterone levels, high prolactin levels; abnormal thyroid hormone levels; systemic disease (diabetes, disseminated sclerosis, tabes dorsalis, peripheral vascular disease); general debility; nutritional deficiency; heavy metal poisoning; drugs including hypertensives, sedatives, amphetamines, diuretics, antacids, e.g. Zantac, Tagamet, antihistamines; check prescriptions in an up-to-date drug guide); alcohol is often a culprit (reduces capacity to make testosterone); nicotine.

DISCUSSION

Two main types of impotence exist. *Primary impotence* implies that the problem has existed since birth (males achieve erections at very early ages). In this case a normal erection does not occur and normal sexual relations have never occurred. *Secondary impotence* is a loss of the ability to gain or maintain an erection adequate for normal sexual relations. Primary impotence shows a greater percentage of abnormal physical problems; however, it does not exclude early psychological trauma or other factors. Secondary impotence points to factors other than physical abnormalities of birth and development. Lack of a morning erection points to organic causes.

The psychological factors influencing normal sexual function in the male are well recognized. Few men have never experienced a lost erection due to an inopportune comment at the wrong moment, stress, fear, anger, insecurity, or some other similar emotion such as fear of failure or various inhibitions. Many men experience these problems in the early periods of their sexual activity, finding that an erection occurs easily and spontaneously prior to actual sexual activity, but melts away as soon as intercourse is attempted. These cases are usually caused by fear of failure, insecurity, or similar psychological factors that ordinarily accompany attempts at performing "skilled tasks" by the inexperienced. The only difference in this case is that the tool used is extremely fickle, being unduly influenced by pre-performance butterflies. The individual's reaction to this fairly normal early failure is extremely important in the development of normal sexual performance. Depending on the level of general psychological adjustment, the individual may conclude quite rightly that the whole embarrassing scenario was simply due to the "jitters" and will be short-lived. The next opportunity with a willing partner probably will prove successful. Others less secure, however, may fear the worst from the outset and assume that they are, or will prove to be, impotent. This fear builds upon normal feelings of insecurity to become a self-fulfilling prophecy.

Similar psychological factors may affect the older, more sexually experienced man. Even one failure due to any number of inter-related factors can set up self-doubt. These initial factors may be psychological or they may be due to any one of several little-recognized physical factors. Many prescription drugs have impotence as a side-effect. If the individual is taking one of these drugs and is not aware, or has been inadequately informed of this possibility, he may wrongly interpret this lack of performance as physiological or senile impotence, which in turn creates psychological stresses that may cause a self-perpetuating condition, even if the drug is withdrawn.

Excess alcohol is a well-recognized cause of impotence as are many recreational drugs (e.g. Ecstasy) Nutritional factors such as extreme vitamin deficiencies or heavy metal poisoning may affect sexual performance, with similar secondary psychological reactions as observed above.

Vascular irregularities such as sclerosis, and low blood pressure may also be a risk factor.

Men with impotence problems should also see Prostate Disorders. These two problems often are cause and effect, and treatment of a troubled prostate often corrects male impotence.

TREATMENT

Diet

All therapy should be preceded by a hair analysis to exclude toxic metal causes. If this proves to be a factor, a heavy metal detoxification program should be started. A general detoxification and rejuvenation regimen is required even in the absence of metal toxicity, since toxicity may be caused by many substances. The best program for impotence is an initial fast on fruit and vegetable juices, followed by a raw foods lacto-vegetarian diet similar to that described under Parkinson's disease. This will encourage toxic elimination and supply essential nutrients often missing in the average diet. Foods to major in are whole grains, green vegetables, fruits, seeds (especially sunflower and pumpkin), nuts, fermented dairy products, free-range fertile eggs, cold pressed oils, sprouted seeds and beans, brewer's yeast, wheat germ, fish, kelp, and other seaweeds. Exclude meat and fowl from the diet totally, unless these are obtained wild or are free from feminizing hormones routinely used as fattening agents. Avoid alcohol, smoking, and drugs.

Physiotherapy

- Alternate hot and cold sitz baths. This is the most effective measure in rejuvenating the sexual organs. Repeat 1–2 times daily, if possible.
- Spinal manipulation: I have seen quite dramatic results with regular spinal therapy in these cases. Repeat 1–2 times per week for 8–12 weeks.
- Ice-cold plunges: these are an excellent tonic for the body generally and pelvic region specifically, if the plunge is confined below the waist. Precede ice plunge with a sauna where possible.

Therapeutic Agents

Vitamins and Minerals— Primary

- Zinc: 30–45 mg 2–3 times daily.
- Vitamin C: 6000–8000 mg daily, in 4 divided doses.
- Vitamin E: 400 IU 2–3 times daily.
- Essential fatty acids: GLA, EPA, flaxseed oil and evening primrose oil.

Vitamins and Minerals— Secondary

- Vitamin A: 25,000 IU daily; vitamin B complex: 25–50 mg 2–3 times daily.
- Vitamin B6: 100 mg daily.

Others—Primary

- Celtic salt (multimineral).
- DHEA.

Others—Secondary

- Kelp: 2–3 times daily.
- Raw pituitary tablets.
- Raw thyroid tablets.
- Raw orchic tablets.
- Wheat germ oil (source of vitamin E).

Botanicals—Primary

Damiana: improves genital blood flow; also a nervine tonic. Very effective. May be used as capsules or as infusion. 2 capsules 3 times daily.

Panax ginseng: adaptogenic, adrenal tonic, aphrodisiac.

Siberian ginseng.

Prickly ash: circulatory stimulant.

Wild yam.

Nettles.

Oats: nutritive.

Botanicals—Secondary

Circulatory stimulants: ginkgo biloba, dong quai, gotu kola and ginger.

Nervine tonics and sedatives: oats, sarsaparilla, saw palmetto, hydrangea root.

INCONTINENCE
(Female: Urinary Stress Incontinence)

DEFINITION AND SYMPTOMS

The involuntary loss of urine in very small amounts, accompanying coughing, sneezing, laughing, walking, running, lifting, or any sudden shock or strain.

ETIOLOGICAL CONSIDERATIONS

- Repeated births
- Failure to do prenatal and postnatal exercises
- Obstetrical trauma
  Tears; instrumental delivery (forceps); large baby; prolonged labor; improper management of labor (failure to empty bladder before second stage)
- Poor pelvic floor tone
- Damage to supports, sphincter mechanisms, and pelvic floor
- Visceroptosis
- Poor abdominal tone
- Bladder prolapse
- Urinary tract infection
- Overweight
- Increased intra-abdominal pressure

DISCUSSION

Stress incontinence is the most common variety of urinary incontinence in females after the childbearing years. It may first be noticed after a prolonged labor where much stretching of the pelvic floor has taken place. In a young and healthy woman this will usually heal, but may return insidiously in later years, especially if postnatal exercises were ignored, or if excess weight becomes a factor. Stress incontinence can occur in the nullipara, or woman never having had a baby, but it is much less frequent. Weak abdominal tone, visceroptosis (a drooping of the entire abdominal contents which puts pressure on the pelvic organs), obesity, and lack of pelvic muscle tone are the major causative factors involved in these cases.

To understand what causes stress incontinence, some knowledge of anatomy is essential. Normally the pelvic contents, in this case the uterus, bladder, and urethra, are maintained in place by ligaments and supported by what is called the pelvic floor. This consists of a group of muscles extending from the pubis to the tailbone (coccyx). This sheet of muscle is pierced by three openings—the anus, vagina, and urethra. Circular muscle layers surround these openings to form two main sphincters, one controlling the anus, another governing the vaginal and urethral openings. Placed just between the anus and vagina is a firm, fibrous area called the perineal body. A strong pelvic floor keeps the pelvic organs well supported in their normal physiological relationships. When it sags, so do the pelvic contents, altering the angle of the urethra as it exits from the bladder and favoring prolapse of the bladder and uterus.

During pregnancy the pressure of the enlarging fetus puts an extra burden on the pelvic floor muscles. Unless proper prenatal exercises are performed regularly, the pelvic floor begins to collapse under the increased weight. During labor the pelvic floor must stretch to allow delivery of the baby. If these muscles are already lax the pelvic floor can become permanently weakened. If postnatal pelvic floor exercises are also ignored, or done for too short a time, stress incontinence may result.

After the menopause, as hormone levels fall, a weakness in this area may become even more evident, resulting in prolapse of the bladder or uterus through the vagina. Women who have had several children, prolonged labors, large babies, large tears, or a forceps delivery are the most severely affected.

Lack of abdominal tone, excess weight, and visceroptosis (drooping abdominal contents) place a further burden and more pressure on the pelvic contents, aggravating a latent incontinence condition. Often, incontinence will only first become apparent as abdominal tone slowly weakens in later years.

TREATMENT

Surgery is often performed to help correct incontinence. Much of this surgery could be prevented by the simple adherence to properly prescribed prenatal and postnatal exercises. This is particularly important when the far-reaching psychological effects of incontinence are considered. Many women seclude themselves from normal activities for fear of losing urine control, with its consequent embarrassment.

Exercises

Pelvic exercises must begin during early pregnancy or before, and continued just after the birth, regularly, for at least 3 months or longer post-partum. All the following exercises are forms of what is commonly called the "Kegal" exercise, named after Dr Arnold Kegal, professor of obstetrics and gynecology at the University of California at Los Angeles. He was the first to popularize the necessity of pelvic floor exercises in preventing and treating incontinence. The pelvic floor group of muscles not only helps support the pelvic contents, but when contracted they restrain

319

urine flow and prevent bowel movements. Since the anal sphincter is already very strong, we are concentrating on the vaginal and urethral sphincter to help exercise the pelvic floor muscles.

Exercise 1

Practice slowing urine flow and eventually stopping it to gain a sense of which muscles are involved. Later, practice stopping urine flow, hold for 1-2 seconds, and repeat 6-8 times as you urinate. Eventually you should be able to stop urine flow quickly, without any leakage. And slowly relax the pelvic floor muscles in stages from full contraction to full relaxation.

Exercise 2

Use the same muscles that you mastered the control of in the first exercise to contract the pelvic floor throughout the day. Do this whenever and wherever possible. This may be repeated 6-8 times during each session and 50-100 times daily. Hold the contraction 2-5 seconds and then relax.

Exercise 3

Contract the pelvic floor muscles while making love. Ask your partner to tell you when he can feel the difference. Repeat many times whenever the opportunity arises.

In these exercises do not hold your breath, bear down (thus pushing down on the pelvic floor), or contract the buttocks, inner thighs, or abdominal muscles. It is best to learn to localize the contraction to the pelvic floor muscles entirely. Do not exhaust the pelvic floor muscles in the early stages. Do only as many contractions at a time as you can do at your maximum contraction, and then 2-3 more. As contractions weaken, discontinue at that time and build the muscle strength slowly, as is done with any other muscular exercise.

Diet

General whole food diet.

Physiotherapy

- Alternate hot and cold sitz baths (postnatal).
- Ice-cold sitz baths (postnatal).
- Abdominal exercises (prenatal and postnatal).
- Swimming: breaststroke/frog kick.
- Bicycling.

Botanicals—Primary

Horsetail: urinary astringent.
Bearberry: urinary tract tonic.
Horsetail: diuretic.
Buchu: urinary antiseptic and diuretic.
Cornsilk and couch grass: urinary tract demulcents

Botanicals—Secondary

Urinary astringents: cranesbill, bearberry, witch hazel, goldenseal, sweet sumach.
Urinary tonics: horsetail, bearberry, and sweet sumach.
Diuretics: dandelion, juniper, clivers, celery seed
Urinary demulcents: marshmallow, comfrey, licorice.

Note: It may also be important to take a nervine sedative such as St John's wort or passion flower.
Note: For a complete book on prenatal and postnatal exercise we suggest *Essential Exercises for the Child Bearing Year,* by Elizabeth Nobel, Houghton Mifflin Co., Boston, 1976.

INFERTILITY

DEFINITION AND SYMPTOMS

Inability or reduced ability to produce off-spring, after 12 months of trying. The condition may affect either male or female partner, or both.

ETIOLOGICAL CONSIDERATIONS

Female

- Immature or abnormal reproductive system
- Uterine prolapse
- Endometriosis
- Failure to ovulate
  Effect of contraceptive pill; low cholesterol; Marathoner's amenorrhea
- Polycystic ovaries
- Fallopian tube incompetence
  Mucus plug; infection
- Uterine cavity infection
- Dry vagina
- Low iron levels
  Menorrhagia; fibroids; polyps; endometriosis; dietary
- Nutritional
  Low protein diets; nutritional deficiency; low cholesterol levels
- Toxicity
- Emotional causes

Male

- Immature or abnormal reproductive system
- Impaired sperm production
- Toxic causes, including heavy metal poisoning (e.g. cadmium from cigarette smoke), radiation exposure, xenoestrogenization, and prolonged drug use including alcohol, marijuana, others; traumatic or infection-related atrophy of testicle; prolonged fevers; undescended testes; varicocele; overheating of testes; endocrine disorders; nutritionally related causes such as pernicious anemia, lack of or increased demand for zinc
- Obstruction of the seminal tract
  Congenital; prostatitis; orchitis; epididymitis; other local inflammatory processes
- Defective delivery of sperm (agglutination)
- Impotence (atherosclerosis; pernicious anemia; testosterone deficiency; low blood pressure; smoking; caffeine excess; low seminal prostaglandin levels, emotional, etc.)
- Reduced sperm motility or viability

DISCUSSION

Due to the large number of physical causes of infertility, patients and their partners should undergo a complete diagnostic evaluation if conception fails to occur within 2–3 years. Once the problem area has been diagnosed, treatment can be directed more specifically. Certainly not all causes of infertility can be influenced by natural therapies; however, the cases that can be are very rewarding. When nothing can be found to prevent conception in either partner, the individualized naturopathic approach represents an excellent approach, and certainly can do no harm, and according to one Australian study, has a better chance of success than IVF programs.

A study done in Australian hospitals compares the success rate of the high-tech, high-expense IVF program with the simple, low-cost natural medicines. The success rate using the IVF program sits at around 20% for clinically infertile couples. And for years, science has applauded itself for such wonderful success. This study shows that natural medicine proves to be about 80% successful.

And at about 5% of the cost to the taxpayer.

The emergence of technological medicine is both expensive and comparatively ineffectual (apart from that used in accident emergencies). The billions of dollars is spent on high-tech equipment and much of it is spent on those suffering chronic diseases, which are often entirely preventable in the first place.

Naturopathic fertility protocols have a proven track record over many decades. Medical diagnosis can work hand-in-hand here; diagnosing specifically what may be the infertility problem will be useful to the naturopathic clinician.

TREATMENT

Pre-Conception Planning

Ideally, conception should be planned for, with both partners aiming for optimal health by the time of the planned conception. Women should stop using contraceptive pills at least 6 months prior, to allow hormone levels to return to normal. Herbal medicines can effectively help with this, particularly black cohosh, chaste tree, licorice and mother's wort as a complex (see Menstrual Disorders). Chaste tree increases serum progesterone levels, thus lengthening the luteal phase of the cycle.

We recommend that both partners, but especially the female, go on a liver detoxification diet for at least 4 weeks, and eliminate any known allergens from food intake, to reduce possibility of transferring them to baby via placenta or breast milk (see Allergies and Food Intolerances). Both partners need a consistently healthy diet, high in vegetarian protein and fish (low in red meats), high in EFAs, vitamins (supplementary vitamins A, B, especially B6 and folate (e.g. wholemeal organic oats) to avoid neural tube defect, and B12, C and E) and minerals (supplement Zinc, Magnesium and Iron).

We recommend an exercise program especially for the female, and an appropriate spinal check. Neither partner should be using any stimulant drugs such as tobacco or coffee.

A very common cause of female infertility is blocked or partially blocked fallopian tubes. This is usually due to previous pelvic infections. Some of these cases may be treated successfully with a combination of strict dietary regimens, nutritional supplementation, and vigorous hydrotherapy. Often the tube is inflamed. These measures may re-establish the delivery route for the ovum. All negative health factors are identified and removed, including coffee, alcohol, drugs, and smoking. Adequate pelvic exercise is encouraged through daily swimming. Local circulation and nutrition is enhanced by twice-daily alternate hot and cold sitz baths. This hydrotherapy is the most important part of the regimen, and is very effective in removing internal inflammation and congestion. Diet should be as wholesome and fresh as possible. Periodic fasting on vegetable juices for 3-5 days is useful, with periods of 2-4 weeks on an adequate protein but mostly vegetarian diet. Soy foods containing phytoestrogens ought to be the protein of choice for the female. Fish, white cheese and organically grown eggs are the only animal proteins allowed. The diet should include plenty of raw and conservatively cooked vegetables, seaweed, seeds, nuts, beans, and whole grains.

Vitamins and Minerals—Primary

Female:
- Vitamin B complex: 50 mg 1-2 times daily.
- Vitamin C with bioflavonoids: take to bowel tolerance.
- Vitamin E: 400-800 IU daily.

Male:
- Vitamin C: 5 g daily. Increases sperm motility as does taurine; reverses agglutination of sperm.
- Zinc: 25-50 mg 1-3 times daily, normalizes testosterone production, increases sperm count in some cases.
- L-Arginine: this is an important food nutrient for males; arginine-rich foods

include nuts, legumes,
- Ginseng, garlic, and whole grains.
- Selenium: 200 mcg daily (essential for sperm production).
- Taurine: improves sperm count

Vitamins and Minerals— Secondary

Females:
- Vitamin A: 50,000 IU 1-2 times daily. (See warning under Vitamin Toxicity, page 56.)
- Vitamin B12: 1 mg intramuscularly per week.
- Folic acid: 1-10 mg daily.
- Iron: 15-50 mg daily.
- PABA: 50 mg daily (works through the pituitary)
- Selenium: 400 mcg daily. Deficiency linked to infertility in both sexes.

Others—Primary

Females:
- Essential fatty acids, especially GLA: (e.g. flaxseed oil, evening primrose oil): 1 tbsp daily.
- Reproductive system functioning.
- Raw ovarian glandular: as directed on label.

Males:
- EFAs: anti-inflammatory, improve levels of seminal prostaglandins
- Brewer's yeast: 1-3 tsp daily.

- L-carnitine: 300-800 mg daily.
- L-lysine: 500-1000 mg daily.
- L-methionine and L-cysteine: 500 mg daily. Antioxidants, chelating agents.
- Vitamin E: 400-800 IU daily.
- Vitamin A and beta-carotene: 25,000 IU of each daily.

Botanicals

Females:
The choice of herbal medicines for a woman contemplating and planning for a healthy conception and pregnancy ought to be guided by a competent herbalist or naturopath, because it will largely reflect her individual requirements determined from an adequate case history, and might change closer to planned conception.

Males:
Panax ginseng: over 3 months can improve: sperm count, total testosterone, free testosterone, sperm motility, and DHT.

Therapeutic Suggestion

Obviously, individual case histories will indicate other, more specific nutrients. Spinal manipulation is a useful adjunctive therapy to help establish better circulation and local nutrition.

INSECT BITES

DISCUSSION

Some people are violently allergic to insect bites and require epinephrine treatment for even minor bites, to prevent severe reactions which can include itching, hives, arthralgia, wheezing and breathing difficulties (even airways swelling and obstruction), anaphylactic shock, unconsciousness and even death.

TREATMENT

The following recommendations are not for these hypersensitive individuals. If you have had a severe allergic reaction to insect bite in the past, you should have access to epinephrine at all times. For the person who develops average or above-average sensitivity to insect bites, inflammation and pain from insect bites may be lessened and shortened in duration through some of the following measures.

Bee or Wasp stings, and other insect bites and stings

- Remove stinger if present; then immediately apply ice to area.
- Apis tincture: 25 drops in a small amount of water 4-6 times daily. Homeopathic dilutions (6×) also used.
- Ledum: (12, 30C) useful for any puncture of the skin.
- Vitamin C with bioflavonoids, especially quercetin: (topical) and internal: 4-5 g just after bite, and 1 g per hour until resolved.

Other:
Tobacco (chew and apply to sting); tea tree oil; ice water plus baking soda soaks; clay packs; charcoal paste; vinegar plus lemon juice applications; onion (topical); green papaya skin; juice (topical); honey poultice; plantain poultice; calendula cream

Tick Bites

Remove the tick as soon as possible. Do not try to burn the tick, or put flyspray, vinegar, kerosene or anything else before removing the tick. Use tweezers, and grasp the tick as close to your skin as possible, rotate the tick anti-clockwise as you pull it out, to give you a better chance of removing the head if it has burrowed in already. Ticks can carry disease, so despatch the tick without hand contact, and wash the bite site with clean soapy water, and apply tea tree or lavender oil.

If the bite is close to lymph nodes, especially around the head and neck areas, tick poison might cause nodal swelling, pain and headache.

Spider Bites

Most spider bites cause no more than local irritation and maybe some swelling. However, several species are potentially deadly, especially to young children, the elderly, and those severely immunocompromised. If you suspect the spider is poisonous, or experience symptoms which can include intense pain at the bite site, nausea, breathing difficulty, profuse sweating, salivation and eye watering, clammy skin and shivering, then seek medical help immediately.

An immobilization bandage should be applied to the site and around the limb, pack ice around the affected area to slow down the spread of the poison, remain calm, and rest as much as possible until you obtain medical care.

For any and all insect bites, large amounts of vitamin C, quercetin and vitamin B5 will help with the detoxification, as will drinking extra amounts of water. Botanical remedies include yellow dock, dandelion, echinacea, thyme.

INSOMNIA

DEFINITION AND SYMPTOMS

Difficulty falling asleep, or awakening from sleep prematurely with subsequent inability to return to sleep. Irritability, depression, emotional disturbances, poor memory.

ETIOLOGICAL CONSIDERATIONS—PRIMARY

- Physical tension
- Emotional or mental stress or preoccupation; over stimulation to nervous system

- Overeating,(especially a large protein meal)
- Caffeine drinks
- Vitamin B complex deficiency
- Irregular sleeping hours
- Lack of adequate ventilation: fresh air can result in oxygen debt
- Lack of physical exercise ("the sleep of the laborer is sweet"); being physically tired contributes to good quality sleep
- Sleep apnea

ETIOLOGICAL CONSIDERATIONS— SECONDARY

- Excess salt: increases blood volume, heart output, and blood pressure
- Food additives, preservatives, and colorings
- Allergy: increased heart rate follows exposure
- Refined carbohydrates, sugar, soda, ice-cream, or other sweets
- Calcium deficiency: poor absorption of calcium or true deficiency
- Iodine excess; out of biorhythm; interference by electrical circuitry, such as electric blankets, waterbed heaters, electrical wiring in or power boxes on bed-head walls, or overhead high-voltage power lines
- Lights left on at night (disrupts the pineal gland producing melatonin, a sleep hormone)
- Becoming dehydrated at night
- Temperature extremes in bed
- Menopause
- Hypothyroidism or hyperthyroidism
- Pain; smoking
- Alcoholism
- Poor mattress
- TV excess
- Heavy metal poisoning
- Unfounded fears, e.g. fear of not falling asleep, fear of not waking; false insomnia: light sleeper syndrome, never sure if sleep occurred; psychological; acute trauma

DISCUSSION

Approximately 20 million Americans are presently taking prescription sleeping pills regularly. An additional $100 million is spent yearly on non-prescription over-the-counter sleep aids. These figures not only emphasize how extensive the problem of insomnia is, but should also be taken as an expression of how drug-oriented our society has become. Apparently, millions of people care so little about their health, or are too lazy to become well enough informed about the insidiously detrimental effects of these medications.

To begin with, over-the-counter sleep aids have been carefully studied in controlled experiments, and it has been found that these medications are no more effective in inducing sleep than a placebo. The medicine tested was Sominex, but many other over-the-counter sleep aids (Nytol, Sleep-Eze, Compoz, Nite Rest, Sure-Sleep, etc.) contain the same "inactive" ingredients. Worse than this multi-million dollar farce, however, is the fact that while these medications do no real good, they certainly may do harm. This really is only the tip of the pill-poppers' nightmare. Sleep studies show clearly that many non-prescription and almost all prescription sleep medications drastically alter sleeping cycles, suppressing REM (rapid eye movement) sleep. This certainly is true for any barbiturates and benzodiazepines, which are the major sleep medication ingredients. To fully understand why suppression of REM sleep is harmful, we must first delve into the normal sleeping cycle.

In the early pre-sleep phase, body temperature falls and alpha rhythm brain waves are prominent. Stage 1 of sleep is usually heralded by "myoclonic jerks", or muscle spasms, followed by a slowing of the pulse and muscle relaxation. Stage 2 is entered after about 5-10 minutes. The brain waves become larger and the eyes roll side to side. After another 20 minutes Stage 3 is entered. Brain waves now become slow and fairly large. Muscles are relaxed and breathing is slow and even. Stage 4 then follows. This stage is called delta sleep and lasts about 20 minutes or so. After this time the sleeper enters the lighter REM sleep characterized by rapid eye movements. The heartbeat is irregular and the brain waves are similar to the waking state. Of the time in REM sleep, 80% or more is spent dreaming. REM sleep lasts 10 or more minutes and then the sleeper enters Stage 2, 3, and finally again delta sleep in a cycle lasting about 90 minutes. Delta sleep lasts longer in the early part of the night, with more REM sleep taking place towards morning. This order of sleep cycles seems to be essential for health. Subjects deprived of REM and delta sleep become irritable, depressed, aggressive, angry, restless and/or apathetic. Once allowed to re-enter REM sleep, subjects spend more time than usual there, apparently making up for lost cycles. If this REM sleep has been suppressed by sleeping pills, health begins to suffer. Once the pills are discontinued the sleeper experiences light, restless, unpleasant sleep with plenty of nightmares. This REM withdrawal sleep, a built-in result of taking medication to *aid* sleep, is usually severe enough to disturb sleep and convince the poor uninformed "Insomniac" that he or she still needs sleep medication, thus starting the cycle all over again.

Insomnia can be properly treated only if its true cause is recognized and removed. Frequently the cause is easy to identify, such as excess caffeine, an obvious stimulant found in coffee, tea, chocolate, and some sodas. More difficult to correct quickly, but usually easily diagnosed, is simple muscular tension due to emotional or mental stress and overstimulation.

Dietary factors other than caffeine may also be involved. The excess use of refined salt has been frequently associated with insomnia. Many sufferers are completely cured by this diet change alone. Overeating before bed is another common fault that is easily corrected. Deficiency of many of the B complex vitamins is associated with general stress syndromes and insomnia. This may be due to the overconsumption of refined carbohydrates which require B complex for their metabolism while being stripped of their own intrinsic B complex components found in the fiber and germ coatings. Stress itself depletes B complex, among other vitamins, as the body's glandular system, particularly the adrenal glands, is over stimulated. Calcium deficiency due to poor absorption or true nutritional deficiency is a common factor in insomnia. Calcium supplementation at bedtime frequently cures sleep disorders. Any food allergy may cause poor sleeping and insomnia. Foods causing allergic reactions are known to increase the heart rate among other actions, causing or aggravating insomnia. Food additives, colorings, preservatives, and pesticides may cause a similar allergic response. Heavy metal poisoning is a well-documented cause of nervousness, mental confusion, irritability, emotional disturbances, and sleep disorders. Many smokers find that their sleeping difficulties are removed once they stop smoking. This is not surprising since nicotine stimulates the sympathetic ganglia and also the adrenal glands, which then secrete adrenalin. This leads to increased heart rate and elevated blood pressure, and hyperreactivity at the neuromuscular junction, the opposite effect desired for sleep.

The use of alcohol as an evening nightcap may not always be either successful or beneficial. Many people respond to alcohol as a stimulant, which it is, at low blood levels. Alcohol also has a similar effect on sleep cycles to that of other sleep aids, reducing the REM cycle. Alcohol also causes dehydration, which can be a cause of poor quality sleep.

Sleep apnea is a condition in which REM sleep is not sustained for more than a few seconds at a time, and causes repeated wakings (can be up to 200 times, often without being aware) throughout the night. Breathing can stop for more than a minute at a time, is irregular, and is associated with snoring. Studies show that sleep apnea causes fatigue and drowsiness throughout the day, and is associated with high blood pressure, increased risk of heart disease and stroke, emotional disturbance and even psychoses.

Another major cause of insomnia is improper or irregular sleeping habits. There is a great deal of evidence detailing the existence of internal biological clocks or rhythms. If we chronically live out of phase with our intrinsic cycles, health begins to suffer. We have all known people who call themselves "day" or "night" people, who claim they think and work best either in the morning or late at night. This may not be simple preference, but our intuitive awareness of the dictates of our biological rhythms. With the advent of electric lighting modern society has placed new and unusual demands on our inner clocks. Many workers now must force their bodies to perform, even in the in middle of their biological sleep time.

Evidence shows that these inner clocks can be made to shift as the need arises, but this takes anywhere from a few days to a few weeks. For workers on rotating shifts, biological rhythms are in constant chaos. This is especially true for pilots and crew members on commercial airlines. Stress, fatigue, and insomnia are the common results of such lifestyles.

TREATMENT

In dealing with a "sleep disorder" it is important to recognize that not all people have the same sleeping requirements. As a person gets to be 50 or 55, he or she usually will require less sleep. Some people can get by quite nicely with 4–6 hours' sleep at night and a catnap during the day. The real criterion as to whether a person is getting enough sleep is his or her general health and energy level. If a person complains that he or she cannot get to sleep until 1 or 2 in the morning, but feels normal, he or she does not have an insomnia problem, but rather a biorhythm misunderstanding. The worst thing for such a person to do is to lie in bed fretting and worrying about why they can't sleep. They must be active until sleep

is desired, as it probably would be if he continued at his normal pace until the time sleep normally came.

Daily tension and stress are major obstacles to failing asleep. Unfortunately, many insomniacs spend time complaining to others about their problem, and little or no time reversing its true causes. The cause of such tension is a complete lack of self-knowledge and self-control. Tension is present only if you allow it to be present.

The only real cure is first to become aware of the problem, find its cause, and then slowly and steadily remove or counteract it. We are dealing here with the basic cause of almost all disease—our improper attitude towards life and lack of knowledge and awareness of ourselves. We often see obviously tense individuals who do not recognize even the gross chronic muscular spasms of their bodies. When asked to be totally relaxed and allow their bodies to go limp like a rag doll, we often find patients completely unable to let go. If we raise their arms, they stay in the air; if we touch their legs they jerk uncontrollably. These people are truly surprised to discover that day in and day out their bodies are in constant muscular contraction, even at so-called rest! Think how much less aware these individuals must be of the mental or emotional causes of this physical tension, and you will begin to understand why sleep does not come easily.

To correct such a situation several avenues are available, depending on the psychological inclination of the patient. Relaxation exercises can help the patient gain an awareness of physical tension and help relax chronic muscular tensions. Several methods are commonly used.

Progressive Contraction/Relaxation Exercises

In this method the subject lies comfortably on a bed and relaxes as much as he or she normally can. Three or four deep, slow breaths aid in reaching this state of maximum normal relaxation. An attempt is made to ignore, or pay no attention to, any thoughts or feelings, with the entire attention gently concentrated on the relaxation procedure at hand. The subject begins by contracting the face and neck into a horrible grimace, holding the contraction for 1-2 seconds, and then suddenly letting go and relaxing. Next the upper arms and chest are contracted, and then relaxed, followed by lower arms and hands, abdomen, buttocks, thighs, lower legs, and finally the feet. End with a final convulsive contraction of every muscle in the body all at once. This whole cycle is repeated 2-3 times. This preliminary exercise should be ended with three slow, deep breaths. Deeper relaxation techniques may then follow.

This technique allows the person who has little knowledge of his or her physical tensions to physically reverse the process by re-educating the various muscles as to what is the state of contraction and relaxation. It is useful for the person who has not yet developed a very subtle awareness of muscular tension, or is unable to release tension by a mental command.

"Draining" Exercise

This technique is an excellent aid to relaxation for the person a little more aware of his or her tension level. Begin by sitting in a comfortable chair and getting as relaxed as normally possible. Imagine that your body is like a bathtub filled with liquid tension, with your fingers and toes being the drain. Start at the very top of your head and imagine that the liquid tension is draining down towards your head and face. Feel the tension as it passes down into your jaws and checks, upper neck, and then shoulders. Sense the freedom from tension and your relaxation as it passes out of your head and neck into your shoulders and upper arms. Keep your mind relaxed and dismiss any other thoughts or feelings. Attend only to the "draining", with a gentle concentration on

the passage of the liquid tension down into the abdomen and lower arms. Feel the tension level lowering and draining into the lower back and buttocks, and beginning to tingle as it enters your hands and fingers. You will feel the tension tingle and flow out of your fingertips, leaving your upper body totally relaxed. Continue observing this draining process into your pelvic region and sex organs, then thighs, knees, calves, and ankles. Finally, feel the tingling as the last bit of the liquid tension drains out of your toes. Finish the exercise with three cleansing breaths, consciously feeling new vitality enter your body with each breath, relieving the old, worn-out, and toxic liquid tension you have just eliminated.

You may find that after you have finished with this exercise, or even part-way through it, tension has once again begun to accumulate in your body. Disregard this and finish the exercise to its end, and then begin all over, if necessary. If this exercise is done twice daily for 15-30 minutes, you will find it becomes easier and more complete. If done regularly, over a period of 3-6 months you will notice deeper and deeper states of relaxation, soon you will notice a steady flow of powerful currents passing through your body at the end of each session. Slowly you will discover that you have learned to recognize your physical tensions throughout the day and you will find it easy to drain them away quickly, even as you sit or stand in your ordinary daily activities.

This draining exercise is an excellent preliminary step before meditation. In meditation you will come more and more in contact with the center of yourself, revealing many things about why physical, mental, and emotional tension exists within you.

Biofeedback

This is a technique used in relaxation therapy and other applications. As applied to insomnia and tension, the subject is taught to recognize tension in the forehead through audible and/or visual feedback from an EM (electromyography). Once the person has learned to control the forehead muscles, he or she then is taught by a similar process with an EEG (electroencephalogram) to produce alpha brain waves that precede sleep.

Hypnosis

This method of curing insomnia works well for many. The usual method is to teach the subject self-hypnosis slowly, allowing him to relax and then sleep.

Exercise

A physically tired body is ready for a good sleep. Daily exercise promotes better sleep, but it is important not to exercise too close to bedtime.

Diet

The diet must exclude all caffeine beverages (coffee, tea, cola) or foods (chocolate). Stimulant drugs, tobacco and alcohol should also be avoided. All refined carbohydrates, especially sugar, are excluded. Food additives, preservatives, colorings, and pesticides may also need to be eliminated, as well as all canned foods or other sources of toxicity or heavy metals. Specific allergies may need to be traced down and eliminated. The evening meal should be moderate in size; overeating at supper may cause sleeping difficulties and nightmares. The foods eaten should be soothing in nature, with simple, compatible food combinations and sufficient sources of B complex and calcium. Bananas, yoghurt, dates and figs, tuna, or (if tolerated) a large glass of warm milk may be helpful just before bed, due to their tryptophan content, an amino acid found useful in inducing a safe, natural sleep without suppressing the REM and delta cycles.

Avoid a large protein component (e.g. red meat) as the digestive system will be working overtime on dealing with it, at a time when you want to rest. Other foods to avoid include ham and bacon, sausages, cheese, chocolate and tomatoes, which contain tyramine, a CNS stimulant.

Sleeping Habits

Try to find out what time sleep comes most naturally and follow the dictates of your body. If sleep is easiest at 2 a.m. don't attempt to sleep sooner. Six hours of sleep taken in the proper cycle are much more refreshing than tossing and turning for hours, waiting for sleep to come. Keep to a regular sleep schedule, always going to bed at the same time to establish a good sleep habit. Make sure your mattress is firm and supportive.

Daily Activities

Try to maintain a relaxed and positive attitude towards life and your daily tasks. Most stress and tension states have their roots in poor attitudes. Most of us tend to blame outside events (our job, our boss, working conditions, the weather, etc.) for our tension. We must slowly come to realize that we have the ability to control our inner state and need not let external factors influence us in a detrimental way. If the conditions in which you live and work are definitely too difficult for you to handle, first try to change yourself. If this is beyond your present abilities, you must make changes in your environment. If necessary, find a new job. Your health is much more important.

The "Power Nap"

Having a sleep during the day can beneficially supplement night time sleep. Studies into what is now known as the "power nap" suggest that early afternoon (siesta) is an appropriate time within the circadian rhythm for a short nap. If you "catch the wave" and have a nap, your body will bring you back to (semi) consciousness after about 15 minutes of deep sleep—you will stir, but don't roll over, and don't just lie there—get up. And you will find that that 15 minutes, called the "power nap", is much more refreshing than if you had 2 hours sleep, from which you can awake feeling worse than before.

Physiotherapy

Play calming music softly as you are going to sleep; hot foot baths: these draw the blood away from the head, making sleep easier; warm baths: these are generally relaxing. make sure the bath is not too hot or it will act as a stimulant; scalp and/or foot massage; general massage; alternate hot and cold showers or head baths (tonic); cold baths (a daily tonic); general exercise, plus fresh air; meditation; candle gazing; relaxation techniques; spinal manipulation; cervical, upper thoracic; hops-filled pillow; breath holding (take three deep breaths and hold as long as possible, repeat three times, and then concentrate on breathing shallowly).

Therapeutic Agents

Vitamins and Minerals—Primary
- Vitamin B complex: 50 mg twice daily, best morning and noon, not night.
- Calcium (chelate form is best): 800–1000 mg daily.
- Magnesium: 400-2000 mg daily.

Vitamins and Minerals—Secondary
- Vitamin B6: 100 mg twice daily.
- Folic acid: important if there is muscle cramping at night (nocturnal myoclonus), or restless legs syndrome.
- Vitamin C: 500-1000 mg 3 times daily.
- Pantothenic acid: 250 mg daily.
- Inositol: 1000-1500 mg taken 2 hours before bed. Enhances REM sleep.
- Zinc: 15-25 mg twice daily.
- Manganese: 1-5 mg daily.

Others—Primary
- Tryptophan: 500-1000 mg 3 times daily with one dose 45-90 minutes before bedtime. Tryptophan is a precursor molecule to serotonin and melatonin
- Melatonin: 1.5 mg to 5 mg, 2 hours or less before bedtime.
- DHEA.

Others—Secondary
- Adenosine.
- Lecithin: 4 capsules 3 times daily and a lecithin protein drink before bed. Blend 50% apple juice, 50% water, 12 almonds, and 1-2 tbsp lecithin granules; or drink milk plus lecithin.
- Brewer's yeast.
- Probiotics.

Botanicals—Primary
Valerian: strong sedative.
Chamomile tea: mild sedative.
Passion flower: sedative: 30-60 drops tincture 45 minutes Before bedtime.
Kava: hypnotic sedative
Zizyphus: sedative, mild tranquilizer, increases sleep time, and time getting to sleep; anxiolytic.
Hops.

Botanicals—Secondary
Chamomile.
Skullcap
Californian poppy.
Catnip and other nervine sedatives.

KIDNEY DISEASE
(Nephritis, Pyelitis, Pyelonephritis, Glomerulonephritis)

DEFINITION

Acute or chronic diffuse, often bilateral inflammation and infection of the kidneys. Each specific term refers to the main area affected, e.g. nephrons, pelvis, kidney, or glomeruli.

SYMPTOMS

Chills, fever, low back pain, bladder irritation, pain on urination (dysuria), frequency, and possibly edema. Each acute episode causes some permanent kidney damage.

ETIOLOGICAL CONSIDERATIONS

- Ascending infection common (cystitis, urethritis)
- Same considerations as cystitis
- Obstruction (stone, tumor, prostate) can cause hydronephrosis
- Systemic disease (diabetes, liver disease, hypertension, SLE, strep throat, and many others)
- Pregnancy
- Diet: excess animal proteins, cow's milk
- Allergy
- Drug damage, toxic insult (heavy metals, pesticides, venom, chemotherapeutic agents)

DISCUSSION

The same considerations that apply to other genitourinary diseases apply to kidney disease (see Cystitis). Always remember that the true cause of disease comes from within. Even Pasteur realized the basic importance of the healing power and vitality of the body when he wrote that "the germ is nothing, the soil is everything". By this he meant that the most important element in the cause or prevention of disease is the state of the tissues of the body, not the presence of pathogenic bacteria.

It is very important to get prompt treatment for all kidney infections since even mild infections can cause some tissue damage. Pyelonephritis is a medical emergency best treated with antibiotics. Antibiotics will usually rid the body of the immediate bacterial infection. Frequently, however, the infection will recur within 2–8 weeks unless the original causes of the lowered tissue vitality are removed. The worst cases we see, and the most difficult to treat, are those which have received multiple courses of antibiotics over a fairly prolonged period of time due to chronic and recurrently acute kidney infections, without an attempt being made to deal with the deeper causes of the disorder.

TREATMENT

Diet

In acute cases the best dietary therapy is to fast on the following liquids:
Cranberry juice—up to 2 pints (1 liter) daily; parsley tea; watermelon seed tea; watermelon juice; mullein tea; barley water; potassium broth

This is followed by a transitional low-protein vegetarian diet. A low-protein (35–40 g daily), low-salt diet must be followed up to 2–3 *years* for complete cure of chronic cases. Adequate protein homeostasis must be monitored during this period.

In chronic cases of kidney disease a different approach is usually necessary. While periodic fasting as above may be useful, a slightly higher protein diet is often more beneficial. Raw goat's milk is an ideal mono diet; or combined with non-citrus fruits and vegetables. Certain foods have proven very beneficial in the healing of kidney disease and should be incorporated into the dietary regimen:

Garlic; horseradish; asparagus; raw honey; parsley; raw goat's milk; watercress; apples; pears; watermelon; potassium broth; celery; cucumber; papaya; mango; potato skins; parsnips; dandelion greens; kale; turnip greens; kidney beans plus pods; carrot, celery, and parsley juice

Spinal Manipulation

Thoracic/lumbar junction T6 to L5, to stimulate nerve, blood, and lymph flow.

Hydrotherapy

- Turpentine stupe: take 2 fl oz (60 mL) spirits of turpentine (Cayce product—not the turpentine in hardware stores). Add to 2 pints (1 liter) hot water. Soak 3–4 thicknesses of heavy toweling in this solution and apply over the kidney area in the back. Keep the towels warm for 15–20 minutes by repeating the application frequently or using a hot water bottle or hydrocolator pack. Do not burn the skin. Repeat 2–3 times and apply 2–4 times daily.
- Trunk packs and/or Hot and cold compresses.

Massage

Massage across the kidney area and abdomen with either of the following:
- 1 fl oz (30 mL) dissolved mutton tallow

with 20 drops spirits of gum turpentine 40 drops camphor 20 drops benzoin 3 drops sassafras added.
- Camphoderm (Cayce product), mutton tallow, turpentine, and camphor.

Therapeutic Agents

Vitamins and Minerals—Primary
- Vitamin B6: 100–250 mg 1–3 times daily; especially where duct blockage by stone is the predisposing cause for the kidney disease; diuretic.
- Vitamin C plus bioflavonoids: 500–1000 mg 2–6 times daily or to bowel tolerance. Any infection needs excess vitamin C; it acidifies urine.
- Magnesium: (citrate form): 400–600 mg daily. Regulates calcium.

Vitamins and Minerals—Secondary
- Vitamin A: 50,000–75,000 IU daily. (See warning under Vitamin Toxicity, page 56.) Helps heal mucous membrane. Larger doses may be needed for a short period.
- Vitamin B complex: 2 5–50 mg 2–3 times daily.
- Vitamin D: reduces aminoaciduria due to defective amino acid reabsorption, due in part to vitamin D deficiency in chronic kidney disease.
- Vitamin E: 400 IU 1–3 times daily.
- Niacin.
- Potassium: 100 mg daily (esp. with nephritis; not if serum potassium is elevated)
- Zinc gluconate: up to 100 mg daily. Stops growth of kidney stones.

Note: With medical or herbal diuretic therapy these supplement doses may need to be increased.

Others—Primary
- Choline: 250 mg 4 times daily. May be made from methionine, but in rapid growth (young children) methionine is needed in large amounts, and so is not

available for conversion to choline. A diet deficient in choline and low in protein in the very young will favor nephritis. Choline causes the body to smell very fishy. Concentrated phosphatidylcholine (lecithin), however, contains much choline and leaves no fishy odor. Use 2-4 capsules 3-6 times daily.

- *L. Acidophilus*: especially important straight after any antibiotic.

Others—Secondary

- Garlic.
- Lecithin: 3-6 tbsp daily helps protect kidneys from atherosclerosis. Contains choline. Especially with nephritis.
- L-arginine: 500 mg, 3 or 4 times daily (esp. with kidney disease).
- Lipoic acid: antioxidant.
- Raw thymus: immune support. 2 tablets up to every 1-2 hours.

Botanicals—Primary

Watermelon seed tea: diuretic, purifies kidneys. 3-4 cups daily.

Bearberry: diuretic, gastrointestinal antiseptic. 20-40 drops tincture 3-4 times daily.

Yarrow: especially if fever is present

Buchu: diuretic, antispasmodic. 10-15 drops tincture 3-4 times daily.

Celery seed: dissolves kidney stones.

Cornsilk: urinary demulcent, and is also antilithic

Uva ursi: diuretic, bactericide.

Cranberry: perhaps the most useful botanical to acidify the urine and promote bladder tissue health. Used as tincture, or juice.

Botanicals—Secondary

Crataeva: antilithic.

Chamomile.

Couch grass: mild diuretic: demulcent.

Echinacea.

High-bush cranberry, or cramp bark: juice.

Marshmallow

Skullcap, St John's wort: nervine sedatives

Horsetail: astringent to urinary tract. 10-40 drops tincture 2-4 times daily.

Parsley: diuretic.

Pipsissewa: renal antiseptic.

Mullein.

Stinging nettle: diuretic. 10-40 drops tincture 3-4 times daily.

KIDNEY STONES
(Renal Calculi, Nephrocalcinosis)

DEFINITION

Gravel or stone formation in the kidneys. Composition of stones is usually calcium oxalate but urates, phosphates, and cystein may be present.

SYMPTOMS

May be symptomless or with intermittent, dull, dragging pain in the upper or lower back, testicle, groin, or leg, usually aggravated by motion. Hemorrhage and renal colic occur when stone enters ureter, causing sudden sharp pain, which may last hours or even days. Sometimes with fever, pallor, frequency of urination, nausea, vomiting, and severe agony occurs.

ETIOLOGICAL CONSIDERATIONS—PRIMARY

- Diet
  Vitamin B6 deficiency or dependency;

calcium deficiency or phosphorus excess; magnesium deficiency; nutritionally induced secondary hyperparathyroidism; excess acid (oxalate plus urate stones); excess alkaline (phosphate stones); excess purines as in gout (uric acid).

- Excess fluid loss, or deficiency of fluids (chronic, often subclinical dehydration causing excessive urine concentration); occupations leading to sweating; living in tropics; runners are at risk; failure to drink water
- Hypercalciuria
  Idiopathic (of unknown cause); prolonged bed rest; excess salt intake; excess protein intake; excessive calcium intake; hyperparathyroidism; Cushing's syndrome; vitamin D excess; sarcoidosis (a chronic disease characterized by nodule formation in lymph nodes, lungs, or bones); multiple myeloma (malignant tumor of plasma cells)
- Excess meat-based protein, and excess soft drinks. Meat and soft drinks contain phosphates, which combine with calcium to form calcium phosphate, which alone or mixed with calcium oxalate form kidney stones
- Excess oxalates
  Chocolate; cocoa; tea; spinach; rhubarb; chard; beet tops; excess sugar and refined carbohydrates; eggs; fish—high in oxalic acid

ETIOLOGICAL CONSIDERATIONS— SECONDARY

- Vitamin A deficiency: some macrobiotic diets
- Excess coffee
- Milk–alkali syndrome (ulcer diet plus treatments—e.g. milk and sodium bicarbonate)
- Chronic urinary infections (stagnation of urine, increased salt concentration, lesion site instigates formation)
- Hereditary (congenital hyperoxaluria or cystinuria)

- Excess aspirin use increases stone formation
- Excess dairy products

DISCUSSION

Normal urine contains many constituents that are present in a supersaturated solution. To maintain this excess solubility, urine also contains certain substances that form complexes to keep these otherwise insoluble salts in solution. Other factors or substances either decrease the output of some of the major constituents of kidney stones or speed their removal from the kidneys. Among these substances are polypeptides, mycoproteins, citric acid, magnesium, and vitamin B6. The amount of urine produced is also a factor and generally the larger the urine output the less chance kidney stones have to form. If a person has a deficiency of the substances that help keep insoluble salts in a solution, or if fluid intake is restricted relative to fluid loss, stone formation is favored.

Recent evidence has appeared to link vitamin B6 and magnesium deficiency with some kidney stones. Vitamin B6 helps control the body's production of oxalic acid and increases oxalate excretion. Magnesium helps increase the solubility of oxalates in the urine. Both factors are important in preventing calcium oxalate stones, which are by far the most common. Although oxalates are found in some foods such as chocolate, cocoa, tea, rhubarb, spinach, chard, and beet tops, this usually amounts to only 2% of the total body oxalates. The rest are endogenous, being produced internally by the body. A 24-hour urine sample will reveal if oxalates are in excess. If so, vitamin B6 and magnesium therapy has proven very effective in preventing future stone formation, especially when combined with proper diet and other naturopathic preventive therapies.

Some diets predispose to stone formation. A strict macrobiotic diet composed primarily of grains and little fruit or vegetables causes the urine to become very concentrated and may cause stones. However, not all or even most people on strict macrobiotic diets get kidney stones.

Much more common than the strict macrobiotic diet in causing stone formation is the typical American diet having an imbalance in the calcium-to-phosphorus ratio. The ideal calcium-to-phosphorus ratio in the diet is near 0.7 parts calcium to 1 part phosphorus. Meat, for example, has anywhere from 20-50 parts phosphorus to one part calcium. Carbonated beverages and refilled foods are also very high in phosphorus. This mineral imbalance stimulates a nutritionally caused secondary hyperparathyroidism that causes increased calcium resorption from bones. This causes weak bone structure and excess calcium being handled by the kidneys, leading to stone formation. Serum calcium levels do not reflect this type of calcium deficiency–phosphorus excess syndrome, since the blood levels are kept in the normal range by the calcium taken out of the skeleton.

Excess dietary intake of protein foods high in the sulfur amino acids also can be a problem. These break down in the body to sulfate and organic acid that leads to an excess acidic environment in the kidney, which causes a reduction in calcium resorption and increased calcium excretion. This further reduces the body's calcium levels, disrupting proper calcium–phosphorus levels.

Refined salt is another common offender, causing an increase in calcium excretion and inhibiting renal calcium resorption, leading to a net calcium loss. Table salt as a condiment is an obvious source; more insidious, however, is hidden salt as found in most refined or convenience foods.

High vitamin C intake for therapeutic reasons has been suggested as a cause of kidney stones. This is disputed by many studies. Anyone on a high vitamin C intake (10 g or more daily) should also increase the supply of magnesium and vitamin B6.

Diets high in sugar and refined carbohydrates increase calcium in urine (by stimulating insulin secretion) and decrease magnesium reabsorption, creating an imbalance between calcium and magnesium, leading to stones. High-fiber diets composed of unrefined carbohydrates lower calcium in urine and reduce the chance of stones.

Gout is associated with uric acid stones that may be aggravated or caused by improper diet (see Gout).

Kidney stones are also common among those who sweat excessively. Occupations that cause extreme water loss or sports such as running can cause the urine to become too concentrated and lead to stone formation.

TREATMENT

With kidney stones, the best results are obtained when the practitioner knows exactly what type of stone is present. A 24-hour urine test will show levels of oxalate, phosphate, urate, cystein, calcium, and magnesium, which will help identify the problem. If the problem lies with uric acid, then a gout-type regimen is beneficial. If, however, oxalate levels are high and magnesium low, in all probability the vitamin B6 plus magnesium plus diet therapy will be very successful. Excess phosphorus and calcium deficiency is best determined by computer dietary analysis.

Diet

The following diet has been very successful in either acute or chronic kidney stones, as well as many other kidney complaints. Stage 1 is to be used in the acute phase until all pain has ceased for at least 24-48 hours.

Stage 1
Follow the diet set out below for 3-14 days:

On Rising
Choose one of the following:
Mullein tea, watermelon seed tea, cranberry juice (unsweetened), potassium broth.

Breakfast
Choose one of the following:
- Watermelon
- 2 fl oz (60 mL) fresh parsley juice in 4 fl oz (60 mL) carrot, celery, and cucumber juice.
- Fresh watercress, parsley, carrot, and celery juice.

Midmorning
Any of the above drinks. Alternate these two groups of liquids at 2-hour intervals. Try to have *at least 2* cups of watermelon seed tea daily in all stages of this diet. Drink as many fluids as possible during this regimen.

Stage 2
Proceed to a diet made up of only raw foods and drink at least 2–3 pints of fresh fruit juice and/or vegetable juices throughout the day.

On Rising
Choose from the following:
Fresh non-citrus fruit juice (especially cranberry juice).
Any drink under Stage 1

Breakfast
Fresh non-citrus fruit, especially watermelon, papaya, banana

Midmorning
Any liquid under Stage 1

Lunch
A raw grated salad composed primarily of leafy green vegetables such as lettuce, celery, watercress, parsley, cucumber, cabbage, etc. You may also include carrots, onions, and cooked asparagus. Alfalfa sprouts or other sprouts may also be added. A simple olive oil, or sunflower oil dressing with plenty of lemon juice, garlic, and herbs may be used. Raw goat's milk yoghurt (in later stages of diet).

Midafternoon
Same as midmorning

Supper
Same as lunch, or in later stages of diet: steamed vegetables, tofu, legumes, brown rice or millet, miso, seaweed, fish, baked potato.

Evening
Same as midmorning.

Potassium Broth
Take the outside ¼ inch (6 mm) of potato with skin, carrots, onions, garlic, cabbage, celery, and any other greens and vegetables on hand. Prepare the broth by washing and chopping the vegetables and then simmer in large covered pot of water for not more than 30–40 minutes. Strain and drink essence only, flavored if desired with pure vegetable concentrate. Excess may be stored in glass containers in refrigerator for up to 2 days.

Watermelon Seed Tea
Grind a handful of watermelon seeds. Steep in hot water for 10–15 minutes, strain. Add a little honey and drink.

Diet—Long-Term

The basis of the long-term diet is eating foods having a better calcium-to-phosphorus ratio. Include plenty of fresh vegetables, fruit, legumes, whole grains, and fermented dairy products. A vegetarian diet is highly recommended, especially to prevent recurrence of stones. Salt is strictly controlled and total protein kept at between 45–60 g daily. Increased fluid intake is encouraged.

Physiotherapy

- Mullein poultice: obtain a large amount of mullein herb. Moisten ¼ inch (6 mm) of herb with very hot water, lay on a large piece of gauze and cover with gauze or cloth. This poultice should be large enough to cover the area from the umbilicus to the pubic region in front, or over the kidney area in back. Apply the poultice and cover with hot wet towels.

Keep these as warm as possible, either by replacing the towels with a second set of heated wet towels, or use a hot water bottle or other source of heat. Keep this poultice on for 30 minutes.

- Spirits of gum turpentine pack.: alternate the mullein poultice with this pack. Mix 2 fl oz (60 mL) spirits of turpentine with 3 pints (1.5 liters) hot water. Saturate a folded towel and apply to the prescribed area (bladder to pubic area in front or kidney area in back). Apply hot wet towels as above. Apply this pack for 30 minutes at the interval prescribed. (Every 1 hour, 2 hours, or 4 hours).
- Hops and lobelia poultice, for severe pain: mix 1-2 oz of the herbs and apply as per directions for mullein poultice.
- Hot Epsom salts compress.
- Hot sitz bath for pain, to help urine flow.
- Alternate hot and cold sitz bath; tonic in chronic cases.

Therapeutic Agents

Vitamins and Minerals—Primary
- Magnesium: 100 mg 2-4 times daily. Helps keep calcium in solution, mobilizes calcium from stone. Take with B6.
- Vitamin B6: 50-200 mg twice daily. Some patients have a biochemical block in oxalic acid metabolism, due to a B6 dependency. These patients need 1000 mg of B6 or more daily to correct this problem. (*Note:* High doses of B6, if taken for a prolonged time by subjects who do not need these very high doses, can be toxic.)
- Vitamin C: less than 10 g daily. Acidifies urine, inhibiting stone formation.
- Vitamin E: 200-400 IU 2-3 times daily.
- Zinc: up to 100 mg daily. Inhibits stone formation.

Vitamins and Minerals—Secondary
- Vitamin A: 10,000-25,000 IU 3 times daily in acute cases; 1-2 times daily for chronic cases. Promotes tissue repair of urinary tract.
- Vitamin B complex: 25-50 mg 2-3 times daily.
- Potassium: 100 mg daily. Inhibits stone formation

Others—Primary
- L-arginine.
- Methionine: 250 mg 2 times daily (before food). Antioxidant, reduces incidence of stones.
- Citric acid.
- Apple cider vinegar: dissolve stones.
- Aloe vera juice: dissolves stones, and is a urinary demulcent and trophorestorative.

Others—Secondary
Essential fatty acid.
Hot water and lemon juice (to dissolve stones).
Olive oil (to help pass stones).

Botanicals—Primary
Gravel root: decoction. 1 cup 2-6 times daily to clear kidneys and dissolve stones.
Bearberry: to ease stone passage.
Couch grass: used for phosphate stones. 5-30 drops tincture 3-4 times daily.
Yarrow: to dissolve stones.
Goldenseal: anti-inflammatory, restores mucous membranes in kidneys.

Botanicals—Secondary
Aphanes.
Birch tea: dissolves stones, removes uric acid.
Chamomile: reputed to help dissolve stones.
Cleavers: to help prevent recurrence. 10-15 drops 2-3 times per day.
Horsetail.
Parsley.
Lobelia tea.
Marshmallow root tea: helps expel stones.
Lemon juice in warm water: 1 cup every half hour to relieve pain.
Other antilithics include wild carrot, celery seed, nettle, pellitory of the wall, stone root, hydrangea and crataeva.

337

Therapeutic Suggestions

The patient must increase liquid intake to 6-8 glasses (1.5-2 liters) daily to prevent a recurrence. More is needed if the person sweats heavily during work or sports, causing excessive water loss. The magnesium supplement with vitamin B6 is the most proven active ingredient of the regimen.

LEAKY GUT

DEFINITION

Leaky gut is an inflammatory condition in which the intestinal epithelial tissues lose their integrity and junctions between cells become semi-permeable, allowing abnormal reabsorption of intestinal contents, causing a wide range of internal disorders affecting the immune system, the autonomic nervous system, digestive system, respiratory and endocrine systems

SIGNS AND SYMPTOMS

Leaky gut is responsible for many signs and symptoms as discussed below.

DISCUSSION

Under normal conditions, the skin of the large bowel or colon (called the enteral mucosa) allows absorption of essential nutrients and fluids while presenting a physical and immunological barrier to the absorption of potentially harmful macromolecules and compounds such as dietary and bacterial proteins and peptides, antigens, intestinal toxins, parasites and microorganisms.

The bowel houses lots of microscopic bacteria (bugs) called "flora". In a healthy bowel, there are between 100,000,000,000 and 1,000,000,000,000, of them, in every milliliter of bowel fluid. There are between 400 and 500 different species we know of residing in the bowel, of which the best known are the *Bifidobacterium bifidum*. They are all friendly, meant to be there; each has its place within this little ecosystem, some live in the mucous lining, some on the right side, some on the left, others in the middle, some at one end, others at the other end of the colon. They communicate with us when there are imbalances, and play important roles in nutrition, digestion, including synthesis of valuable nutrients such as vitamin B5 and vitamin K, and production of valuable acids that actually nourish the enteral mucosa.

Flora also plays a vital role in immune functioning. For example, they produce natural antibiotics and anti-cancer substances. In a healthy intestinal environment, other opportunistic "bugs" cannot survive; our gut flora effectively deals with intruders, parasites, worms, etc., as a natural immunity to these things. They create "natural antibiotics"; substances that keep out unwanted micro-organisms. They are involved in detoxification, and perform a host of other beneficial activities.

There are many things that can affect the health of this floral ecosystem, such as dietary indiscretions, over-prescription of antibiotics and other drugs such as laxatives, environmental chemical exposure to over 70,000 commercially produced chemicals (many deliberately added to food, and chlorine in drinking water which kills good as well as bad bacteria), anal intercourse and stressful lifestyles. This can destroy the balance of the ecosystem, such that one can quickly end up with mucosal inflammation, allergy, and disturbances of the bowel wall barrier.

Breakdown of this barrier (called leaky gut) and consequent inflammation results in increased uptake of antigenic substances across the bowel wall, for example lipid polysaccharides from bacterial breakdown, which can cause the excessive production of nitric oxide, itself an inflammatory mediator and free radical, and this can cause energy depletion at the cellular level. There is also an increased uptake of food chemicals and toxins and increased reabsorption of metabolic wastes into the blood and lymph which contribute to the total body load of chemicals, thus placing greater demands on the body's detoxification reserves and over-stimulation of the immune system. Some of these include cadaverine, putrescine, histamine, indole, skatol, phenol, ammonia, phenyl sulfate, ptomaine, pyrrhol, isoamylamine, which can do many kinds of damage including forming systemic immune complexes and inducing antibodies capable of cross-reacting with normal body tissue. The condition is referred to as autointoxication, or endotoxinemia.

This all puts extra workload on the liver, to detoxify these circulating wastes. Pathological increase in permeability of the intestinal wall tissue is an important factor in the development of a wide range of diseases, especially diseases in which an underlying inflammatory process is part of the etiology, and has been implicated in the following: poor digestion, malnutrition (underweight), fatigue, bloating, iron deficiency anemia, food allergies or intolerances, candidiasis, acute gastroenteritis, chronic urticaria, acne, eczema and psoriasis, Crohn's disease, ulcerative colitis, irritable bowel, constipation and/or diarrhea, juvenile diabetes, cystic fibrosis, exocrine pancreatic defects, bowel and other cancers, AIDS, thyroid disorders, osteoporosis, vasculitis, joint pain and inflammation (including inflammatory joint disease), asthma, fatigue, neurological conditions such as movement disorders, schizophrenia, anxiety and depression, chronic migraine, and many autoimmune disorders such as MS, SLE, RA and ankylosing spondylitis to mention just a few.[34]

Eating yoghurt with *L. acidophilus* and *B. bifidum* daily is good as a maintenance program for ensuring healthy flora, but may not be enough if damage has been caused already. Even one course of antibiotics, or the habit of eating poultry or meat which has antibiotic residue, can be sufficient reason to supplement with Probiotics.

There are some guidelines to follow when selecting probiotics. We recommend a visit to http://www.natren.com. Do not select from the health food shelf, it is best to get a couple of professional opinions.

TREATMENT

Diet

- Dietary corrections must be made, with the elimination of all potential allergens (see Allergies and Food Intolerances).
- Eliminations must be normalized, and enemas or colonic irrigation may be needed initially, to clear out any impacted fecal matter (especially from the transverse colon).
- Worms or other intestinal parasites, if present, must be treated as part of the therapy.
- Chemicals in foods damage the endothelium, so if you can source organically grown foods, even if just for the period of treatment, you will benefit.
- Emphasis is on natural foods that are high in soluble fiber, food for gut bacteria.
- Insulin-containing foods (e.g. onions, asparagus, Jerusalem artichoke), which increase the production of propionic acid, necessary for bowel wall integrity.
- Supplement with digestive and pancreatic enzymes taken with meals.
- Avoid red meat, fish is allowed (3 meals a week) after initial cleansing diet.
- Probiotics are the basis of re-establishing the protective populations of flora.

Note: Specific drugs are known to damage the intestinal barrier, including caffeine, alcohol, aspirin, non-steroidal anti-inflammatory drugs, and antibiotics, so these must be eliminated.

Vitamins and Minerals

- Antioxidant vitamins and minerals: all of these are effective here, especially beta-carotene, C, E and zinc, selenium, oligomeric proanthocyanidins (pycnogenols), as well as vitamins B5, B6.
- Beta-carotene: 100,000 IU daily, or more if required.
- Vitamin B1: 100 mg daily and vitamin B2: 200 mg daily, to help balance the autonomic nervous system (reduce stress, promotes parasympathetic functions—i.e. digestion).
- Folic acid: 75 mg daily. Folic acid helps with DNA repair of intestinal villi.
- Vitamin C and bioflavonoids: 8 g daily, or up to bowel tolerance.
- Vitamin E: 800 IU daily.
- Zinc: 25 mg, 4 times daily.

Others

- Flaxseed oil, bee pollen, fish oils for the essential fatty acids: these down-regulate Inflammatory pathways, especially those which generate nitric oxide.
- Glucosamine: integral to bowel wall integrity.
- L-glutamine: up to 3 g daily. Specific for repair of intestinal wall since it is an energy source for the regeneration of enterocytes, colonocytes, and an immune system nutrient.
- Glutathione: antioxidant, modulates nitric oxide.
- Lipoic acid: powerful fat-soluble enzyme antioxidant, potentiates the effects of other antioxidants, mops up nitric oxide.
- Psyllium powder, slippery elm powder, aloe vera juice, guar gum: excellent sources of mucilaginous fiber from which butyric acid is produced in conjunction with flora. Butyric acid is the principal fuel for the lower intestinal and colon epithelium.
- Detoxifying amino acids: e.g. methionine, glycine, cysteine (especially in Phase 2 liver detox).

Botanicals

Calendula: for tissue repair.

Echinacea: immune system regulation.

Ginger: anti-inflammatory.

Ginkgo biloba: anti-inflammatory, inhibits PAF, reduces neutrophil infiltration and lipid peroxidation, stimulates blood flow to intestinal epithelium.

Goldenseal: mucosal trophorestorative.

Indian barberry: rich source of bio-flavonoids, especially berberine. Berberine-containing herbs can significantly improve gut wall integrity within 10 days, although full healing needs longer.

Licorice: demulcent, anti-inflammatory, anti-allergic, an immune system stimulator of interferon, antiviral, antibacterial, hepatoprotective. Contraindicated in hypertension.

Liver tonics and cholagogues: dandelion, St Mary's thistle; stimulate liver detoxification and bile secretion.

Marshmallow: intestinal demulcent.

LEG CRAMPS

DISCUSSION AND TREATMENT

Leg cramps are an extremely common and disturbing problem. They may affect the young or old, and may occur while walking, or even while in bed. In their simplest form, the cause is a single mineral imbalance. Athletes often get leg cramps due to excessive exercise and sweating, which leads to a mineral depletion. A common mistake is to replace water lost in sweating by drinking water and taking salt tablets. Although salt is lost in perspiration, it certainly is not the only complex of minerals lost. The proper replacement for such mineral loss is fresh fruit and vegetable juice. We know of one marathoner who swears by watermelon juice. Bananas are a good source of potassium. The best prevention of leg cramps due to athletic exertion and exercise perspiration is a diet high in fresh fruits, fresh vegetables, and whole grains. Potassium broth (see Appendix I) is also a useful electrolyte source.

Other forms of leg cramps are more complicated. Older age groups may suffer leg cramps associated with arteriosclerotic changes in the circulatory system and should be evaluated by a doctor well trained in cardiovascular disease. A diet similar to that found under Heart Disease is useful for long-term care. Specifically, vitamin E, 600–800 IU daily, has been found very effective in this type of condition.

Another common cause of leg cramps involves mineral imbalances in the body. Excess phosphorus in the diet from too much meat or soda drinks can be a factor, causing a relative calcium deficiency. To normalize calcium, magnesium, and phosphorus levels, reduce milk and meat proteins and increase vegetables. Hydrochloric acid deficiency may be one reason for poor calcium absorption. Calcium deficiency is often associated with leg cramps, especially when brought on by exercise. Those with dentures who find eating vegetables difficult are especially prone to magnesium and calcium deficiency and leg cramps. The only recourse in these cases is vegetable soups, potassium broth, and raw vegetable juices daily. The following supplements may be of use:

Vitamins and Minerals—Primary
- Magnesium: 500–2000 mg daily, especially for nighttime cramps.
- Calcium: 1000–1500 mg daily, especially if daytime cramps.
- Vitamin E: 600–800 IU daily, to improve vascular circulation.

Vitamins and Minerals—Secondary
- Vitamin B6: 100–250 mg daily.
- Vitamin C: up to bowel tolerance.
- Bioflavonoids: 300–1000 mg daily.
- EPA (eicosapentaenoic acid): 1–2 capsules 2–3 times daily.
- Hydrochloric acid: 5–60 grains with meals.

Botanicals—Primary
Prickly ash: a circulatory stimulant, and peripheral vasodilator.
Wild yam: spasmolytic, anti-inflammatory.
Cramp bark: spasmolytic.
Cinchona: spasmolytic.

Botanicals—Secondary
Pulsatilla: spasmolytic, nervine.
Valerian: spasmolytic, nervine.

LOW BACK PAIN
(Sciatica, Lumbar Disc Herniation or Prolapse)

DEFINITION

Sciatica: neuralgia and neuritis of the sciatic nerve.
Lumbar disc herniation: a bulging of the nucleus pulposus against a weakened segment of the annulus fibrosus.

Lumbar disc prolapse: an actual breach of the annulus fibrosus by nuclear material.

341

SYMPTOMS

Pain or ache in the low back; pain, ache, or altered sensation in the buttocks, thigh, calf, and foot. Muscle wasting may occur late in course, along with reduced reflexes and muscle weakness.

ETIOLOGICAL CONSIDERATIONS

- Poor body mechanics and posture
  Improper lifting, sitting, standing, carrying; lumbar lordosis; weak abdominal muscles; visceroptosis; high heels; insufficient stretching out before working or lifting
- Sedentary life, lack of exercise, weak muscles and excess weight
- Poor nutrition
  Protein deficiency; calcium deficiency; green vegetable deficiency; poor bone, cartilage, ligament, and muscle development
- Bone alterations
  Osteoporosis; ankylosing spondylitis; spondylolisthesis; congenital abnormalities; osteoarthritis; gouty arthritis; rheumatoid arthritis; Paget's disease
- Trauma
  Fracture; ligament or muscle strain; overuse; microtrauma
- Short leg syndrome (real or apparent)
- Spinal dysfunction
  Lumbar, lumbar-sacral, sacroiliac; facet lock syndrome; true disc lesion
- Spinal imbalance
  Flat feet; ankle, knee, hip disorders; iliopsoas, gluteals, paravertebral muscles, plus others; hypomobility or hypermobility
- Referred pain
  Menstrual, gynecological; kidneys; bladder; prostate; colon; ulcer; appendix
- Metabolic (calcium/mineral loss)
  Adrenals; pituitary; parathyroids (hyperparathyroidism); rickets; menopause
- Infection (local or systemic)
- Tumor
- Pregnancy

DISCUSSION

Backache with or without sciatica is one of the most common complaints a doctor deals with in his or her practice. Osteopathic physicians see these cases daily. As you can see from the above list of possible causative factors, back pain is far from a simple disorder. A complete individual case history is essential to allow for proper diagnosis and treatment.

To simplify this discussion we shall concentrate on back pain related primarily to the osteopathic spinal lesion, or "somatic dysfunction" as it is now called (see Spinal Manipulation, page 49), and also that caused by a true disc herniation or prolapse. We will omit back pain due to congenital abnormalities, degenerative arthritis, infection, metabolic disorders, cancer, referred syndromes, and so on. These, however, must always be considered when dealing with acute or chronic back pain.

Although two main syndromes of back pain exist (spinal lesion or "somatic dysfunction" and disc), their causes are often similar. To understand more about why a good back turns bad, first we have to learn a little about how the back is designed to function. The spinal column is basically a stack of specifically designed bones separated by resilient disc cushions. Each disc is made up of a firm, fibrous outer covering, the *annulus fibrosus,* and a softer gelatinous inner core, the *nucleus pulposus.* Each vertebra is uniquely shaped according to its relative position in the spine and its function. There are two areas called *apophygeal facets* where the vertebra approximates the vertebra above and two facets for the approximation below. These facets allow the vertebrae to glide across each other and by their shape and location limit them to certain ranges of motion. Thus, in the neck, these facets allow good overall mobility with relative freedom in rotation, flexion, extension, and side bending, while in the lumbar region the angles of the facets allow free flexion and side bending but severely restrict movement of rotation.

Further controls are placed on spinal movements by strong ligaments that connect adjacent vertebrae together and also bind together groups of vertebrae and ultimately the entire spine. Strong muscles also interconnect the spine to provide both support and the possibility of motion. A series of 31 spinal nerves pass out of spaces between each vertebra.

The problem in the typical bad back involves one of two processes. Either the vertebral functional unit (two adjacent vertebrae and their connective tissue components) is in distress and no longer relating to each other as designed with the disc remaining normal; or the functional unit distress may include disc damage. The difference in severity of these two syndromes is extreme. Any back disorder that includes disc damage is much more difficult to cure and has a higher likelihood of recurring and causing prolonged disability. In reality, disc injuries never heal in the accepted definition of the term. Once they have been damaged, that damage is permanent. That does not necessarily mean, however, that the patient will always be in pain or suffer from disc-related symptoms. Many patients with permanent disc injuries can attain a completely pain-free existence with proper osteopathic care, exercise and a little restraint in their work or play activities.

Many people with bad backs report only trivial motions as the initial cause of their complaint. These include bending over to pick up a sock, touching their toes, opening a window, or even washing their faces. These minor incidences are, however, not the real cause, only the "last straw" in a long list of spinal stress. Except in the case of severe, acute trauma, the real cause of most spinal complaints has less to do with what you did today or yesterday and more with what you have been doing or *not* doing over the last 5–10 years.

The most influential factors in developing a weak back are poor spinal mechanics accompanied by poor muscle tone. The body was designed to function according to clearly defined principles established by the shape of our vertebrae and the manner in which they fit together into three distinct spinal curves. These curves, the cervical (neck), thoracic (midback), and lumbar (low back), allow us to function in the upright position and give us a degree of stability. They are essential to maintain a good center of gravity and to help balance and compensate for carrying our heads erect. Without properly balanced spinal curves, the human frame would be incredibly unstable, capable of toppling over with a strong wind.

In the normal posture, the spinal curves leave the vertebrae and their muscular supports in what can be called a neutral condition. The vertebrae are floating free under no pressure and all supporting muscles are in their gently tonic state. If, through habitual slouching in sitting or standing, walking with high heels, obesity, or by a weakening of the muscles of spinal support, the spinal curves become exaggerated (or reduced), a series of extremely important changes takes places. Muscles which previously were at ease must shorten or lengthen to accommodate for this new position and some must actively contract to counterbalance changes in weight distribution. Ultimately, prolonged contraction of any muscle leads to a shortening and hardening of the muscle fibers, creating ropy fibrous bands instead of healthy flexible muscle.

Over a period of time even the individual vertebra will change in shape in an attempt to minimize stresses. These changes cause localized or referred pains in the manner of the osteopathic somatic dysfunction (see Spinal Manipulation, page 49). The disc also is placed under unusual stresses, which seem to be a factor in its premature degeneration, leading to less elasticity and loss of fluid content. This accelerated wear and tear, along with weakened ligaments and muscles, allows the gelatinous inner nucleus to push against and cause a bulge (herniation) in the outer fibrous covering. Eventually, the inner nucleus breaches this barrier, forming a true disc prolapse when an extra burden is placed on the spine, as in improper lifting or bending. The result is usually an acutely painful and debilitating nerve pinch, most commonly of the sciatic nerve, causing both local and referred pain, or altered sensations in the gluteal region and down the leg.

TREATMENT

Even a normal spine can suffer acute injury due to a fall, auto accident, sudden, unusual or extreme movement, or other traumatic cause. The cause of pain may simply be a result of muscle or ligament strain, in which case rest and proper physiotherapy are all that is needed. Many cases, however, are complicated by what is often called "facet lock syndrome". What occurs here is that the vertebrae become fixed in the extremes of their normal physiological motion and are splinted in place by muscle spasm. Usually it is the very small muscles that control movement of the spine that first go into spasm and then limit spinal movement. Larger muscle groups usually follow into spasm. The pain is usually severe and sudden but often becomes less severe after a week or two if left untreated. Unfortunately, this lessening of pain is often misinterpreted by the patient to mean that full cure is soon to follow. In reality, what is occurring is that the acute "hot" lesion is now "cooling" to become a chronic one. If proper spinal manipulation is not received, this area can be a cause of future distress locally and in referred areas related to the nervous supply of that segment. Muscles that have contracted will begin to shorten and remain a source of spinal movement limitation. Secondary changes in other spinal levels will also occur as the body attempts to re-establish a semblance of spinal balance. For example, if a vertebra in your neck becomes fixed in its rotation to the right, your body might accommodate by fixing one of your other neck, midback, or lumbar vertebrae to the left to keep your head pointing forward. A good rule to go by is that if a minor sore back does not significantly recover with rest after 24–48 hours, then it needs professional treatment. All severe back complaints need to be seen as soon as possible. In general, the longer you wait for treatment, the longer that treatment will take to restore health.

Acute low back pain may also be caused by disc herniation or prolapse. This may have a well-recognized cause, such as attempts at lifting a heavy object, such as a refrigerator or piano, or it may result from trivial motions such as those mentioned earlier. Irrespective of the amount of effort responsible for the actual disc rupture or prolapse, the symptoms are the same. The onset of pain may be gradual over several hours or sudden. The most commonly affected discs are between L3 to L4, L4 to L5, and L5 to sacrum. Common symptoms include pain and numbness in low back, buttocks, thighs, calf, and foot; muscle weakness in thigh, calf, or foot; reduced reflexes; muscle wasting in thigh or calf; and if severe, disorders in function of either bowels or bladder. Most cases of acute disc lesions are preceded by a history of chronic backache. If this structural distress had been listened to and preventive measures begun, no disc rupture would probably have occurred. The only way to prevent back disorders is to keep the body in good muscle tone, and in proper spinal mechanics and use.

The muscles that support the back span from head to toe. If any one group of muscles becomes lax or overtight, other bone and muscle relationships elsewhere in the body will be altered. Even flat feet may be the primary cause in the history of a low back complaint. This is why we recommend full-scale body stretching and toning to prevent back problems. In practice, however, specific muscle groups are more important than others. Certainly, the muscles of the back and gluteal region are important, but most people are surprised to find out that one of the main supports for the back is found in the front—the abdominal muscles. The most common muscular weakness found in the average back patient is weak abdominal tone.

The following exercises have been used quite successfully in treating and preventing back complaints. It is difficult to emphasize adequately just how essential they are. Along with rest, proper physiotherapy, and appropriate spinal therapy performed by a qualified spinal specialist (osteopath, chiropractor, or naturopath), these exercises are responsible for saving millions from extremely expensive, often ineffective spinal surgery.

Back Exercises

Be careful not to overdo these exercises in the beginning, especially if you are presently suffering from an acute low back complaint. Do not be alarmed if the exercises cause some mild discomfort which lasts for a few minutes. If the pain is more than mild and persists for 10–20 minutes, stop their use and consult your doctor. Do the exercises on a firm surface covered with a thin foam cushion or folded towel. As the old proverb says, "Perseverance brings good fortune."

Standard Position

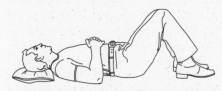

Lie on back with a small pillow under your head and both knees bent.

Knee to Chest

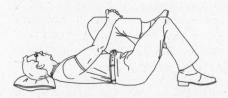

Draw your knee slowly to your chest as far as possible without excessive pain. Hold for 5 seconds and then return to starting position. Repeat four times with each leg individually, and then with both legs simultaneously. Use your legs, not your arms, to

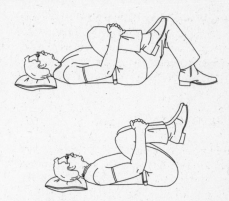

raise legs to chest. The arms are for balance and slight stretching. This exercise stretches the entire low back.

Pelvic Tilt

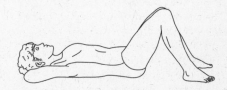

While lying in the standard position simply tighten your buttock muscles and tilt your pelvis up. This will flatten the low back against the floor. Do not try to flatten the spine by contracting your abdominal muscles or legs, but confine the exercise as much as possible to the gluteal (buttock) muscles, squeezing them together tightly.

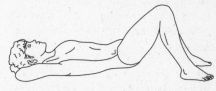

Each contraction is held 5 seconds and then relaxed, gradually working up to 10 or more repetitions. This exercise strengthens the buttock muscles and helps reduce swayback (lordosis). You will also find several other examples of the pelvic tilt exercise in the section on Scoliosis. We often advise patients to contract their gluteal (buttocks) muscles while doing this exercise, to help correct excess lumbar lordosis (sway back) or in

345

cases where the disc degeneration or disc bulge is so severe that it is causing sciatica.

Trunk Stretch

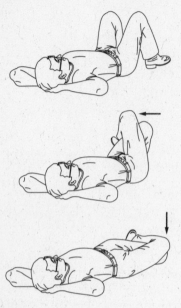

Start in the standard position. Cross right leg over left just above the knee and use this weight as a lever to help rotate leg towards the floor as far as comfortably possible. Hold for 5 seconds. Repeat with other leg. Repeat exercise five times for each leg. Always keep the upper back flat against the floor. This exercise stretches the muscles on both sides of the spine.

Raised Pelvic Tilt

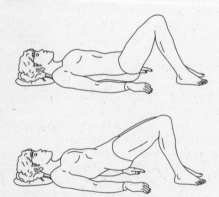

Lie in standard position and perform the pelvic tilt, but continue the contraction to include the buttocks and abdominal muscles so that the hips raise off the floor. Hold for 6-8 seconds and slowly relax. Repeat 5-10 times.

Sit-Ups

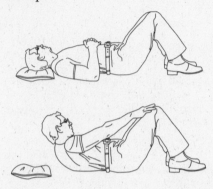

Begin in the standard position and slowly raise head, neck, and upper torso, reaching for your knees. Do not raise mid-back or lower back. Maintain this position with hands positioned gently on the knees for 5-6 seconds and slowly relax. Do not grasp knees. Repeat 5-10 times. As these sit-ups become easier to perform, place your lower legs up to the knee on the seat of a chair, making a right angle with your thighs. Keeping your arms across your chest, do half sit-ups that cause your low back to barely rise off the floor, but no further. You do not have to hold this sit-up. Try to do 150-300 of this type of sit-up daily—half in the morning and half in the evening. Of all the back exercises we know, this is the most effective, if done as pre-scribed. We have seen very bad back complaints improve dramatically. Time and perseverance are essential.

Sit-Up with Chair

Chose a rather low-seated chair and either have an assistant hold you feet securely, or use a strap. This is a more advanced sit-up, but very useful for low back problems.

Initially just do little half sit-ups. Start with 10-15 and gradually work up to 60.

Later as your back improves you can advance to the full sit-up with rotation. Aim at 40–60 repetitions daily.

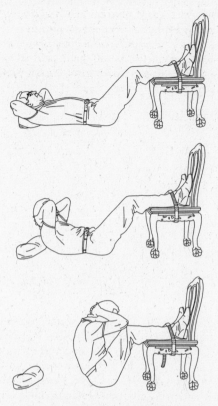

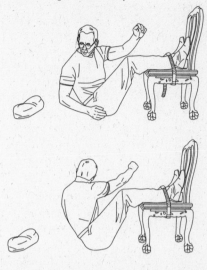

Later as the half sit-ups become easier you may progreess to full sit-ups. Aim to be able to do 40–60 daily.

If you allow your arms to extend back over your head you will mobilize and loosen you midback with each sit-up.

Neck Strengthening

Often patients who also have problems with their neck must first do a few weeks of neck strengthening exercises to prepare themselves to be able to do the sit-up exercises outlined above. You will find no better exercises for this purpose than the ones Sanford advises in his book *Old Age: Its Cause And Prevention*.

Hamstring Stretch

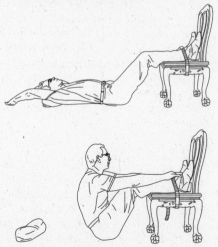

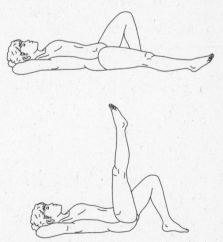

Starting from the standard position stretch out the right leg flat against the floor. Slowly raise the leg as far as you can until a sensation of pain or tightness occurs in the back of your thigh. Hold for 5 seconds and slowly lower leg. Repeat 5-10 times with each leg. Make sure to keep the back flat against the floor and do not use hands or arms as leverage. This exercise helps stretch the hamstring muscles, which get very tight with all back problems.

Knee to Nose

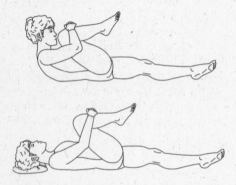

From the starting position bring one knee slowly to the chest, clasp it with both hands and extend the opposite leg until it lies flat on the floor. While keeping the low back flat to the floor, slowly raise head, neck, and upper shoulders forward until the nose touches the knee, or as far as comfortably possible. Hold 5-6 seconds and slowly relax. Repeat with both legs 5-10 times. This exercise helps stretch the flexors of the hip on the opposite side of the leg used and also will help strengthen the abdominal muscles.

Hamstring and Achilles Stretch

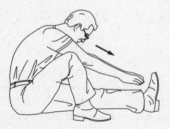

Begin in the sitting position with one knee bent and the other leg flat against the floor with sole of foot firmly placed against the wall. Slowly bend forward until a stretch is felt behind your leg. Hold 5-6 seconds and relax. Repeat 5-10 times with each leg.

Standing Calf And Achilles Stretch

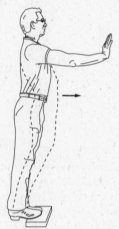

Place front half of foot across a thick book placed 1½ ft (50 cm) from the wall. Place arms against the wall, and with legs kept straight, lean forward towards the wall until the calves and Achilles tendon begin to stretch. Hold 5-6 seconds. Repeat 10-15 times.

Standing Hamstring Stretch

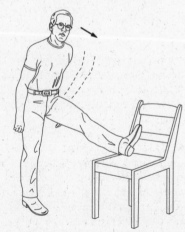

From a standing position place the heel on a low chair. Keeping both legs straight, slowly lean forward until you feel the hamstring muscles stretch. Repeat with both legs 5-10 times.

Iliopsoas Stretch

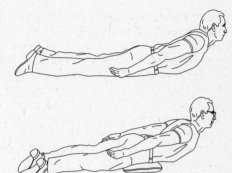

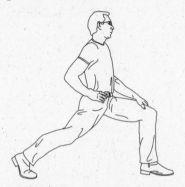

From a standing position place one foot forward as far as you can with knee bent. Make sure front and rear feet point forward. Rock forward, stretching out the anterior thigh muscles, hip, groin, and iliopsoas muscle.

Hyperextension of Hip

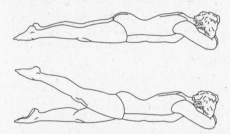

Lie on stomach and raise one leg, with knee unflexed. Hold 4-6 seconds and slowly lower. Repeat 5-10 times with each leg. This exercise helps strengthen low back and buttock muscles.

Low Back Extension

Lie on stomach with hands along the side. Slowly raise the head and chest from the floor. Hold 4-6 seconds and then slowly lower. Rest and repeat 10 times. An advanced form of this exercise is to place a

pillow under the hips and perform the same exercise.

Patients with disc bulges (not prolapsed discs) will often find that extention exercise relieves or entirely eliminates sciatic pain. Many dics problems are the result of forward-bending occupations which gradually cause a weakness in the disc so that it bulges posteriorly, placing pressure on the nerve roots.

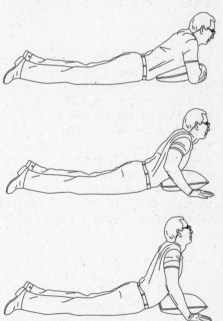

The following extension exercises can be very useful. Begin with about 15 minutes in the first position with a small pillow under your chest. If you find that the sciatic pain gradually becomes less severe, you may progress to the more advanced extension exercises that follow. If your sciatic pains *increase* with this exercise, discontinue.

Hip Roll

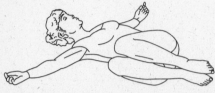

Lie on the back with arms out at your sides. Bend knees with feet close to buttocks. Slowly roll both knees to one side towards the floor while keeping knees close to chest. Slowly return to starting position and repeat on opposite side. Repeat entire exercise 4-8 times.

Physiotherapy

- Interferential electrotherapy: this modality is very useful in acute stages of low back pain either due to simple sprain/strain or disc injuries. It is best applied 2-3 times weekly when back pain is severe.
- Diathermy: Short-wave diathermy is very useful in nearly all types of low back pain, even acute disc injury. It needs to be applied 2-3 times a week in acute cases.
- Ultrasound: this physiotherapy modality has been found very useful in the acute stages of low back pain. Ultrasound is more useful with muscular involvement and best avoided in acute disc injury.
- Ice packs: usually the application of ice in the first 24 hours will be the most beneficial. Make sure not to apply this for too long a period and thus injure the tissues. Ice should be applied for 10-30 minutes with 10-30 minutes between applications. Disc injuries usually respond best to ice or cold application even in later stages of the problem. This acts to help reduce the inflammation around the sciatic nerve.

- Spinal manipulation:
- Complete rest: many acute low back complaints, and especially those with disc lesions, require complete bed rest for the first 24-48 hours after the injury. Do absolutely *nothing* except go to the bathroom. Make sure bowels stay loose and prevent constipation by following a light diet with laxative-type foods. Straining will aggravate the condition. Make sure the bed is extremely supportive, or lay the mattress directly on the floor.
- Heat: local moist heat will help in later stages to loosen tight spinal muscles and give pain relief. Ready-made hydrocolator packs are the most convenient applications but they are not always available. For home use apply hot moist towels, folded several times. These may be placed steaming hot over 2-4 dry layers of towels and then covered with several more layers to retain heat. The thicker the folded wet towel, the longer it will retain its heat. Lie on your back with a large pillow under your knees and a thin one to support your lower back; or on the side with legs drawn up in the semi-fetal position. Care must be taken when applying heat to prevent the tissues from becoming congested with blood. Follow heat applications with the gentle spinal stretching exercises previously described. Excessive use of heat will cause stagnation of fluids and slow healing. In later stages alternate hot and ice-cold applications will be useful to stimulate circulation and healing.
- Hops and lobelia hot compress: for pain relief.
- Warm Epsom salts baths (see Appendix I): very relaxing and antispasmodic.
- Olbas rub.

Therapeutic Agents

Vitamins and Minerals
- Vitamin C: 3000-10,000 mg daily, or to bowel tolerance. Essential for health of connective tissue (disc).

- Vitamin B complex: 25–50 mg twice daily.
- Vitamin B1: 100 mg plus B12, 1 mg intramuscular injection twice per week for 2 weeks, then once a week.
- Vitamin E: 400 IU twice daily.
- Calcium/magnesium in ratio of 2:1 (i.e. 800 mg calcium to 400 mg magnesium).

Others

- Bromelain: 2–3 tablets 3 times daily, taken on an empty stomach only.
- DL-phenylalanine: analgesic, better than aspirin for pain. Increases release of endogenous endorphin-like substances.

General

Lose weight.

MASTITIS (Acute)

DEFINITION

Inflammation of the breast and milk duct system, usually due to infection by staphylococci invading a fissured or cracked nipple. (Not included in this section is fibrocystic breast disease, sometimes called cystic mastitis)

SYMPTOMS

Pain, redness, hard swelling, fever, abscess, and possibly swollen cervical and/or axillary lymph nodes.

ETIOLOGICAL CONSIDERATIONS

- Lack of proper nipple preparation prior to lactation
- Engorged breast, early postpartum or on weaning
- Incomplete emptying in feeding
- Shallow grip on nipple by infant
- Blocked duct
- Nipple fissure with secondary infection
- Poor nipple care and hygiene
- Irritating clothing

DISCUSSION

Acute mastitis is most common during lactation and usually due to invasion of a cracked nipple by bacteria. It occurs frequently in the first week postpartum, due to the combination of poor nipple preparation in the final 2–3 months of pregnancy, breast engorgement due to incomplete emptying, and excessive sucking by the newborn. A further major cause is a blocked milk duct, which may occur at any time during lactation and cause localized engorgement, inflammation, and infection.

Prevention and early treatment of mastitis is essential to avoid the need for antibiotics. Prevention of mastitis begins even before the baby is delivered. For a period of 2–3 months the prospective mother must get her nipples ready for lactation. She should massage her nipples daily with chickweed ointment. Vitamin E also may be used. She should also perform the "nipple pull" several times daily during a shower and dry off with a semi-rough towel.

As soon as the baby is born, the mother must be careful not to feed for overly long periods, to avoid maceration of her tender nipples. Be sure to break suction of infant's mouth on breast by inserting a finger into the corner of infant's mouth, not just pulling nipple out of infant's mouth. After her feeds, she should empty her breast manually or with a breast pump until supply and demand reach an equilibrium. Nipple cleanliness is important and nipples should be gently washed after each feed, if possible. Obviously this is not always possible. Clothing worn next to the breast should always be soft and non-irritating.

TREATMENT

Prompt and energetic treatment is essential to prevent abscess formation and avoid the use of antibiotics. The essentials of treatment involve mostly botanical medications, both internal and external. Apply Phytolacca (poke root) ointment frequently (every 2 hours) externally to all but the nipple itself. Phytolacca tincture should be taken internally. The usual dose is 25 drops diluted in water, 4-6 times daily. Hot compresses of calendula lotion or calendula lotion plus Phytolacca should be applied every 2-4 hours. You may also wish to apply a calendula compress continually for extended periods of 4-6 hours or all night. This may be done by diluting calendula lotion in warm water (50/50 or a higher concentration), saturating a gauze or cotton diaper with the solution, and applying it to the breast.

Other herbal treatments include:

Cabbage leaf poultice: (use fresh cabbage leaves, tuck into brassiere).

Clay packs.

Jaborandi: for blocked duct, internal and external

Castor oil: massage of blocked duct. May also use warm packs.

Dandelion plus onion bulb poultice.

Plantain poultice.

Barberry.

Dandelion and coneflower: internal.

Green onion poultice.

Echinacea: 25 drops of the tincture 3-4 times daily. Best taken with *Phytolacca*.

Therapeutic Agents

Vitamins and Minerals— Primary

- Vitamin C: high doses, 500-1000 mg 4-8 times daily.
- Vitamin A: 10,000-25,000 IU 2-6 times daily.
- Vitamin E: internal, plus external massage.
- Thymus tablets.

Note: Opinion is divided as to the advisability of breast-feeding during the infection. Each case must be evaluated individually; however, continuation of breast-feeding will cause no harm to the infant and is the most efficient method of emptying the breast. Should the breast remain full after feeding, or the infant go off the breast voluntarily, it must be emptied by a breast pump.

MÉNIÈRE'S DISEASE

DEFINITION AND SYMPTOMS

A recurrent and usually progressive disorder characterized by severe vertigo, progressive deafness, ringing in the ears (tinnitus), and a sensation of fullness in the ears.

ETIOLOGICAL CONSIDERATIONS

The cause is considered unknown. Edema of the membranous labyrinth has been found in autopsy. Other postulated factors include disturbed carbohydrate metabolism, excessive salt intake, allergy, stress, viruses, infections, toxic or accumulative, or hormonal intolerances. Symptoms exactly like Ménière's disease can be caused by a cholesteotoma (a tumor-like growth that can erode into the central nervous system from the middle ear if not diagnosed soon enough). Anyone with the symptoms of Ménière's disease should be examined by a specialist to rule out other causes.

DISCUSSION

The only clear pathological condition found in these cases has been swelling of the membranous labyrinth (semicircular canals of the middle ear), with upsets of the balance center. Naturopathic treatments often can help reverse such congestion through diet and lifestyle changes, local physiotherapy, spinal or cranial adjustments, and homeopathy.

One interesting note on Ménière's disease is that occasionally this condition may be a misdiagnosed case of salicylate sensitivity from excessive self-medication of aspirin. This can cause deafness, ringing in the ears, dizziness, headache, vomiting, confusion, and hyperventilation in later stages. It is easy to see how these symptoms could cause confusion. We have seen elderly patients with arthritis who had been diagnosed as also having Ménière's disease, that on aspirin withdrawal had all the symptoms relieved.

High blood insulin levels have also been associated with this disease, and a hypoglycemic diet ought to be followed for 3 weeks to see if there is an improvement in the condition.

TREATMENT

Diet

A general cleansing regimen is usually greeted with rapid results. Fasting for 3–7 days on vegetable juices every 6 weeks is alternated with a diet high in nutrient-rich foods, composed of plenty of raw and cooked vegetables, seaweed, sprouts, seeds, nuts, beans, low-fat yoghurt, and fish. Although this diet is what can be called nonspecific, it is also very effective. We suspect irritants in the diet such as coffee, salt, fried foods, alcohol, and any drugs, and routinely remove these from the diet. The general tonic influence of this diet regimen, along with a better calcium-to-phosphorus ratio,

can only benefit health. Often all that is needed to reverse a health disorder is the removal of obstacles to the body's own self-regulating healing powers.

Physiotherapy

- Exercise: must be gradually increased, to increase circulation to the head. Any exercise will do as long as it aims at increased respiration and improved blood flow.
- Alternate hot and cold head baths: taken once or twice daily will help local circulation and drainage. Use two bowls of water, one very warm and the other ice-cold. Immerse the entire upper head up to and including the ears and jaw area in the warm water for 30 seconds to 1 minute. Follow with the ice-cold immersion. For severe cases, for the elderly, or for anyone with a heart condition, begin with less extreme water temperatures and gradually build up to the ice-cold water.
- Spinal and/or cranial manipulation: should be done once or twice weekly, to help improve local circulation, enervation, and nutrition.

Therapeutic Agents

Vitamins and Minerals— Primary

- Bioflavonoids, especially quercetin: 300–1000 mg, 3–4 times daily.
- Vitamin C: (deficiency problems are often coincidental) 4–6 g daily in divided doses.
- Vitamin E: 400–800 IU daily.
- Vitamin B3 (niacin): 100–200 mg daily, time release (will cause flushing sensation).
- Manganese: 5–10 mg daily.
- Chromium picolinate: 200 mcg daily to help control blood sugar levels.

Vitamins and Minerals—Secondary

- Vitamin A: 25,000–50,000 IU 1–2 times daily.
- Vitamin B complex: 50 mg 1–2 times daily.
- Vitamin B6: 100–400 mg daily.
- Calcium/magnesium: 1:1 ratio. 1000–1500 mg each daily.

Others—Primary

- Coenzyme Q10: 100 mg daily. Improves circulation.
- Essential fatty acids: evening primrose oil and flaxseed oil.

Others—Secondary

- Lithium: 2–3 mg daily.
- Glucosamine.

- Homoeopathic arsenicum, salicylic acid, silicea, and nat. sulf.
- For antinausea: ginger and/or peppermint teas.

Botanicals—Primary

Ginkgo biloba: circulatory stimulant of blood to the head.
Ginger: anti-inflammatory.

Botanicals—Secondary

Ground ivy: anti-catarrhal.
Goldenseal: anti-catarrhal.
Bilberry: contains important OPCs (antioxidants).
Gotu kola.

MENOPAUSAL PROBLEMS
(Change of Life, Climacteric)

DEFINITION

The transitional change in a woman's life when menstrual function ceases. Menopause occurs generally between the ages of 45-55, as a result of reduced estrogen and progesterone production by the ovaries.

SYMPTOMS

These may include amenorrhea, irregularity, increased flow, vasomotor instability, hot flushes and cold sweating, palpitation, vertigo, tingling, chills, nervousness, excitability, depression, fatigue, irritability, insomnia, headaches, muscle and bone aches, and gastrointestinal or urinary disturbances. Later there may be osteoporosis, urinary frequency, stress incontinence, unwanted hair, and drying of vaginal secretions resulting in painful coitus and vaginitis; also, obesity, pruritus, dry skin, reduced breast size, and loss of vaginal elasticity.

ETIOLOGICAL CONSIDERATIONS—PRIMARY

- Adrenal exhaustion
  Hypoglycemia; refined carbohydrates, sugar, coffee, stress
- Diet deficiency
  Calcium, vitamin D, magnesium, and phosphorus; vitamin B complex; vitamin E; others
- Thyroid malfunction
  Thyroid/parathyroid imbalance
- Surgical menopause
  Causes most severe menopausal symptoms, especially if both ovaries are removed.

ETIOLOGICAL CONSIDERATIONS— SECONDARY

Lack of exercise; psychological factors; poor absorption and digestion (Hydrochloric acid deficiency)

DISCUSSION

Much has been written about the female menopause which has turned it into a time of terror, a time of loss, a time of the start of the downhill run home. The whole notion that a woman somehow "loses" something worth keeping at menopause needs to be questioned. After all, fertility hormones are part of her fertility cycle, and the cessation of her cycle ought to be seen as entirely natural, and indeed a welcomed change within her body, a rite of passage, a veritable "passage to power" as Leslie Kenton calls it. The fertility cycle is only one part of a female's life. Hormone changes are the essence of the natural process of leaving fertility behind, and without any treatment, herbal or pharmaceutical, the symptoms of menopause invariably diminish once the body has adjusted to the different and lower level of hormones that after all is appropriate for the non-reproductive years. Menopause is nature's contraceptive. It is not a disease and the whole idea of supplementing or artificially replacing these hormones after the fertility cycle is over is contrary to nature and contrary to health.

The fact is that menopause was intended by nature to be a gradual process of reduced estrogen output by the ovaries with few, if any, side effects. In the normal, healthy, well-nourished and active woman, the pituitary sends signals to the other glands such as the adrenals, and fat tissue to increase their estrogen (estrone) output. This backup system helps to keep some estrogen in the circulation, and helps further maintain a portion of the secondary sexual characteristics. It is only when the adrenal glands are exhausted from poor diet, diet deficiency,

hypoglycemia, and stress that this backup system may fail, leading to the sudden and severe physiological changes now accepted as "normal" for the menopausal western woman.

The psychological symptoms of menopausal distress are caused by previous emotional instabilities present prior to menopause. These may be aggravated by insecurities resulting from much negative education about "the change", and fears of a loss of natural feminine attractiveness.

Estrogen is used in various forms as medication to help halt the menopausal syndrome. Studies have questioned its effectiveness however. In double-blind studies where estrogen was used in one group and a placebo in another, there was no significant statistical difference in the groups, as far as effectiveness in relieving typical menopausal complaints, which led some to suggest that receiving any tablet from the doctor will help relieve many menopausal complaints as long as you believe it will work. This is incredibly insensitive in this context, because for many women menopause can be a difficult time.

New research has challenged assumptions about the importance of estrogen alone in maintaining women's hormonal balance. Rather than being deficient in estrogen, many women produce too much estrogen, or develop increased estrogen sensitivity, which throws out the balance with progesterone and other hormones. Under the influence of anovulatory cycles (where no ovulation occurs, e.g. menopause, stress, malnourishment, anorexia), progesterone production is suppressed, or ceases, and the effect of estrogen dominance can be observed. So over the past decade, estrogen has been variously combined with progesterone (progestogen) and given long-term in the belief it will help prevent osteoporosis (see Osteoporosis). In fact, this is the primary reason given to postmenopausal women, that if they take this stuff they won't get osteoporosis. The truth is, that while low progesterone level is one factor, it is not the primary factor as our discussion of osteoporosis shows.

HRT has not been proven to be safe, and most women are really surprised to learn of the very real and potential hazards of HRT. There has not been a long-term study of the effects of HRT.

Estrogen replacement therapy is contraindicated for women with a history of uterine fibroids, enlarged or fibrocystic breasts, endometriosis, endometrial or breast cancer, liver disease, thrombosis, varicose veins, hypertension or diabetes. Estrogen replacement can also provoke a relative progesterone deficiency, and that is why estrogen therapy is not to be taken for anything other than a short time, no more than 12–18 months. HRT also creates nutritional stress, as it increases the body's need of vitamin B complex, pyridoxine, folic acid, vitamins C and E, and it reduces zinc levels.

There is no evidence that newer HRT drugs are safer than they used to be a few years ago. Today, manufacturers of HRT products give a combined total of more than 124 potential risks and problems, many of which are serious, even fatal (MIMS Annual 1996). The following information has been gleaned from industry literature and warnings by pharmaceutical manufacturers themselves about their products; any one or several of the following can occur in any woman taking HRT.

Adverse Reactions to Pharmaceutical Estrogens

External: skin rashes, irritation, patches, allergic reactions, dark or red pigmentation, spots or lumps, acne, sensitivity to light, hair loss, unwanted hair growth.

Internal: nausea, abdominal pain, bloating, anorexia, vomiting, abdominal cramps, uterine spasm, jaundice, gallstones, changes in liver enzymes, breakthrough bleeding, change in menstrual flow, period pain, pain on urinating, inflamed vagina, uterine growth, fibroids and increase in fibroid sizes, reactivation of endometriosis, change in vaginal secretions, cystitis-like syndrome, breast swelling, tenderness or secretions, changes in libido, PMT-like syndrome,

painful sex, leg pain, tinnitus (ringing in ears), migraine, headaches, depression, nervousness, irritability, inflamed nerve tissue, mood swings, increased appetite, weight change, rise in blood sugar, reduced glucose tolerance (sugar metabolism), rise in blood pressure, thrombosis and other clotting disorders, palpitations, aggravation of varicose veins, muscle and bone pains, spasms, fluid retention.

Adverse Reactions to Pharmaceutical Progestogens

Blood clotting disorders, inflamed veins, cerebral hemorrhage, increase in platelet activity nervousness, insomnia, unusual fatigue, depression, drowsiness, dizziness, headache, tremor, incoordination, rash, itching, acne, unwanted hair growth, hair loss, sweating, fever, liver tumors, abdominal pain, jaundice, hepatitis, gallstones, nausea, appetite changes, breast tenderness, breast secretions, changes in cervical erosion and secretions, Cushing's syndrome, weight gain, swelling of ankles and feet, increase in blood pressure, changes in calcium and potassium levels and liver enzymes, shock reactions.

Getting off HRT

If you want to come off these pharmaceutical hormones—or if you have a medical reason that makes it necessary, there are 3 possible outcomes:

1. You won't notice anything different or unusual.
2. You'll feel better.
3. You'll experience mild to severe withdrawal symptoms of various kinds that could last a few days, weeks or even longer. Your body has been swamped with hormones, and now it has to switch on its own natural production. Flushing is the most common withdrawal symptom.

Generally, it is preferable to taper down the HRT dose over a period of time, for example, over a one month period for each year you have been on the drugs. So if you have been on hormone replacement for 6 years, you might take 6 months to wean yourself off it. However, you may wish to make the transition more rapidly. To make the transition easier, herbal preparations can be of great assistance in reducing any side effects.

Coping with Menopause Naturally

Certain physiological changes do, however, occur in varying degrees as estrogen levels are reduced. The most predictable of these are a slight reduction in vaginal elasticity, and a lessening of its natural lubrication. For some women this can cause some pain with sexual intercourse. This is easily corrected by using an artificial lubricant, and should not limit sexual activity in the least. Far from reducing sexual drive, menopause often increases sexual desire by making the clitoris more sensitive, even though it often does reduce in size. Hot flushes and cold sweats due to vasomotor instability may be corrected by proper diet, exercise, vitamin E supplements, taurine or tryptophan.

These days with the great knowledge of health and herbal medicine that naturopaths can offer, managing menopause naturally and drug-free becomes an adventure into health and happiness for the later years. There are many other health considerations as one goes through "the change", and we present some of these for your consideration.

TREATMENT

The following considerations apply even if you have been on HRT for many years and now want to get off.

The Benefits of Soy Foods

Asian women have traditionally had easy passage through the menopause compared to western women. A primary dietary reason for this is the relatively high intake of soy foods in the Asian diets. Soy foods contain substances known as phytoestrogens. These are plant compounds which are structurally and functionally similar to estrogen, especially estradiol which is the primary post-menopausal estrogen. Gut flora act on these compounds to form phenolic chemicals which bind to and act at estrogen receptor sites throughout the body. Of these phenolic compounds, the flavones, lignans and especially the isoflavones are the most significant. The main isoflavones are genistein, diadzein and equol, and are found only in legumes such as soy, lentils, peas and beans, and are most abundant in the soy foods.

The problem is that estrogens produced as a result of western diets are super-potent, and thus have the capacity to up-regulate the normal effects of estrogen in the body. This problem is compounded by the now widespread influence of xeno-estrogens. Xeno-estrogens are molecules which have chemical structures similar to natural estrogen (from plastic, petroleum and by-products), so they can trigger estrogen-like activity in the body.

Soy isoflavonoids compete with the body's own estrogens, and xeno-estrogens, competitively inhibiting the estrogenization effects at the receptor sites. The net result is a more natural and symptom-free passage through menopause.

See also Osteoporosis.

Diet

As for hypoglycemia: (refer to diet under Hypoglycemia). See also Menstrual Disorders.

Diet should also include:

Seeds and nuts (especially sunflower seeds); wheat germ; foods containing vitamin B complex, iodine, iron and calcium; brewer's yeast; protein supplements, especially soy foods; lecithin granules; seaweed.

Diet should exclude:

Caffeine; refined sugar; alcohol; spicy foods; animal foods, e.g. meat, dairy (yoghurt is OK).

Physiotherapy

- Cold water walks.
- Daily exercises—muscle work.
- Daily walks.
- Hot and cold alternating showers.
- Sauna.
- Wet grass walks.

Therapeutic Agents

Vitamins and Minerals—Primary

- Vitamin B complex: 25–50 mg 2–3 times daily. Intramuscular injections once a week with severe symptoms.
- Vitamin B5: 100 mg, 3 times daily; anti-stress.
- Vitamin B6: 50 mg, 3 times daily; reduces edema.
- Vitamin C: 250–1000 mg 3–6 times daily or more to bowel tolerance.
- Vitamin E: 400 IU 1–4 times daily. Improves circulation, reduces hot flushes. Start with one capsule daily, and increase until symptoms improve.
- Calcium: 800 mg 1–2 times daily.
- Magnesium: 400 mg, 4–5 times daily.
- Vitamin A: 25,000 IU 1–2 times daily.

Vitamins and Minerals— Secondary

- PABA (para-amino benzoic acid).
- Zinc.

Others—Primary

- Essential fatty acids: (GLA, EPA, and evening primrose oil).
- Progesterone cream.
- DHEA.
- Probiotics: an essential component of any regimen, as they help with hormonal balance.

Others—Secondary

- Atomodine (with doctor's prescription) or 636 (Cayce Products).
- Bee pollen.
- Brewer's yeast: 1 tsp 2–3 times daily.
- Kelp: 2–4 tablets 2–3 times daily.
- Raw glandulars (thyroid, pituitary, adrenal, ovarian): with doctor's prescription.
- Royal jelly.
- Taurine.
- L-tryptophan.
- Wheat germ oil: use concentrated forms.
- Lecithin: 1 tbsp 3 times daily, before meals.
- Gamma-oryzanol: 20 mg daily.

Botanicals—Primary

Women have been using herbs for many centuries—different herbs in different places—to assist them through various stages of the reproductive cycle, from puberty to menopause, and everything in between, including fertility control, pregnancy and delivery support, lactation, and the full range of menstrual disorders. The following is a list of some useful herbal remedies.

Black cohosh: estrogenic.

Chaste tree: hormone balancer through the pituitary gland (best taken at 7 a.m. and 4 p.m).

Dong quai: balances hormones; also a blood tonic and emmenagogue; relieves hot flushes.

False unicorn root: contains phytoestrogens.

St John's wort: for neurosis.

Sage: relieves hot flushes (anti-hydrotic).

Botanicals—Secondary

Angelica.

Bladderwrack: thyroid stimulator.

Fennel: estrogenic.

Panax Ginseng: adaptogen.

Fotitieng: adaptogen.

Gotu kola: relieves hot flushes.

Lady's slipper: for anxiety, insomnia, hysteria.

Licorice: estrogen derivative.

Mother's wort: vaginal lubricant.

Oats: nervine sedative.

Passion flower: nervine sedative.

Skullcap: nervine sedative.

Squaw vine: estrogenic.

Wild yam: estrogenic and progesterogenic.

Therapeutic Suggestion

While the female body is undergoing hormonal change, the diet should be as free from foods containing hormones as possible, so organic meat and eggs would be preferred. A vegetarian diet based on soy, nuts and seeds, or with some deep water fish, is ideal. A liver cleansing program would be appropriate at this time, as will attention to the basics such as exercise, lots of water to drink, minimal stress levels, and good quality sleep.

MENSTRUAL DISORDERS
(Amenorrhea, Dysmenorrhea, Metrorrhagia, Oligomenorrhea, Premenstrual Tension)

DEFINITION AND SYMPTOMS

Amenorrhea: absence or suppression of menstruation. Normal prior to puberty, during pregnancy, during lactation, and after menopause.

Dysmenorrhea: painful or difficult menstruation. Cramp-like pains or steady, dull ache 24–48 hours prior to menstruation, persisting for variable periods of time.

Menorrhagia: extremely heavy or prolonged menses.

Metrorrhagia: bleeding between periods.

Oligomenorrhea: infrequent or scanty menstruation.

Premenstrual tension: symptoms occurring just prior to and in some cases during menstruation, abdominal distention, including depression, irritability, edema, sore breasts, and nausea.

ETIOLOGICAL CONSIDERATIONS

* Improper diet leading to nutritional deficiencies

B6; folic acid; B2; B complex; calcium; iron; vitamin K; protein; junk foods (refined foods, coffee, tea, soda, excess salt and excess meat which contains high phosphorus levels causing calcium deficiency) results in nutritional deficiencies.

* Extreme diets:
  Fruitarianism; protein deficiency, excess dieting, anorexia; low/no fat; low cholesterol levels
* Hypoglycemia
* Methylxanthines (coffee, tea, chocolate, cola): these are associated with dysmenorrhea and premenstrual syndrome.
* Stress/psychological
  Anxiety; depression; fear, of pregnancy, of maturity; sudden shock; sexual problems
* Hormonal
  Estrogen therapy; contraceptive pill
* Pathology
  Cancer; endometriosis; fibroids; misplaced womb; salpingitis; cervical lesion
* Other diseases
  Endocrine disorders (pituitary, thyroid, ovary, liver); hypertension; diabetes; blood disorders (including anemia); kidney disease; syphilis; scurvy

ETIOLOGICAL CONSIDERATIONS— SECONDARY

- Abortion or miscarriage; IUD
- X-ray therapy—suppression
- Sudden change of climate
- Poor body mechanics
- Marathoner's amenorrhea
- Puberty, pregnancy, lactation, menopause
- Aspirin: destroys vitamin K (K antagonist)
- Oral antibiotics
- Allergy
- Tumors
- Visceroptosis (dropped abdomen and pelvic contents due to sway back) or weak abdominal tone; spinal lesions have a specific action on pelvic organs or act secondarily through altered spinal mechanics and visceroptosis
- Weak abdominal tone leads to dropped abdominal and pelvic contents, congestion, poor circulation; lack of exercise leads to weak abdominal and pelvic muscles and ligaments, poor circulation.

DISCUSSION

Menstrual disorders have many causes. The first consideration should always be to exclude any pathology or disease process that may be the causative factor. Any bleeding between periods (Metrorrhagia) should be investigated for possible cancer, fibroids, cervical lesions, or other pathology prior to attempting the general therapeutic recommendations. Most menstrual problems can be caused by hormonal imbalances and a 24-hour urine sample may be used as a simple method of evaluating estrogen levels. Evidence of ovulation may also be found by keeping a morning temperature chart. This will aid evaluation and help direct therapy.

Probably the most effective way to upset the entire hormonal balance is to take contraceptive pills. This convinces the body that it is pregnant. After stopping the pill many women fail to regain normal periods for varying periods of months to several years. Amenorrhea following use of the contraceptive pill is very common.

Other hormonal disorders involving the pituitary, adrenals, or thyroid may also produce amenorrhea or abnormal bleeding cycles. This may be physiological, as with hypothyroidism due to iodine deficiency; or psychological, affecting first the hypothalamus then pituitary, thyroid, and ovaries. Stress or the contraceptive pill may also profoundly affect the adrenal glands, which produce 20% of the total estrogen output. These glands are very sensitive to changes in blood sugar levels, so that hypoglycemia may depress adrenal function over time (see Hypoglycemia).

Extreme diets, such as strict fruitarianism, very low protein diets, or repeated strict weight loss regimens, often cause amenorrhea. On these restricted diets, the levels of circulating hormones fall until a normal menstrual cycle is no longer possible and pregnancy unlikely. Many women on these diets have been told and sincerely believe that to no longer menstruate is a sign of purity and is the normal state for women. All we can say is that if this is normal, then so is sterility. If everyone lived on these diets, the human race would probably die out within one or two generations. These people are, unfortunately, led solely by emotion—not intellect or common sense.

Not listed above is anorexia nervosa. This disorder is a psychological problem leading to extreme weight loss and amenorrhea. The strong remarks above are not meant for sufferers of this disorder, who need psychological counseling to cope with their problem, which often results from an inability to adjust to sexual maturity.

Another major cause of menstrual abnormality is poor body mechanics. In the woman with normal posture, with strong abdominal muscles and pelvic supports, the female organs are suspended unencumbered within the pelvis. If, however, the abdominal muscles are weakened, or there is an excess lordotic curve in the low back, the abdominal contents prolapse and put pressure on the pelvic organs. This may result from simple lack of demanding exercises, spinal lesions causing an increase in the lumbar curve, or something as common as habitual wearing of high-heeled shoes, which increases the lumbar curve. Constipation and loaded bowel syndrome may also cause intestinal prolapse.

Failure to do sufficient prenatal and especially postnatal exercises may lead to weakening of the supporting ligaments of the female organs. This is a common finding in menstrual disorders. The resultant prolapse interferes with normal blood and lymph flow, resulting in congestion and reduction in local tissue vitality.

Diet may play a major role in menstrual problems. As previously mentioned, a protein-deficient diet causes amenorrhea and infertility. Hypoglycemia, nutritional anemia, iodine deficiency, and hypothyroidism are some of the more widely accepted nutritional causes of menstrual disorders. Vitamin B complex deficiency and calcium deficiency are also now being recognized. Certainly, calcium deficiency related to cramps is fairly well proven. Vitamin B6 deficiency is also associated with the premenstrual tension syndrome of irritability, cramps, fluid retention, and acne flare.

Stress and psychological problems may profoundly affect menstrual flow. It is not uncommon for amenorrhea to follow a severe psychological and physical trauma. Fear of pregnancy may also be a common factor in menstrual disorders of all kinds. Less obvious psychological problems may also be the cause and should be sought through careful questioning.

An interesting type of amenorrhea has recently been coined "marathoner's amenorrhea", found exclusively among those females who regularly run long distances. Certain levels of body fat and cholesterol are needed for proper hormone production, and when these levels are reduced, hormone production is impaired including those involved in the menstrual cycle.

TREATMENT

Many doctors routinely recommend dilatation and curettage (D & C) for abnormal menstrual bleeding. It is not entirely certain how curettage works, but many hypothesize that removal of a probably hypertrophied endometrium lining the uterus allows a newly formed, normal endometrium to be produced. There is no question that the D & C is effective for some permanently, while others receive only temporary relief, or no relief at all, even after multiple curettage.

Estrogen combined with progesterone will usually stop excessive bleeding. This, however, is not curative and must be repeated at intervals. Estrogen is also routinely used in cases of amenorrhea. This is not reserved for patients with reduced ovarian function, but also commonly used in patients with normal estrogen levels. This has no proven therapeutic results and only induces a menstrual period by what is called "estrogen withdrawal" when the course of medication is stopped. This form of therapy has been much abused by physicians who have accepted the credit for restoring temporary menstrual function without making it clear to the patient that estrogen withdrawal bleeding is not the same as restoration of normal menses.

The naturopathic approach to menstrual disorders attempts to restore normal function by removing the cause and increasing both local and general vitality.

Diet

Although fasting is employed in some cases, especially where toxicity has been a factor, we find a full dietary regimen as for anemia or hypoglycemia the best initial approach. This may be intermixed with short fruit and vegetable juice fasts of 3–7 days. Obviously, amenorrhea due to protein deficiency should not be treated through fasting. The diet should contain foods high in calcium, vitamins A, B complex, C, E, K, and iodine, zinc, iron, and protein. Extra vitamin and mineral supplements are required in the early stages of treatment. The diets outlined under Hypoglycemia or Anemia, stressing vegetarian or fish protein sources with less meat, are best for these conditions.

Physiotherapy

- Alternate hot and cold sitz baths: this is the most effective method of removing pelvic congestion and restoring ovarian and uterine health. Twice daily, if possible. There is no substitute for sitz baths.
- Ice pack to uterus and pubic region or sacral region: for excessive bleeding or pain. Hot compresses may also be applied at the same time to the legs and feet to enhance the action of removing blood from the pelvic region.
- Spinal manipulation: lower thoracic, lumbar, and lumbar/sacral, once weekly for 6-8 weeks. Rest a few weeks and repeat.
- Slant-board exercises.
- Abdominal exercises.
- Prenatal-type exercises.
- Outdoor exercises; swimming.
- Depletion pack.

Therapeutic Agents

Vitamins and Minerals

As with many problems with one's health, the usefulness or otherwise of specific supplements and botanicals will depend on the individual case history, and the presenting signs and symptoms. The following are listed without prioritizing, and selection might best be undertaken in consultation with your naturopathic physician.

- Vitamin A: 10,000-25,000 IU 1-2 times daily.
- Vitamin B complex: 50 mg 1-3 times daily. Intramuscular injection may be useful.
- Vitamin B6: for premenstrual tension and acne; 100 mg 3-4 times daily, initially, then twice daily.

- Folic acid: 25-50 mg daily—especially with abnormal PAP smears.
- Vitamin C plus bioflavonoids: for excess bleeding. 1000-2000 mg 2 or more times per day, up to bowel tolerance.
- Vitamin D: 400-1000 IU daily. Increases calcium absorption along with acidic environment (hydrochloric acid, vitamin C, cider vinegar, lemon juice, etc.). Take care in prescribing extra vitamin D; it is often taken in excess in the diet, and can have toxic effects. A prescription for plenty of sunshine is safer.
- Vitamin E: 400 IU 1-2 times daily.
- Vitamin K: for excess bleeding; antihemorrhagic (alfalfa, seaweed, spinach, cabbage, and other vitamin K foods).
- Calcium: levels are lowest just before menstruation begins. Low calcium may be related to premenstrual tension syndrome, along with vitamin B6. Calcium is especially useful with cramps and heavy blood loss. 1-2 tablets per hour are taken in acute cases. 1000-2500 mg daily as regular dose. Higher doses in individual cases.
- Iron: even one heavy period may use up the entire month's supply of iron. Heavy blood loss always requires iron. 25-50 mg daily.
- Magnesium: 200 mg 2-3 times daily, or 1 mg for every 2 mg of calcium.
- Zinc: 25 mg 1-2 times daily.

Others

- Brewer's yeast.
- Lecithin.
- Choline/inositol.
- Garlic.
- Kelp.
- Alfalfa.
- Essential fatty acids (GLA, evening primrose oil).
- EPA (eicosapentaenoic acid): 3-10 g daily.
- Chlorophyll: 2-3 tbsp 4-6 times daily.
- Protein supplements.
- Tryptophan with doctor's prescription, prescribed according to individual case.

- Atomodine or 636 (Cayce products).
- Raw adrenal tablets.
- Desiccated thyroid.

Amenorrhea (Absence of Menstrual Flow) and Oligomenorrhea (Scant Flow)

Botanicals—Primary
Blue cohosh: emmenagogue.
Dong quai: hormone balancer, blood tonic and emmenagogue.
False unicorn root.
Panax ginseng: adaptogenic.
Ginger: circulatory stimulant, especially if patient is cold (where heat relieves).
Chaste tree: best taken at 7 a.m. and 4 p.m.

Botanicals—Secondary
Angelica.
Black cohosh: ovarian pain; cramps.
Blazing star: for low ovarian function, hypoestrogenism. 10 to 30 drops tincture 3 times daily.
Elecampane.
Licorice root tea.
Life root: uterine tonic; increases local circulation. 10-30 drops tincture 2-4 times daily.
Mother's wort.
Pennyroyal: strong infusion, 3-4 times daily
Pulsatilla: 10 drops 3 times daily; especially if due to stress, apprehension, or other emotional suppression.
Tansy.

Dysmenorrhea (Painful Periods)

Botanicals—Primary
Black cohosh: especially if pain comes before bleeding, with bloating and swollen breasts.
Blue cohosh.
Cramp bark, or high-bush cranberry: spasmolytic, uterine sedative.
Dong quai: uterine decongestant and tonic, circulatory stimulant.
Wild yam root: cramps; ovarian neuralgia.

Botanicals—Secondary
Angelica.
Black haw: antispasmodic; useful with menstrual cramps. 15-30 drops tincture 3-4 times daily.
Chamomile tea: mild calmative.
Corydalis: spasmolytic.
False unicorn root: a uterine tonic used in ovarian dysmenorrhea.
Ginger root.
Lady's slipper: for hysteria.
Life root: uterine tonic; useful in atonic conditions. 15-30 drops tincture 3 times daily.
Mother's wort.
Paeonia: uterine decongestant.
Pulsatilla.
Red raspberry: uterine astringent.
Squaw vine: used in dysmenorrheal especially of menarche.
Valerian: sedative.

Menorrhagia (Prolonged or Heavy Menses)

Take herbs 7 days before due date of period and for first 4 days of period

Botanicals—Primary
Cranesbill: astringent.
Shepherd's purse: anti-hemorrhagic.
Bethroot: anti-hemorrhagic.
False unicorn root: uterine tonic.
Blue cohosh: uterine tonic.
Squaw vine: uterine tonic.
Witch hazel: astringent.

Botanicals—Secondary
Amaranth: astringent. 15-25 drops tincture 3-4 times daily.
Angelica.
Cinnamon: use infusion, 1 cup 2-3 times daily.
Cramp bark, or high-bush cranberry.
Geranium: 15-20 drops tincture.
Life root: uterine tonic, useful in atonic conditions. 15-30 drops tincture 3-4 times daily.
Red raspberry.

Shepherd's purse.
Solomon's seal.
Squaw vine.
Strawberry leaf tea.
White oak bark: astringent.
Yarrow.

Metrorrhagia (Mid-Cycle, Irregular Flow)

It is best to get a medical diagnosis with this condition, as it can indicate serious problems which should be excluded before herbal treatment is commenced. Treatment is the same as for Menorrhagia, with herbs taken for the whole of the cycle, and with less emphasis on astringents.
Pulsatilla.
Blue cohosh.
Chaste tree: best taken at 7 a.m. and 4 p.m.
False unicorn root.

General

Dong quai: all menstrual problems.

MULTIPLE SCLEROSIS (Disseminated Sclerosis)

DEFINITION

A neurological, inflammatory, progressive disease of the central nervous system characterized by scattered areas of destruction of the myelin sheath covering nerves in the brain, spinal cord and optic nerve. Periods of exacerbation and remission occur.

SYMPTOMS

Onset is usually between 20–30 years of age, with peak incidence in the late 20s. First signs are minor and include minor visual disturbances, transient visual loss, double vision, or ocular palsy; fatigue; weakness; slight stiffness or weakness of an arm or leg; minor incoordination; dizziness; temporary

loss of bladder or bowel control; numbness; or mild emotional disturbance. These may come and go with more severe symptoms occurring later, such as tremor; lack of motor coordination; nystagmus; slow, slurred speech; seizures; paralysis; and mental disturbance. Complications of respiratory infections associated with this disease may cause death.

ETIOLOGICAL CONSIDERATIONS—PRIMARY

- Allergy
  Celiac (gluten); yeast; wheat; milk; eggs; any food or chemical
- Leaky gut
- Toxicity
  Pesticides; fungicides; additives; industrial chemicals (acrylics, photolab chemicals, etc.); heavy metal poisoning
- Deficiency of unsaturated fats

ETIOLOGICAL CONSIDERATIONS—SECONDARY

Hypoglycemia; excess saturated fats; refined foods; glandular disturbance (liver, gallbladder, adrenals, pancreas); deficient assimilation; vaccinations; vitamin dependency.

DISCUSSION

Multiple sclerosis is found predominantly in civilized nations. It is most common where the diet is high in saturated fats and refined carbohydrates. The fats involved are not just the obvious ones such as meats, cheese, milk, cream, and butter, but also hidden fats in pastries, baked goods, cookies, cakes, fried foods, and even peanut butters or margarines made with hydrogenated oil. Fats consumed with sugar or other refined carbohydrates are particularly dangerous. Societies such as the Inuits who consume a high amount of saturated fats show no evidence of multiple sclerosis until refined carbohydrates are introduced into their diet. The same fact applies to many other tribal cultures. Hypoglycemia, a condition due primarily to the consumption of refined carbohydrates, is commonly found in subjects with multiple sclerosis.

Not only are refined carbohydrates suspected by naturopaths in the causation of multiple sclerosis, but also in some cases any gluten-containing grain. These include most grains except brown rice and millet. Multiple sclerosis has been arrested in some cases simply by following a totally gluten-free diet (see Celiac Disease). Other food allergies may be a factor, including eggs, milk, or literally any food.

Heavy metal toxicity, especially mercury and lead, but others as well, has been associated with some cases of multiple sclerosis. Toxicity or hypersensitivity to pesticides and food additives, colorings, or preservatives may also be a factor. Glandular disturbances of the gallbladder, liver, pancreas, thyroid, and adrenal glands may be related, causing poor assimilations and interactions between the endocrine and central nervous systems. Many naturopathic physicians suspect that previous vaccination with smallpox, measles, and other inoculations may be associated with multiple sclerosis. These inoculations can cause profound changes within the body years after their introduction.

One hypothesis (which might be viewed as unifying much of the discussion above) is that multiple sclerosis is an autoimmune disease, in which autoantibodies attack the myelin sheath (Schwann cells) which surround and insulate the nerve fibers of the central nervous system. If this hypothesis were correct, then protocols addressing leaky gut would demonstrate clinical success, and this is what naturopathic clinicians tend to find in practice. Such an approach, which addresses suspected causes rather than merely addressing symptomatology, represents possibly the best way to deal with this otherwise insidious disease.

TREATMENT

Multiple sclerosis is a degenerative disease and as such must be treated vigorously, generally, consistently, and over a prolonged period of time before true healing may begin. The first aim of therapy is to arrest the process of the disease, then to build on that foundation and give the wonderful mind-body the opportunity for self-repair, which it can do if the conditions are conducive, with optimal nutrient status. The longer a person has had multiple sclerosis, the less likely is complete cure, since the demyelinated areas of the nerves become scarred and calcified, causing permanent debility. Long-lasting, permanent "remission" (cure by any other name), is the desired outcome of treatment protocols, and are possible with perseverance in some cases. In treatment, refer to leaky gut treatment as well, as this disease is often associated with systemic candidiasis, as is fatigue (often chronic).

Diet

The initial basic diet must be a gluten-free, dairy-less, completely unsaturated fat regimen. This implies complete vegetarianism, even excluding dairy products. Some therapists in the field allow 10–15% saturated fats and dairy products such as low-fat goat's yoghurt. We advise a period of at least 6 months if not a year totally free of saturated fats. This effectively eliminates all meats, dairy foods, eggs, and hydrogenated fats including margarine. The structural lipids the body will synthesize from the essential fatty acids for repair and replacement of the myelin sheathing. Fried foods are also prohibited. Some followers of typical gluten-free diets include non-gluten flour in baking bread. We feel these products are generally abnormal and should be avoided. Since yeast is also highly suspect, we advise absolutely no yeast products. All foods must be free from additives, pesticides, colorings, or preservatives. No coffee, alcohol, salt, or sugar is to be used. No smoking, either! This might sound terribly forbidding, but the diet isn't really that bad. In fact, when the reality of the situation is considered, all we are recommending is a good, wholesome vegetarian diet (can include the fatty fish, e.g. salmon, tuna), without the eggs, yeast, wheat (gluten grains), or dairy products.

There is much about MS which indicates maldigestion, and malabsorption, so "grazing", having 5 or 6 smaller meals daily is to be preferred.

Allergy tests (RAST, cytotoxic, and pulse) should be performed to diagnose any other specific allergens. The foods suggested, all organic and unrefined, are as follows:

- Raw and cooked vegetables, vegetable juices.
- Raw fruits, fruit juices.
- Sprouted seeds, e.g. alfalfa, sunflower, red clover.
- Sprouted beans.
- Cooked beans, tofu.
- Nuts and seeds, especially sunflower and pumpkin seeds; nut butters, stone fruit seeds (e.g. apricot kernels, peach kernels).
- Brown rice and millet.
- Seed yoghurts.
- Cold pressed unsaturated oils.

Periods of raw vegetable juice fasting of 3 days to 2 weeks should be undertaken periodically throughout the regimen.

Physiotherapy

- Spinal manipulation: weekly treatments are advised.
- Massage: use a combination of: 2 fl oz (60 mL) peanut oil, 2 fl oz (60 mL) olive oil, 2 fl oz (60 mL) oil of sassafras, ½ fl oz (15 mL) lanolin, ½ fl oz (7 mL) oil of pine needles. Massage all along spine nightly just after using the Cayce wet cell device (see below).
- Cayce wet cell appliance (with gold): apply 45 minutes daily. For in-depth information see "Two electrical appliances described in the Edgar Cayce readings", available from the ARE Press, Virginia Beach, Va.

Hydrotherapy

- Alternate hot and cold showers daily.
- Alternate hot and cold compresses or sprays to spine.
- Hair analysis: check all cases for toxic metals and then detoxify (see Heavy Metal Poisoning).
- Outdoor exercise without overheating.
- Sunshine (sunbathing, not baking).
- Ocean swimming.
- Outdoor living.

Therapeutic Agents

Vitamins and Minerals—Primary

- Vitamin A and beta-carotene: 25,000 IU and 15,000 IU respectively. Antioxidants.
- Vitamin B complex: 50 mg 3 times daily (non-yeast source if yeast allergy is suspected).
- Vitamin B12: oral dose and intramuscular injections. 1000 mcg up to 3 times daily. Helps maintain myelin sheath.
- Vitamin C and bioflavonoids: up to 10 g or more. Antioxidant, antiedema associated with demyelination.
- Vitamin E: 800–2000 IU daily. Circulatory tonic.
- Magnesium: 1000 mg daily. Anti-stress; calcium absorption; muscular coordination.

Vitamins and Minerals— Secondary

- Vitamin B1: 10–15 g daily, plus 1 g intramuscular injection, 1–2 times per week, with 1 mg B12.
- Vitamin B3: 500 mg up to 20 g.
- Vitamin B6: 100–250 mg 1–3 times daily. Red blood cell production; nervous and immune stimulant; deficiency in some MS cases.
- Folic acid.
- Vitamin B5 (Pantothenic acid): 100 mg daily.
- Vitamin D: 400–1600 IU daily; take care not to exceed toxic levels.

- Vitamin K: 2–5 mg daily; antinausea (alfalfa a rich source, also soy, kelp, spinach, cabbage)
- Calcium/magnesium: in 2:1 ratio.
- Manganese: 2–50 mg daily. Deficiencies common in MS.
- Selenium: 200 mcg daily.
- Zinc: serum zinc levels low in MS; 25–50 mg twice daily.
- Trace minerals, e.g. Celtic salt.

Others—Primary

- Omega-3 essential fatty acids: 2–4 capsules, or 1 tsp flaxseed oil, 2–3 times daily. Fish oils rich in EPA are also advised.
- Probiotics: daily until symptoms subside, then for 6 months thereafter.
- Digestive enzymes, containing HCl: before or during a meal.
- Coenzyme Q10: 90 mg daily. Improves cellular metabolism and tissue oxygenation, as well as being an immune system stimulant.
- L-glycine: 500 mg twice daily on empty stomach. Myelin sheath nutrient.
- OPCs (oligomeric proanthocyanidins): anti-inflammatory, and decrease permeability of the blood–brain barrier.
- Digestive and pancreatic enzymes: take with meals to aid digestion, including hydrochloric acid.
- Phosphotidyl serine: to support myelination.
- Lipoic acid: antioxidant.
- Evening primrose oil-gamma linoleic acid (GLA): 2–4 capsules 3–4 times daily or more.
- SOD (superoxide dismutase): 2–5 tablets 3 times daily.
- Wheat germ oil: large doses. Use octacosanol.

Others—Secondary

- Raw adrenal.
- Atomodine.
- Cod-liver oil: 2–4 capsules 3 times daily.
- EPA: 2–10 capsules 3 times daily.
- Kelp: 2–4 tablets 2–3 times daily.
- Lecithin: concentrated phosphatidylcholine; 3–4 capsules

3 times daily, or more; needed for normal CNS function.
- Inositol/choline (lecithin): soy lecithin contains phosphatidyl serine, nutrient for myelination.
- Psyllium husks or fiber.

Botanicals—Primary

Depurative herbs: e.g. red clover, burdock, pau d'arco, sarsaparilla and blue flag will form part of the treatment protocol to promote detoxification and alkalinizing of the system.

Bilberry and grape seed extract: rich in bioflavonoids and oligomeric proanthocyanidins (OPCs).

Ginkgo biloba: to improve cerebral circulation.

Botanicals—Secondary

Oats.

Rehmannia: relieves side effects of cortisone.

St John's wort.

Albizzia lebbeck: anti-allergic.

Therapeutic Suggestion

MS can become a serious disease when proper treatment is not implemented from the outset. The use of corticosteroidal therapy as either a short- or long-term strategy has problems, and does not address the causative processes.

Our advice is to seek out the services of a naturopathic physician who has had some experience with this disease. One needs a truly holistic approach if one is to reverse this disease. Don't get seduced into the idea that if you've got it, you will probably have it for life, it just isn't true.

NAIL ABNORMALITIES

The condition of fingernails and toenails is a useful diagnostic aid. Healthy nail beds are pink, which indicates a good nutrient and blood supply. The following are some of the more common associations between nail health and nutritional status:

Broken, split, knotted, ridged: calcium deficiency, vitamin A deficiency, check protein absorption

Vertical ridging, white spots, cracking, brittle, rigid: intestinal atony, weak connective tissue

Peeling: vitamin A deficiency

White spots/specks: mineral deficiency (e.g. zinc), thyroid deficiency; hypochlorrhydria

Pitting: iron deficit

Very long: tendency to bronchial disorders

Very short: tendency to heart/vascular pathology

Short, thin, square at base, also bluish in color, no lunule: heart, vascular pathology

Flat, short, no lunule: liver sluggish

Short, flat, deeply sunken into flesh at base: spinal cord disorder/subluxation

Absent moons: protein deficiency

Bent inward at base and curved (also curving over finger edge): positive sign tuberculosis of lymphatics

Yellowish nails: liver/gallbladder problems

Red nails: excess hemoglobin

White nails, poor perfusion pale skin: anemia (iron deficiency)

Thin nails: delicate constitution

Thick: strong constitution

Darkened band (brownish-red) just before separation from finger: kidney disorder (e.g. dehydration)

Poor nail growth: zinc deficiency

Round shaped, white (frog-like): lung disorder (emphysema)

Rounded, like inverted spoons: iron deficiency; neuromuscular coordination problems, hyperactivity

Thin nails, curling up: cell membrane weakness. Anemia

Beau's lines (transverse lines): nail root growth interrupted, as in MI, measles, pneumonia, fever

Onycholysis: nail separates from nail bed (e.g. trauma, psoriasis, drug reactions, fungal, contact dermatitis (nail hardeners). Can also be hypo-/hyperthyroid, iron deficiency anemia, syphilis

Hands

There are some general hand signs which might be interesting.

Swollen, puffy: kidney disorder

Palms yellow: liver

Brown spots on back: liver

Purplish veins, knotted cords: anemia

Pale, colorless fingertips: anemia

Pale folds upon flexion: anemia

Dry, lacy skin: EFA deficiency

Cold, clammy: neural imbalance

Fingers—clubbing: chronic lack of oxygen (in lung problems 80%; heart problems, can also indicate cancer)

NEURITIS AND NEURALGIA

DEFINITION

Irritation or inflammation of a nerve.

SYMPTOMS

Local or referred pain; altered sensation (burning, tingling, numbness); muscle weakness and later atrophy; possible visceral symptoms; sensory, motor, reflex, or vasomotor symptoms.

ETIOLOGICAL CONSIDERATIONS—PRIMARY

*   Spinal lesion
    Cranial; temporomandibular joint (TMJ) syndrome; cervical; brachial outlet syndrome; thoracic outlet syndrome; C7 rib; intercostal neuralgia; sciatica
*   Disc lesion
*   Metabolic disorder
*   Infection affecting a nerve
*   Trauma
    Blow; compression; stretching; exposure to cold
*   Referred from viscera
*   Herpes zoster

*   Nutritional deficiency
    B1 deficiency; B12 neuropathy; anemia
*   Alcoholism

ETIOLOGICAL CONSIDERATIONS— SECONDARY

*   Diabetic neuropathy
*   Optic neuritis (inflammation of the optic nerve)
*   Circulatory (Angina, migraine)
*   Toxic (lead, arsenic, mercury, chemicals, pesticides, others)
*   Vira
*   Lupus
*   Leprosy
*   Cancer
*   Arthritis

DISCUSSION

The most frequent causes of neuritis and neuralgia are conditions related to the bony and other connective-tissue elements of the body where these may put direct or indirect pressure on nerves. In these cases a proper diagnosis by an osteopath, chiropractor, or naturopath is essential to determine if spinal or soft tissue therapy should be applied. This may include spinal manipulation or mobilization, cranial techniques, soft-tissue techniques (massage, neuromuscular therapy, friction, etc.), physiotherapy, exercise therapy, postural re-education, and others. If you need to be seen by a neurologist or orthopedic specialist, they will refer you.

Neuritis and neuralgia may also result from less obvious causes. This includes referred pain from internal visceral complaints such as pain in right shoulder and shoulder blade with gallbladder disease, midback pain with ulcers, or low back pain in menstrual complaints. Post-herpes zoster neuralgia can be a painful problem for months or even years following the original viral skin lesions. Other viruses are also known to cause muscle paralysis and weakness along with nerve irritation.

Severe nutritional deficiencies, especially of the vitamin B complex group, cause well-recognized neuropathies. Vitamin B12 neuropathy is becoming increasingly apparent as many people convert to vegetarian or vegan diets without adequate understanding of essential nutritional requirements. Informed vegetarianism is an extremely healthful diet. However, if proper care is not taken to provide sufficient B12, a severe and permanent nerve degeneration may occur (see Anemia).

Alcoholism and diabetes are also associated with nerve disorders, as are several other systemic chronic degenerative diseases (e.g. lupus, leprosy, cancer, or heart disease). Often an otherwise untraceable neuritis or neuralgia will be found to stem from toxic causes. This may be heavy metal poisoning, chemical exposure, pesticide exposure, or an imbalanced and acidic bloodstream. Similar dietary causes as those found under Arthritis, with which neuritis and neuralgia are often associated, are frequently a factor.

TREATMENT

Diet

Nearly all cases of neuritis or neuralgia will benefit by an initial elimination regimen. A 3-day fast or mono diet on subacid fruit juice or fruit such as apples may be used in some cases, while a longer carrot-based vegetable juice fast may be of more benefit to others. The diet regimen found under Arthritis is an excellent outline to follow to help alkalize the bloodstream in a steady and gentle manner. Emphasis should be placed on raw green vegetables, seaweeds, seeds, and seed or bean sprouts

Physiotherapy

- Spinal therapy, as needed.
- Massage.
- Muscle re-education.
- Hot Epsom salts baths (see Appendix I).
- Alternate hot and cold showers.
- Alternate hot and cold compresses.
- Alternate hot and cold local baths.
- Poultices (mullein, mustard, hops plus lobelia for pain relief—antispasmodic, mullein plus lobelia, chamomile.)
- Myrrh plus capsicum external.
- Menthol ointment external.
- Peppermint oil external.
- Wintergreen oil external.
- Olbas oil combination external.
- Deadly nightshade: *use with medical supervision.* Topical application in neuralgia, 6× dilution internally for pain.

Therapeutic Agents

Vitamins and Minerals—Primary

- Vitamin B6: 250–500 mg 1–2 times daily (carpal tunnel syndrome).
- Vitamin B complex: 25–50 mg 2–3 times daily.
- Vitamin C: to bowel tolerance.

- Vitamin B12: 25 mcg twice daily, plus 1 mg intramuscularly per week.
- Vitamin E: 400 IU 2-3 times daily, especially with post-herpes zoster syndrome.
- Magnesium: up to 2 g daily; chloride form.
- Zinc: 50-100 mg daily; gluconate or sulfate.

Vitamins and Minerals— Secondary

- Vitamin B1: 100 mg 1-2 times daily, plus 100 mg intramuscularly per week.
- Folic acid: 400-800 mcg daily.
- Essential fatty acids: 1-2 tbsp cold pressed oils daily.
- Inositol: 1000 mg 1-2 times daily (diabetic neuropathy).
- Iodine: Atomodine.
- Calcium chelate or lactate: 400 mg 2-3 times daily.
- Magnesium: 200 mg 2-3 times daily.

Others—Primary

- Bromelain: 150-400 mg daily. Anti-inflammatory.
- Essential fatty acids: especially flaxseed oil (2 dsp daily).
- Glutathione: 500-1000 mg daily; important for nerve and brain function.

Others—Secondary

- Brewer's yeast.

- Desiccated liver.
- Kelp: 2 tablets, 3 times daily (not to be taken with Atomodine).
- Lecithin: 4 capsules 3 times daily, or as granules, 1-3 tbsp daily.
- Wheat germ oil.

Botanicals—Primary

St John's wort: specific.
Oats: an excellent nervine tonic.
Willow bark: anodyne.
Bilberry: antioxidant.
Calendula: anti-inflammatory.
Chamomile: nervine tonic.

Botanicals—Secondary

Aconite: homeopathic doses.
Betony.
Blue cohosh.
Bryony.
Catnip.
Celery seed.
Hops.
Jamaica dogwood: for facial or sciatic neuralgia.
Myrrh.
Nettles.
Oregon grape root.
Passion flower.
Peppermint.
Pulsatilla.
Skullcap.
Valerian.
Wintergreen.

NUTRITIONAL DEFICIENCIES

Clinical states of single nutritional deficiencies are, fortunately, fairly rare. This is not to say that even in the developed nations cases of the better known nutritional deficiencies such as vitamin A deficiency (night blindness), vitamin B deficiency (beriberi), vitamin B, deficiency (pellagra), vitamin C deficiency (scurvy), or vitamin D and calcium deficiency (rickets) do not occur.

They do, and in some cases their incidence is on the rise rather than the wane, due to our devitalized western diet. But the relative infrequency of these easily recognizable deficiencies in no way represents the incredible frequency, perhaps as high as 90% or more of the general population (as the latest studies indicate), of subclinical multiple nutritional deficiencies. The average medical doctor looks at the infrequency of reported clinical nutritional deficiencies and draws the false conclusion that our diets are adequate without supplementation.

This oversight is not usually the doctor's fault. The blame lies in orthodox crisis care, medical education and philosophy. Unless something can be shown by a series of tests to be definitively wrong, then everything is presumed to be fine. A disease is not a disease until someone is sick, and sickness is defined clearly in medical texts that do not discuss subclinical nutritional states. Only within the past 20 years or so have some medical doctors expanded their vision of disease to include the early calling cards of disease—the subtle yet significant subjective and objective symptoms and signs of suboptimal nutrition. Health is no longer simply the absence of disease, but rather the perfect freedom of expression of the individual on all his or her three planes of function—the body, mind, and emotions. Any interference and blockage among any of these three facets contain a possible clue to nutritional deficiency. Certainly not all signs or symptoms within the body, mind, or emotions can be traced to nutritional causes; however, all these clues involve nutritional factors. If a person experiences prolonged stress, worry, fear, or anxiety, a close interaction occurs within the body that affects the nutritional state. Think a thought and you invariably move a muscle; feel an emotion and you secrete a host of hormones and initiate hundreds of biochemical reactions. The body and emotions are all connected, and until we can see this, no true healing will take place.

On a more practical level is the purely statistical evidence that a significant proportion of the western population is clearly nutritionally deficient. If we accept the fact that between 1-2% of the population has an increased need over the recommended dietary allowance (RDA) of a particular nutrient (a reasonable assumption, since the manner in which RDAs are established is based on standard statistical evaluation with usually 1-2% of the sample falling either above or below the acceptable range), and if we then multiply this 1-2% by the 50 or so known essential nutrients, vitamins, minerals, and trace elements, we arrive at the conclusion that any given individual has between a 50-100% chance of being deficient in at least one of these life-sustaining factors. This assumes that all of us are already getting the recommended RDAs in our diet, an assumption proven wrong by study after study. Nutritional deficiencies are not the rare, insignificant phenomena we have been led to believe, but rather a prevalent cause of disease in the civilized nations today.

Other studies have made this picture even more grim. In animal studies it has been found that some single nutrient deficiencies (e.g. zinc) in the mother during pregnancy can lead to nutritional deficiencies, nutritional dependencies, and immune malfunction in not only the immediate offspring but to a lesser degree for three generations, in spite of a normal diet. Although these animal studies do not directly apply to humans, they help suggest explanations for several clinical observations. Studies have recorded cases of severe malnutrition in prisoners of war that resulted in vitamin dependency in later years. In one case, they required doses 50 or over 100 times the recommended dose of vitamin B3 to maintain proper physical and mental health.

Depressive/anxiety disorders are becoming more widespread, and epidemiologists suggest over the next 20 years will rival cardiovascular disease as the number one affliction in western civilization. What is interesting is that soils are increasingly deficient in minerals and trace elements, and noteworthy is deficiency of lithium. Lithium is an important modulator of the central nervous system preventing psychoses of various types.

Similar observations have been made with other vitamins. These findings further reinforce the idea that individualized requirements for specific nutrients can be affected not only by genetics as previously recognized, but may also be acquired within one's lifetime. We are sure that more research in this direction will help explain why even the best of diets may no longer supply adequately all nutritional elements for all individuals.

This is a particularly important breakthrough in our knowledge of the possible cause of nutritional dependency disease. It also emphasizes the little understood concept that the pattern for our health and the strength of our immune system may be laid down by our parents or even grandparents. This may explain why, in spite of positive changes for the better in diet and nutrition by many of the population, true health is still hard to obtain. Our health foundation is weak, and it may take generations for this weakness to be corrected.

OBESITY

DEFINITION AND SYMPTOMS

Excess fat storage.

ETIOLOGICAL CONSIDERATIONS—PRIMARY

Obesity occurs when energy in the form of food and beverage nutrient is consumed in excess of the total energy expenditure requirements.

- Excess refined carbohydrates, leading to insulin resistance, syndrome X
- Excess saturated fats
- Improper feeding as infant and child
- Allergy
  Cow's milk; wheat
- Lack of demanding exercise
- Hormonal imbalances
  Hypothalamus; pituitary; pineal; thyroid; adrenal; pancreas
- History of emotional, and sexual abuse

ETIOLOGICAL CONSIDERATIONS— SECONDARY

- Incoordination of assimilation or elimination
- Hereditary predisposition; the contraceptive pill

DISCUSSION

Obesity is not merely a cosmetic problem, but a severe threat to health and longevity. The old proverb stating "The longer the belt, the shorter the life", is entirely accurate. Associated with obesity are diabetes and heart disease, two of the major killers of modern civilization. Our discussion deals with causes of obesity, and then recommendations for healthy weight loss.

The origins of obesity often lie in early childhood. Statistically, children who are overweight by the age of 2 turn into fat adults more frequently than their lean playmates. Early feeding patterns set the stage for adult obesity. The most common mistake is fattening the child with excess starch and cow's milk. Most infants receive starchy foods as their first solid foods, around 4 months of age. This is far too early for proper digestion, and sets the stage for later allergies, as referred to in other sections of this book.

More importantly, however, in causing obesity, these grains cause rapid weight gain. This is in part due to the fact that most grains are of the refined variety of empty calories, stripped of their fiber and bran. Rather than grains being given early and regularly as a first food, they should be introduced relatively late in the weaning process and less frequently, to avoid rapid weight gain. Cow's milk is another cause of rapid weight gain. Its composition was designed for the rapid growth of cows, not children. The fact that most cow's milk given is homogenized, making the fat particles easier to assimilate, is another aspect of milk that favors obesity. Raw unhomogenized goat's milk is a far better food for human infants over 6 months of age and does not cause rapid weight gain since the composition is closer to that of mother's breast milk. Make sure goat's milk comes from a reliable dairy and that the milk has been bottled under proper antiseptic conditions. Prior to 6 months of age, all liquids given to an infant should be boiled to prevent gastroenteritis.

Breast-fed infants have far less chance of becoming obese than formula-fed babies. We have, however, seen enough quite obese infants who were totally breast-fed not to reinforce this commonly quoted statistic too dogmatically. We have seen infants up to 32 lb by the age of one who were totally breast-fed by mothers on "whole food" diets. In most of these cases, but not all, these mothers themselves were, if not obese, at least full-bodied and a little plumpish. Most of the infants demanded the breast nearly every 2 hours day and night, and were allowed fairly unrestricted access. From these observations we feel fairly certain that the cause of such breast-fed obesity is a combination of milk of an unusually fattening nature, and too-frequent feedings.

All mother's milk is not identical and we suspect the mother's own biochemistry goes a long way in affecting the type of food she produces for her infant. we do not generally like the idea of restricting feedings to set times or hours, but see the need for some restraint in these cases. There is also the possibility that the infant is feeding more for psychological reasons than hunger, and pleasant distractions might break the pattern. This is no easy task, but the dangers of obesity make it worth the effort. If the breast-feeding mother is herself on an improper diet of excess refined carbohydrates, sugar, and excess animal fats, she is not only laying the foundation for infant obesity, but also for a generally unhealthy child.

In many cases, the child fortunately passes through childhood without growing fat. Two possibilities can be the cause. The first is that the child, being lucky enough to have parents with some common sense, has been "deprived" of all kinds of sweets, pastries, white bread, soda, sweetened and refined cereals, or other junk foods and given only wholesome unrefined foods. These children then pass into adult life having the least chance of becoming obese and the best chance of a long, healthy life. The second possibility is that the child has been given a typical junk food diet in his or her growing years, but due to an abundance of childhood play and exercise, has been able thus far to avoid weight gain or other obviously noticeable complaints except possibly a tendency to get sick frequently or possibly to have behavior problems.

In fact, if nothing "obvious" is taking place outside, something insidious is taking place inside, as we shall see. As the child passes into adult life the general activity level usually decreases markedly, but the diet does not, except maybe to include alcohol, which is certainly not an improvement. The body has already become accustomed to a diet of quickly absorbed refined carbohydrates and internal biochemical changes have been made to deal with these more or less as demanded. The pancreas now knows it must act fast at the first signs of sugar in the system since from experience it knows a flood of it will soon be in the bloodstream. Refined carbohydrates are, after all, very quickly absorbed. This increased sugar sensitivity may then progress into a clinical case of hypoglycemia (low blood sugar), especially with the added burden of alcohol, which, next to refined sugar, is the ultimate refined carbohydrate. Couple these dietary influences with the addition of stress from a job or new family life, which depletes the adrenal glands, the co-manager of our blood sugar level along with the pancreas, and we see how profoundly our internal chemistry has been abused.

It is no small wonder then that the chemistry of an obese person is found to differ from the average person of normal size. Most obese people show abnormal glucose tolerance and have raised blood levels of cholesterol, triglycerides, and free fatty acids. Many overweight people report quite honestly that they do not eat any more than other people and yet still gain weight. Although this statement is occasionally born out of a lack of awareness of true eating habits, more often than not it is true. Fat people often don't eat more than thin people. Often, the reverse is true with some thin people eating far more without gaining weight. This does not necessarily mean that the thin person has a healthier biochemistry, but he or she certainly has a different one. Often, both are suffering from the insidious results of the same refined diet, but have made different biochemical adjustments, depending in part on hereditary predisposition, or the state of their organs of elimination, endocrine system, or nervous system.

The basic problem in obesity then is an abnormal biochemistry caused by a diet of excess refined carbohydrates and saturated fats, and a reduction in activity level when reaching adult life.

The common answer to this problem is usually "eat less and exercise more". This advice is both right and wrong at the same time. Certainly, weight loss can be obtained by a calorie-restricted diet and an increase in exercise. The problem, however, is in preventing weight gain after the diet is over. If an obese person stores fat better than a thin person on the same diet, something must be done to change the inner controls or else the obese person will be doomed to a lifetime of ridiculously limited diet and self-reproach for each minor incident of leniency.

No real progress will ever be made along these lines unless the actual biochemistry of the obese person is changed. The answer to the dietary aspect of obesity is not necessarily to eat less, but to eat properly. Certainly, refined carbohydrates will cause weight gain and these must be totally excluded from the diet and replaced by unrefined high-fiber carbohydrates such as brown rice, millet, barley, buckwheat, wheat berries, bulgur, corn, and other whole grains. These should be cooked only enough to make them chewy but not soft. In the early stages of weight loss and weight maintenance they should not even be ground up or used in flour form, as in bread. The reasons for these changes are simple. A person can eat a much larger amount of refined starches and grains than their whole grain counterparts. The refined grains are also much easier to digest and absorb. By eating whole grains cooked very conservatively one can eat only a fraction of the amount previously eaten and can thoroughly digest even less. The difference is obvious if we compare the stool contents after several meals of cornbread as opposed to corn on the cob. A similar difference exists between white rice and brown rice, or between white bread and whole wheat bread. With unrefined grain the person eats much less but the stools are much larger. To prove this, first eat an entire loaf of white bread at one meal and try to eat an entire loaf of whole wheat bread at another meal. You will soon see what we mean.

One step further than the concept of refined vs. whole food is the concept of "unaltered whole grains", which works even better with the obese. A similar comparison between bread made from white flour and bread made from whole wheat flour can be made between whole wheat bread and whole wheat berries. If the whole grain itself is eaten and has not been ground up into flour by powerful grain mills, much less can be eaten and still less digested and absorbed. For this reason the best diet approach for the obese is a balanced diet of fresh fruit, raw vegetables, protein, especially vegetarian protein, and unaltered, unrefined, high-fiber carbohydrates.

Healthy Weight Loss

To change the biochemistry exercise is needed, but not as usually suggested. Weight loss due to caloric benefits of exercise is not all it is made out to be. Walking may use up to 120 calories per hour while actual jogging burns only 440 calories per hour. The average obese person is incapable of doing enough exercise to expend sufficient calories to affect profound weight loss. In reality, the best way to lose weight would be to exercise and play as actively as when we were young children—in other words almost constantly, but this is clearly impossible. The second best is to exercise as if one were to train for a demanding sport such as football or boxing. Clearly this is also pretty impossible for the average person with a job or a family.

As explained in the excellent book *Fit or Fat?* by Covert Bailey (Bailey, Covert, *Fit or Fat?* Houghton Mifflin Co., Boston, 2001), and which we recommend to everyone who is overweight, the only type of exercise of real significance for the obese is aerobic exercise. Bailey points out clearly that only through a regimen of sufficiently prolonged aerobic exercise can the biochemistry of the body be altered. He shows the futility of most of the weight loss diets, since the real problem is not one of overweight, but "over fat". What this means is that an obese person has more fat, not only in the normal subcutaneous fat reserves, but also more fat content in the muscles. The average percentage of fat in muscles is somewhere from 12–22%, depending on body type, occupation, and sex. Athletes tend to have much lower muscle fat, even down to 5–6%, while females tend to be on the upper part of the scale. The obese person, however, has a higher than normal percentage of muscle fat. What seems to occur in the fattening process is that as we grow out of our active childhood into adult life, we use less of our muscles in our daily duties. If the diet is improper and the body has developed abnormal responses to dietary carbohydrates, alcohol, or fats, these unused muscles begin to accumulate fat. Initially, no weight gain is noticed since fat is merely being substituted for muscle, but eventually obesity begins to develop. Normal diets to lose weight only reduce fat stores or even worse, protein weight, and do not significantly

affect muscle fat. For true weight loss a biochemical change is necessary, and once again the way is through aerobics.

What are "aerobic" exercises? To quote Bailey:

The word aerobic means air, but more specifically refers to the oxygen in the air. The muscles need oxygen to function and their need for oxygen goes up dramatically when we work them. We can measure how hard a muscle is working by how much oxygen it is using (or burning). As you exercise harder, you need more oxygen and the heart rate goes up. Increases in your heart rate due to exercise are an indirect measure of how hard your muscles are working."

We recommend steady, non-stop aerobic exercise for a duration of not less than 12–20 minutes, depending on the exercise, at 80% of the maximum heart rate, providing there are no health complications to make this inadvisable.

The type of exercises considered "aerobic" are non-stop exercises such as those performed in aerobic exercise classes, fast walking, jogging, running, rope jumping, calisthenics, jumping jacks, bicycling, rowing, cross-country skiing, roller skating, etc. Swimming is an aerobic exercise but is not advised for weight loss since the water temperature is usually colder than body temperature and signals the body to store fat for insulation, clearly not what is desired. As a cardiovascular exercise, or for the entire body tone, however, it is excellent.

Many people feel that they get plenty of exercise on their job or about the house, but this is not "aerobic" exercise and therefore has little or no real effect on true weight loss. Even if you work with your body all day long (as a carpenter, for instance), the activity is usually intermittent and rarely calls for 100% use of your muscles.

True aerobic exercise changes the body on a biochemical level, altering the deeply ingrained way the obese handle carbohydrates and fat. These exercises also stimulate the endocrine system, which may be a factor in weight gain in the first place. Certainly, thyroid disorders have been implicated in obesity, as have disorders of the hypothalamus, pituitary, pineal, pancreas, adrenals, and sex glands.

Patients often ask what their ideal weight should be, or how much weight they need to lose for their height. All the height vs. weight charts that have ever been written are totally useless in determining proper weight, since they in no way take into consideration what proportion of the body is fat, and which is toned muscle. Two people of the same height can weigh the same, while one is composed of muscle and the other of fat. Even if you start with fat and through dieting end up fitting into the weight charts, what good is it if you look skinny with sagging skin? What you need is to replace fat with muscle. Get in shape rather than just get out of a bad one.

In the final analysis all you need is a mirror and a large water source to judge your weight accurately. The mirror will show general body shape. If you look more like a blob than a figure eight, you have a way to go. You don't need a medical degree to know what a shapely body looks like. If you float easily in water, it means you still have plenty of fat. When you begin to sink easily on exhalation you are getting there.

TREATMENT

Diet

The basic diet includes the following:
Raw fruit: moderate amounts of raw citrus and subacid fruits are allowed. No sweet fruits such as grapes or dried fruits should be consumed. Fruit juices are also forbidden since these are in essence "refined", being devoid of their pulp and roughage. The only exception is diluted red grape juice taken an hour before all meals. This helps decrease the appetite, allowing the subject to eat less, and does not signal a weight gain. Bananas also are not allowed.
Raw vegetables: allowed almost without restraint. A raw salad meal should be taken once or twice each day, alone, or with other compatible foods such as protein or unrefined starch.
Cooked vegetables: the only cooked vegetables allowed are fresh and conservatively cooked (steamed, stewed, lightly sautéed, or baked, but not fried) fresh vegetables. No frozen, fried, or canned vegetables are to be used. The proportion of cooked vegetables consumed should be less than raw. Vegetables properly cooked are still slightly crispy. Potatoes are allowed 2-3 times per week but only if eaten with the skin.
Proteins: beans, sprouted beans, sprouted seeds, nuts in moderation, fish, chicken and turkey (wild, if possible), low-fat yoghurt, and poached eggs are the major proteins with the vegetarian sources stressed. No meat is allowed unless it is from wild game, which has far less fat content. Most meats you find in the supermarkets have been raised with the use of hormones which can trigger weright gain and should be avoided.
Carbohydrates: all refined carbohydrates are absolutely forbidden. This means sugar, alcohol, white flour and its products (bread, pastry, macaroni, etc.), quick oats, most packaged cereals, and any other processed starch. Eat only conservatively cooked, unrefined brown rice, millet, barley, rye, buckwheat, wheat berries, bulgur, corn, and any other whole grain. These should be taken in their natural state and not ground into flour for bread or cooked cereal. Let your teeth do the grinding.
Fats: cold pressed unsaturated oils are allowed for salad dressings with lemon juice and/or apple cider vinegar plus herbs, or when needed in cooking in very small amounts.

Obviously, one should not overeat, a tendency that may be carried over from days of eating unrefined carbohydrates. Until the stomach adjusts to its proper size, some restraint in the diet is obviously required. It is also far better to eat four to five smaller meals than 2-3 large ones. A useful rule to eliminate habit snacking is to eat only while eating. In other words, when eating, concentrate only on the meal or snack at hand. No talking, reading, listening to the radio, watching TV, or any other mental distraction is allowed. This eliminates the tendency to munch incessantly and requires that the person be hungry enough to discontinue all other activities to eat. A simple diet might be as follows:

Half an hour before breakfast
6 fl oz (190 mL) glass of diluted grape juice, 2:1 with water, sipped slowly.

Breakfast
Fresh raw fruit (especially citrus) or fresh raw fruit with low-fat yoghurt
Choice of:
- Fresh raw fruit and a small handful of nuts.
- Poached eggs and fruit.
- Poached eggs and whole grain such as brown rice or millet.
- Salad.
- Salad and nuts.
- Salad and low-fat yoghurt.

Midmorning
Fresh vegetables such as carrot or celery sticks.
Apple.
1 fruit plus 8–12 almonds.
Herb tea.
Dandelion coffee.
Raw or baked tofu (teriyaki tofu or other).

Half an hour before lunch
Diluted red grape juice.

Lunch
Always have a raw mixed salad composed of at least three vegetables that grow above the ground for each that grows below. In addition, choose from:
- Beans.
- Fish.
- Turkey or chicken (twice per week only).
- Wild game meat.
- Tofu.

- Whole grain.
- Baked potato with skin (2–3 times per week only, in any meal).
- Nuts or seeds (pumpkin, sunflower, etc.).

Midafternoon
As midmorning.

Half an hour before supper
Diluted red grape juice.

Supper
Raw salad or cooked vegetables.
Protein and whole grain (1 cup cooked) individually cooked and served as acasserole dish.
We suggest obtaining several good salad and whole food cookbooks. Variety and interest must be maintained. With a little experience you will learn to make nearly anything out of whole foods. Use your imagination, but use whole foods. In addition to the basic diet, take 1 tbsp raw bran with 1–2 glasses of water 10–15 minutes prior to each meal. This tends to reduce appetite.

The Modified Protein-Sparing Fast/Diet

Another approach to weight loss for relatively short terms (1–3 months) is the modified protein-sparing fast/diet. During the normal fasting state the body first mobilizes glycogen stores in the liver and tissue stores. These are converted to glucose and supply the brain and tissues with this vital energy source for the first 12–24 hours of the fast. Following this period, the body begins to convert both fat and protein into glucose to maintain an adequate supply in the blood to sustain life. Without a steady supply of glucose the brain cannot function, and general lethargy can set in.

Unfortunately, with the conversion of fat to glucose, by-products are produced, which, if allowed to build up in the blood, cause a state of acidosis and toxicity. This is one of the reasons many people suffer varying degrees of unpleasant symptoms such as headaches, mental lethargy, and foul breath during the first 2–3 days of a fast. Fortunately, the body has the ability to stimulate the release of hormones not normally present in the brain that are capable of utilizing as a new source of energy the previously toxic substances (ketones), resulting from the conversion of fat to glucose. This biochemical trick occurs during the fasting state and is the reason why most people experience a feeling of renewed vigor and even a slight euphoria on or shortly after the third day of a fast. Finally, the brain has guaranteed itself a steady supply of glucose. This new source of energy is not, however, sufficient for the total body need for energy and therefore protein from the muscular system, and much later from organs, is utilized to fulfil this need. This protein conversion to glucose causes muscle wasting, certainly not the desired result of a weight loss regimen, which is aimed at fat deposit mobilization.

To prevent this protein loss and still mobilize fat from its stores, causing generalized weight loss without at the same time losing muscle, the modified protein-sparing diet is used. On this regimen a person fasts on a well-balanced instant protein powder. We recommend a non-dairy (non-whey) protein powder, such as soy. This is consumed three times daily in 6–8 fl oz (190–250 mL) of diluted juice or low-fat soy milk, oat or creamy rice milk. 2–3 tbsp of the protein powder are taken with each liquid meal, to equal approximately 50 g of protein daily. This satisfies the body's protein need and spares the body mobilizing its own protein sources. By not consuming large amounts of glucose directly in the form of carbohydrate, the brain continues to produce enzymes capable of utilizing ketones for energy and this fat is still mobilized. The urge to eat is very small since hunger is partly controlled by the blood glucose levels which will remain fairly constant throughout the diet.

Being "in ketosis" can be measured by sampling first morning, mid-stream urine using a ketostick, available from pharmacies and drug stores. We recommend aiming for a more mild, rather than a severe ketosis, as measured by the color chart.

To maintain bowel function in the absence of solid food, a hydrophilic bulking agent (for example, psyllium powder, linseed meal, oat bran, etc.) is taken 2–3 times daily, with a glass of water. This swells in the stomach as water is absorbed, providing a non-digestible "meal" that not only keeps the bowels functioning regularly, but also provides a sensation of fullness in the stomach. This is felt by the stomach, which sends impulses to the brain, basically saying, "I'm full, thank you, no need to feel hungry right now."

Water should be taken regularly to total 6–8 large glasses daily. This helps the bulking agent swell adequately and helps dilute the many toxins provided by the breakdown of proteins and fats for energy; also toxins stored within the fat stores which are liberated as the fat stores melt away. One salad meal daily is eaten with a home-made dressing of 2 tbsp flaxseed oil (essential fatty acids for structural maintenance of the brain, skin, hormones, etc.) and 1 tbsp apple cider vinegar to aid digestion.

If constipation does occur, we recommend the use of the herb cascara (*C. sagrada*) to ensure the problem is only a temporary one.

A good multivitamin, multimineral supplement should be taken on this diet. It would also be beneficial to drink three cups of warm potassium broth (see Appendix I) daily, and eat as much celery or raw mushrooms as desired.

On this regimen you should expect to lose 4–5 lb (2–2.5 kg) per week, possibly more initially. This regimen should be followed by a calorie-reduced high-fiber diet coupled with aerobic conditioning. A weight loss of 20 lb in 4–5 weeks is not uncommon. The diet may safely be continued to 1–3 months with proper supervision. It is essential to have medical supervision on such a diet if it is followed for over 3 weeks. In the past, several deaths have resulted because overzealous dieters have followed a liquid protein diet from nutritionally inadequate sources for extremely prolonged periods of time.

Another short-term diet that has been used for weight loss is the so-called "high-protein" diet made famous by Dr Atkins (*New Diet Revolution*) This diet, and versions since, is based on the fact that if you reduce your carbohydrate intake below that needed for daily energy needs your body naturally will convert to burning fat for fuel. There is no question that this diet works. The only problem in following this diet is to do so in a manner consistent with naturopathic principles of good health. A great deal of research supports the view that whole grains are positive health factors that help protect us from a whole host of diseases. Unfortunately the high-protein diet makes the consumption of any significant part of our diet as whole grains impossible. It doesn't take very long on the high-protein diet to begin to notice problems of constipation due to fiber deficiency. We're not saying that this diet is not useful, because it is. You just need to modify it a little to make sure the choice of carbohydrate you are allowed on this diet is of the best possible unrefined kind. You also need to obtain free range meats, eggs and poultry, since a large portion of this diet will be these proteins. Try to have as much fish on this diet as you can. Make sure you have a large salad meal each day. With these provisions you should be able to lose weight on Dr Atkins' diet safely if you desire. Once you reach your ideal weight you should convert to a more traditional naturopathic diet with whole grains as the foundation.

Physiotherapy

- Aerobic exercise: continuous for 12–20 minutes minimum at 80% maximum heart rate (see *Fit or Fat?* by Covert Bailey), 6 times per week.
- Saunas to be taken whenever possible 1–6 times per week.
- Alternate hot and cold showers stimulate the circulation and endocrine system.
- Spinal manipulation and massage: 1–2 times per week.

Therapeutic Agents

Vitamins and Minerals— Primary

- Vitamin B complex: 50 mg 1–2 times daily.
- Multiminerals: e.g. Celtic salt.

Vitamins and Minerals— Secondary

- Vitamin B6: 100 mg 1–2 times daily for fluid retention problems.
- Vitamin C.

Others—Primary

Chromium tablets: for energy.

Kelp: (diuretic), to assist with getting rid of edema

Essential fatty acids (GLA, EPA, evening primrose oil, flaxseed oil)

Bran: 1 tsp with 1 glass water 10–20 minutes before meals; reduces appetite.

Others—Secondary

- Refer also to Hypoglycemia for herbs such as gymnema and goat's rue.
- Amino acids: taken before meals will reduce hunger and total intake.
- Atomodine (Cayce product): hypothyroid.
- DL-phenylalanine: appetite suppressant, 100–300 mg daily.
- Garlic.
- Lecithin.
- Raw pancreas tablets.
- Raw pituitary tablets.
- Raw thyroid tablets.

Botanicals—Primary

Garcinia cambogia: reduces appetite, reduces fat mass.

Bilberry: antioxidant.

Dandelion: liver tonic, cholagogue.
Siberian ginseng: adrenal tonic.
Refer also to Hypoglycemia for herbs such as gymnema and goat's rue.

Botanicals—Secondary

Fucus (bladderwrack): for obesity due to
hypothyroid condition, especially
where there is edema.
Poke root (highly toxic, see p. 60): infusion
of poke berries twice daily or poke
berry tablets, 2–3 times daily.
Lymphatic decongestant.

Therapeutic Suggestion

If you are contemplating a high-protein—low carbohydrate diet to lose weight, we recommend you do it in cycles. Continue one for no longer than 5 weeks, then revert to a "maintenance" program as suggested above for a further 5 weeks, then if you have more weight to lose, do another 5 weeks on the weight loss program, and so on. This way you minimize the negative impact of prolonged ketosis.

OSTEOPOROSIS

DEFINITION

Decrease in bone mass and density with loss of mineral and protein components.

SYMPTOMS

Back pain, pain on weight-bearing (T8 and below), kyphosis, loss of height, spontaneous fractures, muscle spasms.

ETIOLOGICAL CONSIDERATIONS—PRIMARY

- High-protein diet: induces calcium deficiency if the protein excess is animal in origin.
- Poor calcium absorption: calcium absorption decreases with age.
- Menopause
- Excess sweets and refined carbohydrates: stimulate alkaline digestive juices, making calcium insoluble (calcium is more soluble in an acid medium).
- Lack of exercise
- Magnesium deficiency: 80% loss in refining of grains.
- Phosphorus excess (excess meat, soda drinks, processed foods)

- Hydrochloric acid deficiency, enzyme deficiency

ETIOLOGICAL CONSIDERATIONS— SECONDARY

- Lactase deficiency
- Postoperative ulcer, stomach removal, dumping syndrome
- Prolonged stress
- Alcoholism
- Pregnancy, lactation, menstruation, repeated births
- Heavy metal toxicity: excess aluminum or cadmium is associated with bone loss
- Hormonal imbalance (parathyroid, thyroid)
- Phytic acid
- Oxalic acid
- Drugs; steroids; antibiotics
- Vitamin D, magnesium, calcium, and protein deficiency
- Poor dentures, leading to reduced green vegetable intake
- Distilled water, soft water
- Extreme vitamin C deficiency
- Sodium fluoride in water binds calcium
- Excess bicarbonate of soda
- Malabsorption syndromes

- Cushing's syndrome
- Hyperparathyroidism
- Acromegaly
- Smoking
- Bedridden: lack of movement and disuse leads to atrophy
- Aluminum excess: causes pseudohyper-parathyroidism

DISCUSSION

Bone is not, as many people believe, an unchanging material. In fact, each of the body's bones is constantly being remade. No single bone strut is ever permanent. Osteoblast and osteoclast cells are constantly dissolving and reforming bone. In addition, bone acts as a reservoir of calcium plus other minerals. When the blood level of calcium begins to fall, calcium is mobilized from the bones.

It has been estimated that over 30% of the American population suffer from calcium deficiency. The recommended adult minimum daily requirement (MDR) for calcium has been set at 800 mg daily. Some people, especially the aged, get 450 mg or less. To maintain calcium balance, the body mobilizes calcium from the bone by the action of parathyroid hormone (PTH). This mobilization is most pronounced at night.

Pregnancy, lactation, and growth also demand extra amounts of calcium. In pregnancy and lactation the MDR is raised to 1200 mg. With infants it is 540 mg.

Calcium need increases with age due to multiple factors, including poor digestion, lack of dentures which results in an altered diet (lack of green vegetables), hydrochloric acid deficiency, lack of exercise, and others. Calcium absorption is fairly inefficient, with up to 70–80% being excreted in the gut. This percentage is even greater in cases of hydrochloric acid lack in the digestive juice.

Unfortunately, calcium lack does not show itself early. Often the first sign of osteoporosis is a broken bone, or is seen on a routine chest x-ray. Calcium deficiency will show itself on x-ray only after 30% of the bone is lost.

Excessive consumption of meat is another factor leading to calcium deficiency. Meat contains 20–50 times more phosphorus than calcium. This leads to a loss of calcium from the bones to keep a proper phosphorus/calcium ratio in the blood. Aggravating this situation even more is the excessive meat eater who also smokes. Smoking increases the acidity of the blood, which inhibits conversion of vitamin D into its active form, leading to a pseudohyperparathyroidism with bone demineralization.

Many people believe they consume enough milk and cheese to prevent calcium deficiency. Unfortunately, however, calcium absorption from these sources may be very poor in cases of dairy intolerance. A far better source of calcium is to be found in raw green vegetables which are high in both calcium and magnesium. It is the general lack of raw vegetables in the diet that predisposes many people to osteoporosis. Vegetarians have less incidence of osteoporosis. The calcium-to-phosphorus ratio is much more favorable in vegetables than in dairy or meat products. This may be one factor explaining this observation.

Certain foods have also been implicated in inducing calcium deficiency and osteoporosis. Foods containing calcium oxalate bind calcium and thus make it unavailable. These foods include spinach, chard, beet greens, and chocolate. Recent research, however, questions this conclusion. The amount of calcium oxalate in these foods appears only capable of binding approximately the amount of calcium within these foods themselves, and not other foods taken in the same meal. Still, caution is suggested, to avoid excessive use of these foods in the diet. Phytic acid found in wheat and oats also will bind calcium. Wheat, however, contains the enzyme phytase, which acts in the leavening process to split phytic acid, rendering it incapable of binding calcium. This occurs only in the leavening process. A diet high in unleavened bread can inhibit uptake of zinc and calcium and cause rickets or osteoporosis. This seems to be a problem only for those on severely restricted diets.

Oats, however, contain very little phytase and some studies have associated a high incidence of rickets and osteoporosis in Scotland with habitual consumption of porridge. Other studies, however, stress the ability of the gut to acquire the capability to split phytic acid if accustomed to oats over several generations.

An interesting note on milk in relation to calcium absorption is that lactose, the sugar in milk, has been found to favor calcium absorption in people of northern European stock. These people seem to have a larger amount of lactase, the enzyme needed to digest milk. This seems to be a survival factor in countries with little exposure to sun.

Other research has provided more insight into causes of osteoporosis. The largest ever investigation on diet shows that in populations where the dietary intake of calcium and dairy products is high, the level of osteoporosis (as well as many other diseases) is the *highest*, and populations which have lower intakes of calcium actually have a stronger skeleton. For example, 25 million American women over age 40 have been diagnosed with osteoporosis and arthritis. These females have been drinking in excess of 2 pints (1 liter) of milk daily for their entire adult lives. Scandinavians are among the world's heaviest milk drinkers and they have the highest rates of osteoporosis.

African Bantu women take in only about 350 mg of calcium daily (the average Australian woman—600 mg per day). They bear nine children on average which they breast feed each for 2 years, and they rarely (if ever) suffer calcium deficiency or osteoporosis. Stone-age people did not consume animal milk; they had large, strong bones. We now know that if we adapt to (or have been brought up on) a relatively low-calcium diet, the body becomes more efficient with it; less calcium is excreted in the urine, and increases its rate of calcium absorption from the gut, in other words the body becomes more efficient in calcium absorption. Of course, calcium is contained in many foods,

including vegetables, nuts and seeds, legumes, and fruits. The calcium in milk is not our only or even best source. It is largely unable to be absorbed. Pasteurization (heat) destroys enzymes needed for absorption of dairy-based calcium by the human gut. The evidence points to the conclusion that drinking milk does not prevent osteoporosis.

What Are the Causes?

Perhaps the most significant causative factor of osteoporosis is a high intake of acid-forming foods, such as dairy foods, red meat, refined sugar, and grains. These foods create a more highly acidic environment in the system, especially tissues and the blood. This causes calcium loss from the blood through the kidneys, which in turn causes calcium loss from the bones. Because of the body's requirement for strict acid-alkali control (for example, blood pH has to be kept within the very narrow range of 7.35–7.45—alkaline, or else tetany, coma and death would follow rapidly) the body's homeostatic control mechanisms will pull calcium from the bones when it has to, calcium being an alkali mineral, in order to buffer against the threat excess acidity causes to the whole system. It is a case of a part of the body being sacrificed for the benefit of the whole.

Osteoporosis is caused by a number of things, the most important of which is excess intake of protein. The overall metabolic effect of dairy foods is acid-forming, whereas vegetable proteins contained in soy, nuts, brown rice, green leafy vegetables, is not acid forming, and does not pull calcium out of the bones.

The problem is further complicated by the fact that most people who consume milk products (cheese, butter, etc.) tend also to consume high levels of other protein, such as meats and grains, which are also acid-forming. These high-protein diets which regularly include animal proteins such as red meat, white meats, fish, dairy foods, actually increase secretion of calcium from the body in the urine. Red meat contains anywhere from 20–50 times more phosphorus than calcium. This excess phosphorus stimulates the parathyroid glands which mobilize calcium from the bones, and this extra calcium is then deposited around the joints, explaining the common finding in osteoporosis of less dense bones with calcium build-up around the joints. Vegetarians have less osteoporosis than meat eaters; a good vegetarian diet will have a much better phosphorus-to-calcium ratio. Another source of excess phosphorus is soft drinks.

Lack of magnesium in the diet can also be an important factor. Through its involvement in the normal activity of the parathyroid hormones controlling calcium, adequate serum levels of magnesium are necessary for proper calcium metabolism. Hypomagnesemia can result in hypocalcemia and peripheral resistance to the effects of vitamin D. In fact a high calcium intake intensifies magnesium deficit, so people who have calcium-enriched foods or supplements to an extent that the calcium-to-magnesium ratio of 2:1 is exceeded, a relative or absolute magnesium deficiency will also exist. Especially given that a stressed person requires more magnesium, and given that the dietary trend in the west is away from dietary magnesium sources such as fresh, raw green vegetables, it is not surprising to see osteoporosis on the increase. The best dietary sources of magnesium are the fresh leafy green vegetables.

While on the subject of vitamin D and the parathyroid hormones, remember that vitamin D is synthesized by direct exposure to the sun. There is an increasing unhealthy phobia about getting sun on the skin (see Cancer), and women who demonstrate higher rates of osteoporosis tend to get less sun on their bodies.

Several drugs definitely cause osteoporosis. These include the steroids and many antibiotics. Of these, steroids are the most important, since these are frequently taken over a period of years, and create an acidic environment. A frequent finding in cases of rheumatoid arthritis with steroid medication is osteoporosis with spontaneous fractures.

Reduction in estrogen levels at menopause is also a factor, but it is a relatively *small* factor in the onset of osteoporosis, as you would expect since low postmenopausal estrogen is an entirely natural, designed occurrence. Although estrogens are frequently used as therapy for osteoporosis in postmenopausal women it is the opinion of many experts that not only does estrogen therapy have many dangerous side effects, including cancer, but many studies reveal that it has no more effect in correcting osteoporosis than do simple calcium and mineral supplementations, and calcium has no dangerous side effects, especially if taken in dietary forms. (see Menopausal Problems).

It appears that the best preventative of postmenopausal osteoporosis is a proper diet in which acid and alkaline foods are more balanced, along with proper exercise in the sunshine, drinking lots of water, and adequate (not excessive) calcium levels prior to menopause. This means careful thought long before menopause begins.

PREVENTION AND TREATMENT

Diet

The diet should have an excess of green leafy vegetables and adequate sources of protein, especially vegetarian in origin. A meat-free diet is best, with plenty of fruits, vegetables, legumes, whole grains (such as brown rice, barley, and millet), nuts, sprouted seeds and beans, and fermented dairy foods such as kefir and yoghurt; in short, a vegetarian or lacto-vegetarian unrefined diet. Taking extra calcium foods just before bed is useful. Salads should contain lemon juice or cider vinegar dressing to increase calcium absorption. Contrary to popular belief, milk and dairy sources are not a very good source of *absorbable calcium* and should not be increased in the diet. In fact, some cases may require reduction of dairy intake to establish proper mineral balance and reduce tissue acidosis.

Physiotherapy

- Daily exercise.
- Sunbathing daily if possible.
- Sea bathing.

Therapeutic Agents

Vitamins and Minerals— Primary

- Chondroitin sulfate with MSM.
- Zinc: (for bone alkaline phosphatase) 25-50 mg, 2 times daily.
- Magnesium: 2000 mg twice daily.
- Vitamin E: 400-800 IU daily.
- Vitamin D: 400-1000 mg daily.
- Silica: to ensure adequate collagen synthesis.

Vitamins and Minerals— Secondary

- Vitamin B complex: 25-50 mg 2-3 times daily.

- Boron.
- Vitamin C: 1000-2000 mg 2-4 times daily.
- Copper.
- Calcium orotate: best source, 1000-1500 mg daily
  or: calcium lactate: with no milk intolerance.
  or: calcium glucomate.
  or: chelated calcium: 800 mg twice daily.
- Manganese.
- Osteoapatite.
- Pancreatic enzymes.
- Hydrochloric acid: if hypoacid.
- Cod-liver oil.
- Apple cider vinegar, water and honey: 1-2 times daily before meals.

Botanicals
Comfrey.
Horsetail.

PARKINSON'S DISEASE

DEFINITION AND SYMPTOMS

A chronic, slowly progressive disorder of the central nervous system characterized by hypokinesis (impairment of movement); muscle weakness; rigidity; tremor ("shaking palsy"); unsteady, shuffling gait; and an expressionless look on the face (Parkinson's mask). First sign is usually a hand tremor which is present at rest, but may disappear during purposeful movement. Speech is monotonous and handwriting is cramped. Muscle cramps and pain often occur.

ETIOLOGICAL CONSIDERATIONS—PRIMARY

- Liver damage.
- Nutritional deficiency.

- Environmental Toxins.
- Food allergy.
- Reduced dopamine levels in central nervous system.
- Encephalitis may precede disease.
- Cerebrovascular disease.
- Oxidative damage to nerve cells (free radicals, especially hydroxyl radicals).
- Excessive iron concentration in the substantia nigra.
- Chronically excessive amounts of serum cortisol.

ETIOLOGICAL CONSIDERATIONS— SECONDARY

Trauma; syphilis; tumor; drugs; heavy metal poisoning; chronic states of inflammation.

DISCUSSION

Parkinson's disease and Parkinson's-like symptoms may occur following encephalitis, trauma, cerebrovascular disease, or drug usage, or may accompany syphilis or tumor. These cases, however, cannot explain the large proportion of Parkinson's sufferers who show no apparent cause for their disorder.

Most cases show a clear abnormality in the brain. The areas of the brain affected are the globus pallidus and substantia nigra. This damage interferes with central nerve connections responsible for visual and proprioceptive information essential for normal postural maintenance and movement.

On the biochemical level the brain has been found to show a reduced level of dopamine, usually found in high concentration within the substantia nigra. The drug L-dopa has been used therapeutically. This precursor to dopamine penetrates the brain, is converted into dopamine, and helps relieve some of the symptoms of Parkinson's disease, such as slowness in movement, rigidity, and tremor. Other biochemical factors are probably involved, also, since L-dopa does not correct all the disease's symptoms.

There are some authorities that suspect that brain cells are damaged by toxins, either environmental or those from pharmaceutical or recreational drugs, food additives or pesticides that are not detoxified by the liver. Poor liver function therefore is a possible contributing factor in these cases as is toxic overload.

Some promising results come from the clinical application of strict naturopathic principles to Parkinson's disease. Like some other difficult-to-understand degenerative diseases, a drastic lifestyle change and internal detoxification often have shown remarkable results. With so much to gain and absolutely nothing to lose, the naturopathic approach given below should be tried for at least 6 months to 1 year, or longer. The only side effect will be improved health.

The treatment of Parkinsonism is best managed by or with a neurologist, or well-trained internist, and the patient must be referred if the symptoms persist or worsen.

TREATMENT

Begin therapy with a hair analysis test and any allergy tests available. Specifically test favorite foods.

Diet

It is always best to begin any treatment of a serious degenerative disease with an initial period of rebuilding. The best rejuvenation regimen in these cases is the raw foods lacto-vegetarian diet. This includes unlimited fruits, vegetables (especially greens), vegetable juice (carrot), seaweeds, sprouted grains, raw seeds (e.g. sunflower, pumpkin), and yoghurt. The object of this diet is to supply an abundance of vitamins, minerals, trace elements, essential fatty acids, and proteins to replenish the weakened body and strengthen the general vitality.

After this rejuvenation regimen is followed for a period of 4–6 weeks the patient will be ready for his or her first major elimination, which takes the form of a 7–14-day vegetable juice fast emphasizing carrot, beet, and green vegetable juice combinations. Spirulina, wheat grass and other green drinks and juices may also be added. Enemas should be taken on days 1, 2, 3, 5, 7, etc. This fast is broken by 1–2 days on grated apple and yoghurt and followed by a diet similar to the initial rejuvenation regimen, with the addition of seafoods. Shellfish are not allowed, only small ocean reef fish. It is essential to obtain organically grown foods whenever possible, and to avoid all canned, frozen, preserved, or otherwise poisoned or devitalized foods. Over the next 6–12 months alternate this rejuvenation diet with periods of fasting for 3–7 days every 4–6 weeks.

Physiotherapy

- Alternate hot and cold showers.
- Alternate hot and cold head douches.
- Saunas followed by massage and spinal therapy.
- Outdoor exercise.
- Sun and ocean baths.
- Wet cell appliance (gold)—(Cayce product).

Therapeutic Agents

Vitamins and Minerals—Primary
- Vitamin E: 400 IU 2-3 times daily. Antioxidant.
- Vitamin C: 500-2000 mg 3-4 times daily (helps counteract the side effects of L-dopa). Must be accompanied by vitamin E and selenium.
- Selenium: 200 mg daily. Antioxidant
- Vitamins and Minerals—Secondary.
- Vitamin A: 25,000 IU 1-2 times daily. (See warning under Vitamin Toxicity, page 56.)
- Vitamin B complex: 50 mg 2-3 times daily.
- Vitamin B1.
- Vitamin B3: 100-500 mg daily, to improve blood circulation to the brain. Start with 50 mg 3 times daily and slowly increase. Niacinamide does not cause flushing.
- Vitamin B6: 150 mg to 2 g daily (Do not take B6 if you are taking L-dopa, since it will interfere with its action).
- Vitamin B12: 1000 mcg intramuscularly 1-2 times per week.
- Iron: up to 20 mg daily, best as fumarate or phosphate.
- Zinc: 25-50 mg 1-2 times daily.
- Magnesium: 400-2000 mg daily.
- Calcium: 800-1000 mg daily.
- Manganese.

Others—Primary
- Acetyl-L-carnitine and coenzyme Q10: 240 mg daily Improves neuronal mitochondria energy output.
- Tyrosine and d-phenylalanine: Precursors to dopamine. Take between meals, not with carbohydrates. 1500 mg of each daily.
- Adenosine: 200 mg daily; a neuro-regulator
- Glutamine: up to 6000 mg daily. Precursor to GABA, catalyst for formation of acetylcholine. Detoxifies ammonia. Not for cancer patients.
- Essential fatty acids: use GLA or evening primrose oil.

Others—Secondary
- SOD (superoxide dismutase)—to inhibit free radical damage to neurons, spares dopamine.
- GABA to stabilize brain cell activity.
- Lecithin: as concentrated phosphatidylcholine: 4 capsules 3-4 times daily, or more; raw pituitary tablets.
- Raw adrenal tablets.
- Raw brain tablets; kelp: 2-3 times daily.

Botanicals—Primary
Hawthorn: circulatory stimulant.
Yellow dock: depurative.
Burdock: depurative, liver detoxification.
Cayenne: lymphatic stimulant.
Poke root: lymphatic stimulant (highly toxic, see page 60).
Yarrow: lymphatic stimulant.
Ginkgo biloba: improves blood circulation to the brain.

Botanicals—Secondary
Dandelion.
Siberian ginseng.
Sarsaparilla.
Nervine sedatives and tonics, e.g. skullcap, valerian, and St John's wort.
See Heavy Metal Poisoning if aluminum toxicity is a factor.

PEPTIC ULCER
(Gastric Ulcer, Duodenal Ulcer)

DEFINITION

A circumscribed erosion of the mucous membrane of the stomach and/or the duodenum.

Gastric ulcer: usually found on the lesser curvature of the stomach.

Duodenal ulcer: usually occurs on the duodenal side of the pyloric region.

Peptic ulcer: a common name for either of the above. The word "peptic" comes from the enzyme pepsin, which digests protein.

SYMPTOMS

Localized gnawing, burning pain (the pointing sign), heartburn, local tenderness, pain referred to the interscapular area, nausea, vomiting, diarrhea. Pains are related to food. Duodenal pain comes on 2-4 hours after meals and is relieved by food. Patient wakes around 2-4 a.m. with pain. Gastric ulcer begins just after eating, or within 20 minutes.

ETIOLOGICAL CONSIDERATIONS—PRIMARY

- Refined diet: protein stripping of carbohydrates (acts as buffer to stomach).
- Improper diet: coffee, tea, tobacco all stimulate excess acid production. Highly seasoned and fried foods stimulate acid production. Excess sweets, and beverages such as soda and soft drinks cause excess acid; overconsumption of sweets with no protein buffer a factor.
- Acidosis: excess acid and/or decreased mucus protection.
- Hypochlorhydria (diminished levels of hydrochloric and gastric acids).
- Stress: upsets normal digestive process.

ETIOLOGICAL CONSIDERATIONS— SECONDARY

- Constipation (gastric stresses, chronic purging).
- Chronic gastritis plus indigestion (reflux of bile, alcoholism, low blood sugar, iron deficiency anemia, aspirin, steroids, parasites, spinal T4 to T9).
- Food allergy.

DISCUSSION

The long-held view that the primary causes of ulcers are excess acid and stress is losing favor. While these factors often are present in many patients and may be contributing factors, it is becoming increasingly obvious that improper dietary habits are the primary cause in nearly all ulcer patients. Although naturopaths for years have stressed the importance of an unrefined diet in preventing disease, it took the efforts of a medical doctor, Dr T.L. Cleave, to present these ideas in a form acceptable at least to a significant minority of the scientific medical community. Although we feel Dr Cleave's insights into the causation of peptic ulcer and what he coins "the saccharine diseases", that is, diabetes, coronary heart disease, diverticulitis, obesity, and dental caries, are incomplete, they explain the role of diet and the refining of carbohydrates in the causation of peptic ulcers quite clearly.

Studies of the African Zulus of Natal, Ethiopian peasants, and natives on the Gold Coast in Africa (Ghana), where the incidence of peptic ulcers was exceedingly low or non-existent, led Dr Cleave to conclude that the main dietary difference between these people and ourselves is that we generally tend to eat highly processed, refined foods rather than whole grain foods. Refined foods such as white rice and white flour are all made by removing the outside germ and bran of the whole grain. This leaves mostly carbohydrate, or starch. The germ and bran, however, contain a large amount of fiber and protein. These are very important in normal digestion and also contain valuable minerals and vitamins necessary for good health.

During digestion the stomach produces hydrochloric acid which provides the proper conditions for the enzyme pepsin to break down protein in foods. The stomach itself is protected by a mucous layer, also made up of protein. Normally, the stomach acid does not affect the stomach wall and digests only foods. The protein in our diet helps protect us form the acid in our stomach, where it acts as a buffer. This is the main reason many doctors advise a high-protein milk diet for people with ulcers. The protein in milk helps, temporarily, to neutralize or buffer the stomach acid, and gives relief from ulcer pains. Refined grains, which have lost their outer coverings, no longer contain such a large amount of protein, so that when white rice or white bread is consumed, the stomach is exposed to much acid and very little protecting protein. If this is done repeatedly for a period of months or years, the stomach slowly gets eaten away and an ulcer is the result. Coffee, tea, smoking, and alcohol may aggravate this condition since each of these stimulates hydrochloric acid production.

The protein stripping of carbohydrates is even more of a problem when we consider the enormous consumption of sugary sweets in the civilized nations today. Unlike wheat, which may have lost 30% of its protein contents in refining, these products are completely devoid of all buffering protein. The result of their use is the stimulation of acid production for digestion, with literally nothing to be digested, except of course the stomach or duodenal walls!

Other factors in civilized nations also affect digestion. Stress certainly is a factor, in conjunction with a refined diet, causing digestion to halt and allowing food and digestive juices to lie for long periods in the stomach. The parasympathetic nervous system, which is responsible for the function of the digestive organs, ceases to act when the sympathetic nervous system, which is very responsive to danger and stress, is stimulated. This is the main reason all naturopaths emphasize eating only when relaxed and stress-free. Overeating or eating when not really hungry will cause indigestion and predispose a person to gastritis and ulcers. The peristaltic movements are decreased and gastric emptying time is increased.

Certainly all the other etiologic considerations have their influence, but diet, as you can see, plays the major role.

TREATMENT

Diet

There are no hard and fast rules in the dietary treatment of ulcers. Initial therapy depends on individual considerations, such as the severity of the ulcer, its duration, chronic or acute, vitality of the patient, weight, previous ulcer diets, dependency on antacid medication, etc. In general, if the patient has not already lost much weight a period of liquid dieting is very useful. This allows the ulcer to heal, especially if the liquids used are all specifically prescribed with this aim in mind. The fast may continue anywhere from 3–21 days, depending on the case. The following liquids have been found especially beneficial:

Stage 1
- Cabbage juice: contains metioninic acid and other undiscovered ingredients. This juice helps to normalize the mucous membrane in both stomach and duodenum. Drink 4–5 cups of half fresh cabbage juice and half celery or carrot juice daily.

- Comfrey tea: contains allantoin, a cell proliferant. The tea is very mucilaginous.
- Slippery elm tea: soothes and heals mucous membranes. Also very mucilaginous.
- Licorice root decoction: 700-1400 mg of deglycyrrhized licorice daily.
- Carrot, celery, and cabbage juice.
- Carrageen moss tea.
- Marshmallow decoction.
- Raw potato juice.
- Alfalfa tea.
- American saffron tea.
- Potassium broth.
- Fenugreek tea or decoction: heals and soothes inflamed mucous membranes.

Stage 2

This liquid diet should then be followed by the introduction of nourishing, easily digested foods, such as the Concord grape and raw goat's milk diet, taken at frequent intervals. The previous liquids in Stage 1 are also continued in this diet.

The following foods are useful at this stage if introduced slowly: ripe banana, okra, raw goat's milk, parsnips, beef juice, baked apples, cooked carrots, soy milk, papaya, raw goat's yoghurt, avocado, raw egg, yams, gelatin.

After this interim diet, finely grated raw vegetables are added to the regimen, as well as thoroughly cooked grains. The emphasis at this stage, as with previous diets, is to completely masticate each mouthful until it is liquefied; even liquids should be "chewed".

Physiotherapy

- Trunk or abdominal packs.
- Ice compress (for hemorrhage).
- Hot moist compress (for pain, apply front and back)
- Spinal (T4 to T9).
- Avoid sugar, refined foods, refined grains, alcohol, gum, chocolate, nicotine, tea, coffee.
- Salt, hot spices, red meats.

Therapeutic Agents

Vitamins and Minerals—Primary

Use with discretion, depending on case. Be careful with their introduction. As with all ulcer prescriptions, *go slow*.

- Vitamin A (micellized): 10,000-25,000 IU 4-6 times daily. Nourishes and protects stomach and intestinal lining.
- Vitamin B complex (liquid): 50 mg 2-3 times daily. Intramuscular B complex and B12 in early stages.
- Vitamin C (buffered): dose depends on condition and response to use. Facilitates wound healing.
- Bioflavonoids, especially quercetin: to inhibit histamine release.
- Vitamin E: 400-800 IU daily, helps reduce excess acidity, relieves ulcer pain, helps with healing.

Vitamins and Minerals—Secondary

- Vitamin K: 100 mcg daily.
- Pantothenic acid.
- Zinc: 25-50 mg 2-3 times daily.
- Iron.

Others—Primary

- Glucosamine: to restore mucous membranes
- Acidophilus powder.
- L-glutamine: 1.5-2 g daily, heals ulcers.
- Pectin: demulcent in the duodenum.
- Bromelain and papain: to improve digestion.

Others—Secondary

- Duodenal substance: 1-2 tablets with meals.
- Chamomile tea.
- Essential amino acids.
- Kelp.
- Pancreatic enzymes.
- Spirulina: 1 tsp 3 times daily.

Botanicals—Primary

Aloe: fresh juice. 1-11/5 fl oz (30-45 mL) 2-3 times daily. Reduces pain, promotes healing.

Comfrey: trophorestorative, demulcent.
Cat's claw.
Marshmallow.
Goldenseal: anti-microbial (against *Helicobacter pylorii*), and trophorestorative; specific for ulcers.
Slippery elm: demulcent; $^1/_2$ tsp in warm water 4–6 times daily.
Licorice root: promotes gastric and duodenal healing.

Botanicals—Secondary
American saffron.
Chamomile: nervine sedative, and anti-inflammatory.
Chickweed succus.
Geranium: bleeding ulcer.
Licorice: deglycerrhized.
Meadowsweet.
Myrrh.

Plantain.
Poke root (highly toxic, see p. 60).
White oak bark.
Wormwood: antimicrobial.

Therapeutic Suggestions

We usually do not advise any nutritional supplements in the early stages and rely on diet changes and mild demulcent herbs such as slippery elm. Later, as the condition improves, we advise supplements according to need. Intramuscular vitamins are useful in early stages and in severe cases. Vitamin C intravenously also may be useful to accelerate healing. Severe cases with blood in the stool; severe anemia; black, tarry stools; or severe epigastric or back pain should be referred to a sympathetic M.D.

PHLEBITIS AND THROMBOPHLEBITIS

DEFINITION

Phlebitis: irritation and inflammation of a vein.
Thrombophlebitis: presence of a thrombus (clot) in a vein with irritation of the vein wall.

SYMPTOMS

May be symptomless or show redness, edema, tenderness, heaviness, aching, slight fever, embolism. Sudden death is possible.

ETIOLOGICAL CONSIDERATIONS—PRIMARY

- Blood stasis
  Prolonged sitting (e.g. long plane trips); Prolonged bed rest; inactivity
- Heart disease
- Toxemia
- Excess animal-based protein and saturated fat diet
- Injury to endothelium of blood vessels
  Trauma; intravenous lines; bacteria; chemicals
- Increased coagulation of blood
  Contraceptive pill; malignancy

ETIOLOGICAL CONSIDERATIONS— SECONDARY

- Allergy
- Obesity
- Varicosities
- Fracture
- Postsurgical
- Debility
- Pregnancy (enlarging fetus may cause

pressure on blood vessels, reducing flow)

- Smoking may lead to vasoconstriction; stress may lead to vasoconstriction

DISCUSSION

Phlebitis and thrombophlebitis are extremely serious conditions. A clot in a vein tends to form at areas of irregularity, trauma, or inflammation due to injury, intravenous lines, bacteria, or irritating chemicals. It begins as dense layers of platelets and fibrin, and later may become a large, friable, jelly-like mass, which may break off to form an embolism, or free-floating body in the bloodstream. Embolisms may travel to the lungs, heart, or brain and occlude small blood vessels. This may have disastrous and even fatal results. Thrombophlebitis most commonly develops in the deep veins of the lower leg, but it may occur elsewhere.

Conditions causing blood stasis, which allows a thrombus to propagate, are the major causes of thrombophlebitis. Faster-moving blood helps to clear the blood vessels effectively and helps prevent thrombus formation. Postsurgical or postpartum thrombophlebitis is particularly common. Any other condition that restricts blood flow, such as prolonged bed rest, sitting, inactivity, obesity, varicosities, or heart disease may be a contributing factor. There has been much discussion in the press of deaths following long plane flights caused by clots forming from prolonged sitting in confined seats.

The use of oral contraceptives has now been recognized as carrying an increased risk of thrombophlebitis and embolism. For some as yet unknown reason many malignancies show an increased coagulation of blood, causing an increased chance of thrombus formation.

A little-recognized factor, but extremely important, is the influence of toxicity in the bloodstream. This factor, along with nutritional deficiency, is probably the primary cause of the phlebitis in the first place. The worst combination of factors is a nutritionally deficient, toxic bloodstream in a sedentary individual who smokes and is under stress.

TREATMENT

All cases of phlebitis and thrombophlebitis must be under the care of a physician. They are serious and possibly life-threatening problems, not to be taken lightly.

Diet

The main dietary aims are elimination and blood cleansing. Begin with a 3–7-day fast on citrus juice (grapefruit) and vegetable juice (carrot and others). Nightly enemas should be taken. For those unable to fast the all-fruit diet (see Appendix I) will be adequate. The initial fast is followed by a raw foods diet still stressing citrus and carrot juice, but also including a large amount of green salads and sprouts. The basic diet should be as follows:

On Rising
Hot water and lemon.

Breakfast
Grapefruit.

Midmorning
Carrot juice.

Lunch
Mixed raw green salad with plenty of sprouted seeds and beans, and a large portion of steamed onions.

Midafternoon
Carrot juice.

Supper
As lunch.
Five to 10 days on this gentle blood-cleansing regimen should help alleviate the problem. This diet is followed by an unsaturated fat

vegetarian diet, stressing citrus, green vegetables, sunflower seeds, soy protein (lecithin), and whole grains, until the condition is completely removed. Absolutely no sugar, refined carbohydrates, fried foods, coffee, tea, alcohol, or smoking is permitted during this regimen.

Physiotherapy

- Alternate hot and cold compresses and showers
- Hot Epsom salts baths (see Appendix I).
- Mild exercise.
- Papaya poultice.
- Mullein tea poultice.
- Plantain and witch hazel poultice.
- Elevate foot of bed 4 inches (10 cm) if thrombosis is in leg.
- Avoid: crossing legs; prolonged sitting; inactivity; constipation; garters, girdles, or restrictive clothing
- Be sure to get up and move about on planes at least once every hour

Therapeutic Agents

Vitamins and Minerals—Primary
- Vitamin C: 6-10 g daily; helps keep capillaries strong.
- Bioflavonoids, oligomeric proanthocyanidins.
- Vitamin E: 400 IU 2-3 times daily. With adequate calcium it is an antithrombic agent. Helps strengthen blood vessels.

Vitamins and Minerals—Secondary
- Vitamin A: 25,000 IU twice daily.
- Vitamin B complex: 50 mg 2-3 times daily.
- Niacin: 200-600 mg daily (helps dissolve fibrin).
- Pantothenic acid: 100 mg daily.
- Rutin: 100-200 mg daily.

Others—Primary
- Essential fatty acids: flaxseed oil, GLA or evening primrose oil; helps decrease adhesiveness of platelets.
- Mucopolysaccharides: contain hyaluronic acid, heparin, and chondroitin sulfate (foods high in these "protein sugars" include oats, okra, shark fin soup, NZ green-lipped mussels, comfrey, raw oysters, aloe vera, ginseng, slippery elm).
- Bromelain: 2 tablets 3 times daily taken on an empty stomach: proteolytic, dissolves clots.
- Garlic: 2 capsules 3 times daily.
- Lecithin: 3-4 capsules 4 times daily (helps inhibit clotting).
- Orthophosphoric acid: blood thinner.
- Acetyle L-carnitine: 500 mg daily. Protects blood from accumulation of fat.
- Coenzyme Q 10: 200 mg daily. Improves circulation.
- L-histidine: 500 mg daily. Blood vessel dilator.

Others—Secondary
- Raw spleen: anticoagulant.
- Chlorophyll.
- Wheat germ oil.

Botanicals—Primary
Gotu kola and paeonia: both have specific antifibrin activity, and are specific for this condition.
Ginger: vascular anti-inflammatory.
Horse chestnut: reduces edema associated with this condition
Ginkgo biloba: anti-PAF (platelet aggregation factor) to reduce abnormal clotting of platelets.
Clivers: lymphatic stimulant

Botanicals—Secondary
Comfrey: poultice.
Mullein tea: internal.
Plantain: poultice.
Note: The above therapies are mostly for use with superficial venous thrombophlebitis. Phlebothrombosis of a deep vein is a life-threatening situation and requires treatment in an inpatient facility.

POISON IVY

DEFINITION AND SYMPTOMS

A contact dermatitis resulting from irritation of the skin by the resin of the poison ivy plant. Within hours, or sometimes several days, the skin begins to itch or burn, followed by the eruption of small blisters which may coalesce to cover large portions of the body. As the vesicles rupture, crusting forms, overlying a raw, oozing surface.

TREATMENT

Wash skin with antiseptic soap as soon after exposure as possible. Apply antipruritic skin lotions such as calamine lotion. Cooling compresses with cold water and vinegar are very useful every 1-2 hours. A bath in potassium permanganate may help relieve itching, as will oatmeal baths. A plaster of baking soda moistened with water is also useful. Other treatments include plantain poultices and goldenseal infusion wash.

Rhus toxicodendron and *Urtica urens* tinctures taken internally at frequent intervals will shorten the course of the rash. Saltwater swimming is very effective therapy.

Therapeutic Agents

Vitamins and Minerals
- Vitamin C: 1000 mg per hour.
- Vitamin A: 25,000-50,000 IU 1-2 times daily.
- Vitamin B complex: 50 mg twice daily.
- Zinc: 25-50 mg 2-3 times daily.

Others
- Rhus tox: 12×; 30C.
- Calamine lotion: apply 4-6 times daily.
- Chlorophyll: bowel detoxicant.
- Raw adrenal: 2 tablets 3 times daily.

Botanicals
Aloe vera: apply sap or gel to rash every two hours.

PREMENSTRUAL TENSION SYNDROME

DEFINITION AND SYMPTOMS

A cyclic condition related to the menstrual cycle, characterized by tension, irritability, sudden mood swings, depression, hostility, emotional disturbances, anxiety, crying, lack of energy, sleeping difficulties, headaches, sinusitis, vertigo, faintness, fluid retention, swelling and soreness of breasts, abdominal bloating, abdominal cramps, acne flare, craving for sweets or alcohol. Onset is usually 4-10 days prior to menstruation and ends abruptly after onset of flow.

ETIOLOGICAL CONSIDERATIONS

- Hypoglycemia.
  Excess sweets; excess coffee, tea, soda, chocolates, alcohol.
- Essential fatty acid deficiency
- B complex deficiency
- Vitamin B6 deficiency
- Contraceptive pills (fibrocystic breast disorder)
- Glandular imbalance
  Estrogen excess; progesterone deficiency

ETIOLOGICAL CONSIDERATIONS— SECONDARY

- Magnesium deficiency
- Stress.
- Adrenal exhaustion.
- Stress-induced hypoglycemia
- Vitamin B deficiency
- Vitamin C deficiency
- Water retention
- Lead or copper toxicity

DISCUSSION

The premenstrual tension syndrome has been recognized for centuries. Most sufferers of severe premenstrual tension are aware that they have a problem. Cyclic outbreaks of uncontrolled emotions cause distress to other family members and are often a source of deep remorse once the "witch cycle" is passed. Many women readers may be bristling with animosity at this point. We think it fair to mention very early in this discussion that certainly not all women suffer from the premenstrual syndrome, and of those that do, many experience only the physiological symptoms and not the more advertised psychological ones. Much evidence, however, does support the fact that these psychological symptoms do exist for some women. The highest number of violent crimes committed by women occur in the premenstrual period, 4–7 days prior to menstruation. This period is the peak for women being admitted to both prison and psychiatric institutions. There also is an increased percentage of female accidents and suicide attempts during this part of the menstrual cycle. Brain waves in the premenstrual period are increased in frequency and amplitude compared to those of midcycle, another indication of a true psychological alteration.

For years premenstrual tension was considered to be entirely psychosomatic in origin. Later authorities gave women a little more consideration and blamed the condition on the normally fluctuating female hormones, estrogen and progesterone. Although the exact role of these hormones in causing common premenstrual symptoms is as yet not clearly defined, certain overall patterns have emerged in PMS sufferers. The female hormone estrogen has been found elevated in the late luteal phase, reaching its maximal point 1–5 days before menstruation. By contrast, progesterone in PMS patients shows a reduction in the midluteal phase, compared to non-PMS control subjects, reaching its lowest relative deficiency 5–10 days before menstruation. Other studies have implicated increased levels of follicle-stimulating hormone (FSH), aldosterone, and prolactin. Of these hormone abnormalities, those most significantly associated with the symptoms of PMS seem to be the late luteal estrogen excess, and midluteal progesterone deficiency.

Although repeated studies show a correlation between elevated estrogen and elevated estrogen/progesterone ratios with premenstrual anxiety, irritability, and depression, the actual mechanism by which these hormonal changes influence moods and how they may interrelate with known micronutrient deficiencies is still unclear. We know that elevated estrogens interact with brain enzymes to cause an elevation of adrenalin which is known to trigger anxiety; with noradrenalin, known to promote hostility and irritability; and with serotonin, which helps cause nervous tension, fluid retention, and inability to concentrate. Dopamine, which is believed to balance the effects of these three amines by enhancing relaxation and mental alertness, is found to be at reduced levels.

Irrespective of exactly which hormone or combination of hormones, vitamins, and minerals initiates the physiological or even psychological symptoms of premenstrual tension, the usual implication being made is that "women are just made that way".

Obviously, this explanation is incorrect. It completely fails to explain why some women have severe premenstrual symptoms while others have mild or even no symptoms whatsoever. We do not doubt that this syndrome is mediated by one or more of the female hormones described above. Whatever the glandular "cause", which as yet is still not specifically known, the general condition of premenstrual tension is due to a hormone imbalance and this imbalance, like most other imbalances within the body, is due, we feel, to an improper mode of living. Hypoglycemia, stress, and nutritional deficiency due to improper diet seem to be the main factors causing this hormonal imbalance.

Hypoglycemia, caused by an improper diet of refined carbohydrates, sweets, pastries, coffee, and alcohol, is well known to cause bouts of emotional instability and clouded thought. PMS patients have been shown to consume more refined carbohydrates and 2.5 times the amount of refined sugar than normal non-PMS controls. It is not the hypoglycemic state itself that causes premenstrual tension. Low blood sugar affects the individual in relation to food, and not the menstrual cycle. Its symptoms disappear after food is eaten and are never prolonged for days on end. What hypoglycemia does, however, is to overburden the adrenal glands as they struggle to keep up with the roller-coaster ride of the drastically fluctuating blood sugar level. This is significant for several reasons. The adrenal glands require large amounts of vitamin B complex and vitamin C, among other nutrients, to maintain their functioning. They literally burn off a great deal of the body's supply of these vitamins when overstressed, depriving the rest of the body of these essential substances at the same time.

The typical diet that produces hypoglycemia in the first place is composed of highly refined carbohydrates which are stripped of their B complex in the refining process. Vitamin B complex in turn is essential for carbohydrate metabolism. Thus we have a vicious cycle of B complex-deficient foods consumed in excess that require B complex for metabolism (therefore B complex must be obtained from elsewhere in the body for this purpose), producing hypoglycemia, creating adrenal exhaustion.

The adrenals in turn require excessive amounts of B complex for their own function. If we now couple this catastrophic scenario with habitual consumption of coffee and alcohol, both of which further stimulate the adrenal glands violently and deplete B complex even further, we begin to see why B complex and B6 in particular have been found useful to some degree in preventing and treating premenstrual tension.

Stress-induced adrenal exhaustion is another common finding in these cases. If severe, this may even lead to stress-induced hypoglycemia. Stress also is important since emotions play such a strong role in the female endocrine system, affecting first the hypothalamus, then the pituitary, ovaries, and adrenal glands. Prolonged stress is also known to cause a relative dopamine deficiency. The combination of improper diet and stress is the most detrimental of all.

All of this abuse to the adrenal glands has particular importance in relation to hormonal balance. The adrenal glands also function as a backup for the ovaries, producing about 20% of the total estrogens.

Several other nutritional factors have been associated with this symptom. PMS patients consume 4.5 times more dairy products than normal controls. This correlation is interesting since it is known that saturated (animal) fats inhibit the formation of PGE1, an anti-inflammatory prostaglandin found deficient in PMS women. PGE1 synthesis is also inhibited by *trans* fatty acids as found in processed or heat-treated vegetable oils and margarine, alcohol, and stress-induced catecholamines. Animal fats also contain large amounts of arachidonic acid, which acts as a precursor to PGE2, PGF2, and thromboxane, which function antagonistically to PGE1. This may be the reason that sources rich in *cis*-linoleic acid and gamma-linolenic acid (GLA), such as evening primrose oil, which enhance PGE1 production, have been found useful therapeutically with PMS.

Magnesium deficiency is also associated with PMS and is known to cause a depletion of brain dopamine levels. Erythrocyte magnesium levels taken from PMS patients in the midluteal phase have been shown to be significantly lower than in control groups. Magnesium and zinc are required for the synthesis of PGE1, from the cis-linoleic acid pathway. Magnesium deficiency may result from lack of whole grains and vegetables in the diet, or may be the result of stress-induced adenocorticoid secretion, or prolonged diuretic use. A little tip here; if you crave chocolate, it may be the expression of the body's need for magnesium.

Interestingly, the supplementation of vitamin B6 (pyridoxine) has been reported to normalize low erythrocyte magnesium levels. B6 deficiency may also be a factor in low dopamine levels, since this vitamin acts as a co-factor in dopamine biosynthesis.

Other neuroactive substances that are vitamin B6-dependent are alpha-amino-butyric acid, a brain neurotransmitter producing sedation, as well as serotonin and tryptophan. The earliest reports that vitamin B6 therapy was useful in PMS were found in relation to women on the contraceptive pill, which is known to be associated with vitamin B6 deficiency. Later studies showed its effectiveness with many PMS patients not previously on oral contraceptives. Still other reports found that vitamin B6 was not as effective for some of the class of PMS patients whose symptoms were primarily depression. In cases where an acne flare occurring premenstrually was a symptom, vitamin B6 was found to be up to 72% effective. Once again, the precise therapeutic mode of action of vitamin B6 is not yet clear. Preliminary findings demonstrate that it increases midluteal serum progesterone and reduces elevated estrogen levels. It is suspected that B complex deficiencies, and in particular vitamin B6 deficiency, may cause a lowered hepatic clearance of estrogen, causing an elevated serum level to occur.

Another very interesting nutritional factor related to PMS is the use of essential fatty acids. In double-blind placebo trials, evening primrose oil has been proven effective in significantly relieving PMS symptoms. The postulated mode of action is the enhanced synthesis of PGE1 from the increased supply of cis-linoleic and gamma-linolenic acid.

Vitamin E has also been found useful in the treatment of PMS with most improvement in cases where benign breast disease was a major problem. Vitamin E plays a role as antioxidant, and may help prevent adverse inflammatory reactions to dietary fats by preventing rancidity. Vitamin E may also play a role by inhibiting the formation of PGE-antagonist derived from the arachidonic acid found in animal fats. Other antioxidants, such as vitamin C or selenium, may play a role, as well as vitamin A and zinc.

TREATMENT

Diet

The most effective dietary regimen is an integration of the diet regimens found under Hypoglycemia and Heart Disease. These emphasize elimination or drastic reduction of refined carbohydrates and simple sugars, a reduction of animal-based proteins, and an increase in unrefined whole grains and essential fatty acids. This diet combination is aimed at normalizing the blood sugar level, healing the overburdened adrenal glands, and providing a proper supply of vitamins, minerals, trace elements, and essential fatty acids. It is important to exclude coffee, tea, cola, chocolate, salt, alcohol, cigarettes, and heated or processed oils.

Stress Reduction

Even a good diet will not totally protect the body from the devastating effects of prolonged stress. Stress is often the result of an improper attitude or approach to life and its problems (challenges). Many times we hear patients say that they simply have no time to devote to relaxation exercises or meditation, even when they recognize stress as a real health problem. This attitude comes from a completely inappropriate value system and lack of self-knowledge.

One of the most valuable assets a person can have in life is the ability to be relaxed, poised, and centered. This "centering" or concentration can bring even the most difficult of tasks within your capabilities. To obtain and maintain this desirable state of being, a certain amount of effort and time is required; however, the effort, time, and energy saved throughout your day by more efficient and productive action more than compensates for this expenditure. In reality, most people waste a phenomenal amount of time and energy each day. Fifteen or 20 minutes once or twice daily devoted to relaxation exercises or meditation can be set aside by even the busiest person. The truth of the matter usually is that people have the time, but have so little control of their thoughts, feelings, and actions that they are *unable* to sit quietly, until completely exhausted by their day. This is all the more reason to begin disciplining the mind.

You will find a list of relaxation exercises under Insomnia. These are very useful in stress reduction, as are many forms of meditation.

Physiotherapy

- Spinal manipulation: once weekly for 4-6 weeks and then once or twice per month until two normal premenstrual tensionless months pass.
- General exercise: exercise helps stimulate and regulate the hormonal system. It also helps reduce stress.
- Outdoor fresh air walks and sunbathing.
- Ocean swimming.

Therapeutic Agents

Vitamins and Minerals—Primary
- Vitamin B complex: 50 mg 2-3 times daily.
- Vitamin C: 1000-2000 mg 3 times daily or more to bowel tolerance.

- Vitamin B6: 250 mg twice daily, especially when an acne flare occurs with the premenstrual tension syndrome. Also used for its diuretic characteristics when fluid retention problems are severe.
- Vitamin E: 400 IU 2-3 times daily.

Vitamins and Minerals—Secondary
- Vitamin A: 10,000-20,000 IU daily; 40,000-100,000 IU 10 days premenstrually in difficult cases.
- Calcium lactate or chelate: 2-3 times daily (total 800 mg).
- Magnesium: 400 mg 1-3 times daily.
- Zinc: 25-50 mg daily.
- Others, as found under Hypoglycemia.

Others—Primary
- Probiotics.
- Evening primrose oil: 1000 mg 3 times daily. GLA may also be used.

Others—Secondary
- Brewer's yeast.
- Desiccated liver.
- EPA (eicosapentaenoic acid): 5-10 g daily.
- Parsley tablets: diuretic.
- Raw adrenal tablets; raw ovary tablets.
- Raw pituitary tablets.
- Tryptophan: with depression.
- Reduce liquids premenstrually; no coffee, tea, cola, chocolate, sugar, or refined carbohydrates.
- No alcohol until cured, then only in moderation.
- Salt: fluid retention is the major cause of physiological symptoms. Avoid salt-containing foods such as dried fish, dried meats, soy sauce, hot dogs, pickles, salted popcorn, monosodium glutamate (MSG), cheese, bacon, ham, canned foods, butter, salted nuts, etc. Use only an unrefined sea salt such as Celtic salt.

Botanicals—Primary
The following herbs are specifics for the related conditions:

PMT-P (with cramping pain)
Dong quai
Poke root (highly toxic, see page 60)
PMT-A (with anxiety)
Chaste tree: best at 7 a.m. and 4 p.m.
True unicorn root (*Aletris farinosa*)
and false unicorn root (*Helonia
luteum*)
Wild yam
Squaw vine
PMT-C (with cravings)
Gymnema silvestre
Bitter herbs: (help stabilize blood sugar
levels)
Goat's rue
Bilberry
Globe artichoke
Fringe tree: specific for the pancreas
PMT-D (with depression)
Blue cohosh
Withania
St John's wort
Panax ginseng

False unicorn
Liver herbs such as St Mary's thistle and
dandelion
PMT-H (with hyperhydration, or edema)
Red clover
Dandelion
Chaste tree
Other diuretics such as bladderwrack
might be useful
General PMT symptoms can include:
Headaches: chaste tree
Digestive upsets: chamomile
Acne: chaste tree

Therapeutic Suggestions

When fibrocystic breast disease is present
with PMS, it is essential to stop all coffee
and use high levels of GLA (gamma-linolenic
acid) as found in evening primrose oil along
with vitamin E, and vitamin B6.

PROSTATE DISORDERS
(Benign Prostatic Hyperplasia, Prostatitis and Prostate Cancer)

DEFINITION

Benign prostatic hypertrophy: enlarged
prostate gland.
Prostatitis: inflamed, swollen prostate
usually due to infection. May be acute or
chronic.
Prostate cancer: cancer of the prostate
gland.

SYMPTOMS

Dysuria (painful urination), painful defeca-
tion, frequency of urination, inability to
empty bladder fully, desire to urinate, incontinence of urine, possible fever, impotence,
back pain, painful orgasm.

ETIOLOGICAL CONSIDERATIONS—PRIMARY

- Cancer must always be considered first,
  to exclude this as a possibility.
- Diet: too little alkaline foods, constipation, too little fiber, excess alcohol, tea,
  coffee, spices, essential fatty acid deficiency, zinc deficiency.
- Congestion: sluggish bowels, poor
  lymph and blood flow, toxicity of blood,
  poor abdominal tone.
- Sedentary occupation
- Lack of exercise

ETIOLOGICAL CONSIDERATIONS—SECONDARY

- Spinal lesions
- Excess exposure to cold surfaces
- Infection (gonorrhea, foci spread from elsewhere)

DISCUSSION

The prostate is a chestnut sized gland that lies just below the male bladder and surrounds the urethra. The prostate secretes a lubricating fluid that helps prevent infection and aids in sperm motility.

Having a "prostate problem" does not mean you have got cancer, or that you will die from prostate cancer. There are several different conditions, and one needs careful diagnosis to know just what might be happening.

Prostatitis involves inflammation of the prostate, by some infectious agent, such as a bacterium, even gonorrhea, or a non-bacterial agent, and the symptoms of urinary dysfunction in these cases are usually accompanied by chills, fever, low back pain, and burning upon urination.

Most prostate problems however involve a benign (meaning non-cancerous) swelling of the prostate gland, and it is estimated that in western society over 50% of men between 40 and 60 years old have an enlarged prostate gland, a condition known as *benign prostatic hyperplasia* (BPH).

A more serious condition is *cancer of the prostate*, the second most common malignancy in men, and in men older than age 55, is the third most common cause of cancer death.

Nutritional research now supports the view that all of these conditions are often preventable and the increasingly common benign prostatic hyperplasia responds very successfully to simple dietary changes and nutritional supplementation.

All of these conditions are serious and cause very uncomfortable symptoms and a cancerous prostate can become the site from which more disseminated cancer originates, which can be life threatening.

Once the prostate is the site of infection or cancer, it's a bit late to consider prevention. While there are still benefits from nutritional supplementation in these instances, you definitely need to have proper medical care and advice. Non-bacterial and benign prostatic hyperplasia, however, respond very well to changes in diet, reduced toxic exposure and nutritional supplementation.

When enlarged, the prostate pinches off the flow of urine, causing the characteristic symptoms of progressive urinary frequency, urgency and difficulty in voiding urine, or a small urine output. A classic sign is waking frequently at night with an urge to urinate but finding it difficult to do so. These symptoms gradually increase in severity over time until urine flow becomes extremely difficult and limited. The retention of urine can irritate the bladder creating the conditions suitable for infection and in later states may also irritate and damage the kidneys. Symptoms of bacterial and non-bacterial prostatitis include the above but there are the added symptoms of chills, fever, low back pain and burning upon urination. Cancer of the prostate unfortunately often has very few symptoms although any of the above symptoms may be present. Diagnosis is usually made by digital exam and needle biopsy.

Orthodox medicine considers prostate enlargement to be a normal consequence of the aging process. Certainly its occurrence is so frequent in the 40–60 age group to support this view. However, just because something is common does not necessarily mean it is normal. There is a great deal of evidence obtained by studying differing populations, animals and human subjects, that prostate problems are not a normal part of aging, but in fact related to diet and environmental toxicity.

In the case of benign prostatic hyperplasia, current knowledge of the mechanism that causes the prostate to enlarge with age is now fairly well accepted. The prostate tissue is very sensitive to the hormone dihydrotestosterone which is converted from the male hormone testosterone. As men age, although their testosterone levels decrease, dihydrotestosterone begins to accumulate in the prostate, triggering diffuse prostatic enlargement. The reason for this paradox (i.e. less testosterone and five times more dihydrotestosterone in prostate tissue) is due to two main factors: increased uptake of testosterone by the prostate and decreased removal of dihydrotestosterone from the prostate tissues.

Increased uptake of testosterone is linked to another hormone, prolactin. If prolactin levels increase, testosterone levels increase in the prostate as does the conversion from testosterone of dihydrotestosterone. Some drugs used in treating prostate enlargement are used because they lower prolactin levels, but this class of drugs has severe side effects and is not used frequently. We now know that prolactin levels are increased by beer and alcohol, pointing to a lifestyle change that if enacted, could be helpful with some prostate problems. The trace mineral zinc taken with B6 also reduces prolactin levels and is a safe alternative to these toxic drugs.

Decreased removal of testosterone and dihydrotestosterone from the prostate is linked to another hormone, estrogen. Estrogen, normally thought of as a female hormone, is also present in men and its relative proportion to testosterone increases as testosterone levels fall with age. Estrogen inhibits enzymes that metabolize testosterone and dihydrotestosterone and these hormones are left accumulating within the prostatic tissue, activating prostatic growth.

Unfortunately the medical treatment for most prostate disorders is not usually curative. With bacterial infection, bed rest and antibiotics are prescribed. Often the infection becomes chronic or recurrent and is very difficult to eliminate. In non-bacterial inflammation, the doctor may attempt prostatic massage several times a week. Occasionally drugs are used to manipulate the hormone levels, but tend to have many undesirable side effects. Often the inflamed prostate does not return to normal.

The treatment for prostate enlargement is usually surgery to remove the enlarged prostate tissue. Although most who have this operation still retain some sexual ability, it is definitely altered by the operation. Therapy for prostate cancer is the use of female hormones and castration. Obviously anything that will help prevent these problems is the best course.

While the hormonal changes outlined above occur to some extent in all men as a natural process of aging, there is a great deal of nutritional and clinical research that clearly shows that most, if not all, prostate problems are preventable, and often reversible by simple lifestyle changes, diet and nutritional supplementation.

Studies of population groups that naturally live different lifestyles and have differing eating habits are often used to show that these factors are important in preventing disease. It has been observed for example that the frequency of prostate cancer varies in different parts of the world. While the United States has a rate of 14 and Sweden 22 deaths per 100,000 population, Japan's rate is only 2 per 100,000. However, Japanese immigrants to the United States develop prostatic cancer at a similar rate to the country they migrate to suggesting an environmental or local nutritional factor as the principal cause for these population differences. Two such factors that have been suggested in the literature are exposure to toxic chemicals and pesticides such as dioxin, polyhalogenated biphenyls, exachlorobenzene and dibenzofurans and diethylstiboestrol. Cadmium excess as a result of cigarette smoking, second hand or passive smoke exposure and air pollution is also linked to prostatic enlargement. Cadmium excess increases the conversion of testosterone to dihydrotestosterone.

It is quite possible that part of the cause of the sudden increase of benign prostatic hyperplasia and prostatic cancer over the last two decades is a result of the ever increasing toxic load of chemicals and pesticides in our environment and food. This

401

points us towards avoidance of these chemicals when reasonably possible and protecting ourselves from their toxic effects by natural detoxifying and antioxidant supplements to our diet to help our body protect itself against this excessive toxic load. As we will see later there is ample clinical evidence that various nutritional factors such as zinc, essential fatty acids, flavinols and saw palmetto extract to name just a few, help prevent and reverse the most common prostatic disorder, benign prostatic hyperplasia. Other studies relating to cancer prevention in general give us evidence that many types of cancer are also preventable by proper diet and adequate or supplemental antioxidants such as beta-carotene.

As in most diseases found more frequently in "civilized" countries, proper diet is the single most important preventative to prostate disorders. Research now points to a diet composed of plenty of fresh fruits and berries, raw and conservatively cooked vegetables, whole grains (high in fiber), seeds and nuts (especially pumpkin seeds), beans, fermented dairy products, fish, and few added fats and oils. High cholesterol levels are associated with prostate enlargement. The oils consumed should be cold pressed and high in essential fatty acids (e.g. sunflower oil).

Advances in nutritional research now enable us to understand why many traditional folk remedies have been so effective in treating prostate problems. The following type of diet will protect against the development of disease of the prostate, and will enable the body to provide an environment in which healing can occur.

Diet

Initially, we recommend a totally saturated fat-free, vegetarian diet, using plant protein combinations, and soy foods. The diet should be a high-fiber, non-citrus, alkaline-reacting diet, containing large amounts of raw green vegetables, essential fatty acids, and zinc. The fiber content will help correct habitual constipation and adding 1 tbsp raw bran (psyllium powder) to each meal further aids in this process.

Essential fatty acids as found in cold pressed unrefined vegetable oils such as sunflower, safflower, and sesame should be included in the diet regularly. Nuts and seeds are also important sources.

Zinc foods such as oysters, herrings, clams, wheat and rice bran, wheat germ, molasses, eggs, nuts, pumpkin seeds, peas, carrots, corn, beans, brown rice, garlic, onions, and brewer's yeast should be included in the diet whenever possible. Due to the unreliability of present food sources of zinc, however, additional zinc supplements will also be needed.

It is wise to begin the dietary regimen with an internal cleansing regimen, the length and severity depending on the patient. The apple mono diet is an ideal cleansing regimen in this condition and involves eating four meals of organic apples and drinking diluted (50/50) apple juice and water periodically throughout the day when thirsty. This may be followed for 3–7 days or longer. 1 tbsp cold pressed olive oil should be taken on the evening of the final day of this diet.

Specific Nutrients for Prevention and Cure

Nutritional research has pinpointed certain foods and nutritional substances that are particularly beneficial in the prevention and treatment of prostate disorders.

Vitamins and Minerals— Primary

- **Zinc:** Adequate zinc intake and absorption is the single most important prevention and treatment for the condition of benign prostatic hyperplasia. Adequate zinc in the diet and the use of supplemental zinc has been shown in clinical studies to reduce the size of the prostate and to reduce the symptoms of prostatic enlargement in the majority of patients. Zinc has also been shown to inhibit the enzyme that converts testosterone to dihydrotestosterone, the culprit that accumulates in the prostate to trigger enlargement of its tissues. Zinc also makes these male hormones less available by inhibiting their binding to prostate cells. This makes these hormones more available for removal from the prostate.

Zinc also inhibits prolactin secretion which we saw earlier plays a role increasing testosterone in the prostate. Although zinc is found in a variety of foods such as meats, liver, eggs, seafood (especially oysters), grains, seeds and wheat germ, its percentage is variable depending on the soil these foods grow in or the animals forage in.

The efficiency of zinc absorption, even if present in adequate amounts in the diet, reduces with age. The main reason for this seems to be a decrease in output by the pancreas of picolinic acid which, when present in the intestine, forms a complex with zinc to aid in its absorption. Since picolinic acid is made in the body from the amino acid tryptophan with B6 acting as a co-factor for this conversion, one way to enhance picolinate manufacture, and thus zinc absorption is to also supplement the diet with B6. Tryptophan supplementation enhances prolactin levels and is therefore not recommended.

Attention should also be given in cases of pancreatic insufficiency to the overall pancreatic enzyme production which may need to be supplemented by pancreatic enzymes to aid in digestion of starch, fats and proteins. This helps prevent and treat the multiple nutrient deficiencies which may be found in the aged, zinc deficiency included.

Alcohol consumption reduces zinc absorption and increases its excretion which leads to zinc deficiency. Vitamin B6, needed for zinc absorption as seen above, is also reduced by alcohol use. These are just a few of the ways diet and zinc are related to prostate problems. As you can see, if you are a modern man, you probably need zinc supplementation.

Dose suggestion: zinc citrate, gluconate, sulfate, chelate or picolinate to equal 25-30 mg elemental zinc twice daily.

- Vitamin B6: necessary for adequate zinc absorption. Dose suggestion: 50-100 mg 2 times daily.
- Beta-carotene and antioxidants: recent research clearly shows that beta-carotene and other antioxidants (e.g. vitamin c, zinc, vitamin E and selenium) provide a protective function in preventing damage by free radicals and can help prevent cancer. Up to 200,000 IU daily.
- Vitamin C and bioflavonoids: 6-8 g daily in divided doses.
- Vitamin E: 400 IU 2-3 times daily.
- Selenium: 100-300 mcg daily.
- Calcium: 800-1000 mg daily.
- Magnesium: 400-2000 mg daily.

Others—Primary

- Essential Fatty Acids (EFA/GLA): supplementation of EFA/GLA complexes containing alpha-linolenic acid (omega-3) has resulted in significant improvement with prostatic enlargement. This positive effect is due to the correction of an essential fatty acid deficiency commonly found in patients with prostate disorders and may also be due to the ability of these supplements to stimulate prostaglandin formation (PGE1). Prostaglandin competes with testosterone for binding sites and a reduction of this type of prostaglandin has been observed with age and in cases of benign prostatic hyperplasia. Flaxseed and evening primrose oil are good sources of the essential oils. Dose suggestion: flaxseed oil may be taken 1 tsp twice daily or the equivalent in capsule form or use evening primrose oil capsules, 1000 mg capsules twice or 3 times daily.

- Raw pumpkin seeds (pepitas): pumpkin seeds are high in zinc and essential fatty acids. Their use in the treatment of prostate enlargement has been recommended in folk medicine and has been proven by clinical experience to be effective. Dose suggestion: 1-2 handfuls of raw seeds daily.
- Bee/flower pollen: contains flavinols, anti-inflammatory. 100 mg 3 times daily.

Others—Secondary
- Brewer's yeast.
- Chlorophyll.
- Garlic.
- Kelp: 2 tablets 3 times daily.
- Lecithin: 1-2 tbsp 1-2 times daily, or in capsule form.
- Probiotics.

Botanicals—Primary

Saw palmetto: a herb with a long history as a successful treatment for the relief of prostate disorders. The berry and its extract have been extensively researched in Europe and the US. Clinical trials show these extracts dramatically reduces the size of the prostate and the associated symptoms of benign prostatic hyperplasia. The mode of action appears to be its ability to prevent conversion of testosterone to dihydrotestosterone and interfere with dihydrotestosterone's binding to receptor site S7 within the prostate. Saw palmetto berries and extracts are very safe. No toxic effects have been shown. Dose suggestion: 100-200 mg twice daily, or in tincture complex.

Pygeum: a large evergreen tree found in tropical Africa. Research has shown extracts of the bark of this tree to be a very effective treatment for benign prostatic hyperplasia. The action is to reduce inflammation by inhibiting the body's production of inflammatory prostaglandins. The same active ingredients are found in saw palmetto and pumpkin seeds which have a long history of use in folk medicine and naturopathically for the treatment of prostate disorders. Dose suggestion: 100 mg twice daily.

Panax ginseng: has a long use in oriental medicine as a male rejuvenator. Studies have shown ginseng increases testosterone levels and decreases prostate size. Zinc absorption is also increased. Dose suggestion: 50-100 mg once or twice daily

Horsetail: a herb used for centuries to increase urine flow. It is now recognized to also have anti-inflammatory and antibiotic properties. Its use is indicated with prostatitis and subsequent irritation of the bladder.

Grape seed extract: a very good source of biologically active flavinols. Flavinols are widely dispersed in the vegetable kingdom, however their concentration is fairly low. They are non-toxic and extremely effective anti-inflammatory substances very useful with non-bacterial prostatitis and benign prostatic hyperplasia.

Botanicals—Secondary

Bearberry: diuretic.
Buchu: diuretic.
Couch grass: diuretic.
Echinacea: anti-infective.
Fenugreek: tea soothes and cleanses mucous membrane of urinary tract.
False unicorn root.
Geranium: astringent.
Gravel root: diuretic.
Juniper berries: diuretic.
Marshmallow: diuretic and demulcent.
Parsley root: diuretic.

Other Therapies

- Hot sitz baths are useful to help relieve pressure on the urethra and allow the bladder to empty fully. Chamomile tea may be added to the water to increase this effect. Used primarily in acute conditions.
- Hot compresses have an effect similar to the hot sitz bath, and are also used in acute conditions.

- Alternate hot and cold sitz baths are used to reduce congestion and increase circulation in a chronic condition, or just after the acute stage has reduced in severity.
- Alternate hot and cold perianal sponges are used with an effect similar to the hot and cold sitz baths, but are employed more in chronic conditions and as maintenance therapy, once cure has been established.
- Cold perianal sprays.
- Ice-cold retention enemas.
- Ice applied to perineum for pain in acute prostatitis.

Physiotherapy

- Abdominal exercises to correct visceroptosis (a sagging condition of the internal organs due to weak musculature).
- Prostatic massage exercise: lie on back with legs extended. Bend knees and hips to draw knees to chest. Spread knees apart and press soles of feet together firmly. Keep soles of feet pressed together firmly as you extend your legs to floor. Get up to 75–100 times daily.
- Spinal
  Lumbar; lumbosacral; sacral.
- Internal massage to the prostate: done by a physician will help reduce the swelling of the prostate, reduce acute retention problems, and help break down any fibrous buildup on and around the gland. This must be done repeatedly for proper results. (*Note:* This is contraindicated in acute prostatitis due to infection.)
- Sex life
  Avoid coitus interruptus; avoid prolonged intercourse; avoid abstinence; avoid excitation without natural climax.

Hydrotherapy

- When the prostate is inflamed or enlarged and it is difficult to pass urine, a warm sitz bath will make the tissues relax, easing the flow. Just place warm water in a bath and sit immersed in the warm water for 15–30 minutes.
- To increase the circulation and aid in reducing the size of the prostate, alternate hot and cold sitz baths are very useful. You may use two large plastic tubs, large enough to accommodate your bottom and still retain enough water to cover you from your upper thigh to your lower abdomen. Fill one tub with hot water, as hot as you can comfortably bear, and the other with ice cold water. First sit in the hot water for 3–5 minutes then switch over to the ice cold tub for 2–3 minutes. Repeat this process 3 times, ending with the cold water. This technique is very effective and one of the best tonics you can use for your prostate. Repeat 1–3 times daily.

PSORIASIS

DEFINITION

A chronic relapsing skin disease.

SYMPTOMS

Skin lesions with silvery scales found most frequently on knees, elbows, and scalp. However, any skin area may be involved, including the nails. The symptoms tend to flare up acutely with remissions. Arthritis in the smaller joints is commonly associated with psoriasis.

ETIOLOGICAL CONSIDERATIONS—PRIMARY

- Thinning of walls of small intestine, especially the jejunum or lower duodenum.
- Thinning of walls of the large bowel (leaky gut).
- Faulty essential fatty acid utilization.
- Acid/alkali imbalance.
- History of constipation.
- Vaccination after-effects.
- History of antibiotic use.

ETIOLOGICAL CONSIDERATIONS— SECONDARY

- Poor eliminations.
- Emotions may play a part.
- Malfunction of liver, kidneys.
- Excess meat-eating: associated with the amino acid taurine.
- Possible copper excess and zinc deficiency.
- Faulty diet.
- Food allergy.

DISCUSSION

Psoriasis has been considered practically incurable by orthodox methods. Various external applications such as coal tar, zinc paste, tar plus ultraviolet light, and steroids have been advised for years, with little success. The latest treatment in severe cases is a combination of the drug methotrexate with special ultraviolet sessions. This therapy carries the severe danger of toxic effects to the liver and bone marrow, and although somewhat successful in the short term, must be repeated frequently due to remission.

The reason these methods all fall miserably to cure this tenacious disorder is that no attempt is made to remove its cause. This is primarily due to the fact that the cause is considered unknown. Psoriasis can never be cured by external applications without removing the cause. The real cause or causes of psoriasis are internal, not external, according to the Edgar Cayce readings. The most common factor seems to be a thinning of the small intestinal walls. This allows toxins to enter the circulation system and lymph, which sets up irritations on the skin. This thinning may be due to constipation, faulty utilization of fats, food allergy, spinal lesions, malfunction of liver and kidneys, previous vaccinations, Candida overgrowth, or other factors.

Treatment of psoriasis takes much time and perseverance for the best results. Allergy tests such as RAST, cytotoxic, or pulse tests may reveal common foods that cause allergic reactions. Rotation diets, where suspected foods, especially grains, proteins, and any other suspected foods are not consumed more frequently than every 4–7 days, are also very useful to desensitize the individual. Milk and wheat may also act in ways other than true allergy by means of intestinal incompatibility or enzyme deficiency. It is wise to exclude these foods for 6 months, even if allergy tests are negative. Improper weaning to cow's milk and wheat is often a major cause.

Many naturopathic physicians have observed that previous vaccinations seem to be another cause of allergic skin conditions, including eczema and psoriasis. Other drugs such as antibiotics can cause long-term allergic skin reactions.

TREATMENT

The aim of therapy is to remove conditions that result in a loss of intestinal villi with thinning of the bowel, to remove allergens and irritants from the diet, and to provide a diet and herbs that help soothe these delicate membranes. In most cases balancing the body fluids' pH (acid/alkaline ratio) is a major aim.

Diet

Food consumed should be primarily alkaline in reaction, with at least one meal daily consisting of raw vegetables. Yellow foods are especially useful in the long term. Soybeans, tofu, and lecithin are also very useful due to their cholesterol-lowering capabilities. In general, citrus fruits should be avoided, as well as tomatoes, red meats, saturated fats, hydrogenated fats, sweets, alcohol, pastry, or carbonated beverages. If food allergy is suspected, several tests are available to help confirm this. Some commonly offending foods are meat, wheat, eggs, citrus, and dairy products. These often are excluded in initial phases of the diet.

A good procedure with which to begin therapy is the 7–21-day vegetable juice fast, emphasizing carrot juice. With this, if possible, add ultra-green substances such as Spirulina. Therapeutic herb teas should be taken frequently in addition to the vegetable juices. These include slippery elm tea, mullein tea, and American saffron tea. During this fast enemas or colonics are to be taken and a series of colonics are to follow the fast, 1–2 times per week for 2–6 weeks, in some cases.

Following the initial fast, the high-fiber, high-raw-vegetable, no-acid, no-meat diet begins. Psoriasis sufferers seem to have extreme difficulty handling saturated fats and these should be reduced to a minimum or excluded entirely from the diet. These patients often have been found to have high serum cholesterol levels. Repeated fasts may be necessary to aid further recovery and correct the lesions of the small intestine. At all times eliminations must be kept regular. This may require herbal purification, colonics, and spinal manipulation to achieve permanent results. See section on Yeast Infection if this is a suspected cause.

Foods especially useful are: soy; yellow foods; green vegetables; seaweeds; 10-day brown rice diet.

Physiotherapy

- Castor oil packs: apply to lower abdomen nightly for 45 minutes to 1½ hours. Use 3–4 thicknesses of undyed wool. Saturate this with castor oil and wring out lightly. This is then heated in a special pot used for this purpose only. You may reuse the same cloth 20–40 times. just store in the pot and add more castor oil as needed with each use. This cloth is applied as hot as the body can bear to the area from the lower right rib border over the entire right side of the abdomen, down to just above the pubic bone. The pack is then covered with an oiled cloth or plastic and kept warm with a heating pad. If necessary, the bed may also be protected by plastic. After the application, wash the area with a weak solution of bicarbonate (1 tsp to 1 quart of warm water).
- Alternate hot and cold showers to stimulate the circulation.

Other

- Ocean swims and sun: as often as possible.
- Ultraviolet light. Be careful, however, not to overuse the ultraviolet lamp as skin cancer has been associated with chronic overexposure. Natural sun rays are best and most effective.
- Enemas.
- Colonics.

Spinal Manipulation

To correct constipation. Adjust midthoracic through sacral region, 1–2 times per week.

Therapeutic Agents

Vitamins and Minerals— Primary

- Vitamin A: 25,000 IU twice daily or more with supervision. Use any dose of vitamin A over 50,000 IU daily with medical supervision only.

- Bioflavonoids (anti-inflammatory) Quercetin especially down-regulates the 5-lipoxygenase inflammatory pathway, modulates calmodulin activity, and increases cyclic AMP levels.
- Essential fatty acids: 2–4 capsules GLA (gamma-linolenic acid) 3 times daily.
- Flaxseed oil:, 2 tbsp daily.
- Glucosamine: (inhibits psoritic cell proliferation)
- Zinc: 25–50 mg 3 times daily (if bowel upset occurs, reduce dose).
- EPA (eicosapentaenoic acid): 2–4 capsules 2–3 times daily.

Vitamins and Minerals— Secondary

- Vitamin B complex (yeast-free, if allergic to yeast): 25–50 mg 2–3 times daily.
- Vitamin B12: 1 mg, IM injection once weekly.
- Folic acid: 25–75 mg daily.
- Vitamin C: ascorbates may be tolerated best.
- Glutamine.
- Evening primrose oil: 1–2 capsules 3 times daily.
- Hydrochloric acid: 5–20 grains per meal if hypoacid.

Others—Primary

- Chondroitin sulfate: improves synthesis of ground substance in skin.
- Probiotics.
- Lecithin (phosphatidylcholine): soy lecithin is the most important additive to the diet; soy products are also beneficial.

Others—Secondary

- Cod-liver oil: 2–4 capsules 3 times daily.
- Elixir of lactated pepsin: to regularize eliminations.
- Homoeopathics: arsenicum, sulfur might be useful starting points.
- Pancreatic enzymes.
- Sulfur (organic colloidal sulfur): 6–8 drops 3–4 times daily for 4 weeks;

4 drops 3–4 times daily until symptoms improve.

- Spirulina: 1 tsp 2–3 times daily.

Botanicals—Primary

Coleus forskolii: is known to increase cAMP

Yellow American saffron tea: (Cayce product). Dilute tea in water 4 times daily to help heal thinned intestinal walls.

Slippery elm tea.

Botanicals—Secondary

Bergamot oil: apply oil to lesion, then expose to sun or ultraviolet lamp. Sensitizes skin to ultraviolet light.

Bloodroot extract.

Burdock root: as decoction, or 20–40 drops of tincture 2–4 times daily.

Chamomile.

Common figwort: 1–3 mL of tincture 1–2 times daily.

Mullein.

Oregon grape root.

Sarsaparilla.

Wild clover.

Yellow dock.

Therapeutic Suggestions

Psoriasis is an extremely difficult condition to cure, and great perseverance is required. This disorder in particular must always be dealt with on all levels of the person, especially emotional. Look deeply into what irritates you on a psychological level, to see what may be irritating you on a physical level. Each patient responds to the regimen uniquely, and individual modifications are required. Many cases respond well to vitamin A topically, followed by sunlight, or ultraviolet exposure. Sunlight is best, whenever possible. This must be done in conjunction with the suggested nutritional changes. Essential fatty acids also are useful, including EPA (eicosapentaenoic acid) and GLA (gamma-linolenic acid) and primrose oil.

The question of essential fatty acid malabsorption or faulty metabolism is of particular interest in relation to psoriasis. Essential fatty acid deficiency in humans causes skin rashes resembling eczema and psoriasis. Some patients receive favorable results by reducing saturated fats and increasing unsaturated fats in the diet, while avoiding commercially transformed or overheated unsaturated fats (such as margarine or fried foods), which contain harmful trans fatty acids known to interfere with normal essential fatty acid metabolism. Other patients appear to have a block in normal essential fatty acid metabolism, and can bypass this fault by using evening primrose oil, high not only in linoleic acid as are the vegetable oils of sunflower, safflower,

corn, soy, and flaxseed, but also containing significant amounts of gamma-linolenic acid. The only other dietary source of this is human milk, which may explain why breast-feeding seems to be protective against many cases of infantile eczema.

The use of various oils in the form of EPA (eicosapentaenoic acid) is also another way to help bypass this biochemical fault along a closely related pathway. It is our feeling that significant advances will soon be made in better and hopefully less expensive forms of essential fatty acids and their metabolic products, to help correct these very tenacious skin disorders.

SALPINGITIS AND SALPINGO-OOPHORITIS

DEFINITION

Salpingitis: inflammation of the fallopian tubes.
Oophoritis: inflammation of the ovaries.

SYMPTOMS

May be acute or chronic. Tenderness of fallopian tube; severe (in acute cases) abdominal pain, usually bilateral, but may affect only one ovary or tube; fever; coated tongue; vaginal discharge common; swelling; abscess possible, with later peritonitis; pain with sex; infertility common.

ETIOLOGICAL CONSIDERATIONS—PRIMARY

* Ascending infection more common due to Menstruation; postpartum; postabortion; IUD
* Congestion
  Spinal; diet; lack of exercise; psychological; constipation; appendicitis

* Diverticulitis of sigmoid colon, causing left salpingo-oophoritis

ETIOLOGICAL CONSIDERATIONS— SECONDARY

* Appendicitis direct spread
* Tuberculosis of Fallopian tubes
* Mumps (oophoritis)

DISCUSSION

The fallopian tubes and ovaries are anatomically open to the outside world with all its foreign infective agents by access through the vagina and uterus. Physiologically, however, these delicate inner passageways and glands are protected by built-in self-defense mechanisms and barriers. The vagina, with its acidic nature (see Vaginitis), helps protect pathogens from flourishing. The thick mucous plug of the cervix further acts as a mechanical barrier to invasion. Hair-like cilia in the uterus and fallopian tubes

409

themselves constantly waft any debris or bacteria downward towards the cervix and vagina (muco-ciliary escalation).

These protective measures are normally effective in preventing infection from outside. However, during menstruation, several of the mechanisms fail to operate. The mucous plug is not effective and the vagina becomes relatively alkaline. Normally, infection is still prevented, especially with a healthy flow. In the postpartum period, again, similar self-defenses are reduced. In addition there is the possibility of infection introduced from outside during delivery, from retained products of conception only slowly being eliminated or entirely retained, or tissue trauma and congestion. Coupled with the prolonged vaginal discharge that normally follows childbirth (2-6 weeks), these factors make the possibility of an ascending infection extremely likely. In fact, most cases of salpingitis due to ascending infection either follow birth or abortion.

An IUD is also a major cause of ascending infections, due either to septic inoculation at the time of insertion, or to mechanical irritation and congestion, creating a more favorable environment for bacterial growth.

Congestion is a little-understood cause of salpingitis. Any organ or tissue that suffers poor circulation of blood, lymph, or nerve supply will lose the ability to resist infection. It is this loss of resistance that is a central factor in so many internal infections. In the case of salpingitis, congestion may be strictly local due to a spinal lesion; confined to the pelvic/abdominal region due to constipation, diverticulitis, appendicitis, or poor abdominal tone; or more systemic because of improper or deficient diet, lack of exercise, psychological causes, or other general health factors.

Salpingitis usually is accompanied by involvement of the ovaries due to direct spread of infection, and also via the lymphatics. It may be either acute or chronic, and is classified into two types, *catarrhal* or *suppurative* (pyogenic or infective). In the catarrhal form an excess of mucus is associated with congestion of the fallopian tube walls. In the suppurative form actual infection is found. Either form may, and usually does, permanently damage the delicate inner linings, leading to adhesion formation and possible occlusion of the tubes. In many cases the fimbriated end will swell with the infection and adhesions may permanently close this opening. Any of these damaging results may lead to infertility by hindering the passage of the egg from the ovary through the fallopian tubes, where it is fertilized, and on into the uterus where implantation occurs.

Surgical repair of the tubes when possible is unfortunately only about 30% successful. Even if the tubal blockage is removed and the tubes are reunited, adhesions may later form due to the surgery itself, creating a new barrier. The only possibility of pregnancy left for a woman with blocked fallopian tubes is test tube impregnation.

TREATMENT

Antibiotics are the usual course of treatment prescribed in salpingitis. We have mixed feelings about their use in this instance. The danger with salpingitis, as previously explained, is damage to the fallopian tubes. This damage may be best prevented by quick and appropriate treatment that removes the inflammation or infection as fast as possible. In a case of suppurative or pyogenic salpingitis, if an antibiotic can quickly remove the infection to prevent damage, we are in full support. Unfortunately, this is not always the case. Too often we see women who have received antibiotic therapy for acute salpingitis, only to suffer from incredibly stubborn cases of chronic salpingitis because the true causes were never removed and antibiotics could only have a short-term effect. These cases are extremely difficult to treat, either with further courses of antibiotics or natural therapies. Whatever the cause of such a situation, the result is the same—a woman with damaged fallopian tubes and probable infertility.

The decision whether or not to use antibiotics must include a careful consideration of the patient, past history, and present complaint. In all cases where antibiotics are used, naturopathic treatments should also be used to help remove the primary causes. These methods are outlined below and are very effective, though they may appear extremely simple in design. In acute cases, where the patient is in general good health and has no previous history of similar pelvic disorders, the decision to use antibiotics is no easy task. These patients make the best response to both antibiotics and naturopathic treatment. If the woman is in a downgraded health condition generally, then antibiotics may be needed as the body's vitality may be too low to respond rapidly enough to prevent damage.

For a patient with a chronic condition, especially one who has a history of previous antibiotic prescriptions, little can be lost from an extended application of naturopathic treatments. This is probably the patient's only hope, short of surgery, of removing her disorder. After a reasonable period of treatments, if little response is forthcoming, antibiotics may be tried in conjunction with therapy, in the hope of preventing surgery.

Diet

Depending on the patient and the condition, varying periods of vegetable juice fasting or fruit juice fasting are beneficial. With the catarrhal type of disorder short periods on the mucus-cleansing diet may also prove beneficial. These cleansing fasts may then be followed with periods on an all fruit or an all raw fruit and salads diet, followed by a good blood-building, primarily vegetarian protein, diet.

The following fasts or simple elimination diets may be used:
- Carrot juice: the high vitamin A content is useful to heal mucous membranes.
- Carrot mono diet.
- Fruit juice diet.
- Apple mono diet.
- Raw fruit diet.
- Raw fruit and salads diet.
- Mucus-cleansing diet.

These fasts will need to be continued until, in an acute condition, all symptoms are gone, or alternated with other less severe diets for the prolonged treatment necessary in the chronic condition. Acceptable interim diets are the anemia diet with only vegetarian proteins, or the asthma Stage 2, low-carbohydrate, mucus cleansing, high-fruit-and-vegetable diet. In general, all mucus-forming foods such as dairy products and concentrated starches are to be avoided, as well as all animal products or irritants such as coffee, alcohol, and any other negative health factor, until all symptoms have been removed.

With proper diet and supportive therapies an acute case should resolve in 5-10 days, but will require a further 2-3 weeks therapy to prevent recurrence. The chronic case may take months of vigorous treatments, but once cure has been established, and providing the patient stays on a healthy regimen, the problem usually does not return.

Physiotherapy

- Sitz Baths
  The use of alternating hot and cold contrast sitz baths is the most effective measure in removing pelvic congestion and inflammation.
  Directions: obtain two containers or utility tubs 1 ft (30 cm) or more deep. These should be big enough to allow immersion from midthigh to the umbilicus, including the entire pubic and pelvic regions. Fill one container with very hot water (as hot as comfortably bearable) and the other with ice-cold water. First sit in the hot tub and place your feet in the cold tub. After 3 minutes reverse so that your bottom is in the ice-cold tub and

feet in the hot tub. In 3 minutes reverse again and repeat the cycle 3 times, beginning with bottom in the hot water and ending with bottom in the cold water. Then briskly dry off with a rough bath towel. Repeat 2-3 times or more daily, depending on the severity of the condition. The alternate hot and cold bath will pump blood vigorously through the pelvic region to remove congestion and speed nutrition to these areas to hasten healing.

- Depletion pack (with doctor's supervision only):
Apply to the upper third of a tampon and insert into vagina twice daily (morning and evening), retaining for 3-6 hours. This formula may be obtained premixed from Eclectic Institute.
- Alternate hot and cold compresses:
These are applied directly over the painful pelvic region, 2-3 minutes hot, 2-3 minutes ice-cold. Thick toweling folded in four thicknesses should be used to retain heat or cold. A hot water bottle wrapped in moist toweling will help prolong the hot application, and an ice bag wrapped in moist toweling will prolong the cold.
- Cold compresses:
In the acute stage, repeated cold applications 20 minutes on, 5-10 minutes off, will be very beneficial (heat is often contraindicated with acute inflammation).

- Abdominal or full trunk packs:
These should be applied nightly in acute and chronic conditions.

Therapeutic Agents

Vitamins and Minerals—Primary
- Vitamin C: 500-1000 mg 4-8 times daily.
- Bioflavonoids: anti-inflammatory.
- Zinc: 15-45 mg 1-2 times daily (aids in healing).

Vitamins and Minerals—Secondary
- Vitamin A: 25,000 IU 3 or more times daily for 6 weeks (under supervision).
- Vitamin E: 400 IU twice daily (prevents scarring).

Botanicals—Primary
Poke root: decongestant (highly toxic, see page 60).
Goldenseal: mucous membrane tonic.

Botanicals—Secondary
Bearberry.
Black cohosh.
Black haw.
Coneflower: 20 drops of tincture 4-6 times daily.
Saw palmetto.
Wild yam root.

SCHIZOPHRENIA

DEFINITION AND SYMPTOMS

Mental illness characterized by abnormal or disturbed associations, a reduced range of emotional response, detachment from reality, and severely mixed feelings that can become incapacitating. Hallucinations and delusions are also present in some cases.

ETIOLOGICAL CONSIDERATIONS—PRIMARY

- Altered biochemistry in the brain Genetic enzyme deficiency
- Genetic excessive requirement of certain vitamins, minerals, essential fatty acids, or enzymes
- Toxicity

Heavy metal poisoning; drugs (recreational—excess use of marijuana, cocaine, LSD); pesticides; chemicals
- Nutritional deficiency
- Excess need
Deficient diet; excess of some minerals (copper); deficiency of some minerals (zinc, manganese); vitamin B deficiency, e.g. B6, and/or subclinical pellagra—B3
- Hypoglycemia

ETIOLOGICAL CONSIDERATIONS— SECONDARY

- Gluten intolerance, dairy product intolerance; alcoholism; pep pills, prolonged weight reduction diets
- Cerebral food allergy (allergic reactions affecting behavior or perception); stress, nervous exhaustion
- Traumatic event; glandular imbalance (pineal, pituitary, thyroid, adrenal); deficient brain circulation; spinal lesions (coccyx to occiput, incoordination of spinal centers); destructive, self-condemning thoughts

DISCUSSION

Schizophrenia is a fairly common disorder affecting about 3% of the population at some time in their lives. Patients may show no previous symptoms until a severe trauma suddenly initiates symptoms (reactive schizophrenia) or the condition may be the end result of slow deterioration in an individual with a history of being shy and withdrawn.

The orthodox approach to schizophrenia is the use of various tranquilizers, all with severe side effects, electro-convulsive shock therapy, and psychotherapy. Within the past 20–30 years a great deal of research and clinical trials have led many in the psychological world towards diet and nutrition as a factor in the cause and cure of some cases of schizophrenia and other mental illnesses. The main conclusion is that psychoanalysis alone, or combined with drug therapy, is of little or no use in the actual cure of mental disease in most cases, since the real cause involves an abnormal brain biochemistry due to a genetic or acquired condition involving one or many nutrients, or in some cases, toxins. In spite of the rather large body of evidence supporting these views, the average psychiatrist still denies that nutrition plays any part whatsoever in mental illness. This belief that nutrition has no bearing on mental disease, or any disease for that matter, is prevalent among many physicians.

It has long been known that severe deficiencies of some of the B complex vitamins cause psychological symptoms which in some cases are strikingly similar to schizophrenia. Severe vitamin B12 deficiency causes difficulty in concentration, poor memory, hallucinations, agitation, and manic or paranoid behavior. Biotin deficiency, another B complex member, will cause depression, lassitude, panic, and hallucinations. Severe vitamin B3 (niacin) deficiency (pellagra), with its characteristic nervousness, loss of memory, confusion, paranoia, insomnia, depression, and hallucinations, so closely resembles schizophrenia that in 1966 Dr Abram Hoffer suggested that schizophrenia may be a vitamin-dependency disease. He cites several examples where experimental animals and prisoners of war were kept on diets deficient in vitamin B3 for prolonged periods, only to find that when B3 was again available in the diet, the body then required up to 60 times more B3 than the average person to prevent pellagra. As in other typical vitamin-dependency diseases, these victims had developed an increased need for a particular substance, greater than could be derived on a diet containing ordinary amounts

Dr Hoffer also describes B6-dependent pellagra and schizophrenia, although occurring less frequently. It was found that schizophrenics excrete a highly toxic pyrrole known as KP (kryptopyrrole), which reacts chemically with vitamin B6, forming a complex which binds strongly with zinc,

413

producing not only a severe vitamin B6 deficiency, but also one of zinc. Supplemental B6 and zinc in these pyroluric patients produces favorable results.

Dr Carl Pfeiffer, of the Princeton Brain Bio Center in New Jersey, is another pioneer in the brain biochemistry of schizophrenia, as well as in the nutritional implications of these findings. Dr Pfeiffer has recognized two major sub-groupings depending on their blood histamine levels.

The low-histamine (histapenic) group is characterized by symptoms including thought disorders, grandiosity, paranoia, over-arousal, hallucinations, hypomania, and mania. Associated with this grouping are low zinc and folate levels, and a high serum copper. The elevated copper may cause depression or paranoia. Treatment for this group includes supplementation of folic acid, vitamin B12, niacin, vitamin C, with zinc and manganese taken to reduce elevated copper levels.

The less frequent high-histamine (histadelic) group Dr Pfeiffer characterizes by "fast oxidation, little fat, long fingers and toes, severe depression, compulsion and phobias". He has found that folic acid aggravates these patients severely, turning mild depression into severe agitated depression.

Other aspects of diet and nutrition are associated with schizophrenia. Hypoglycemia is a common concurrent finding. Although it is not entirely certain that low blood sugar precedes schizophrenia, it is well accepted that hypoglycemics experience many emotional and perceptual changes, similar to other mental diseases.

Dr Cleave, in *The Saccharine Diseases*, made similar conclusions about the effects of a refined diet, independently implicating refined carbohydrates in the cause of schizophrenia. Dr Cleave found schizophrenia uncommon in tribal Africans living on a traditional unrefined diet, but found it a common psychosis among their urbanized brothers consuming refined carbohydrates. It is significant to note that consumption of carbohydrates is involved in the causation of both hypoglycemia and pellagra.

Cerebral allergies also may be a factor in schizophrenic behavior. Literally any food may be the cause of learning disabilities, manic depressive states, hyperactivity, confusion, lethargy, and other abnormal perceptual states such as those seen in schizophrenia. Gluten-containing grains are particularly suspect and contain neuroactive peptides.

Other recent research has implicated faulty essential fatty acid metabolism or deficiency as a cause of some psychotic and neurotic mental disorders, schizophrenia included. Pioneering research by D.F. Horrobin suggests a genetic biochemical defect in essential fatty acid metabolism. Whether or not there exists a genetic defect, the therapeutic value of linseed oil, a rich source of the essential fatty acid alpha-linolenic acid (omega-3), with a variety of "mental" problems is being confirmed in clinical trials. In 1981 Donald O. Rudin, of the Department of Molecular Biology, Eastern Pennsylvania Psychiatric Institute, Philadelphia, Pa., reported very favorable response to 2–6 tbsp daily of linseed oil in divided doses with cases of schizophrenia, manic depression, and agoraphobia. Other essential fatty acids such as evening primrose oil, sunflower seed oil, and eicosapentaenoic acid (EPA) also may be of use (see Allergies and Food Intolerances for diagnosis and treatment).

Another major cause of schizophrenialike symptoms is heavy metal poisoning. Although the physical and psychological symptoms of lead, mercury, or copper excess are well documented, it is very rare for a schizophrenic patient to be tested for elevated levels as a possible cause of this condition. In our patient files we have one well-documented "schizophrenic" patient who had received the typical gamut of psychological therapy and drugs for over 2 years with no benefit. We discovered a severe lead poisoning due to his occupation as an auto body repairman. With detoxification and proper diet, his symptoms were gone completely within 3 months.

In another case a young man, age 21

suffered delusional symptoms, and he was eventually diagnosed by psychiatrists as schizophrenic. His history suggested this problem could be traced to typical patterns of stress and nutritional causes. He had suffered severe workplace burns to his hands and was placed in hospital for several weeks. He was placed on an antibiotic drip (altering bowel flora leading to leaky gut) and given lots of pain killers (which put extra detoxification stress on his liver). While convalescing at his home for months afterward, his diet fell away to consist of lots of junk food (fatty foods and sugar predisposing to poor brain chemical production) and he was sleeping till midday then going partying and smoking marijuana till the wee hours of the morning (disturbed wake/sleep cycle, and mind-altering substance abuse). This, together with some personal emotional stress, led him to develop schizophrenia (as diagnosed by psychiatrists).

When he came to stay with his father he was shocked at his poor general state of physical health, as much as by vacant stare, the preoccupation with and the mumbled responses to "the voices", and the loony effects of the full moon. The psychiatrists wanted to start him on antipsychotic drugs (e.g. haloperidol). It seemed to him quite clear that his son had not become schizophrenic because he had lacked the proffered drugs in the first place, so it was equally clear to him that he would not be cured by taking them. He refused to allow it (and was berated and called irresponsible in so doing), and persuaded his son to trust the natural way and follow a naturopathic health regime His own understanding of what healing requires, is that unless one deals effectively with causes of a process, and looks at reversing these, then anything else whether natural or synthetic, naturopathic or allopathic, cheap or expensive, will at best be merely palliative. He wanted cure. Fortunately this man was well versed in naturopathic philosophy and he knew that Naturopathic law states that if we exclude those things from the body (and the brain is a physical body organ) which predispose to

imbalance and disease, and supply all the right nutrients in the right amounts, then the mind-body will re-establish homeostasis. This is the fundamental starting point for any type of healing the body needs to do.

The treatment plan that was instituted aimed firstly at getting the patient's sleep cycle normalized, reducing the amount of fast foods he seemed to crave in favor of fresh salads and vegetables, get him drinking lots of water, and taking herbal medicines prescribed to address aspects of hypoglycemia, digestion, and liver detoxification. Also prescribed were probiotics, zinc and glutamine to help reverse the damage the antibiotics, soft drinks, stress and other things had caused in his gut, and aimed to get his circulatory systems working by encouraging him to exercise in the ocean (boogie boarding) in the sunlight, and provided opportunity to talk with a counselor about his flagging levels of self-esteem.

Despite the difficult compliance problems, there were signs of progress virtually from the first month. Within 7 months there was no sign of the schizophrenia, and there has been no relapse since. The message here is, that naturopathic principles really do work. As seen in the case above they can work without resorting to antipsychotic drugs which in themselves are not curative.

TREATMENT

Standard treatments for schizophrenia have an exceptionally low success rate, deplete many essential vitamins, and are highly toxic. If these facts alone were not enough for the average psychiatrist to try nutrition, specifically mega-niacin therapy, the evidence of the carefully conducted medical trials of niacin should be. As early as 1939, nineteen schizophrenic psychiatric patients were treated successfully with niacin. In 1949 one study showed 29 schizophrenic cases cured with niacin, none of which showed any physical signs of pellagra. Ten-year double-blind studies of niacin in 1962 showed a 75% success rate in schizophrenics with no rehospitalization as compared with 31% of the control group not receiving niacin therapy. These are just a few examples.

Although niacin therapy has been found extremely useful, it is important to remember that in most cases the best results can only be obtained by first minimizing all negative health factors and optimizing the positive. Dr Hoffer recognized this need and as a first course of action advises an optimum diet to lay the foundation for further therapies.

Diet

The best maintenance diet for schizophrenia is the hypoglycemia regimen outlined under Hypoglycemia. This helps keep the blood sugar level under control and minimizes symptoms while the rest of the nutritional therapy takes effect. Best results will be obtained, however, if this diet is modified to be gluten-free and dairy-free (see Celiac Disease for complete details of a gluten-free diet).

Some practitioners have obtained excellent results with prolonged fasting of 7–14 days in the treatment of schizophrenia. If done properly, a prolonged fast normalizes blood sugar levels and removes toxic substances from the body. In practice we have found that the major barrier to progress with nutrition for the average schizophrenic lies in the patient's family environment. It is absolutely impossible to enforce or suggest dietary changes unless the entire family is willing to modify their diets at the same time. Absolute consistency is required, to get the desired results. All persons in the family do not necessarily have to follow the details of the hypoglycemic regimen, but all must eat only the best of unrefined whole foods and these alone should be made available in the house for consumption. All sweets, pastries, refined foods, canned foods, soda drinks, and other devitalized products should be

removed from the home. Hair analysis and allergy tests (RAST, cytotoxic) should be performed early in therapy and repeated at 6–12-month intervals.

Physiotherapy

- Spinal massage: use peanut oil, olive oil, and lanolin.
- Spinal manipulation: treat generally once a week.
- Meditation: encourage meditation or relaxation exercises twice daily by example, and with guidance.
- Kindness and love: give plenty of both daily.
- Home environment: look internally to see the internal chaos you as parent, sibling, or partner represent.
- Sunshine, ocean, peace, and quiet: all will be helpful.

Therapeutic Agents

Vitamins and Minerals

The following list reads like a dictionary of vitamins; the purpose here is to focus attention on the need to ensure that there is no nutrient deficiency standing in the way of recovery.

- Vitamin A: with allergy, lung, or mucous membrane disorders.
- Vitamin B complex: 50 mg 3 times daily.
- Vitamin B3: 3–30 g daily. 3–6 g mixed niacin/niacinamide as initial dose.
- Vitamin B1: with depression.
- Vitamin B2: with vision problems and cracked corners at the mouth.
- Vitamin B6: with flat glucose tolerance curve, allergies, hyperactivity, convulsions, or malabsorption, indicated in kryptopyrrhole (KP) syndrome schizophrenia, with B3. 80 mg daily or 1 mg for each 15 mg of B3 used. Higher doses may be needed.
- Pantothenic acid: with fatigue or allergy; 200–600 mg daily.

- Vitamin B12: 1 mg intramuscularly once per week or more in some cases.
- Vitamin C: 6-40 g; low C in urine of schizophrenics.
- Vitamin D.
- Vitamin E: 800-1600 IU daily; reduces anxiety.
- Inositol: 200-1000 mg daily.
- Vitamin B6: 250-1000 mg daily with supervision.
- Folic acid: especially needed where anti-convulsants have been used since these deplete folic acid stores. Also needed in histamine type schizophrenics (see C. Pfeiffer, *Mental and Elemental Nutrients*); up to 2 mg daily.
- Biotin.
- Zinc: especially with elevated copper levels. Reduces anxiety; particularly indicated with other skin rashes. 30-50 mg 2-3 times daily.
- Magnesium.
- Manganese: also helps restore raised copper levels and helps remove the Parkinson's-like side effects resulting from long-term use of strong tranquilizers.
- Methionine: detoxifies histamine (useful in high-histamine-type schizophrenia).

Others
- Atomodine (Cayce product).
- Brewer's yeast (contains inositol and B complex): 4-6 tbsp daily.
- Choline (as concentrated phosphatidylcholine lecithin): 6-12 g daily.
- EPA (eicosapentaenoic acid): 1-2 g 3 times daily.
- Glutamic acid (glutamine).
- Liver tablets, liver infections: contain inositol plus B complex.
- Evening primrose oil: 3-6 g daily.
- Taurine.
- Tryptophan: 1-3 g daily.
- Tyrosine.

Botanicals
Chamomile: mild sedative.
Passion flower: sedative.

Therapeutic Suggestions

Not all cases of schizophrenia are nutritionally related, and even when they are, many other variables play a role. It is, however, in the best interest of the patient to seriously try the nutritional approach prior to drug therapy being relied on completely.

SCOLIOSIS

DEFINITION

A functional or structural lateral curvature of the spine.

SYMPTOMS

Fatigue in low back after prolonged standing, sitting or exercise; muscular aches in low back or mid-back. Back or neck pain are later symptoms. Asymmetry is observed in standing position (i.e. one shoulder is higher, pelvis appears rotated or twisted, a visible hump is present on one side of the spine when standing or appears when bent over to touch toes.

ETIOLOGICAL CONSIDERATIONS

- Leg length differences
  Prior leg or pelvis fractures
  Severe knee or ankle injuries
  Muscular imbalances (e.g. psoas spasms, tight hamstrings, tight tensor fasciae latae or iliotibial band, weak hip adbuctors—especially gluteus medius), weak oblique abdominals unilaterally)

417

Congenital or developmental hip disorders (e.g. congenital hip distraction or Perthe's disease)

Congenital asymmetry of pelvis

Congenital abnormal formation of vertebrae

- Injury or muscular imbalance

Severe sprain/strain of pelvis, lumbar or thoracic ligaments and muscles

Somatic dysfunction of the spine

Postural causes

Work related

Heavy book bags

Dominant hand syndrome

Mother's back syndrome

Disc prolapse

Tissue contraction from extensive burns

Poor muscle tone

Nerve damage

Nutritional: deficiency (e.g. rickets), osteoporosis/osteomalacia

- Neuromuscular disorders

Cerebral palsy

Charcot Marie tooth syndrome

Poliomyelitis or other viral causes

Muscular dystrophy

Spinal cord tumor or trauma

Congenital hypotonia

DISCUSSION

Scoliosis is defined as a lateral curvature of the spine but since the mechanics of the spine do not allow side bending without some rotation, scoliosis always involves both lateral side bending and rotation.

Diagnosis is initially made by physical examination. Observation of the subject from behind and bent over usually reveals the presence of asymmetry. It is often useful to take a standing x-ray that includes the upper part of the femur (thighbone), pelvis and low back and thoracic spine. Often the scoliosis extends well into the neck and full spine x-rays are used.

Classic C-shaped curves show one side of the pelvis to be elevated and the shoulder on the same side to be depressed. In S-shaped curves, the shoulder on the same side is usually higher as well. Some cases of scoliosis can be seen on x-ray to begin very specifically at one individual joint level and motion palpation will easily reveal the limited direction of its motion. If the cause is not congenital due to abnormal bone formation, or due to an injury that has damaged the disc which then blocks movement in one or usually in several directions, the problem may be successfully resolved by osteopathic treatment to the dysfunctional segment and treatment of the secondary effects of the problem area. Usually the cause of the scoliosis is more complex and involves muscular imbalances or leg length differences. Leg length differences are easily corrected, once diagnosed, by inserts into the shoe of the short leg, or added to the heel and sole in cases where the difference is in excess of $1/2$ inch (8 mm), that being the outside limit that can be accommodated inside most shoes. Runners may be made to accommodate $1/3$ inch (1 cm) in some cases.

Muscular imbalances must be specifically diagnosed. The most common sites to cause scoliosis are the hip flexors, hamstrings, tensor fasciae latae, iliotibial band, teres and latissimus dorsi. If weak, the following muscles will contribute to scoliosis: oblique abdominals, hip flexors, hip extensors, hip abductors, hip adductors, upper and lower abdominals, back extensors and middle and lower trapezius.[35]

You can easily screen your own child throughout early growth and puberty to detect any asymmetry of spinal development, and you should. It is constantly a source of amazement when we examine a teenager who has obvious curvature of the spine and that neither the patient or the parent has ever noticed. Simply have your child stand upright but naturally in bare feet on a hard flat surface. Stand behind the child and observe. Look to see if one shoulder is higher than the other. This is the most obvious usual sign of a C or S type curve. Look to see if one scapulae bulges out more than the other. Look to see if there is a bigger gap between the lower back and the arm on one side or if you see a skin fold on one side and not the other in the low back region on the side. Bend down so the pelvis is at eye level and place your level hands on the top of the pelvic bones just at the waist. Is one higher than the other? Is one side more forward than the other? Stand back and have the child touch their toes. Is one side of the spine higher, forming a hump? Lay the child down on the floor. Have them bend their knees, lift their bottom off the floor and then down again. Grab both ankles and extend the legs. Bring the legs together. Do the ankles meet at the ankle bone that sticks out? If you see any irregularity, you need to have your child properly evaluated by a trained specialist for the cause of these asymmetries to prevent a spinal curvature from becoming a life long problem.

TREATMENT

The treatment for spinal curvature problems varies depending on the cause and age at which it is diagnosed.

"Short leg" scoliosis is the simplest to correct and usually to diagnose. If one leg is actually shorter than the other, the pelvis will tilt and rotate, causing the lumbar spine to curve, becoming concave on the side of the longer leg. Usually the vertebrae will then rotate towards the convex side. A secondary curve will then often develop in the thoracic spine, making an S-shaped curvature of the spine. This isn't the end of it as usually the neck will have some degree of lateral curvature and a final accommodation to forward viewing will be made at the occiput/C1/C2 complex. Muscles on the concave side will shorten and those in the convex side will lengthen.

A short leg may arise from congenital causes, a leg may simply not grow as fast as its partner, diseases of the hip such as Perthe's disease may cause the leg to be shortened, fracture of the leg or ankle may alter its growth or length (longer or shorter, but usually shorter especially if it has occurred in a bone not fully developed), or even a knee injury or ankle sprain may be

the original cause. In each case, all that is needed is an accurate diagnosis and a properly measured lift to the shoe of the short leg. Standing pelvic view x-rays are usually needed for accurate diagnosis and a scanogram x-ray is ideal. This gives exact measurement of the leg length differences.

Even these measures are not absolute since the standing posture can be affected by muscular imbalances that mimic leg length discrepancies. We have seen many standing x-rays that clearly show one leg being longer than the other that had muscular/postural causes rather than a real short leg.

A similar cause of scoliosis is the "apparent short leg". In this case, the legs are not actually uneven in length, but appear to be so due to spinal imbalances. The pelvis is a common site for these dysfunctions, which can be fairly complex. Although an osteopath may phrase these problems in terms of positions of bones, this is for convenience only. The problem is rarely if ever just "bone out of place" as is the common lay understanding, but in reality a functional problem of the structural framework which includes not only the bones but also the ligaments, surrounding musculature and fascia.

This is a point that must be constantly remembered to avoid treatments directed at only part of the problem (i.e. just the bone positioning), and thus not ever addressing the real cause. In reality osteopaths think in terms of limitations to function, and it is through restoring proper function that asymmetry of the spine is best corrected.

There are many causes of pelvic and lumbo/pelvic dysfunction. Obviously, slip and fall type injuries can have serious long-term complications if left untreated, or even when treated if they have been traumatic enough

Since the leg itself is attached to the large pelvic bone, the ilium, any injury that leaves this bone rotated forwards or backwards will alter the apparent length of the leg, cause the pelvis to twist, the lumbar spine to rotate and a spinal curve to result. Muscular imbalances will also cause the position of the pelvis to alter and affect apparent leg length. Common examples of this are tight hamstrings on one side pulling on the ilium restricting its movement forward, or tight psoas muscles limiting movement of the hip backward and pulling the ilium forwards thus limiting its rotation backward.

As a general class, muscular imbalances are the most common cause of scoliosis. The most striking examples of this were the result of the polio epidemic of the 1950s. When the polio victims recovered, it was observed that paralysis of large muscle groups on one side of the body caused the spine to twist and rotate.

Similar, if less dramatic, spinal curvatures are the result of muscular imbalances. A benign form of this arises out of "hand dominance" as a result of using one side of the musculature of the upper torso more frequently for daily tasks. The common pattern for strongly right-handed individuals is a concave right thoracic, concave left lumbar scoliosis. Usually noted is a pronated left foot, tightness of the left iliotibial band and weakness of the right gluteus medius, left hip adductors and left oblique abdominals. In left-handed individuals, the reverse findings are common.

Not surprisingly, faulty postural habits are a common contributing factor in the origin of scoliosis pattern. It is important to observe your children (and yourself) for improper body mechanics when standing, sitting and lying. Habit patterns of standing on one leg with the other bent or lying on one side supported by the elbow to head to watch TV or do homework are common problems. Sitting on one leg habitually is another. The position for writing at a desk often causes problems. For example, right-handed individuals usually sit with their upper torso counter-rotated to write.

Simple daily tasks like driving an automobile often leave one hip flexed for long periods. Carrying heavy bags often causes muscular imbalances of the spine as does carrying heavy babies for long periods while doing housework or chores. Another common problem is the position we sit in at work at computer stations, causes chronic spinal rotation.

Obviously, from the list of causes and the complexity of this problem, you are going to need some expert help in diagnosis and therapy. Make sure you incorporate a specific exercise program to help deal with the muscular imbalances that are almost always a major or *the* major factor causing this problem. Do not expect someone else to reverse scoliosis for you. This is one condition that, without your help, probably will *not* be solved. The following general exercise program has been proven effective in reversing lateral curvatures of the spine and is a wise addition to most rehabilitative programs for scoliosis.

Konstancin Exercises

This exercise program is one of the few proven methods shown to help reduce the severity of scoliosis. Obviously the earlier the spinal curvature is diagnosed, hopefully prior to the end of the growth phase, the better is the result. However, even long-standing curvature of the spine can benefit from this exercise program. As with all other forms of self-improvement, regularity is essential for optimum results.

1. Hip Abduction

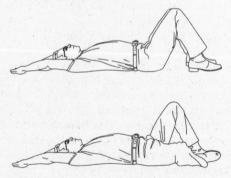

Begin on your back with knees bent and arms over your head. Slowly allow the right knee to drop to the floor, or as close to the floor as is comfortable, then slowly rise back to center. Repeat this 10 times and then repeat exercise with the left leg.

2. Pelvic/Lumbar Roll

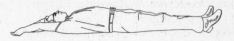

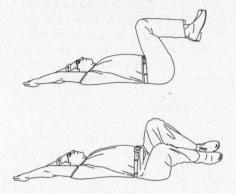

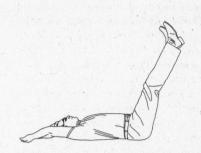

Begin as with exercise number one. Slowly bring both knees towards your chest at about a 45° angle. Allow both legs together to roll to the side towards the floor as far as comfortably possible (do not over-twist initially; gradually increase this exercise's excursion over a period of weeks). Slowly raise both legs back to center. Repeat towards the other side. Repeat entire exercise 10 times.

3. Right Angle Pelvic Tilt

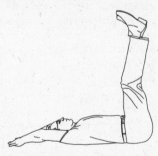

From the starting position as in exercise one, raise your legs to a 90° angle or until the lower back (small of back) touches the floor. Hold this position for a count of 10. Return to starting position and repeat exercise 10 times.

4. Straight Leg Raise
This is a fairly advanced exercise that must be done carefully and slowly. If this exercise causes lower back pain or leg pain gradually increase the degree of elevation until 90° angle can be obtained. Do not do this exercise if you have a disc related injury. Begin on your back with the arms over your head. Slowly raise legs to a 90° angle. Try not to arch your back while doing this exercise. Repeat slowly 10 times. (If this exercise is difficult or painful, only do 1–2 repeats and gradually increase to 10 repeats over a period of a month or two).

5. Straight Leg Raise with Head Flexion

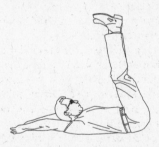

Begin on your back with arms over your head. Slowly raise legs to 90° and flex head forwards. Hold this position according to the timetable below:

1st week: hold 30 seconds and repeat exercise 3 times.

2nd week: hold 45 seconds and repeat exercise 3 times.

3rd week: hold 60 seconds and repeat exercise 4 times.

4th week: hold 75 seconds and repeat exercise 4 times.

421

5th week: hold 90 seconds and repeat exercise 4 times.

6th week: hold 105 seconds and repeat exercise 5 times.

7th week: hold 120 seconds and repeat exercise 5 times.

6. Low Back Extensions

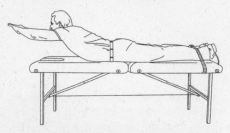

Begin on your stomach with your legs restrained by a strap, or have someone hold them down. Raise your upper body and hold according to the time schedule in the previous exercises. At first raise your upper body only a few degrees and gradually increase the amount of extension.

7. Low Back Extensions (Advanced)

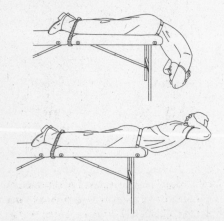

Begin with face down on a table with upper half or your body overhanging the edge at 90° and lower legs restrained by a strap or assistant. With arms clasped behind your neck, slowly raise (extend) your back to level or slightly beyond into extension. Slowly lower back to starting position. Repeat 10 times. (*Note:* This is an advanced

exercise and you may need to slowly build up to it with the other back exercises and begin with only 2 or 3 repetitions and slowly increase over a period of weeks before 10 repetitions are possible.) You will also find a specific back apparatus, the "roman chair" at most exercise equipment supply outlets, which accommodates this very useful exercise with maximum efficiency and comfort. If there is known disc thinning or instability in the lumbar region, do not do this exercise.

8. Standing Squat

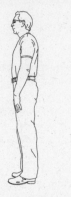
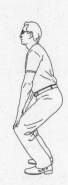

Begin standing, knees straight and palms on thighs. Lean forward slightly and slide hands down to knees, keeping the back and neck as straight as possible, then return to upright position slowly. Exhale while going down and inhale while going up. Repeat 10 times.

9. Standing Pelvic Tilts

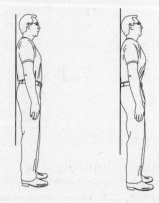

Begin standing with back against the wall and hands at sides. Keep knees slightly bent and feet two inches away from wall. Tilt pelvis and flatten your low back against the wall. Hold for count of five and relax. Repeat 10 times.

10. Standing Pelvic Tilts/Arms Raised

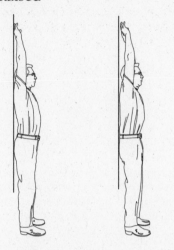

Same as previous exercise, except with arms held above head. Repeat 10 times.

11. Standing Flexion Towards Toes

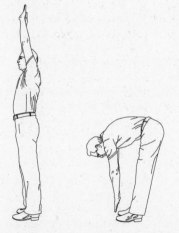

Begin standing with hands on thighs. Forward bend with knees straight and slowly attempt to touch toes. Obviously some people may not reach this goal and only get to knees. The aim is to increase this range slowly and safely. Repeat 10 times. Known disc sufferers beware this exercise. Extreme flexion exercises can cause posterior disc bulges to aggravate.

12. Sitting Flexion

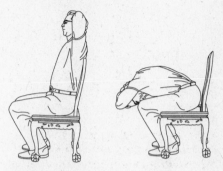

Begin sitting with arms behind neck and knees at 90°. Slowly lean forward until abdomen and chest rest on thighs and then slowly raise upright. Repeat 10 times.

13. Sitting Side Bending

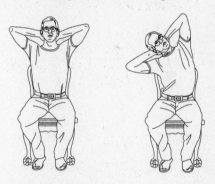

Sitting with hands behind the neck as above, lean slowly to the left as far as possible, then raise upright slowly. Repeat to right. Do this exercise for 10 cycles.

14. Sitting Trunk Rotation

Sitting with hands behind neck, rotate left as far as possible slowly and return to neutral, then rotate to the right and return. Repeat cycle 10 times.

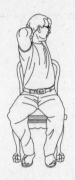

Begin on hands and knees. Do pelvic tilt by rotating your pelvis and hold for 6 seconds. Repeat 10 times.

16. Classic "Pointer"

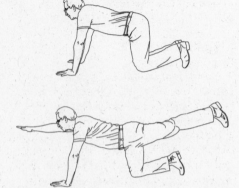

15. Kneeling Pelvic Tilt

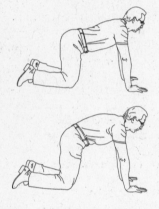

Begin on hands and knees. Lift right arm and left leg and stretch as far as possible. Hold for count of 5. Repeat with opposite leg and arm. Repeat cycle 10 times.

SENILE MEMORY LOSS
(Age Related Memory Impairment)

DEFINITION AND SYMPTOMS

Loss of normal ability to think and remember present and past facts, events, names, places, etc.

DISCUSSION

Senility is nearly synonymous in most people's minds with old age and yet we all know or have heard of someone 80, 90, 100, or older whose mind has remained sharp as can be. So ingrained is the idea of senility, however, that many businesses require those over 65 to retire on the assumption that they must be getting a little befuddled. Nothing could, or should, be further from the truth if the person has taken reasonable care of himself or herself.

Common causes of senility include poor circulation to the brain, cerebral arteriosclerosis, prolonged nutritional deficiency, heavy metal toxicity, prolonged drug use, and lack of exercise.

There is so much demand on our attention in today's increasingly complex world. We are exposed to literally thousands of pieces of information every day, whether via print, the spoken word, TV and computer screens. It is impossible to remember everything that begs our attention; so we need to develop new skills so we can firstly ascertain just what we ought to remember, then commit it to memory and then selectively discard the rest, without "throwing the baby out with the bathwater".

TREATMENT

Prevention of senility must begin early in life. The diet must be composed of plenty of uncooked foods. Daily exercise to the point of breathlessness is essential to maintain adequate circulation. Heavy metals must be avoided by refraining from using aluminum pans or canned foods. A diet similar to that found under Heart Disease is probably the best form of prevention and treatment.

Therapeutic Agents

Vitamins and Minerals—Primary

In addition to the diet and exercise regimen and supplements recommended under Heart Disease, the following will be specifically useful:

- Vitamin A: 25,000–50,000 IU daily.
- Vitamin B complex: 50 mg 1–2 times daily.
- Vitamin C: up to bowel tolerance.
- Vitamin E: 800 mg daily.
- Bioflavonoids: 300–1000 mg daily.

- Choline: needed for production of acetylcholine (lecithin, a good source of choline): 2–4 capsules 3–4 times daily.
- Silica 6×: (4 tablets daily) if aluminum toxicity is suspected.
- Zinc: 25–50 mg 1–2 times daily.

Botanicals—Primary

Ginkgo: circulatory stimulant especially for the brain.

Bacopa: combines well with schisandra as a brain tonic, good when revising for exams too!

Panax ginseng: reduces the demand for cortisol

Gotu kola: to improve cerebral circulation.

Oregon grape: antioxidant.

Botanicals—Secondary

Garlic.

Nettles: good source of silica.

Horsetail: good source of silica.

Withania.

Oil of rosemary: mental stimulant.

Others—Primary

- Tyrosine and d-phenylalanine: both are precursors to dopamine. Take between meals, with water, 1500 mg of each.
- Glutamine: precursor to GABA; detoxifies ammonia; catalyses acetyl-choline.
- Taurine: brain nutrient.
- Ice-cold head baths daily.

SINUSITIS

DEFINITION

Inflammation of the accessory nasal sinuses.

SYMPTOMS

Nasal congestion and postnasal discharge, headache, pain behind eye, tenderness, fever, loss of smell.

ETIOLOGICAL CONSIDERATIONS—PRIMARY

- Diet
  Excess milk and dairy products; milk allergy; excess carbohydrates; raw vegetable deficiency; acidity
- Allergy
  Food; inhalants
- Suppressive

Poor treatment of previous colds
- Toxemia
  Bowel stasis; poor eliminations; liver congestion

ETIOLOGICAL CONSIDERATIONS— SECONDARY

- Cervical spinal lesions: lower cervical; upper thoracic
- Vasoconstriction
- Poor circulation
- Poor lymph elimination
- Obstruction: enlarged turbinates, deviated septum
- Polyps
- Emotional
  Stress; irritants; adrenal exhaustion

DISCUSSION

The typical patient with chronic sinusitis characteristically follows an acid-reacting diet, having an excess of starches and dairy products and lacking in sufficient raw green vegetables. It is well known by naturopaths that this type of diet causes an increase in the amount of mucus produced by the body and favors tissue congestion. One of the most common signs of this is sinus congestion and irritation. Mucus is not only produced in excessive amounts, but can contain irritating elements accumulated. This may be due simply to the over-consumption of foods that render the body fluids more acidic, or due to actual toxic eliminations from chemicals, pesticides, or other causes of toxemia, such as poor eliminations. These irritants set up inflammation and discharge in the mucous membranes of the sinuses. A secondary infection may then settle into the downgraded congested tissues, resulting in acutely painful sinus headaches.

Most of these patients also have a history of treating previous acute eliminations such as the common cold with sup-pressive or improper treatments. Often, causes similar to those under Allergies are found in these cases. Invariably, either cervical or thoracic spinal lesions will be found to aggravate these upper respiratory complaints.

TREATMENT

Acute sinusitis is extremely painful. Fortunately it is also fairly easy to relieve rapidly by natural methods. Even stubborn cases of the more chronic sinus conditions usually respond well. One patient in particular who had received every orthodox treatment available for a period of 6 months with no relief came for naturopathic treatments out of desperation. She had already made plans to fly overseas to see a specialist she had heard of, if our treatments failed to give her relief within a week. She was free of pain within 3 days! We are constantly amazed at the effectiveness of the simple methods that follow.

Diet

It is always best to begin the dietary regimen with a 3–5-day mucus cleansing diet as follows:

Stage 1
Breakfast
Citrus fruit (especially grapefruit).

Midmorning
Fresh vegetable juice (carrot).

Lunch
A large plate of boiled or steamed onions; a little vegetarian seasoning may be used to flavor, but no salt. An orange for dessert.

Midafternoon
Fresh vegetable juice (carrot).

Supper
Same as lunch.

Evening
Potassium broth, or as midmorning.
Take 2 garlic capsules three times daily.

This diet may be followed with 1–2 days on fresh citrus fruit, or if desired you may go directly to a raw food diet for 3–7 days. Eat plenty of fresh fruit, fruit juice, fresh vegetable juice, and raw salads with onions. Follow this with the Stage 2 asthma diet (below) until all residual symptoms are cleared. In many cases repeated mucus-cleansing diets may be needed to correct the condition. It is absolutely essential to avoid all irritants in the diet during this process. This includes coffee, tea, alcohol, strong spices, salt, sugar, and smoking.

Stage 2
Breakfast
Choose between:
- Any fresh fruit, raw or stewed.
- Stewed or baked apple with soaked or simmered raisins.

Lunch
A large, varied, raw salad composed of vegetables that grow mostly above ground, in the ratio 3:1 (e.g. lettuce, cabbage, celery) plus carrots and onions; (peppers, watercress, cucumber). Also have a large plate of boiled or steamed onions topped with vegetarian seasoning or miso. A few walnuts, almonds, or hazel nuts may be added to the salad. Tofu may be added to the meal.

Evening
Choose between:
- Same as lunch.
- A vegetarian protein meal excluding eggs and cheese, plus steamed or baked vegetables. Fresh or stewed fruit as desired.

Later in regimen
Lean meat, fish, or poultry (not fried) with vegetables. Fresh or stewed fruit as dessert.

Drinks
When thirsty, choose from fruit juice, vegetable juice, potassium broth, or herb teas.

Take 2 garlic capsules with meals. Always include raw onions in the salad meals.

If allergy is the cause of repeat attacks, follow regimen for Allergy.

Physiotherapy

- Glycothymoline packs (Cayce product) Soak 3–4 thicknesses of gauze or cotton cloth with glycothymoline (very warm). Apply to painful and congested sinuses for 15–20 minutes, renewing the compress as it cools, and repeat the application until passages clear. (*Note:* In some cases heat may cause more pain. Use ice-cold compresses while doing a very hot foot bath. Another alternative is heat to the back of the head and very cold to forehead.)
- Alternate hot and cold compresses.
- Inhalations: hot water steam with oil of eucalyptus (or leaves), oil of pine (or pine needles), and thyme or cloves.
- Nasal irrigations: beet juice: in ice-cold water
  Borax nasal douche
  Chlorophyll nasal douche
  Lemon and water douche plus nasal spray
  Thuja oil nasal spray
  Warm water and dissolved Celtic salt
  Specific nasal technique (for congestive cases only) performed by many naturopaths and osteopaths.
- Spinal manipulation:
  Cervical; cervical/thoracic; upper thoracic.
- Neck exercises
- Daily vigorous exercise
- Epsom salts baths (see Appendix I) or compresses, locally.
- Alternate hot and cold baths locally (in chronic condition, but not during acute stage).
- Olbas inhalation.

Therapeutic Agents

Vitamins and Minerals— Primary

- Vitamin A: 25,000 IU up to 6 times daily in acute cases; 2-3 times daily in chronic cases. Anti-infection, mucous membrane nutrient.
- Vitamin C and bioflavonoids: 500-1000 mg hourly in acute cases. Anti-infection, anti-inflammatory.
- Zinc: 25-50 mg, 2 times daily.

Vitamins and Minerals— Secondary

- Vitamin B complex: 25-50 mg 2-3 times daily.
- Vitamin B6: 100 mg twice daily.

Others—Primary

- Digestive enzymes between meals, especially if they contain papain and bromelain, which are mucolytic.
- Garlic: 2 capsules 3 times daily.
- Onions: cooked and raw.
- Onion syrup: 1 tsp per hour in acute cases.
- Cayce expectorant (Product 49): 1 tsp 3-6 times daily.

Others—Secondary

- Cod-liver oil.
- Glycothymoline: internal antiseptic. 2-3 drops daily.
- Horseradish.

- Horseradish plus lemon juice.
- Raw adrenal.
- Raw thymus: 1-4 tablets per hour in acute cases.

Botanicals—Primary

Goldenseal: specific for mucous membranes, anti-catarrhal, astringent and trophorestorative.

Albizzia: anti-allergy.

Horseradish: anti-infective, mucolytic.

Eyebright: anti-catarrhal, and anti-inflammatory.

Prickly ash: circulatory stimulant.

Botanicals—Secondary

American elder
Autumn crocus
Barberry
Beech leaf tea
Cayenne
Comfrey
Echinacea
Dandelion
Fenugreek
Golden rod
Juniper berries
Mullein
Mustard seeds
Nettle
Poke root (highly toxic, see page 60)
Queen of the meadow
Red eyebright
Sarsaparilla

SKIN CANCER

DEFINITION AND SYMPTOMS

From time to time lesions can appear on the skin in a variety of shapes, sizes and colors. Some are harmless, such as warts, moles, skin tags and a variety of others. But some are "cancerous", in the sense that they behave, or have the potential to behave, as cancer cells do, with uncontrolled division of cells which can spread to other parts of the body.

There are many different categorizations for skin cancers such as basal cell carcinoma (BCC), squamous cell carcinoma (SCC), melanoma. The differences between various types have to do with factors such as how deep the lesion appears, how quickly it can grow, and other factors.

ETIOLOGICAL CONSIDERATIONS—PRIMARY

- Sun and ultraviolet exposure: excessive exposure to sun is the most recognized risk factor
- Free radical damage
  Trans-fatty acids (e.g. margarine); environmental chemical pollution (external); pharmaceutical, agricultural and other chemical pollution (internal)
- Improper diet: deficiency of fresh vegetables
- Nutritional deficiency: beta-carotene and antioxidants
- Sunscreen and sunblock use: many contain chemicals harmful to the skin

DISCUSSION

Medical diagnosis of skin cancer ultimately depends on a microscopic analysis of a tissue sample from the lesion (called a biopsy). Anything else is a guess.

A skin cancer is called a "primary lesion". As the cancer gets more mature, single or multiple cells break away from the primary lesion, and travel in the blood or lymph circulation, presumably in an attempt by the body to excrete these cells to sustain life. The danger is if these cells become "stuck" in places such as the liver, pancreas, lungs or other organs. This leads to these cancer cells starting another lesion, this time called a "secondary tumor" within or attaching to an internal organ. This process is called "metastasis", and as these secondaries grow, they can cause obstruction leading to organ failure and death. This is why it can be important to deal with a skin cancer sooner rather than later.

Mostly authorities blame the sun and the ultraviolet (UV) rays as the single most important risk factor in the causation of skin cancer. It does seem to be a major contributing factor, as epidemiological correlations of incidence suggest. However, sunshine is an integral part of healthy living, and so many aspects of our health depend on regular exposure to it.

Certainly, there is mounting evidence that ozone-layer deficiency is not good for the skin, allowing through more damaging sun rays. And repetitive sunburning can predispose some individuals to certain carcinomas. So one must take care especially in tropical climes to protect one's skin from sun damage.

Medical studies on the effectiveness of sunscreens and sun blocks are not conclusive. A recent study of 10 other studies, however, has concluded that a person has a significantly *increased* risk of getting skin cancer if sunscreens are regularly used. It is clear that these studies are as yet inconclusive and various interpretations of the currently available data are possible. On the pro-sunblock side one of the interpretations of these conflicting studies is that people who regularly use sunblock tend to overestimate the effectiveness of these products and still receive damaging doses of UV. A recent Norwegian study, however, has found that the common UVB filter, octyl methoxycinnamate, actually killed skin cells on contact and that this effect was magnified with sunlight exposure. These studies come as no surprise to naturopaths who have consistently advised against their use with the caution to avoid prolonged sunbathing sufficient to cause burning. It is not entirely unreasonable to suspect that sunscreens can actually cause skin cancers. Most sunscreens contain benzophenone (or derivatives) as an active ingredient. It is a potent free radical, and is activated by sunlight. Such activity could certainly cause melanomas and other skin cancers, and there is growing concern within the scientific community with this prospect. Other common constituents such as

TREATMENT

Skin cancers are serious, possibly life-threatening health problems that are best prevented if possible. Diet seems to play a major role in preventing skin cancer and recent studies indicate that a diet low in fat and high in foods that contain beta-carotene is your best defense. Antioxidants are another class of nutrients that act as preventatives to the development of skin cancer. Reduction of UV exposure by limiting sunbathing hours and avoiding midday sun is essential.

Clinics in the US and Australia have been legally (and sometimes illegally) using herbal anti-cancer creams now for many years, to successfully treat skin cancers. These herb-based creams, in which herbal constituents act synergistically (together), effect an outcome that none of the herbs in isolation could.

The combination of herbs involved exhibits highly active anti-cancer properties. From clinical experimentation and observation, it is evident these creams have the quality of being cancer cell specific. That is, they only act on cells that are cancerous; they do not affect non-cancerous tissue.

There are some major problems with the orthodox approach to skin cancer.

Diagnosis

Lets say you complain of a skin lesion which might have been changing, say in size, or color (especially spread of red/white/blue pigmentation to surrounding normal tissue), or there is some change in the surface characteristics, consistency, or shape, maybe some itchiness, and signs of inflammation in the surrounding healthy tissue. Any lesions that weep must be suspect. You go to a doctor, he might make a guess at what it is, or he may refer to a dermatologist, and to be sure of what it is (*if* it is cancerous, and *what type* of cancer it might be), a biopsy is taken, and sent to the laboratory for microscopic analysis.

Cutting through a skin cancer to obtain a biopsy sample exposes cancerous cells to the blood and lymph in a way nature does not do. Large numbers of cells (a clump) can be released into circulation all at once, and such clumps are much more likely to become "stuck" in tiny capillaries somewhere, and thus more readily cause secondary tumors. Surgeons say they need the data a biopsy provides in order to know how large an area to cut out "to get it all". However, clinically we see many patients who have had biopsy and surgery, only to have the cancer come back again. So a biopsy does not ensure success of the surgical attempt.

Surgery

Surgery is the standard approach for the "more dangerous" types of skin cancers. Surgery attempts to excise every cancer cell associated with that lesion.

In spite of knowledge gained from the pathology report on the tissue sample, the surgeon will still be guessing at where he or she should cut, and as to how much tissue he ought to take. So surgery cannot guarantee removal of the lesion. We see many people coming into the clinic who have had surgical attempts to remove a lesion, with several effects.

One result is that the cancer recurs (after a couple of years). Another result is that we find that the surgical excision has actually disseminated cancer cells along the margins of the cut. These cells form little colonies around where the original lesion was, and often getting caught up in scar tissue as well. Another risk of surgery is the potential for damage to nerves; a risk that is significant when it comes to important facial nerves for example. A further "side-effect" of surgery can be scarring. Some surgery is quite extensive and deep, invasive of underlying structural tissue such as fascia. Scarring can be subtle, or radical, often requiring skin grafting and/or cosmetic surgery.

OTHER MEDICAL TREATMENTS

Radiation therapy is sometimes used to try to "mop up" cancer cells the surgeon missed. It has been shown to be largely ineffective; we have seen evidence where recurrence has occurred following surgery and radiation. Besides being unreliable, and promoting a false sense of security, radiation has the potential to cause massive free radical damage which itself is potentially carcinogenic.

Chemotherapy is a highly controversial adjunctive skin cancer treatment. Flourouracil has been used topically, but it has been found to cause local metastasis. It has also been shown to inhibit normal cell division.

Cryotherapy, the common procedure of freezing lesions off is usually reserved for more harmless (non-cancerous) lesions. While the procedure itself is relatively safe, it does leave scarring, and more often the lesion recurs.

Accessing the Skin Cancer Alternative

Access can be difficult, but there is "underground" knowledge that is worth finding out. Queensland, Australia, is said to be the "skin cancer capital of the world". In Queensland, naturopaths are legally permitted to treat skin cancers in their clinics, using herbal creams, but may not be able to sell the cream as such.

Preventative Agents

We are designed to get sunshine on our skins for many health-promoting reasons.

But in certain places, there is a culture of fear about sunshine. We recommend sunbathing, not sunbaking. Use protective clothing and cover up when in the sun for prolonged periods. White zinc paste is the only safe sunscreen cream we know about; most proprietary sunscreens contain benzophenones, nitrosamines and cinnamates, all known generators of free radicals which cause oxidative tissue damage and are carcinogenic agents.

Vitamins and Minerals

- Vitamin A: 50,000–100,000 IU daily in emulsified form with medical supervision for toxic effects. Antioxidant.
- Beta-carotene: 10,000 IU twice daily. Precursor to vitamin A and a known anti-cancer agent.
- Vitamin C with Bioflavonoids: 5000–30,000 mg in divided doses daily to bowel tolerance. Enhances immune function and is an anti-cancer agent.
- Vitamin E: antioxidant and to promote tissue repair.
- Zinc: 50 mg daily. To aid immune function and skin health and repair.
- Selenium: 200 mcg daily. Protects against UV and free radical damage.

Others

- Grape seed extract: antioxidant, protects against UV damage.
- Coenzyme Q10: 100 mg daily. Improves cellular oxygenation.
- Kelp: 500–1000 mg daily.

SMOKING

DEFINITION

The addictive habit of smoking tobacco for physical and psychological causes.

SYMPTOMS

Pallor, premature aging, discolored teeth and skin, bad breath, coated tongue, frequent colds, bronchitis, emphysema, lung cancer, and many others.

ETIOLOGICAL CONSIDERATIONS

- Emotional insecurity
- Stress
- Improper diet
- Hypoglycemia
- Peer group pressure
- Oral gratification
- Nicotine addiction
- Alcoholism

DISCUSSION

The tobacco industry has to be given credit for the effectiveness of its advertising campaigns over the years. They spend more money than any other industry in advertising and have succeeded in creating the impression that when you smoke, sophistication, independence, and the macho look are yours, along with good times, beautiful companions, and success in your career.

Peer pressure has created most smokers, along with the industry's seductive advertising. The first cigarette is usually very unpleasant. Poisons are introduced into the body, which rebels with nausea and perhaps a headache. After a few attempts at smoking, however, the body slowly becomes accustomed to the poisons and the addictive effect of nicotine takes hold. Nicotine is a highly addictive drug, and once the addiction is implanted, the body continues to demand its "fix". The smoking habit is then established. The usual physiological demand of the body is at least the nicotine content of 10 ordinary cigarettes daily. Often it is much more.

As public awareness of the dangers of smoking grew, the industry produced low-tar, low-nicotine cigarettes. However, since the body has developed a need for a certain amount of nicotine daily, more of these low-tar cigarettes are usually smoked than regular ones. Low-nicotine cigarettes also produce more carbon monoxide than regular ones. In an effort to produce satisfactory taste for these low-tar, low-nicotine cigarettes, various additives are used, which in themselves may be carcinogenic. Recent research shows that nicotine metabolites in the blood are related to the number of cigarettes smoked, low-tar or not. Low-tar cigarettes do not lower the risk of heart disease or lung damage.

Besides the physical addiction, which is very real, smoking quickly becomes associated with positive actions, such as a good meal or conversation with a close friend. People attempting to stop smoking have great difficulty due to these associations, as well as not knowing what to do with their mouths and hands, which were busy in the process of smoking.

Each cigarette is estimated to take away 8 minutes of life. This means that for the one-pack-a-day smoker, every year he or she gives up 1 month of life. For the two-pack-a-day smoker, this totals up to 12–16 years less of life, and the much greater possibility that the quality of the shorter life will be severely diminished. Cigarettes contain over 4000 known toxic poisons, any one of which in sufficient quantity can kill. Only 1 drop of pure nicotine (which may be obtained from 145 cigarettes) is sufficient to kill an adult.

Smoking is a causative factor in many diseases, reducing not only the length of life, but also the quality of life. Smokers as a group have more colds, sinusitis, bronchitis, emphysema, heart attacks, strokes, and other upper respiratory and circulatory problems than non-smokers. Smoking aggravates diabetes, ulcers, high blood pressure, Burger's disease, and glaucoma, and may help cause osteoporosis, smaller babies, miscarriages, stillbirths, and lung cancer.

Smoking affects the circulatory system in several ways. After only one cigarette the heartbeat is increased 20–25 beats per minute. This increases the load on the heart and increases the blood pressure. The heart itself requires more oxygen due to the increased work load. However, at the same time the carbon monoxide from the cigarette forces the oxygen from the bloodstream, depriving the heart of oxygen it needs.

Smoking also constricts the peripheral blood vessels, reducing blood flow to the hands and feet. After the last cigarette 6 hours must elapse before the circulatory system returns to normal. For the smoker who has the last puff just before going to bed, and the first puff on awakening, the circulatory system is normal for only a short 2 hours out of the entire 24-hour day.

The lungs and respiratory system are the most directly affected by smoking. The lung of a smoker is dark gray and less elastic than the pink, healthy lung of the non-smoker. The natural cleaning mechanisms of the lung, the cilia and macrophages, are unable to do their necessary work due to the tar deposited within the lungs. This effect is even worse for smokers in cities with poor air quality. Lack of cilia action, which normally propels mucus and residues out of the lung in a wave-like action, and reduced functioning of the macrophage cells, which engulf irritants and unwanted material, lead to an increase in the cough reflex to expel this accumulated matter. Local irritations and a drying of the mucous membranes further stimulate the cough reflex. This smoker's cough may settle into chronic bronchitis, then emphysema. Shortness of breath is characteristic of most smokers.

Lung cancer is the end result of the local irritation and exposure to the carcinogenic components of cigarettes. Smoking also appears to have a deleterious effect upon the immune system. Circulating immunoglobulins and antibody responses to antigens are depressed. The immunosuppressive effects of smoking take 3 months to reverse once smoking has been stopped.

The effect of smoking on the skin is that of premature aging. The skin becomes very dry, has an unhealthy pallor, and wrinkles markedly. The irritation of cigarettes, pipes, or cigars on lips and tongue leads to an increase in cancer in these areas. Taste, smell, and even vision are affected by smoking. Most former smokers report an increased acuity of all senses once smoking has been discontinued. Smoking also produces an insulin reaction which creates low blood sugar, resulting in fatigue, irritability, and the desire for another cigarette, setting up a vicious cycle.

Osteoporosis, or loss of minerals from bone, with its consequent weakening, is either aggravated or caused by smoking. Other diseases such as ulcers usually will not heal while the patient continues to smoke. Smoking increases the acid secretions in the stomach.

Women smokers may suffer more severe menopausal symptoms as well as premature onset of menopause; male smokers suffer more prostate problems.

Smoking destroys the body's supply of vitamin C. Each cigarette will destroy up to 25 mg of vitamin C. At one pack daily, this far exceeds the normal intake of this vitamin, which is essential for so many psychological processes. This prolonged vitamin C deficiency may be a factor in the increase in cancer of heavy smokers.

In general, smokers are sick more often, are absent from work more often, and spend more money on drugs, doctor's bills, and hospitals. Smoking workers usually are less efficient than non-smokers, and get less work done in an average day.

Smoking while pregnant leads to smaller babies and more stillbirths. The babies suffer from drug withdrawal symptoms when born and for several days will cry more often than other babies. Nicotine passes through breast milk and affects the nursing infant by dosing it with nicotine. Children of smoking parents generally are sick more often and do less well in school. They are also more likely to become smokers at an early age.

Anyone in the same room with a smoker suffers damaging effects even though they are non-smokers. The smoke causes tearing of the eyes, constriction of the mucous membranes of the nose, as well as constriction of the blood vessels. Non-smokers are affected by the tar, nicotine, and carbon monoxide as well as many of the other poisons. It is now thought that second-hand smoke is more toxic than that which is inhaled directly by the smoker. For anyone suffering from a heart condition, emphysema, stroke, or any other weakened body condition, the results can be aggravated with possibly fatal results. Inhaling smoke in a confined area such as a closed car can be particularly dangerous. The smoke from a smoldering cigarette is the most dangerous type, producing three times the amount of tar and five times the amount of carbon monoxide.

Clearly, smoking is not a benign social habit. If the tobacco industry were not so strong an influence in politics, and if legislators themselves were not so addicted to its use, as is a good portion of the general population, tobacco would probably be a controlled drug. There is also the huge revenue from high tobacco taxes to be considered. One has to suspect that in spite of all the talk, governments do not want to lose this large revenue. Any drug or other substance that caused this many harmful effects would surely be made illegal.

TREATMENT

Many smokers have tried unsuccessfully to stop smoking many times. They have sometimes tried by cutting down, but this is almost impossible since the body makes its physical addiction demand of at least 10 cigarettes as seen above. Each time the effort fails, the addiction becomes even more deeply entrenched. Frequently, depression and a lack of self-respect follow these failed attempts. A series of these unsuccessful attempts often leads the person to feel he or she will fail in other facets of life as well.

Many rationalizations are used by smokers to defend their smoking habit, which they know is very dangerous and yet which they are unable to control. "I like to smoke" is a frequent excuse. (What they really like is the "fix" or nicotine lift without which they would suffer the pains of nicotine withdrawal.) Or: "I think better with a cigarette!" (Actually, smoking constricts the blood flow and oxygen to the brain, making thinking less clear.) Or: "A cigarette calms me down." (After only one cigarette tremors

in the fingers increase 39%. The insulin response with consequent irritability and fatigue causes adrenal exhaustion and nervousness, not calmness.)

The ingrained habits and associations in smoking are so deep that only a definite campaign to recognize and change these habits can have a chance to succeed. Only a fortunate 3% are able to stop smoking on their own. The remainder either continue smoking or seek help.

No program will be effective, however, unless a person is properly motivated and each person has to provide that motivation himself or herself.

After a person stops smoking, however, he or she must realize that they can never have another cigarette or the habit is reinstated, and nicotine will once again latch its addictive hold on the individual.

Diet

The best diet for most smokers is found under Hypoglycemia. This diet helps maintain a constant blood sugar level and prevents many of the ups and downs that often stimulate the desire to smoke. Very high doses of vegetables, carrots, and citrus fruits are advisable for their detoxifying effects, and as a valuable source of vitamins and minerals. High fluid intakes help to detoxify nicotine in the early stages. When possible, dilute fruit and vegetable juice fasting may be tried. These help overcome the nicotine craving a little and of course detoxify the body rapidly. These fasts may be anywhere from 7-21 days, with supervision. This is a very effective way to stop smoking and get over the nicotine habit, if the patient is willing to follow it.

Habitual coffee drinking is frequently associated with excess smoking. Coffee consumption needs to be slowly reduced if great quantities have been taken, to avoid a toxic effect. The aim should be to reduce coffee from 6-10 cups every day to 1-1½ in the first 3 days of pre-therapy, and to stop altogether by the start of any behavior modification and aversion therapy, or any other therapy for that matter.

Physiotherapy

- Sweat baths, saunas: daily In the detoxification regimen to get nicotine out of the system.
- Colonics: twice per week for 1–3 weeks.
- Exercise: increase all activity.

Therapeutic Agents

Vitamins and Minerals

- Vitamin A: 25,000 IU 2–3 times daily for 1 month. Beta-carotene sources are best in this instance (necessary for proper health of mucous membranes).
- Vitamin C: 3000–10,000 mg daily, to detoxify nicotine. Up to 30 g intravenously to aid withdrawal.
- Vitamin B complex: 50 mg 3 times daily.
- Vitamin B3 (niacin): 100 mg up to 1 or more grams, 2–3 times daily.
- Vitamin B1: 50–100 mg daily.

Botanicals

Lobelia (Indian tobacco): contains lobeline, which is very similar to nicotine. It helps wean the patient off nicotine and is non-addictive, so once the habit is broken, lobelia may then be discontinued. Smoke, or take 5–15 drops 6 times daily.

Aversion therapy with lobelia: procedure— no smoking is allowed except for a concentrated period of 1 hour daily when 15 drops of lobelia are taken internally ½ hour and then 15 minutes before the first cigarette is lit. With each 15-minute period, a further 15 drops diluted in water are taken while cigarettes are smoked end to end. The result will be nausea, which soon becomes associated with smoking. In 5 or 6 days the desire for cigarettes will probably have disappeared. (Unfortunately lobelia is not allowed to be sold in Australia. You can still order it from the US and import it for personal use.)

Calamus: chew root, then smoke. Will also cause nausea as a negative feedback.

Chamomile: take 3–6 times daily to relax.

See Stress for specific herbs indicated for calming the nervous system.

SPRAINS

DEFINITION AND SYMPTOMS

Trauma to a joint (ankle, knee, back, wrist, etc.) with varying degrees of ligament injury or tearing, causing rapid swelling, pain, and discoloration.

DISCUSSION

All sprained joints should be treated along the same lines. Most people think of ice application for a sprained ankle, but for some reason the average person feels at a loss when other joints are sprained. We are always surprised to see how many people will put heat and not ice on a sprained or severely strained back. A joint is a joint. Obviously, some joints cannot be easily treated with the standard RICE treatment (rest, ice, compression, and elevation), but ice and rest are the mainstays of such treatment and should always be employed.

TREATMENT

The general treatment for all sprains, where possible, is discussed below.

Rest

Do not use the affected joint from the first moment of injury for at least 2 days. If the ankle is involved, use no weight-bearing. Crutches are to be used when you must be upright, but avoid as much moving about as possible these first few days. Severe shoulder injuries require a sling to allow full rest. Severe back sprains require 24–48 hours of *complete* bed rest. Only after 24–48 hours, once pain and swelling has begun to subside, can you begin to mobilize the joint within the pain margin, taking care not to reinjure the joint.

Ice

As soon as possible after the injury, hopefully within minutes, apply ice to the area. Swelling begins immediately, so it is essential to reduce this as rapidly as possible to minimize pain, reduce possibility of adhesions, and speed healing. Apply ice over one layer of toweling to prevent burning the skin or immerse joint in ice water. Keep ice on for 30 minutes. Ice is also used in the recovery period as long as there is any sign of inflammation.

Compression

To further prevent swelling, cover crushed ice with a plastic wrap and apply an adhesive bandage. Leave on 30 minutes, unwrap for 5-15 minutes, and rewrap. After the second ice compression wrap, apply a standard compression bandage which consists of a layer of cotton, a layer of elastic, another layer of cotton, and a final elastic wrap. Keep toes or extremities exposed to make sure of adequate circulation. If toes turn blue, unwrap and rewrap less tightly. This compression bandage may stay in place for a full 24 hours when the joint is checked, or it may be removed every 2 hours for an ice application.

Elevation

Elevate the injured joint to prevent effusion into joint and surrounding tissues. As healing progresses over the first 24–48 hours, and swelling and pain are reducing, the joint is now ready for mobilization. Place the joint in hot water, or use a hot compress. Slowly move the area in all its normal movements to the point of pain, but not beyond. Some joints may require passive mobilization where the joint is taken through its movements without the patient's muscular assistance. Ice should still be used periodically throughout the day to speed healing and prevent the joint from swelling. If for any reason the joint swells after an activity, apply ice.

Physiotherapy

* Interferential electrotherapy: apply electrotherapy 3 times the first week or two depending on the severity of the sprain.
* Short-wave diathermy: Apply short-wave for 20 minutes 3 times per week for two weeks.
* Ultrasound: use ultrasound applied under water 3 times per week for two weeks.
* Alternate hot and ice cold foot baths: fill one container large enough to cover foot and ankle with hot water and another with ice cold water (including ice cubes) Place the injured foot in the hot water for 3 minutes then into to ice-cold water for 3 minutes. Repeat cycle 3 times ending with the ice-cold. You will find the ice-cold bath is very painful for the first few days. If you cannot bear the whole 3 minutes in the ice-cold, take your foot out when it gets unbearable, wait 15 seconds and then reimmerse. This therapy is the single most valuable part of your recovery so do not exclude it simply because it is painful. Do this alternate foot bath twice daily until all pain is resolved.
* Exercise: it is essential for you to regain mobility as soon as possible. By day 3 you

need to begin to move your ankle slowly both passively and actively. With your hands, move you ankle slowly up and down, then side to side. Be careful to avoid reinjuring any torn ligaments. Using your muscles, do the same movements, also with extreme care. After a few more days you can begin to stretch the injured muscles. Fold a towel so that it is about 3 inches (8 cm) wide. Place this towel under the front one-third of you foot and *very gently* pull you foot towards your head (flexion). Only pull as far as your foot will go without pain. Do not be concerned if this movement is very limited. Now very gently push down against the resistance of the towel. Hold this effort for 6 seconds, stop pushing slowly, wait half a second, and the pull on the towel so that the front half of the foot comes more into flexion. Repeat this cycle 5 times. Do this exercise twice daily. You also need to do the same type of stretch for inversion, eversion and extension.

Therapeutic Agents

Vitamins, Minerals and Others

- Bromelain: 2–3 tablets 3–4 times daily, taken only on an empty stomach This is the best anti-inflammatory medication available for soft tissue trauma.
- Arnica tincture (topical): apply 4–6 times daily.
- Vitamin C and bioflavonoids: 4–5 g at time of injury; 1 g per hour for first 2–3 days.

Homoeopathics:

- Hypericum 12, 30C, every 10 minutes until pain is managed.
- Arnica 12, 30 C to minimize bruising, hourly for 6 hours, then 2 times daily for several days.

Note: all severe sprains should be checked for fracture. If severe effusion into the joint has occurred, it may best be aspirated to prevent adhesions.

STAPHYLOCOCCAL INFECTION
(Staph, Impetigo, "School Sores")

DEFINITION

Staphylococcus: a small round bacteria growing in clusters. May infect any area of the body.

Impetigo: a highly contagious, superficial skin infection usually caused by staphylococci, or occasionally *Streptococcus*.

SYMPTOMS

Staphylococcal infection: pimples, furuncles, boils, carbuncles, abscesses, osteomyelitis, enterocolitic pneumonia, bacteremia, occasionally fatal.

Impetigo: red swellings becoming pustules or large pus-filled bullae which rupture and form a yellow crust. May rapidly spread in infants with risk of fatal systemic infection, although this is rare. May complicate other skin lesions such as eczema, scabies of fungus infections, or other types of dermatitis.

ETIOLOGICAL CONSIDERATIONS—PRIMARY

- Poor hygiene
- Diet
  Toxic; low-protein; excess sweets, fruit; excess acidity; green vegetable deficiency; milk or other allergy with staph infection secondary

- Allergy with staph infection secondary
- Post antibiotic staph infection
- Postsurgery staph infection

ETIOLOGICAL CONSIDERATIONS— SECONDARY

- Polluted bathing water (especially ocean, swimming)
- Insect bites
  Cuts at site of entry, poor care
- Predisposition (staph sensitivity, newborns, nursing mothers, skin disorders, diabetes, lung conditions

DISCUSSION

Staphylococcus bacteria are found almost everywhere in the environment. They live quite happily on the nasal membranes and skin of most healthy people. Normally, however, they cause no problem and go unnoticed.

An interesting fact about staphylococcal infections (and most other infections for that matter) is that some people seem more susceptible than others. In studying the differences between those who are very susceptible and those practically immune to staph infection, we can find both the cause and the cure.

Poor hygiene is considered a major cause of staph infection. This may be the cause in a few extreme cases where gross neglect leads to infection, especially where there is an abrasion or cut present. In general, however, with the exception of lack of attention to superficial injuries and neglect of basic sanitation or cleanliness, hygiene is probably one of the least significant causes of staph infection in the average situation. Exceptionally clean and hygienic people do indeed get staph infections.

Diet and its effect on immunity and general vitality is a significant causative factor. Contrary to the popular "new age" belief that all disease may be cured by fruit juice fasting, staph is a disease frequently found to be precipitated by excess fruit, or at least some form of sugar, along with a pronounced protein deficiency.

As with most other diseases, we do see many with staph infections on a refined, devitalized, and toxic diet, but a large number are "new age" fruitarians or fairly strict vegetarians. These people often eat excess fruits in the belief that fruit is health-giving, and very little protein in the belief that protein is dangerous to the health.

Both beliefs are right and wrong. Fruit and fruit juice are excellent purifiers and may be used medicinally to encourage eliminations. It is superb as a medicinal agent. As a luxury food or source of vitamin C and a few other vitamins and minerals, again, it is superb. As a staple food, however, it fails miserably. The taste of fruit, we all know, is delectable. Most succulent fruits, however, contain little more than sugar, water, a few vitamins and minerals, and little, if any, protein. Not only is fruit in excess not particularly good for you, it may even be quite bad. Too much quickly absorbed sugar as found in most fruits can seriously upset the glucose-regulating system in the body, adversely affecting both the pancreas and adrenal glands (see Hypoglycemia).

Excess sugar in any form favors staph growth and multiplication. Staph doesn't care if your sugar comes from cane sugar, alcohol, honey, grapes, or apples.

Protein is another example of a misunderstood food. All the negative publicity concentrated proteins have received in the past 20 years has turned many towards protein avoidance. It has become obvious that excess animal proteins are hazardous to health. The link between saturated fats and heart disease is now fairly well accepted. It is now clear that a partial or even total vegetarian diet is more conducive to long life and a reduction of many health complaints. But many people have rejected nearly all proteins to live exclusively on fruits and vegetables, even to the exclusion of nuts or beans. While it is possible to live on this diet if extreme care is taken to supply vegetable matter with high protein content, any severely restricted diet of this nature may become a health risk. Staph infection is one of those risks.

We think it fair to point out that some people do follow these strict regimens with good results. If proper care is taken the result may be a healthy and strong vitality. We are more concerned with those who obviously are not well suited to this regimen, proven by their lack of vitality. Staph infection is not a cleansing process. The boils are not removing toxins from within in most cases, but result from reduced vitality and are a disease process. The end result of ignoring a staph infection or treating it through extended fasting could lead to bacteremia and death. Others who commonly contract staph infections are on no specific diet regimen but habitually eat little protein and eat excessive amounts of fruits and fruit juices, other sweets, or refined carbohydrates.

Antibiotics, so often used with even minor infections, are both a blessing and a curse as far as staph infection is concerned. We are strongly against the habitual and routine use of antibiotics for any and almost all infections, colds, fevers, etc., as they are routinely prescribed by most physicians. Not only is the natural way quite effective in these minor to moderate problems, but the over-use of antibiotics is rapidly creating a world health crisis.

The longer we use antibiotics regularly, the more resistant strains of bacteria emerge. Many diseases that were all but wiped out are now re-emerging even stronger than ever and are almost impossible to kill off. Not only is an individual these days exposed to antibiotics as medicine from cradle to grave, but they are even found in milk and meat products, to name just two.

Our objection to this abuse in this particular case is threefold. The first is that antibiotics destroy not only the target pathological bacteria, but also destroy the entire ecology of the body, which in many cases depends on friendly bacteria for our health and pro-

tection. Once these allies are destroyed, *Staphylococcus* may take a strong hold.

Our second objection is that the use of antibiotics for minor staph infections tends to cause antibiotic-induced yeast infections that may be very difficult to treat, especially if there is systemic spread.

Lastly, antibiotics used even for the most trivial infection often cause a chronic case of allergic dermatitis which may in turn become infected with a secondary staph infection, complicating an otherwise simple problem. Infants seem particularly sensitive to antibiotics. One of the saddest and most difficult problems that confront most naturopaths is seeing an infant who, upon receiving antibiotics for one or two small skin infections or a mild case of impetigo, develops an antibiotic dermatitis which then settles into a chronic eczema, covering the entire body. This then commonly becomes infected with a secondary staph infection.

It may now seem strange, after writing about the evils of antibiotics, for us to say how life-saving antibiotics can be in severe staph infections. If the infection is allowed to get out of control and enter the bloodstream and the patient has swollen glands and fever, or other signs of systemic infection, the time has arrived for antibiotics. At this point the infection has established too strong a hold to be treated with natural therapy safely. General vitality cannot defend the body's borders and needs help.

It is unfortunate that something as useful and lifesaving when used with discretion as antibiotics should become one of the major threats to world health because of indiscriminate use. Antibiotics should be reserved for the few times of true health crises that most people do encounter within their lifetimes. With proper diet, preventative care, and simple natural treatments, even these few crises may often be avoided.

TREATMENT

To treat staph infections and impetigo properly with natural therapies, the infection should be caught early and treated vigorously. Haphazard treatment will not be curative and only allows the infection to spread.

Diet

Susceptibility to staph infection may be due to excess sugar in one form or another. The best therapeutic regimen in these cases is one high in green vegetables and vegetarian protein, with absolutely no sugar, honey, refined carbohydrates, or alcohol. Fruit consumption is severely restricted or eliminated until the infection and rash are gone. Protein supplements are recommended 2–3 times daily. In the case of impetigo, the child is usually on a diet high in fruits, fruit juices, and carbohydrates with a deficiency of vegetables other than potatoes and other starches. For these children, the best diet is one of raw and cooked vegetables, especially green and yellow or orange foods, no fruit or fruit juice, and only unrefined carbohydrates, along with adequate protein.

Hygiene

The skin and mucous membranes normally function as a protective barrier for the body. Subtle qualities of pH, cilia hairs, bacteria flora, and quality of secretions help prevent infection. Once these barriers are breached by an abrasion or cut, the internal immunological defenses act as secondary protective mechanisms. The integrity of the immunological system may be affected by diet, nutritional deficiency, glandular disorders, stress, and many other factors. Some people seem virtually immune to staph infections. They can receive deep gashes and give them little or no attention, even to the extent of leaving the wound dirty and unattended, and it will still heal quite happily without infection. Other people can get the slightest prick and will develop a staph infection almost overnight. It is obvious that individual resistance is very

important and varies from individual to individual. Once again we see that it is not the germ that causes disease, but a favorable environment that allows ever-present germs to flourish.

It is not wise to allow a wound to go untreated. Clean cuts need less attention than jagged ones. Any situation that causes the skin to lose its normal circulation is more likely to lead to infection. Deep, penetrating punctures or wounds that cause much tissue damage always need to be treated. Dirt and foreign matter must be removed and the area washed with soap and water and flushed with hydrogen peroxide. Although alcohol and iodine do kill bacteria, they also destroy healthy cells and should not be used. Tea tree ointment or oil is the best application for a cut or wound. It is much more effective than other antibiotics such as bacitracin and is also an antifungal agent.

Goldenseal or calendula tea may be used as a wash. Give the wound fresh air and sunlight, and avoid prolonged immersion in water. Avoid salt water contact as this delays healing and may encourage spread. Expose to strong sunlight if possible.

Local Treatments

Wash area with full-strength tincture of green soap. Crust should be removed for rapid healing. Apply warm goldenseal tea compresses to firmly adherent crust. Flush with hydrogen peroxide and then apply full strength tea-tree oil. Repeat every 2 waking hours. Apply tea tree ointment at night. Ultraviolet exposure daily as an antibacterial agent is encouraged where possible. Another approach is to follow the same procedure as above, but instead of using a tea tree oil application, use castor oil, 3 parts; to eucalyptol, ½ part. This may be more useful in some cases of impetigo, where the skin is so raw that the tea tree oil causes severe pain or aggravation. Another useful topical application is the combination of herbal tinctures of myrrh, calendula, and echinacea, and add a couple of drops of tea tree oil if handy. Change pillow covers and sheets nightly. Take care to disinfect these along with any towels, washcloths, or clothes that may cause reinfection, or spread to other family members.

Therapeutic Agents

Vitamins and Minerals—Primary
Vitamins A and C are lowered by infections.
- Vitamin A: very high doses (for short term): 10,000–20,000 IU daily (infant), 20,000–60,000 IU daily (child), 75,000–200,000 IU daily (adult).
- Vitamin C: very high doses: 500–1000 mg daily (infant), 1000–3000 mg daily (child), 3000–20,000 mg daily (adult).
- Zinc: necessary for healing.

Botanicals—Primary
Echinacea
Garlic: internal, external to lesion; external as foot compress (see Appendix I).
Tea tree oil: external; antifungal, antibiotic, specific.
Goldenseal.

Botanicals—Secondary
Burdock.
Comfrey.
Gentian violet: apply twice daily (1%).
Oil of bitter orange: antibiotic.
Eucalyptus.

Others—Primary
Probiotics: topically and internally, double recommended dose.

Others—Secondary
Raw thymus: 2 tablets 4–6 times daily.
Essential fatty acids.

STRESS

The human mind-body has developed ways of attempting to deal with the stressors of everyday life. If the individual is successful, the internal environment is able to maintain homeostasis (harmony, balance). But if the cumulative effects of stress are too great, if too unusual, or long-lasting, then a series of biochemical and other changes can occur. Hans Selye in 1956 defined these changes in what he referred to as the general adaptation syndrome (GAS). He identified three stages in GAS:
1. Alarm reaction, or the fear/fight/flight response, in which the hypothalamus triggers the sympathetic nervous system and adrenal medulla, and adrenalin and cortisol are secreted into general circulation
2. Resistance reaction, in which the hormonal response diminishes, only appropriate organs "battle" the stressor
3. Exhaustion, which reflects prolonged stress, in which organs and systems "wear out"; the mind and body now "draft" other organs and systems, initiating further adrenalin and cortisol secretion (often adrenal cortex becomes enlarged); most organs and systems are affected and harmed; there is shrinkage of the thymus, spleen, lymph nodes; there is a decrease in white blood cell production, sex hormones decline; blood pressure increases; all of which leads to immune system illnesses, chronic hypertension, impaired mental function, cardiovascular disease, and cancer.

Nearly every disease we know can be aggravated or even caused by stress or destructive emotions. We have discussed stress-related hypoglycemia, headaches, colitis, ulcers, enuresis, fatigue, high blood pressure, and a whole host of other conditions.

TREATMENT

Stress management has to do with:
- Identifying stressors (external and internal—physiological)
- Minimizing exposure to stressors
- Effectively managing *response* to stressors (i.e. coping skills, and relaxation response)

How to Take Control

Loss of control drastically increases stress.
- Know when you are *really* out of control, not just *feeling* as though you are (e.g. don't jump to negative conclusions, don't over-generalize, don't just go along with others just to fit in
- Realize that although you can't always control what happens, you can always control how you respond or react (e.g. deep breathing, sit down and think first)
- Make lists of your goals (for today/week/month/year...prioritize/do difficult first). Make it your number one goal to be happy
- Expect much, but be realistic; goals are challenges, not stressors
- Don't be afraid to fail
- Internalize goals (e.g. *feeling* rich vs. *being* rich)
- Make work your play, in other words, you either love your work, or you should find something else to do
- Carefully consider what other people in your life expect of you. Are these expectations realistic, do they accord with your goals?
- Learn to say no and be true to yourself
- Simplify your life and don't be a slave to technology

How Support Vanquishes Stress

Research shows all the time that having close personal relationships/friends and family/church/a sense of community/being a member of a club, will mean a sense of self, and feeling part of a group is prerequisite for managing stress and for good health. The "Rosetta Study", based on a small New Jersey town with a close-knit population of mostly Italian Americans who adhered to old country traditions and customs, demonstrated that living within this supportive network of camaraderie led to remarkably good health. In all other ways, the townsfolk demonstrated statistical normality with the control groups. They did not practice conventionally healthy lifestyles, for example they ate lots of red meat, had normal rates of obesity and high blood pressure, and were typical in drinking and smoking habits.

The significance of this study was that the Rosetta population demonstrated extraordinarily low rates of stress-related diseases, including cardiovascular disease and ulcers. The study also showed that when individuals moved away from this family community, this supportive network, they quickly succumbed to the signs of stress.

Here are some things to consider, to help one reduce the negative impacts of stress in one's daily life.
- Enjoy the human touch, hugs, massages.
- Ensure you have someone you can talk to about anything.
- Have an animal pet; pets love their owners unconditionally.
- Loving others increases one's perception of being loved (altruistic egoism); love stops stress; love heals.

Stress Release: The Regenerating Power

Don't "bottle it up". There are four ways of releasing stress (outlets):
- Physical action (burn it off), with especially aggressive exercise, e.g. power walking; martial arts; vigorous gardening.
- Verbal releasing, e.g. talking, crying, laughing, yelling, writing. NB the composition of tears varies, for example

emotional tears can include adrenalin, endorphins, neurotransmitters.

- Displacement: take out frustrations on a pillow (scream, hit, etc.).
- Meditation is perhaps the best possible way, a so-called "magic bullet" to reduce stress. The spaces between the thoughts feel timeless, and help one regain perspective on one's life.

How to Meditate

For beginners:
- Find a quiet place, no interruptions.
- Allow 10–20 mins, 2 times daily, preferably before breakfast, before dinner.
- Sit comfortably, consciously, close eyes, be calm, breathe slowly and deeply.
- Stop internal dialogue (stop thinking in words, don't plan, don't recall).
- (to help) repeat a mantra, e.g. "peace", "love", "om nama shiva", "shalom".
- Don't worry if thoughts intrude (they will); allow, dismiss, mantra, breathe.
- When finished, sit quietly for a few mins, and merge with normality.

More advanced (for a sensation of continuous energy flow)
- Sit comfortably, cross legged, spine straight, hands together (right resting in left) palms up thumbs touching in lap.
- Close eyes; visualize all tension leaving body
- Focus all mental energy on the pineal gland (the 3rd eye)
- Silently chant.
- Continue for 10 mins (ignore distractions).
- Inhale deeply, hold for 15 seconds, exhale and relax.

There are other ways to help one let go of emotional stress, such as *autogenic training*: lie down in quietness, become passive, eyes closed, feel heavy in arms, legs, imagine limbs are becoming warm, imagine heart beat slowing, concentrate on deep breathing, imagine forehead becoming cool.

You can also learn how to progressively relax individual muscles. Lying down, start with a conscious movement of the toes and feet, then relax the toes and feet; move onto the calf muscles, knees, thighs, hips and so on, each time consciously moving then relaxing each muscle group. Cover every area of the body, front and back, and the face and head muscles. See also the stress release exercise under Hypertension.

There are many other forms of stress management such as prayer, biofeedback, self-hypnosis.

The physiological beneficial effects of these types of meditation and relaxation are:
- A slowed metabolism, i.e. a hypometabolic state (only other way, sleep, hibernation).
- Decrease in blood lactate.
- Decrease in heart rate, blood pressure, breathing rate.
- Melatonin is increased, and there is a decline in the production and circulation of the stress hormones, such as adrenalin and cortisol.

Therapeutic Agents

No list of supplements will cure stress if the cause is primarily emotional, or due to external conditions. The following list of supplements will help deal with physiological and biochemical *results* of stress, and if taken in conjunction with efforts to deal with the cause of stress, will be instrumental in the overall therapy.

Some cases of stress are solely due to nutritional deficiencies or excesses and these will be corrected by dietary changes and nutritional supplementation alone. For instance, animal products are naturally high in phospholipids, arachidonic acid and other potent mediators of physiologic stress and inflammation. During the slaughtering of animals, the beasts are subjected to the stress and the organs of these animals (mainly the adrenal glands) secrete large amounts of stress hormones, notably adrenalin and cortisol into their bloodstream and into their tissues. Elevated levels of stress hormones remain present in the meat eaten by us. They act as stressors in our bodies. A largely vegetarian diet, with some fish perhaps, is recommended for those who suffer from stress. Caffeine in excess adds to biochemical stress, as does excessive cigarette smoking.

How one eats when one is stressed is just as important as *what* one eats. When stress is prolonged, as for people who are constantly "stressed out", then it means that digestion becomes chronically very poor, we start to miss out on vital nutrients, we become malnourished, which in turn creates further physiological stress, and disease sets in. Fasting, or a regime of water, juices and broth during times of stress are extremely beneficial, even curative in their effects.

Have you ever noticed an animal that is stressed? It will not eat, it drinks lots of water, and tries to escape the stress, and rest. We seem to have lost the wisdom of nature. When we keep on eating when stressed, the problems only become exacerbated. Digestion requires a lot of energy, and when the energy is focused elsewhere, food (especially lots of food, or complex foods) is impartially digested, we can become constipated, or diarrheic, causing toxins to build up in our systems, causing further problems than we would have had if we had not eaten and dealt with the stressors properly.

So we need to honor the parasympathetic nervous system, the system of rest/digest, not merely at mealtimes, but in more general terms. We need to ensure we have a balanced lifestyle, one which adequately deals with stress so that it does not impact on our digestive system, thus creating disease. When stressed, we recommend eating slowly, grazing, and choose simple foods which are easily digested, such as salad and cooked vegetables, and fresh fruit.

Vitamins and Minerals—Primary

- Vitamin B complex: 50 mg 2-3 times daily.
- Vitamin C: to bowel tolerance.
- Magnesium: 600-2000 mg daily.

Vitamins and Minerals—Secondary

- Vitamin A: 25,000-100,000 IU daily.
- Pantothenic acid: 25-50 mg 1-2 times daily.
- Vitamin E: 400-800 IU daily.
- Calcium: 800-1000 mg daily.
- Potassium: to 8 g daily.
- Zinc: 25-50 mg 1-2 times daily.

Others—Primary

- Probiotics.

Others—Secondary

- Essential fatty acids, especially flaxseed oil.
- Evening primrose oil.
- Hypothalamus: 1 tablet 2-3 times daily.
- Raw adrenal: 1 tablet 2-3 times daily.
- Thymus: 1-3 tablets 2-4 times daily.

Botanicals—Primary

Astragalus: adaptogenic.
Ginseng (Panax and Siberian): adaptogenic, adrenal support, anti-stress.
Withania.
St John's wort.
Schisandra.
Gotu kola.
Nervine sedatives and tonics such as skullcap, passion flower, hops, kava kava, valerian, bacopa, zizyphus.

Botanicals—Secondary

Consider also herbs as for Anxiety, Depression, Insomnia, Hypertension.

Therapeutic Suggestion

Stressed out people often "live on their adrenals". It is important to support the adrenal glands in times of stress, and some tips from the section on Digestive Disorders will help. Above all, reduce your coffee intake slowly over a week or two, to 2 cups daily at most.

TEETH AND GUM DISEASE
(Caries, Periodontal Disease: Gingivitis and Pyorrhea)

DEFINITION

Caries: gradual dissolution and destruction of tooth enamel and dentin, eventually involving the tooth pulp.
Periodontal disease:
Gingivitis: inflammation of the gums surrounding the teeth.
Pyorrhea: inflammatory enlargement and degeneration of the soft tissue and bone surrounding teeth, leading to recession of gums and loosened teeth.

SYMPTOMS

- Dental caries
  Frequent cavities; irregular enamel
- Periodontal disease
  Bad breath; foul taste in mouth; red, swollen, bleeding gums; sensitivity to hot or cold; receding gums; loose teeth; loss of teeth

ETIOLOGICAL CONSIDERATIONS—PRIMARY

- Refined carbohydrates (foods stick to teeth)
- Vitamin deficiency
- Sugar
- Poor hygiene
  Improper brushing; lack of flossing
- Vitamins A, C, D, calcium, magnesium, phosphorus, trace mineral, or protein deficiency
- Soft drinks
- Phosphoric acid in soft drinks dissolves enamel, and they contain up to 13 tsp sugar, as well

ETIOLOGICAL CONSIDERATIONS— SECONDARY

- Overcooked foods
- Excess meat-based protein and/or processed foods
- Heredity (some families show poor tooth calcification)
- Excess hot or cold foods lower gum vitality
- Prolonged bottle feeds, especially at night (milk or fruit Juice bottle syndrome)
- Poor diet of mother during pregnancy or lactation
- Severe infection in infancy leaves poorly developed layers of enamel
- Diabetes

DISCUSSION

Both caries and periodontal disease are diseases of civilization related to abnormal dietary habits. Archeological findings show clearly that Stone Age peoples had remarkably little of either tooth or gum disease. Further findings show that the peasant classes of ancient Egypt who could afford only simple whole grains had far fewer cavities than the ruling class, who lived on more refined foods. Recent studies of rural populations eating unrefined foods show very strong gums and teeth but once they are exposed to a more modern diet containing sucrose and refined cereal grains, a rapid deterioration takes place.

Healthy gums and teeth begin early in gestation and depend to a large extent on the diet of the mother. Strong teeth specifically require adequate supplies of vitamins

A, C, D, calcium, magnesium, phosphorus, trace minerals, and protein. If the mother's diet was marginal in any of these nutrients prior to pregnancy, the deficiency would be magnified by the increased needs of the fetus. In most cases, nutrients needed by the growing infant will be leached from the mother to the extent they are available. This is the reason for the old adage, "a tooth lost for every child". Calcium and other minerals are extracted from the mother's bones and teeth to provide for the growing needs of the infant. This obviously sets the stage for dental problems in the mother. Evidence also suggests that nutrient-deficient mothers make babies with poor teeth.

Rats fed on a good diet give birth to baby rats with teeth strongly resistant to disease. Poorly fed nutrient-deficient rats, however, produced offspring with teeth highly subject to decay. Repeated pregnancies closely following each other is another factor in dental problems for the mother and infant. Studies show that later siblings have statistically more dental disease than the first-born child.

Although the mother's diet during pregnancy is very important in the subsequent development of strong teeth in her newborn, the baby's diet in early infancy and childhood is equally important. It is important to remember that teeth are made from within and require not only a few vitamins and minerals, but a generally good diet. A sound diet makes sound teeth and is a child's best guarantee that he or she will have little or no dental problems. No amount of external cleaning measures will be of much benefit if the diet produces weak teeth.

Once the teeth are formed and hopefully have an even, tough layer of hard, impervious enamel, proper diet is essential to prevent tooth decay and gum disease. The biggest enemy of healthy gums and teeth is plaque. Colonies of micro-organisms form difficult-to-remove plaque, which then causes fermentation of carbohydrates, producing acids that dissolve away minerals in the tooth's enamel. The enamel becomes brittle and ultimately is breached, allowing destruction of the inner pulp.

Although carbohydrates are implicated in the process, it is the ultra-refined carbohydrate of sucrose (sugar), along with other refined grains such as white flour or white rice that are the main offenders. A glue-like substance called dextran is produced by a specific *Streptococcus* in the mouth, and is necessary to fix the plaque in place on the tooth margin. Dextran can only be produced from sucrose. Other refined carbohydrates such as white bread are very sticky and become easily lodged between teeth and gum margins, providing ideal fuel for plaque to ferment. This leads to erosion of the enamel and irritation of the gums. The gums may develop pockets, which act as further reservoirs of impacted food materials, creating an ideal environment for bacterial proliferation. Eventually the gums become inflamed (gingivitis) and begin to recede (pyorrhea), leaving the tooth root exposed. Finally the tooth loosens and falls out or must be removed due to infection. Gum disease also creates infection which may have profound effects on the general health.

Another possible factor in tooth loss is periodontal disease where alveolar bone surrounding the tooth becomes weakened and less dense. According to present statistics, two-thirds of the population of the US suffers some degree of periodontal disease. Recent research has implicated modern diet in both periodontal disease and osteoporosis, or a generalized bone loss. A diet high in phosphorus and low in calcium seems to be a major factor. The typical western diet high in red meat has a ratio of between 1 part calcium to 25–40 parts phosphorus. The normal ratio should be 0.7 calcium to 1 part phosphorus. Other foods high in phosphorus are refined foods and carbonated soda beverages. As the phosphorus level increases in relation to calcium, the parathyroid glands are stimulated to produce a hormone, parathormone, which acts to withdraw calcium from bones. This causes a weakening and shrinking of the alveolar bone surrounding teeth and allows bacteria to proliferate in these spaces, initiating gum disease and tooth loss.

PREVENTION AND TREATMENT

Diet

Since a high-phosphorus and refined diet is the major cause of tooth and gum disease, the best prevention and treatment is a diet high in raw fruits, raw and conservatively cooked vegetables, nuts, fermented dairy products, and whole unrefined grains. Such foods are very rough and chewy, cleaning the teeth and massaging the gums as they are eaten. Excess meat, sugar, soda, candy, refined cereals, and over-cooked foods are to be strictly avoided. In several studies where sweets were replaced after a meal with an apple, dental caries in subjects were reduced drastically. If this single dietary change could do so much to reduce dental problems, imagine how few cavities children would have if everyone avoided all the refined foods that make up such a large proportion of our diets today. Periods of restricted diet on all fruit or all raw foods will speed recovery in cases of established pyorrhea.

Local Hygiene

Proper brushing and flossing of the teeth helps prevent plaque build-up and removes food residues. The proper brushing technique now recommended is to use a soft, rounded-end nylon brush, and with the edge of the brush applied at a 45° angle at the gum–tooth junction, gently massage the gum in small, circular, vibrating movements. The object is to massage the gum–tooth margin and loosen plaque and food particles. Later, the typical tooth polishing and stroke/brushing from gum to tip of tooth is used. Follow with dental flossing.

Recently an old Edgar Cayce treatment for gum disease has become popularized by several prominent dentists. Several modifi-cations of this are advised, but the original Cayce recommendations advise brushing 1–2 times daily with an equal combination of baking soda and salt. Some dentists recommend rinsing with hydrogen peroxide. We have never used this rinse with any of our patients and so cannot comment on its effectiveness. The baking soda brushing, however, is effective in removing plaque. In addition, we find the following procedure very effective if followed regularly:

- Daily dental flossing
- IPSAB massage
  After the baking soda and salt brushing, massage the gums vigorously with IPSAB (Cayce product) twice daily. IPSAB is anti-infective, astringent, a glandular tonic, and increases local circulation. It contains prickly ash bark, sea water, calcium chloride, sodium chloride, iodine trichloride and essence of peppermint. Apply IPSAB to loose teeth with cotton.
- Glycothymoline, myrrh, and goldenseal rinse: follow IPSAB massage with mouth rinse from a mixture of:
  $\frac{1}{2}$ fl oz (15 mL) glycothymoline
  30 drops tincture of myrrh
  30 drops tincture of Hydrastis (goldenseal).

As instructed on every bottle of IPSAB, have at least one large salad each day.

Other local therapies sometimes used are:

- Gum massage.
- Ipsident: (Cayce product).
- Eucalyptus oil: massage once daily.
- Witch hazel massage once daily.
- Vitamin E massage 1 fl oz (30 mL) goldenseal, 1 fl oz (30 mL) myrrh, 1 pint (500 mL) water. Infusion: rinse 3 times daily.

Therapeutic Agents

Vitamins and Minerals

- Trace minerals: e.g. Celtic salt.
- Vitamin D: 400–1000 IU daily.
- Vitamin A: 25,000 IU daily.
- Vitamin B5.

- Vitamin C plus bioflavonoids: (buffered, and with reduced ascorbic acid) 500–1000 mg 3 times daily.

Vitamins and Minerals— Secondary

- Vitamin B complex: 25–50 mg 1–2 times daily.
- Vitamin B6.
- Folic acid: 800 mcg daily.
- Vitamin B12.
- Vitamin E: 400 IU daily (chew); plus local application to gums.
- Zinc: 15–25 mg 1–2 times daily.
- Calcium and magnesium in a ratio of 2:1. Usual dose is calcium, 800 mg daily, magnesium 400 mg.

Others—Primary

- Green vegetables, sea vegetables, e.g. Spirulina.
- Probiotics, especially Lactobacillus.

Others—Secondary

- Cod-liver oil.
- Hydrochloric acid, cider vinegar: acid helps calcium absorption.

Botanicals

Cayenne
Echinacea
Goldenseal
Myrrh

THORACIC OUTLET SYNDROME AND BRACHIAL NEURALGIA

DEFINITION

Compression of the lower cord of the brachial plexus of nerves as it passes between the first rib and clavicle, due to a lowering of the shoulder girdle, the presence of an abnormal seventh cervical rib, enlarged seventh cervical transverse process, or strong fibrous band.

SYMPTOMS

Pins, needles, numbness, and pain in one or both hands, occurring 2–3 hours after falling asleep, which usually wakes the patient due to discomfort. Wasting of small muscles in hands may occur, as well as coldness or swelling.

ETIOLOGICAL CONSIDERATIONS

- Lowering of the shoulder girdle Muscle weakness in middle age

(weakness of shoulder elevator muscles, upper trapezium, and levator scapulae); general fatigue; carrying excess heavy weights; over-use of arms; poor posture
- Seventh cervical rib abnormality
- Enlarged seventh cervical transverse process
- Strong fibrous band

DISCUSSION

Thoracic outlet syndrome is a fairly common problem, occurring due to compression of the lower branch of the brachial plexus of nerves which exit from the lower cervical vertebrae to pass underneath the clavicle and on into the arm. The lowest cord of the brachial plexus lies in close proximity to the first rib, where it is subject to compression between the first rib and the clavicle, if the muscles that help support the shoulder girdle in elevation become weakened. This is the common adult-onset syndrome which usually progresses gradually, causing pins and needles sensations and numbness and pain in one or both arms. The discomfort usually occurs in the middle of the night.

Other structures in the region, such as an abnormally developed transverse process, cervical rib, or a hard fibrous band, may compress the lower brachial nerves or in some cases restrict blood flow in the subclavian vessels and cause circulatory symptoms similar to Raynaud's disease with resultant coldness, pallor or redness, and some swelling.

Cervical rib syndrome or that of an enlarged transverse process usually differs from thoracic outlet syndrome of muscular weakness origin in that the former conditions are more frequent in younger persons and the pain or paresthesia occurs shortly after heavy lifting, wearing a heavy coat, or simply having the arms hang in a dependent position. Nocturnal pain is not usually present. X-rays will clearly show the abnormal bony development of the seventh cervical vertebra in most cases; however, even a strong fibrous band in this area may cause compression which will not be noticeable with a routine x-ray.

Typical adult-onset thoracic outlet syndrome is almost always caused by poor muscular tone. The average patient is middle-aged, with a lowered shoulder girdle due to the cumulative effect of weakness of the upper trapezium and levator scapulae muscles along with gradual reduction of disc space, normal with the aging process, and consequent changes in spinal curves. The patient complains that he or she is awakened by pronounced pins and needles sensations, numbness, and pain in one or both hands, 2–3 hours after having fallen asleep. Getting up into a sitting or standing position helps relieve the disagreeable symptoms. These symptoms may recur, leaving the hands literally numb on awakening. During the day few symptoms are present unless heavy lifting is performed. In some cases even a heavy overcoat will instigate symptoms of pins and needles. Over time the symptoms may include the lower arm, upper arm, and even the shoulder, and are usually worse on days where heavy lifting or exertion has been performed.

Nocturnal symptoms are usually the result of prolonged nerve compression occurring during the day and are a nerve recovery phenomenon. Only when the nerve compression caused in the shoulder weight-bearing position is relieved, in this case by lying down to sleep, can the nerve recover. This recovery takes time in the case of a prolonged compression, which is the reason it takes several hours before symptoms are sufficiently strong to wake the patient.

TREATMENT

The basis for therapy in the muscle weakness type of thoracic syndrome relies on muscular and postural re-education. The following exercises must be repeated twice daily until the muscles gain strength. The number of repetitions may be increased as well as the weights used.

Shoulder shrugs

Stand with arms at sides, with a 2 lb (1 kg) weight in each hand, shrug shoulders upward and forward. Hold 1–2 seconds and relax slowly. Repeat 10 times. Shrug shoulders upward and backward. Hold 1–2 seconds and relax slowly. Repeat 10 times. Shrug shoulders upward. Hold 1–2 seconds and slowly relax. Repeat 10 times. Gradually increase weights as these exercises no longer

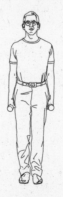 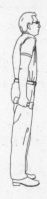

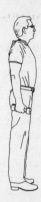

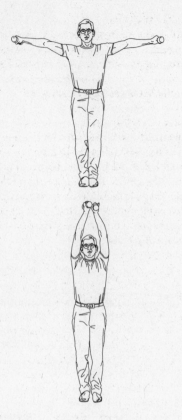

cause fatigue. The weights used may be the standard barbell type or sandbags, cans, jars, etc., as long as the weight is known.

Corner press

Stand facing the corner of a room with feet 2-3 ft (60-100 cm) from the wall, one hand on each wall at shoulder height and arms outstretched. Slowly allow the chest to press forward into the corner as you inhale, and press outward back to the original position while exhaling. Repeat 10 or more times.

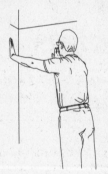

Arm lift

Stand with arms held out at shoulder level, palms downward, holding 2 lb (1 kg) weights. Raise arms sideways over the head until back of hands meet, keeping arms straight at all times. Slowly lower arms to shoulder level. Repeat 10 times. Increase weights to 5-15 lb (2.3-6.8 kg) as muscles become stronger.

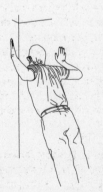

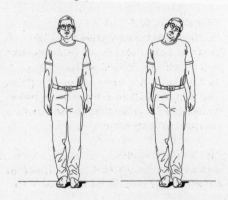

Neck exercise

Stand erect with shoulders very slightly shrugged. Slowly bend head to right, attempting to come as close to your shoulder with the ear as possible, without shrugging the shoulder. Repeat to the left.

Upper trunk raise

Lie face down with a small pillow under the chest and hands clasped behind the back. Raise the head and chest as high as possible off the floor, pulling the shoulders backward while keeping the chin close to the chest. Inhale while going up. Hold 3-5 seconds, exhale as you return to the starting position. Repeat 10-20 times.

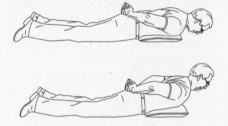

Spinal Manipulation

Twice a week initially; later 1-4 times per month.

Others

* Swimming: 3 times per week.
* Medicine ball throwing: keep ball shoulder high or higher.
* Evening armchair sitting: sit with elbows supported on an armchair and shoulder girdle elevated for 20-40 minutes each evening to allow for nerve recovery while awake. Continue session until usual night-time symptoms of pins and needles appear and then cease. This will prevent night-time symptoms from occurring.
* Avoid heavy lifting and heavy overcoats.
* Lifting advice: shrug shoulders first prior to lifting and keep in partly shrugged position while lifting proceeds. This will prevent nerve compression.

THYROID DISORDERS
(Simple Goiter, Hypothyroidism, Hyperthyroidism)

DEFINITION

Simple Goiter

An enlargement of the thyroid gland. This may be due to iodine deficiency in foods or due to natural goitrogens in foods such as cabbage or kale that block synthesis of thyroid hormone and therefore stimulate thyroid-stimulating hormone (TSH) production via the hypothalamus and pituitary centers.

Hypothyroidism

Myxedema: low thyroid function due to atrophy of thyroid, following radioactive iodine therapy for hyperthyroidism or secondary to hypofunction of anterior pituitary. *Cretinism:* juvenile hypothyroidisrn due to a deficiency of thyroid hormone during fetal period or early development. Causes are inborn errors of iodine metabolism, abnormally developed thyroid, enzyme blocks in thvroid hormone production, and dietary deficiency. The thyroid may be absent, reduced in size, or greatly enlarged.

Hyperthyroidism

Thyrotoxicosis, Graves' disease: excessive production of thyroid hormone with growth or atrophy of thyroid gland, increased metabolic rate, and possible bulging of the eyes (exophthalmos).

SYMPTOMS

Hypothyroidism

Cretinism: physical and mental development is retarded. Tongue is enlarged, lips thickened, and mouth is held open and drooling. Umbilical lesion common with pot belly. Apathy, constipation, sallow skin.

Myxedema: large tongue; slow; deep speech; thickened dry skin; puffiness of hands, face, and eyelids. Baldness of scalp and outer one-third of eyebrows. Mental apathy, sensitivity to cold, constipation, menstrual disorders, low blood pressure, weight gain, insomnia.

Mild hypothyroidism: a wide range of symptoms is associated with this most common thyroid condition. These include easy fatigability, headaches, chronic or recurrent infection, eczema, psoriasis, acne, menstrual disorders, painful menstruation, depression, cold sensitivity, psychological problems, and anemia.

Hyperthyroidism

Thyrotoxicosis, Graves' disease: insomnia, nervousness, weakness, sweating, over-activity, sensitivity to heat, weight loss, tremor, stare, and exophthalmos (eye bulge). The heart is over-active and enlarged, with systolic hypertension and possible heart failure. The thyroid is usually enlarged or nodular. Psychosis occurs in severe cases of "thyroid storm", when all symptoms are severely aggravated due to stress, infection, surgery, or other causes, which may have a fatal outcome.

Hypothyroidism

ETIOLOGICAL CONSIDERATIONS—PRIMARY

- Iodine deficiency, or defect in iodine metabolic pathways

- Autoimmune disease (Hashimoto's thyroiditis)
- Post-radioactive iodine therapy
- Post-hyperthyroid surgery
- Excess of Brassica foods (Brassicas have goitrogenic activity)

ETIOLOGICAL CONSIDERATIONS— SECONDARY

- Vitamin E deficiency; vitamin A deficiency
- Selenium deficiency
- Zinc deficiency
- Pituitary disorders
- Diet pills
- Emotions
- Spinal lesions
- Hereditary predisposition
- Medical drugs (e.g. estrogen; some anticonvulsants and rifampin increase thyroid hormone production to exhaustion)
- Cigarette smoke, chlorinated compounds, e.g. pesticides

Hyperthyroidism

ETIOLOGICAL CONSIDERATIONS—PRIMARY

- Autoimmune disease (Graves' disease—affects eyes also)
- Excessive intake of iodine rich foods, e.g. kelp
- Excess of thyroid hormone, whether over-medication, or endocrine changes

ETIOLOGICAL CONSIDERATIONS— SECONDARY

- Liver damage: insufficient enzymes being produced to deactivate thyroid hormones
- Vitamin A deficiency

- Vitamin E deficiency
- Vitamin B6 deficiency
- Pituitary tumor (causing an increase in TSH)
- Emotions
- Spinal lesions
- Diet pills

DISCUSSION

The thyroid gland plays a key role in controlling the body's metabolic rate. It is in turn controlled directly by secretions from the pituitary and hypothalamus in the brain. The hypothalamus is affected greatly by strong emotions. For these reasons the thyroid is especially susceptible to the emotional state. When the eastern understanding of body centers is studied, we find the thyroid to be in the throat *chakra* or energy center. This center may be hindered by emotions such as fear or inability of self-expression, sexual excess or frustration, and general frustration. Spinal lesions from C3 to T1 or T2 may affect the thyroid gland as well, producing either hyperthyroidism or hypothyroidism.

Since the thyroid has a major effect on metabolism and the blood glucose level, it also has a strong effect on the mental state, causing mental depression, lethargy, fatigue, and psychosis. This may play a role in abnormal mental states in puberty, pregnancy, postpartum depression, and menopause.

Dietary causes of thyroid disorders may work hand-in-hand with their emotional counterparts, or independently. The most obvious is iodine deficiency. Iodine may be deficient in foods grown in certain localities, creating what is called endemic goiter. This is easily corrected by consuming iodine-containing foods. The incidence of endemic goiter is now reduced due to the addition of iodine to condiments. Unfortunately, the condiment is table salt, which is on its own a health hazard and avoided by those aware of its harmful effects or by those on a salt-restricted diet. Certain foods called goitrogens actually hinder iodine utilization. These include kale, cabbage, peanuts, soy flour, brussels sprouts, cauliflower, broccoli, kohlrabi, and turnips.

Vitamin E deficiency reduces iodine absorption by the thyroid by 95%, causing the thyroid to become over-active and enlarge to compensate. This may be part of the reason thyroid disorders are so common in pregnancy and menopause where vitamin E deficiency is common.

Of specific importance in the causation of thyroid disorders is long-term use of "diet" pills. Various forms of "speed" or dexedrine are often used to increase the metabolic rate and reduce the appetite. Used frequently, these upset the normal control mechanisms of the entire hormonal system and may permanently alter thyroid function, predisposing either to hyperthyroidism or hypothyroidism.

Surgical or radioactive iodine treatments for hyperthyroidism often cause a permanent case of hypothyroidism that requires lifelong use of the hormone prescription thyroxine. The best course of action when possible is to strengthen the weakened glands, remove the causative factors, and promote healing from within. The basal body temperature test (see page 455) can be used, not only for diagnosis but also as a gauge of treatment effectiveness. If the treatment is working properly the basal temperature will return to normal.

TREATMENT

The general treatment for thyroid disorders is based on a gentle stimulation of the thyroid through proper diet, physiotherapy, food supplements, and herbs to raise the local and general vitality and allow the imbalanced hormones to reach a proper equilibrium.

Diet

Some thyroid patients benefit from foods especially high in iodine, vitamins E, A, C, and B complex. Raw foods are generally excellent for the glandular system. Foods of specific usefulness in some cases are: Seaweed; seafood; kelp, dulse; egg yolks; garlic; wheat germ; radishes; mushrooms; watercress; brewer's yeast; soy foods; lima beans.

At all times the food eaten should be unrefined and as close to its natural state. Two to 4 weeks or longer on a raw foods diet of raw green salads, seaweed, nuts, seeds, sprouted seeds, sprouted beans, and vegetable juices will have a strongly tonic effect.

All treatments, even dietary, for thyroid disorders should be undertaken with the assistance of a qualified nutritionally minded doctor in conjunction with an endocrinologist. Some of the therapeutic agents could become detrimental if taken in improper doses for a particular patient or thyroid condition.

Physiotherapy

- Sauna baths.
- General exercise until vigorously sweating.
- Sea bathing and sun baths.
- Meditation.
- Spinal manipulation: C3 to T1 or T2.
- Yoga exercises specific to thyroid disorders: shoulder stand, plough.

Therapeutic Agents for Hypothyroidism

Vitamins and Minerals—Primary

- Selenium: is required to convert T3 to T4, and is absent in many soils.
- Vitamin E: increases iodine uptake by thyroid and heals scars in gland. 400-1200 IU daily.
- Tyrosine: a precursor to thyroid hormone synthesis, and helps activate thyroid in hypothyroid cases. 1000-1500 mg daily, before meals.
- Iodine: 100-1000 mcg daily.
- Zinc: 25 mg 2-3 times daily, stimulates thyroid function.
- Iron (to 50 mg daily) stimulates thyroid function

- Vitamin A (preformed): 10,000-25,000 IU, 1-3 times daily. (Hypothyroid patients do not convert beta-carotene to vitamin A efficiently).

Vitamins and Minerals—Secondary

- Vitamin B complex: 25-50 mg 1-3 times daily. Intramuscular injections may be useful.
- Vitamin B6: 50-100 mg 1-2 times daily.
- Vitamin B1, B2, B3, B5 (increased need in hyperthyroidism): 50-100 mg once daily.
- Vitamin C: 250-1000 mg 2-3 times daily.
- Copper: 1-3 mg daily.

Others

- Atomodine (Cayce product): all iodine-containing medications should be taken only with a doctor's prescription. They can be toxic if taken in excess.
- Brewer's yeast.
- Calcium fluoride.
- Calcium and magnesium.
- Garlic.
- Kelp.
- Raw adrenal tablets (with doctor's prescription): 1 tablet 1-3 times daily.
- Raw hypothalamus tablets (with doctor's prescription): 1 tablet 1-3 times daily.
- Raw pituitary tablets (with doctor's prescription): 1 tablet 1-3 times daily.
- Raw thyroid tablets (with doctor's prescription): 1-2 tablets 1-3 times daily.
- Desiccated thyroid (prescription).
- Thyroid (homeopathic dilutions). Thyroid 6× very useful in thyroid complaints.
- Wheat germ oil.

Botanicals—Primary

Bladderwrack and coleus: both stimulate the thyroid to secrete thyroid hormones.

Bugle weed, melissa and mother's wort: inhibitors of thyroid function.

Botanicals—Secondary

Blue flag
Barberry
Irish moss
Lettuce
Oak
Poke root (highly toxic, see page 60)
Yellow dock
For exophthalmos:
American hellebore
Bugle weed
Cactus
Hawthorn
Pheasant's eye
Strophanthus

Note: A useful home test for hypothyroidism or hyperthyroidism is the basal body temperature test as first suggested by Dr Broda Barnes. Axillary temperature (under the arm) is taken for 10 minutes first thing, before getting out of bed in the morning. Do not record if menstruating. Test on five successive mornings, then average the findings (add each of the five readings together, then divide by 5). Normal range is from 97.8-98.2°F (36.4-36.7°C). Temperatures below this range are suggestive of hypothyroidism, and those above, of hyperthyroidism.

Therapeutic Suggestion

In autoimmunity (Graves' disease), need to check for food allergy, and test and treat for leaky gut, and reduce inflammation with essential fatty acids (e.g. fish oil), bioflavonoids, and vitamins C and E, B2 and B3.

TONSILLITIS AND ADENITIS

DEFINITION

Inflammation and possible infection of tonsils and/or adenoids.

SYMPTOMS

- Acute
  Fever, chills; sore throat, swollen, red; difficulty swallowing; tender swollen lymph nodes
- Chronic
  Mouth breathing, foul breath; lassitude, frequent colds; poor hearing; Eustachian tube blockage

ETIOLOGICAL CONSIDERATIONS—PRIMARY

- Toxins
- Diet
  Excess starches; milk allergy; excess dairy products; excess sugar; green vegetable deficiency; improper weaning
- Poor eliminations
  Skin; constipation; deranged stomach

ETIOLOGICAL CONSIDERATIONS— SECONDARY

- Spinal (impairment of local circulation, accumulation of toxins)
- Suppressive treatments to previous acute colds

DISCUSSION

The tonsils and adenoids are lymphoid structures designed by nature to act as filtering agents for viruses, bacteria, and toxins. Not only do they protect us from external agents, but they also act as sensitive barometers of our inner health. When the blood or lymph fluids become overburdened with toxic waste or bacteria, these organs become inflamed and infected. These toxic overloads are usually due to an improper diet and poor stomach, bowel, skin, kidney, and liver function.

The typical child with recurrent tonsil infection and enlargement has been weaned to a diet high in milk and carbohydrates and very low in green vegetables. This causes a relative acidity and toxicity in the system. Excess mucus is produced by the imbalance of consumption of mucus-forming foods, such as milk, cheese, and bread, and an almost complete lack of the elimination and cleansing elements in the vegetable kingdom. Junk foods, sweets, and other highly processed or devitalized foods lower the body's vitality and congest the system so that elimination is required.

Food allergy may also cause tonsillitis. The two most commonly involved foods are milk and wheat. Thus, a child on even a small amount of these foods might suffer severe physical distress if an unsuspected allergy exists. The incidence of milk allergy is very common. True milk allergy, however, need not be the only process by which dairy product consumption may aggravate the system. Milk contains the sugar lactose which requires the enzyme lactase for complete digestion. This enzyme is commonly found in the digestive system of young children. However, in many cases this ceases to be produced as a child becomes older. This causes the milk to be incompletely digested, causing gastric irritation and mucus production. The incidence of milk intolerance due to digestive enzyme deficiency alone is somewhere around 15–25% in Caucasians and up to 85% in Orientals.

Wheat also may cause physical distress in ways other than strict allergy. The protein gluten found in wheat and other related grains can cause intestinal irritation and loss of the small villi which line the intestinal walls, necessary for proper absorption. The result is a thinning of these areas, inefficient absorption, toxic reabsorption, and systemic irritation which may lead to tonsillitis among other disorders. These two allergies or digestive incompatibilities are so common that a diet restricting dairy products and gluten-containing grains is usually the first course of treatment in these cases.

Poor eliminations are another major cause of tonsillar enlargement and infection. The highly refined diet of white bread, white rice, overly cooked vegetables, refined sweets, and other fiber-deficient foods causes the body to lose its regular natural eliminative function. This can cause serious health problems and almost always is involved in cases of tonsillitis (see Constipation).

Spinal lesions in the neck may also reduce blood and lymph flow to these vital structures, causing reduced tissue vitality and congestion.

As with other diseases, tonsillitis is also usually the result of suppressive treatments to other acute diseases such as the common cold. These eliminative efforts by the body have been suppressed by improper diet and drugs, leading to a toxic build-up finally expressed by tonsillitis, asthma, and other more serious diseases.

The old medical approach to a case of tonsillitis was tonsillectomy. Its routine use has been abandoned ever since it was observed that the incidence of Hodgkin's disease was slightly increased in patients who have had a tonsillectomy. This procedure did nothing to remove the basic causes of the condition and only denied us the service of a faithful defender. It made no more sense to routinely remove tonsils than it would to remove the red oil-pressure warning lights in a car. Only on rare occasions, when the condition of the tonsils has become chronically enlarged, fibrotic, and pustular, may it be best to have them removed. In such an instance, the tonsillar infection can be very difficult to heal and continues to act as a reservoir of infection to pollute the entire body. With this in mind, it becomes increasingly obvious that proper attention should be given to the first acute attacks of colds, sore throats, or tonsillitis, to prevent a chronic condition from developing.

TREATMENT

Simple acute tonsillitis, although very uncomfortable and disturbing, is relatively easy to treat. Once a throat culture eliminates strep throat (for which antibiotics may be required), the acute inflammation and infection is not difficult to remove within 3–10 days by natural methods. Chronically enlarged tonsils and adenoids, however, take much more time. Once the adenoids have enlarged to the extent they interfere with nasal breathing and cause the patient to breathe through his or her mouth, there is a serious problem. This can totally change the developing features of the face, leaving it permanently altered. It also may severely reduce the normal hearing range in the critical learning years. It therefore becomes extremely important to reduce the size of these structures as much as possible, and as soon as possible. By the time the child is 9 or 10, enlarged adenoids are usually much less of a problem anyway, but we cannot afford to wait for the body to slowly grow out of the problem. Vigorous treatment is required.

Diet

The simplest initial treatment for children to follow with either acute or chronic tonsillitis is the all-fruit diet (see Appendix I) or fruit juice fast. Fasting may be very difficult for young children to handle, except when the throat is so sore and painful that no solid food is possible anyway. If fasting is possible, it should be continued at least as long as pain exists and then the all fruit diet may be instituted. This allows any fruit or fruit juice except banana. When fasting do an enema nightly or on days 1, 2, 3, 5 and 7.

An alternative approach, which is very effective, is the 3–5-day mucus cleansing diet, as follows:

On Rising
Hot water, lemon, and honey.

Breakfast
Citrus fruit.

Midmorning
Carrot juice or citrus juice.

Lunch
A large plate of boiled or steamed onions. Natural soy sauce may be used. Citrus as dessert if desired.

Supper
Same as lunch.

Evening
Same as midmorning.

In chronic cases short periods of fasting should be rotated with longer periods of the all-fruit diet, mucus-cleansing diet, and Stage 2 of the asthma diet, which stresses non-allergic, non-mucus-forming foods with plenty of vegetables (see Asthma).

All these diets must also be accompanied by the internal and external treatments suggested below.

Physiotherapy

- Goldenseal, myrrh, and glycothymoline. Mix 1 oz (30 g) of the two herbs (as alcohol tincture) with 16 fl oz (500 mL) of glycothymoline. Gargle daily 4–6 times.
- Epsom salts baths (see Appendix I).
- Enemas.
- Gargles.
- Hot water, salt, and lemon: gargle 3 times daily.
- Lemon juice
- Goldenseal.
- Myrrh.
- Fenugreek tea.
- Chlorophyll.
- Throat sprays or swabs Goldenseal, myrrh.
- Throat compress.
  Three parts mullein, 1 part lobelia for

457

pain relief. Alternate hot and cold.
- Throat pack
  Soak a small towel in ice-cold water. Wrap around throat and pin. Leave on 1-3 hours. Repeat twice daily and at night.
- Endonasal technique (see Appendix I)
- Spinal manipulation: cervical and upper thoracic. Frequently in acute cases, weekly in chronic.

Therapeutic Agents

Vitamins and Minerals—Primary
- Vitamin C and bioflavonoids: 250-500 mg chewable every hour in acute cases, or 6 times daily in chronic cases. To bowel tolerance.
- Vitamin A: high doses are required. 10,000 IU 3 times daily for child if acute; 25,000 IU 3 times daily in adult if acute.
- Vitamin B complex: 25-50 mg 3 times daily; best in liquid form.

Others—Primary
- Onion syrup: 1 tsp 3-6 times daily.
- Vegetable juice: especially carrot, parsley, celery, ginger and garlic all-in-one juice; 2-4 daily.

Others—Secondary
- Caldwell's syrup of pepsin (laxative)

- Fenugreek tea.
- Garlic: 2 capsules 3 times daily.
- Glycothymoline: 2-3 drops (internal antiseptic).
- Herbal laxatives (gentle).
- Lemon juice.
- Lymph glandular.
- Pineapple juice.
- Spleen glandular.
- Syrup of figs (laxative).
- Thymus: 2 every hour.
- Zinc: 15-30 mg 3 times daily.

Botanicals—Primary
Clivers: lymphatic decongestant.
Echinacea: internal and topical.
Myrrh: local swab.
Marigold flowers: tincture, or as throat swab.
Poke root: very useful and effective lymphatic decongestant (highly toxic, see page 60. For painful, hard, glandular enlargements. 25 drops in water 4-6 times daily in acute cases; 3-4 times daily in chronic cases.

Botanicals—Secondary
Eucalyptus.
Goldenseal: local swab and gargle.
Pleurisy root.
Red raspberry tea.
Sage tea.
St John's wort.

UNDERWEIGHT

DEFINITION AND SYMPTOMS

Failure to maintain optimal weight for height.

ETIOLOGICAL CONSIDERATIONS—PRIMARY

- Digestive disorders

  Hydrochloric acid deficiency; pancreatic enzyme deficiency; malabsorption syndromes
- Hormonal imbalance
  Hyperthyroid
- Improper diet
  Low-energy foods; junk foods; restricted diets (e.g. fruitarianism); protein deficiency
- Excess exercise or energy output
- Lack of appetite

Zinc deficiency; cancer or other wasting disease
- Emotional
- Stress, anxiety; anorexia nervosa; bulimia

ETIOLOGICAL CONSIDERATIONS— SECONDARY

- Drug use
- Hypoglycemia, diabetes
- Allergy
- Parasites, worms

DISCUSSION

We all know someone who can eat and eat while still remaining extremely slim. Although this may make an overweight person envious, it does not nearly equate with optimum health. Frequently, these individuals have a very inefficient digestive system and are absorbing very little of the food eaten. Digestive enzyme deficiency or failure of food absorption is very common. Malabsorption syndromes due to allergy or food insensitivity are also very common.

Endocrine imbalances involving the thyroid, pancreas, and adrenal glands can make weight gain impossible. Hypoglycemics and diabetics have a particularly difficult time maintaining proper weight.

Occasionally we see very emaciated patients as a result of a specific dietary regimen. We once saw a 76 lb (35 kg) woman who had been living on fruit exclusively for 14 months. She had about 2 months more before she would have died on such a diet, had she not added protein to her regimen. Some strict vegetarians who have no knowledge of complete proteins can have plenty of calories per se but inadequate protein, causing their body's own protein to begin breaking down.

Zinc deficiency has been known to reduce the appetite as can some wasting diseases, such as cancer. Stress or emotionally based weight loss may require psychological help.

TREATMENT

The actual cause must be diagnosed, if possible. We always suspect digestive enzyme deficiency and allergy or food sensitivity. The consistency of the bowel movement, and a check for undigested foods, can be a valuable diagnostic aid. The diet most useful for weight gain is similar to that found under Hypoglycemia or Diabetes. Adequate and complete proteins are essential: $2^1/_2$-$3^1/_2$ oz (70–100 g) of dietary protein should be adequate, along with a diet of 60 or 70% unrefined carbohydrates and 50–60 g of dietary fat, most of which should be from unsaturated sources.

Therapeutic Agents

Vitamins and Minerals—Primary
- Zinc: 25–50 mg, 1–2 times daily.

Vitamins and Minerals— Secondary
- Vitamin A: 25,000 IU daily.
- Vitamin B complex: 50 mg, 1–2 times daily.

Others
- Probiotics: especially *L. acidophilus* which specifically helps with the absorption of nutrients across the walls of the small intestine.
- Arginine: increases protein metabolism
- Digestive enzymes: to include hydrochloric acid and pepsin.
- Pancreatic enzymes.

Botanicals
Bitter herbs: promote release of gastric juices, increase appetite, protect gut tissue, promote bile flow, enhance pancreatic functioning, so these are important in the treatment of being underweight.

Damiana: anabolic in action (builds muscle)
Meadowsweet: aids in restoring gastric acid
Gentian: digestive bitter
Oats: nutritive

Therapeutic Suggestion

Sometimes the underweight client is one who is "stressed out", running on the sympathetic nervous adrenal energy, and tends to "gobble" his or her food. Herbal adrenal tonics and adaptogens are of use in these instances, and nervine sedatives might be indicated to "calm" one down and balance the autonomic nervous system. See suggestions under Digestive Disorders as to how to approach the art and practice of calm, unhurried and happy eating.

VAGINITIS
(Thrush or Candidiasis, Trichomoniasis)

DEFINITION

Vaginitis: inflammation and irritation of the vagina.
Thrush: infection caused by *Candida albicans* fungus. May affect the vagina, anus, mouth, skin, or nails.
Trichomoniasis: protozoal infestation (by *Trichomonas vaginalis*) of the genitourinary tract, either in the male or female.

SYMPTOMS

Vaginitis: irritation, redness, intense itching, odor, discharge, painful sex.
Thrush (vagina): profuse, offensive, curdy discharge with inflamation, burning, itching, and painful sex.
Nails: painful red swellings leading to hardened, grooved nails.
Mouth: creamy white patches on inflamed mucosa.
Skin: inflamed, with red rash.
Trichomoniasis (female): frothy, thin, non-bloody vaginal discharge; rash; burning irritation; itching; and painful sex.
Trichomoniasis (male): usually symptomless carrier.

ETIOLOGICAL CONSIDERATIONS—PRIMARY

- Antibiotics (damaged ecology).
- *Candida albicans* overgrowth.
- Raised vaginal pH (contraceptive pill, pregnancy, diabetes, menstrual period, after miscarriage, or abortion).
- Diabetes.
- Corticosteroids.
- Tight-fitting synthetic underwear (poor ventilation; warm, moist environment).
- Diet (deficiency in vitamins B complex, B6; excess sugar and refined carbohydrates).

ETIOLOGICAL CONSIDERATIONS— SECONDARY

- Poor hygiene.
- Coitus transmission.
- IgA immune deficiency.
- Stress.
- Spinal.
- Allergy.
- Congestion.

- Postmenopausal hormone changes causing dryness of vagina and lack of lubrication during sex.
- Debilitation.

DISCUSSION

The normal vaginal ecology is a balance between many commensal organisms normally found in the vagina. These consist of a very large number of microorganisms, fungi, bacteria, and protozoa. Certain of these coexisting organisms are essential to normal vaginal health, such as Döderlein's bacillus, a species of Lactobacillus. This diversity of flora is controlled by several factors. The most important of these are the amount of glucose present in vaginal secretions, the acid–alkaline balance, and the hormonal state. Clinical infections such as candidiasis or trichomoniasis only occur when this natural balance is upset, allowing these fungi or protozoa to flourish and multiply in a more favorable environment.

Role of Sugar and pH

Normal vaginal secretions contain a large amount of glucose. This gives a high pH (basic or alkaline) quality to these discharges. The organisms that cause vaginal infections thrive on glucose. Fortunately, the Döderlein's bacteria, a normal inhabitant of the vagina in its mucous membrane, convert this glucose to lactic acid. This lowers the pH (making it more acid) just enough to keep other microorganisms from taking over.

Role of Menstrual Cycle, Pregnancy, and Contraceptive Pill

During the normal menstrual cycle estrogen rises to a maximum at ovulation. This causes an increase in thin, sticky, alkaline mucus produced by the cervical glands. As this mucus passes down the vagina it gathers vaginal cells which break down and release their sugar content. This raises vaginal pH, making infection more probable. The actual menstrual flow further raises alkalinity. During pregnancy these alkaline changes are more sustained and encourage the common vaginal infections that often occur at this time. Use of the contraceptive pill, which simulates pregnancy, provides the ideal environment for vaginal infection.

Role of Antibiotics

Antibiotics kill disease-causing bacteria and friendly flora indiscriminately. These friendly bacteria exist all over the body, but their most important sites are the intestinal tract, where they help synthesize B vitamins; and the vagina, as described above. The widespread use of antibiotics has led also to a widespread epidemic of vaginal infections in all ages. Vaginal and systemic Candida infections are an increasing concern following antibiotic use. It has been frequently observed that the most common after-effect of antibiotic use in women is a vaginal yeast infection. With repeated antibiotic use, the fungi that are normally present in the colon in controlled numbers may begin to proliferate and colonize the entire gastrointestinal tract. This can be a very serious problem, and has been associated not only with repeated vaginal infections, but also with panallergic conditions where the patient develops multiple allergies. The actual mechanism that causes these allergic-like symptoms is as yet not entirely clear. It is suspected that either the yeast produces a toxic substance that acts on remote tissues and organs, or, what seems to be more likely, that the fungus alters the structure and functions of the small intestine, causing a thinning of the wall, which allows larger allergenic protein molecules to pass into the bloodstream.

Other Factors

- Stress: stress upsets normal hormonal balance and reduces blood flow to parasympathetically innervated organs such as female organs.

- Spinal imbalances: L1–5: disturbs normal blood and nerve flow to pelvic organs.
- Congestion: poor blood flow due to stress, spinal imbalances, lack of exercise, poor adrenal tone, diet deficiency, or any other reason will downgrade tissue health and encourage infection.
- Diet: excess sugar, fruits, refined carbohydrates, or alcohol will lead to excess sugar in vaginal secretions. Strongly alkaline diets increase vaginal pH. Excess acid diet will favor simple vaginitis with rash and itching.
- Toilet: frequent douching will upset vaginal ecology. Children should be educated to wipe front to back to prevent infecting vagina.
- Clothes: tight-fitting synthetic underwear reduces ventilation and creates a warm, moist environment ideal for infection.
- Sex: excess sex or intercourse without proper lubrication will irritate vaginal walls.
- Age: senile changes in vaginal walls can lead to irritation and rash.

TREATMENT

Simple vaginitis and thrush respond quite readily to natural therapies. Trichomoniasis, however, can be very stubborn. Occasionally, orthodox treatments (e.g. flagyl) fail to eliminate the infection, leaving a deep-seated problem very difficult to relieve by any means. In such a stubborn case we sometimes recommend following the treatments outlined below with one final series of metronidazole (flagyl) for both male and female partner. This will often succeed where the orthodox approach alone has repeatedly failed. Unfortunately we know of no other regimen that will be as effective and know of few naturopathic alternatives for the male partner. This does not necessarily mean that natural alternatives do not exist, but simply that we are at present unaware of them. Recent reports, however, show

that trichomoniasis in males responds to high levels of zinc. Certainly, for the female with simple vaginitis, thrush, or less entrenched trichomoniasis, the simple therapies below are sufficient without drug medication.

Diet

During the 2 weeks of intense vaginal treatments aimed at establishing a normal internal ecology, the food eaten needs to be at least 80% raw, with an abundance of fresh vegetables. Salads are recommended for the main course for both lunch and supper. This is necessary to provide the proper healing influence on the mucous membranes; however, the urine needs to be artificially acidified by drinking 3–4 glasses of unsweetened cranberry juice each day. This is very important. Garlic and onions should be part of each meal.

In general, the type of diet regimen found under Cystitis will be adequate. With thrush, one must stop taking both contraceptive pills and brewer's yeast and make sure that the vitamin B complex used is from a non-yeast source.

Therapeutic Agents

Vitamins and Minerals—Primary
- Vitamin C: 1000–6000 mg daily.
- Vitamin A: (high dose): 25,000 IU 2–3 times daily.
- Vitamin B complex (high dose): 25–100 mg 2–3 times daily.

Vitamins and Minerals—Secondary
- Vitamin B6: 50–100 mg twice daily.
- Vitamin E: 400–800 IU daily.
- Zinc sulfate: 200 mg twice daily (trichomoniasis).
- Garlic: 2 capsules 3 times daily.
- Lactobacillus: 1 tsp 3 times daily.
- Thymus tablets: 6–10 tablets daily.

Douches

- Yoghurt, lactic acid, or acidophilus: 1 tbsp added to 2 pints (1 liter) warm water, twice daily.
- Yoghurt with powdered acidophilus added, straight.
- Apple cider vinegar douche: 2 tbsp to 1 quart warm water twice daily.
- Goldenseal: $1/2$–1 tbsp to 1 quart warm water twice daily.
- Tea tree oil: 1 tbsp to 1 quart warm water douche twice daily.
- Bay leaf or barberry tea douche.
- Oxysulfate plus Hydrastis (goldenseal) douche: 2% copper sulfate solution. 1 tsp to 1 pint of warm water.
- Glycothymoline douche: 1–2 tbsp to 1 quart water. Alternate with: Atomodine douche: 1–2 tbsp to 1 quart water.
- White oak bark douche: for leukorrhea.
- Hemlock douche: for leukorrhea.
- Douche: use just enough permanganate of potash to color warm water. Add 1–2 drops myrrh tincture.
- Iodine: 1/1000 solution retention douche once daily (trichomoniasis).

Suppositories

- Lactic acid wafers.
- Boric acid: 2 capsules inserted nightly for 2 days; 1 per night for 1 week, 1 weekly maintenance dose.
- Goldenseal and cocoa butter: 1 inserted nightly.
- Gentian violet plus tampon.
- Cabasil garlic inserted nightly.

Baths

- Salt water bath: $1/2$ cup to a tub of water. Allow to enter vagina.
- Fume sitz baths: add 5 drops of myrrh tincture and 10 grains of balsam of tolu to 6 liters ($1\frac{1}{2}$ gallons) of boiled hot water. Sit over basin and expose irritated membranes to the rising steam fumes.

Local Applications

- Calendula lotion: apply to irritated vaginal walls full strength or 50/50 with water.
- Calendula powder, calendula ointment.
- Goldenseal powder.
- Goldenseal and witch hazel tincture diluted: applied locally.
- Calendula, goldenseal and berberis.
- Thuja, tea tree oil, and calendula.
- Ultraviolet ray: internal application.
- Ichthyoll 20%: local application.
- 0.5–1% gentian violet: painted inflamed mucosa.
- B6 vitamin salve.
- Goldthread and goldenseal.
- Witch hazel.
- Chickweed ointment.

Thrush

Oral:

Acidophilus: $1/3$ tsp 3 times daily by mouth.
Niacinamide: 100-mg tablet crushed and put on infant's tongue; plus 100 mg twice daily to breast-feeding mother.

Nails:

Tea tree soaks (water-soluble tea tree): dilute with hot water. Soak twice daily for 15 minutes, then apply tea tree oil or cream. Urine soak is particularly effective also.

With the large number of possibly useful therapeutic agents, the following outline of a suggested procedure may be of benefit:

Trichomoniasis

Days 1–3:

Atomodine or iodine douche, morning.
Tea tree oil douche, afternoon and evening.
Calendula lotion applied locally to irritated membranes.

Days 4–6:

Oxysulfate and Hydrastis (goldenseal) douche, morning.
Atomodine or iodine douche, afternoon.
Goldenseal and cocoa butter suppository, evening.
Calendula lotion locally.

Days 7–11:

Apple cider vinegar douche, morning.
Yoghurt or acidophilus douche, afternoon.
Boric acid suppository, evening.

Days 11–18:
Boric acid suppository, evening.

Thrush

Days 1–3:
Tea tree oil douche, morning.
Oxysulfate and Hydrastis (goldenseal) douche, afternoon.
Goldenseal and cocoa butter suppository, evening.
Calendula lotion, locally.

Days 4–6:
Oxysulfate and Hydrastis (goldenseal) douche, morning.
Apple cider vinegar douche, afternoon.
Goldenseal suppositories, evening.
Calendula lotion, locally.

Days 7–9:
Apple cider vinegar douche, morning.
Yoghurt or acidophilus douche, afternoon.
Goldenseal suppository, evening.
Another regimen that works well with vaginal yeast infections is as follows:

Days 1–2:
Tea tree oil douche, morning and afternoon.
Boric acid crystals suppository, evening (One 00 capsule).

Days 3–4:
Tea tree oil douche, morning.
Apple cider vinegar douche, afternoon.
Boric acid suppository, evening.

Days 5–7:
Apple cider vinegar douche, morning.
Yoghurt or acidophilus douche, afternoon.
Lactobacillus capsule suppository, evening.

Days 8–14:
One 00 capsule mixed boric acid plus Lactobacillus suppository each evening. Some cases may require oral nystatin therapy for a period of up to 6 months if the Candida has overgrown throughout the entire intestinal tract. Also useful is oral probiotics, garlic, biotin, caprilic acid, and a yeast-free, refined carbohydrate-free diet.

VARICOSE VEINS AND VARICOSE ULCERS

DEFINITION

Abnormally dilated, lengthened, and sacculated superficial veins of the lower extremities. May cause ulceration in later stages.

SYMPTOMS

Muscle cramps, fatigue of leg muscles, sore calf muscles, ankle swelling, eczema, and ulcers.

ETIOLOGICAL CONSIDERATIONS—PRIMARY

- Diet
  Refined carbohydrates; deficiency of vitamins E and C
- Constipation
- Obesity
- Pregnancy
- Lack of exercise, sedentary occupation

ETIOLOGICAL CONSIDERATIONS— SECONDARY

- Posture, poor body mechanics
- Poor circulation
- Spinal (lumbar, sacral, coccyx)
- Acidity, improper eliminations
- Congenital valve insufficiency
- Leg crossing
- Prolonged sitting or standing
- Liver damage
- Abdominal tumors
- Blood clot

DISCUSSION

The veins are equipped with a series of one-way valves that allow blood to enter in the direction towards the heart and away from gravity. This is a necessary function since veins, unlike arteries, do not have a positive pumping action exerted by the heart itself, nor any intrinsic muscular activity. Venous pumping is performed by the leg muscles massaging the veins during muscular activity. This action slowly pushes the blood uphill through the series of valves towards the heart. This muscular venous pumping action is aided by the diaphragmatic action sucking blood up against gravity.

Weakening of the vein wall leads to dilation of the vein with subsequent damage of the valves. Once the valves have been severely damaged or destroyed, the increased blood stasis leads to the bulging veins so often the visible sign of varicosity; there is no cure. If circulation to the superficial skin becomes reduced, a gradual process of tissue starvation occurs, leading to difficult-to-heal varicose ulcers.

Surgery has been performed to remove, and even replace the dilated, damaged veins with veins from other parts of the body. This does remove the unsightly dilated veins and improves local circulation, but does nothing to prevent a recurrence, which is common.

Here again we have an extremely common ailment which can be considered one of the "diseases of civilization". Varicose veins are found very rarely in undeveloped nations whose inhabitants still live on unrefined foods. The same dietary factors that lead to constipation and hemorrhoids (which in fact are a form of varicose veins) also cause varicose veins (see Constipation, Hemorrhoids). Our diet in developed nations includes a very large proportion of devitalized, fiber-deficient, refined foods. These nutrient-deficient foods cause the tissues of the body to become weakened and low in vitality. A low-fiber diet also slows the bowel transit time of foods, leading to toxic reabsorption and hard, difficult-to-pass feces. Often this process becomes so extreme that actual pressure from a loaded bowel can restrict the venous return of blood from the legs, leading to varicosity. In these cases it is usually the left leg which is most affected, since the descending colon, splenic flexure, and lower rectum are the areas most likely to be overloaded. Obesity has a similar action, but its effects are usually bilateral. Girdles and other restricting clothing may be a cause. Poor spinal mechanics and posture can affect venous return, especially with a severe lumbar lordosis leading to visceroptosis, or a drooping of the entire abdominal and pelvic contents that restricts venous return.

Prolonged standing has, in the past, been cited as the major cause of varicose veins. However, recent studies find little difference between those whose occupations require standing or sitting. The key factor seems to be lack of demanding exercise and a sedentary existence.

Spinal lesions are a common cause of reduced circulation and tissue malnutrition, and may lead to valve degeneration or favor constipation and act indirectly, as discussed.

In women, pregnancy is commonly the time when varicose veins are first a problem. The hormones present during the latter part of pregnancy cause all the involuntary muscles to become lax, favoring constipation and dilated varicose veins. In the final states of pregnancy, the pressure of the baby's head lower in the pelvis may also act as a mechanical barrier to proper venous return.

TREATMENT

Diet

The first objective is to establish proper bowel eliminations. Patients usually have a history of chronic constipation and a laxative habit. The best initial approach is either a 3-day fruit juice fast with enemas nightly (and no further laxatives or enemas taken in

465

the future), or a 3-day apple mono diet where all that is eaten are apples and apple juice. On the evening of the third day, 1-2 tbsp of olive oil are to be taken. Follow this with the full constipation diet (see Constipation). *Cascara sagrada* tincture is taken in tonic doses over a period of 4-6 weeks, beginning with 25 drops in water four times daily and gradually reducing to three times, twice, one time, and then stopping altogether as the bowels show renewed regularity. Cascara, when taken in this way, becomes a tonic rather than a laxative to the bowels.

Follow this diet with a high-fiber one based on the constipation diet, but more flexible in nature once regularity is established. A large amount of citrus fruit and salads is encouraged. Fruits such as berries and cherries are rich in OPCs (proanthocyanidins) and improve vein wall strength. Pineapple and papaya contain enzymes which protect against clotting disorders, as do garlic, capsicum, onion and ginger. We also advise 1 tbsp psyllium powder with a glass of water is to be taken 3 times daily, both during the initial diets (except when fasting) and later as a bowel regulator on a permanent basis.

Physiotherapy

- Slant board abdominal exercises.
- Upper leg and calf exercise.
- Wet grass walking.
- Salt water walks knee deep in the ocean.
- Walking, bicycling, swimming, etc.
- Headstands.
- Elevate foot of bed 4 inches (10 cm).
- Keep affected leg elevated whenever possible.
- Alternate hot and cold leg sprays.
- Alternate hot and cold sitz baths.
- Alternate hot and cold showers.
- Spinal manipulation.
- Dry body brush (see Appendix I).
- Flex and extend ankles frequently.
- Local massage upward (not over thinned veins) with warm olive oil and myrrh.

- Massage feet in fluid from old coffee grounds; also apply over thinned vessels.
- Mullein poultice.
- Hot sage tea compress.
- Witch hazel compress.
- Slippery elm poultice to ulcers.
- Vitamin E to ulcers.
- Clay poultice to ulcers.
- Comfrey poultice to ulcers.
- Ultraviolet light to ulcers and varicose veins.
- White oak bark tea compress.
- Bayberry tea compress.
- Stone root tea compress or ointment.
- Pressure bandage.

Therapeutic Agents

Vitamins and Minerals—Primary
- Vitamin C plus bioflavonoids: 1000-6000 mg daily. To bowel tolerance.
- Quercetin: 600 mg daily. Improves vascular integrity.
- Vitamin E: 400-1200 IU daily. Reduces clots, and pain of varicosity.

Vitamins and Minerals—Secondary
- Vitamin A: 25,000 IU 2-4 times daily.
- Vitamin B: 25-50 mg twice daily.
- Folic acid.
- Calcium.
- Zinc.
- Copper.

Others—Primary
- Digestive enzymes between meals: reduces fibrin activity.
- Glucosamine: supports collagen synthesis in the veins themselves.
- Proline, lysine, glycine: the major amino acids involved in collagen and elastin production
- Essential fatty acids: GLA, EPA, fish oil and evening primrose oil.
- Chondroitin sulfate: supports ground substance synthesis.
- Witch hazel cream: topically, astringent.

Others—Secondary

- Arnica cream, and Arnica homoeopathics (6×, 12C)
- Blackstrap molasses.
- Psyllium powder: 1 tbsp with water 3 times daily.
- Chlorophyll.
- Garlic: 2 capsules 3 times daily.
- Lecithin.
- Rutin: 2 capsules twice daily.
- Wheat germ.
- Zinc.

Botanicals—Primary

Bilberry: high in proanthocyanidins.
Horse chestnut: vascular tonic.

Hawthorn: vascular tonic.
Globe artichoke: portal hypotensive.
Fringe tree: portal hypertensive.
Ginger: circulatory stimulant and anti-inflammatory.
Prickly ash: peripheral vasodilator, circulatory stimulant.

Botanicals—Secondary

Fringe tree: circulatory stimulant.
Mullein tea.
Stone root: 1–4 capsules daily.
Buckwheat: vascular tonic.
Sweet clover.

WARTS
(Verrucae)

DEFINITION

Benign epithelial tumors caused by a virus. They may affect the hands, arms, face, body, feet, and anal or genital region. The three most commonly seen types are common, venereal, and plantar warts.

SYMPTOMS

Raised, irregular (common, venereal), or flat (plantar) growths on the skin. These may be symptomless or cause pain and discomfort, especially in areas of constant contact, such as the sole of the foot.

ETIOLOGICAL CONSIDERATIONS—PRIMARY

- Viral infection (HPV—human papilloma virus)
- Lowered resistance (reduced immunological state)
- Deficiency of vitamins A and C, and zinc

ETIOLOGICAL CONSIDERATIONS— SECONDARY

- Glandular development
- Trauma
- Psychogenic causes

DISCUSSION

Warts are virus infections. Naturopathically, the causes of warts are no different from any other bacterial, viral, or parasitic infection or infestation of the body. These infections occur due to a lowered vitality and lack of resistance on the part of the host.

A key factor with warts in particular is a state of lowered immunological activity. This may be due to an improper diet of nutrient-deficient refined foods. Certainly, deficiencies of vitamin A, vitamin C, and zinc have all been related to an increased incidence of viral infections. These often lower the body's ability to fight off even everyday viruses such as those that cause warts.

Warts tend to appear at times when general glandular development is occurring. Thus they are fairly infrequent in the very young, but common in the puberty and teen years. Coincidentally, these are also the years that nutritional deficiencies of vitamins A and C, and zinc are most common. Warts are much less common in the aged when glandular systems are no longer functioning as actively.

Warts are most frequently found in areas exposed to trauma or repeated friction. They rarely cause anything more than a cosmetic problem, except with the case of plantar or venereal warts. Plantar warts can cause severe discomfort, making normal walking very painful. Genital warts can totally upset normal sexual relations, causing physical discomfort and severe psychological depression. Women with venereal warts should get a Pap smear and also be examined by a gynecologist. External condylomata are sometimes accompanied by internal warts (cervical human papilloma virus has been recently linked to an increased risk of subsequent cervical cancer with an estimated increase in the range of 200 times as likely).

Psychogenic factors are well recognized in relation to warts. They seem very susceptible to all types of suggestion, either in their creation or cure.

TREATMENT

The usual methods of removing warts by acids, surgery, burning, electrotherapy, and freezing carry a high percentage of recurrence over a much larger area than previously affected. The reason this occurs is that attention has not been placed on the major causative factors. Warts are like signs, that the immune system is weak. Best results are obtained when internal, external, and psychological measures are taken simultaneously. Vigorous treatment is needed especially with venereal warts, which may be very contagious, and spread rapidly to cover the entire anogenital region.

Diet

The nutritional state has a great deal to do with general host resistance and a strong immunological system. Dietary changes, however, may take 6 months or longer to alleviate the condition. Foods high in vitamins A, B complex, C, and in zinc in particular should be stressed. The diet should have a large proportion of raw foods. The internal dietary and nutritional approach is especially necessary where warts are so widespread and numerous that topical therapy is practically impossible.

In these cases, along with the general upgrading of the nutritional status, it may be necessary to acidify the entire system artificially for a 2-week period by the use of 20–30 drops of orthophosphoric acid taken in water daily. This has a very strong effect on systemic warts. It may be repeated 2–3 times after a 2-week interval. High doses of vitamins A, B complex, C, and of zinc are used with all warts for 1–2-month periods, with care not to extend vitamin A therapy at too high a dose for too long, causing toxic results. Generally, 50,000–100,000 IU for up to 6 weeks is non-toxic for adults, especially if the emulsified form is used.

Psychotherapy

Hypnosis for warts is very effective.

External Applications

All the following local therapies have been used with success for some people. Several may need to be tried to get results.

- Garlic: apply thin section over wart as continuous poultice. Avoid healthy tissue.
- Castor oil and baking soda poultice: mix castor oil and baking soda into a paste and apply to wart; keep covered with band-aid each night. Do not pick at wart during the day, but let it slough off within 3–6 weeks. This may at times

cause some pain. If so, stop the application and then apply again on the following evening.

- Castor oil: apply 3 times daily and at night. Cover with band-aid. May take 2 or more months to be successful.
- Vitamin E: apply 400 IU capsules 3 times daily and cover with band-aid. Takes approximately 2 months.
- Vitamin A (micellized): 25,000 IU applied topically 3 times daily and night. Cover. Especially useful in plantar warts.
- Podophyllum tincture (May-apple or American mandrake) (highly toxic—see p. 60): antimitotic, caustic: simmer ordinary tincture until reduced to one-fourth. Apply 1 drop carefully to wart once daily. Protect surrounding skin with vaseline, paraffin, or sticky plaster to prevent tissue damage. Keep covered with adhesive tape. Repeat daily for 2–3 weeks. Care must be taken in treating multiple warts simultaneously with Podophyllum since it is toxic, even by absorption through the skin. *Never use Podophyllum unless under medical supervision.*
- Podophyllum tincture 20% and compound tincture of benzoin 80%: apply to anogenital warts.
- Thuja tincture: especially useful in anal and genital warts. Thuja oil is also used topically.
- Salicylic acid and thuja: apply with care. Protect surrounding skin. Repeat application 2–3 times daily.

Other Treatments Suggested by Some

- Powdered vitamin C: topical as paste and covered with band-aid; black walnut tincture.

- Comfrey ointment, root poultice, or leaf poultice; plantain poultice for plantar warts; fresh dandelion juice. Apply locally and then cover; oil of sulfur; chickweed juice or poultice; sassafras oil; tormentil oil; oil of gaultheria; thymol; fresh greater celandine juice; green fig juice.
- Green papaya juice; aloe vera; onion and salt compress.

Internal Botanicals and Dilutions

- Castoreum 30×.
- Nitric acid 30×.
- Thuja tincture, thuja 30×.

Therapeutic Agents

Vitamins and Minerals— Primary
- Vitamin A (emulsified): 50,000–100,000 IU daily for 6 weeks.
- Vitamin C: maximum dose to bowel tolerance.
- Zinc: 50–100 mg daily.

Vitamins and Minerals— Secondary
- Vitamin B complex: 25–50 mg 2–3 times daily.
- Vitamin B6: 50 mg twice daily.
- Vitamin C: 1500–6000 mg daily.
- Vitamin E: 600–1200 IU daily.

Others
Garlic: 2 capsules three times daily.

WORMS

DEFINITION

Infestation with various types of worms, including pinworms, roundworms, hookworms, and tapeworms.

SYMPTOMS

None, or local irritation of anus, weakness, fatigue, lack of vitality, grinding of teeth at night, loss of appetite, irritability, frequent colds, brittle and hard fingernails with ridged longitudinal lines, anemia, loss of weight.

ETIOLOGICAL CONSIDERATIONS—PRIMARY

- Poor diet
  Sugar; refined carbohydrates; excess dairy; excess acidity; raw green vegetable deficiency; excess meat; excess cooked foods; constipation; lowered resistance; poor hygiene; lack of exercise
- Upset internal ecology

DISCUSSION

The human body supports many life forms, both externally and internally. Some of these do little or no harm, and in fact are usually never noticed. Others are actually beneficial, such as the bacteria that normally inhabit the intestine and vagina. These help to protect the body from invasion of other more detrimental viruses, bacteria, or parasites.

Worms of various kinds can enter the body through several avenues and, if conditions are favorable for their development, may multiply. If this colony is not kept in check by the body's own defenses, the infestation soon becomes a burden on the body and health is downgraded.

Threadworms, Pinworms (*Oxyuris* or *Enterobius vermicularis*)

This is the most common of worm infestations. The infection rate among children is often close to 100%. Most people have had, have, or will have a pinworm infestation at one or more times in their lives. Many have pinworms right now but do not even know it.

Pinworms are spread by inhaling or ingesting their eggs, which are widespread in the environment, especially where children live or play. These eggs are extremely tiny. The female worm emerges from the anus at night to lay her eggs in the external anal folds. This causes irritation and itching. The area is then scratched and the eggs pass from the fingernails to others directly or via food. If left on the anal region they hatch, re-enter the anus and mature. The eggs also gather on the bedclothes and enter the air as the sheet or blanket is shaken out, spreading throughout the room and infecting by ingestion or inhalation. The worms may be seen as tiny, thread-like, maggot-sized worms in the stool, or at the anus at night. They infest the large intestine and may cause appendix irritation, leading to false appendicitis. A single female may lay 10,000 eggs, which then mature in 2 weeks.

Parents seem to suffer most, psychologically, when their child gets pinworms. We have seen parents completely beside themselves with disgust when they discover such an infestation. We would like to reassure you that pinworms are not that bad. Certainly a large infestation can be a negative health factor as the worms do compete for the body's food supply, but much less so than with the other worms discussed below. The first infestation is usually the worst, and then the body slowly develops an immunity so that a low-threshold infection is maintained without much detriment, even without treatment. Drug therapy for worms is very appealing to the parent, since it offers a quick solution to a distressing condition. One dose of Povan is usually very effective in killing the worms. The reinfection rate, however, is nearly 100%. The problem, of course, is that the real causes were never removed and re-exposure for a typical child is practically certain no matter how many precautions the parent may take.

As with other infections, pinworms develop best if vitality is low. It is clear from studies of children in the same classroom that some develop a strong immunity to worms and get either light or no infections, while others never seem to develop immunity and harbor large infestations indefinitely. The most documented difference between these two groups is not general hygiene, as some might expect. It is diet. Those who are most susceptible generally eat more refined carbohydrates and sugar than their classmates, and have much less fiber in their diet.

Roundworms (*Ascaris lumbricoides*)

Ascarids have been humanity's constant companions probably since we began domesticating pigs. Where soil pollution, warmth, and moisture are common, so are roundworms. Ascarids are large nematode worms reaching 8–14 inches (20–36 cm) in length. They have a narrow tapered head and the females have a blunt tail. They normally inhabit the small intestine where they feed on undigested food and have also been known to bite the mucous membranes of the intestine and suck the host's blood.

A single female produces about 200,000 eggs each day. These eggs pass out of the body with the feces and develop or remain viable wherever moisture and oxygen exist. They are very resistant to chemicals and can even survive long exposure to seawater. Complete drying is lethal, but with moisture the eggs may remain alive for years. When the eggs are swallowed the larvae then hatch in the small intestine and penetrate their mucous membrane. From here they are carried by the blood to the liver, heart, and lungs, where they burrow out into the trachea, esophagus, or throat, to be swallowed. They then settle down and develop in the small intestine where they reach maturity in 2½ months.

They are commonly spread by hand-to-mouth contact. This emphasizes the importance of hygiene in restaurants and is one of the main reasons it is a state law for employees in the food-handling industry to wash their hands after a visit to the toilet. Contamination is also spread readily in areas where human manure is used for fertilizer. Vegetables or fruit grown on such soil then spread the infection. Young children may also spread them by defecating where others may then easily be infected.

Infection with *Ascaris* is not nearly as benign as with pinworm, and a serious health risk occurs with heavy infestations. As the worms pass through the lungs, a severe and possibly fatal pneumonia may result. Abdominal symptoms include diarrhea, abdominal discomfort, or vomiting. The worms may become tangled, causing intestinal blockage requiring surgery, or may block various organs or ducts such as the gallbladder, or even the appendix. There is some evidence that these worms may produce toxic substances causing delirium, nervousness, convulsions, or coma. They may even cause poor digestion of proteins by interfering with the digestive enzyme trypsin, leading to malnutrition. The body reacts to these worm infestations with antibodies which may be responsible for a number of allergies.

Prevention depends mainly on proper nutrition, as with all infections, proper disposal of human feces, good hygiene, and proper washing of vegetables, especially where "night soil" is used.

Hookworms (*Ancylostoma duodenale* and *Necator americanus*)

These worms cause much injury to humans. Hookworm infestations, however, are rarely spectacular, but year after year insidiously drain the vitality and undermine the health. Many so-called worthless or lazy people are suffering from hookworms that stunt them mentally and physically.

Hookworms are rather fat and about $1/2$ inch (1 cm) long. They possess powerful teeth that latch onto the bowel walls and allow the parasite to inflict severe damage to the intestine while sucking large amounts of blood. Each female produces 5000–10,000 eggs each day. The eggs pass out in the feces and develop into larvae in moist, warm soil. These free-living larvae then feed on bacteria and other small matter in the excreted feces until they either die from lack of moisture, or are stepped upon by a barefooted host. They then bore into the skin, pass into the lymph channels or blood vessels, making their way to the heart and lungs, where they burrow out into the air spaces and are passed upward towards the throat by the action of cilia hairs within the lungs themselves. Here they are either expectorated and then die in the sun or are swallowed, to pass into the intestine to mature and grow. Each worm lives anywhere from 5–15 years. Hookworms are primarily tropical in origin. Cold and dryness will kill the larvae as will salt within the soil. Animals such as pigs, dogs, and cattle may eat the eggs and aid in the spread of infection by voiding these eggs unharmed in areas most likely to affect humans. Infestations are more common among agricultural workers, or those living in rural areas, especially where shoes are not often worn, or where human feces is used as a fertilizer.

Diet has a profound effect on hookworm infestation and host resistance. Most of the injury done by these worms results from the consequent anemia and protein deficiency from the blood lost to the parasites. This lowers host resistance and reduces the body's capacity to produce antibodies. It is well proven that patients recover best from hookworms on a diet high in protein, iron, and other blood-building elements. This diet is also essential in the prevention of large infections. The severity of hookworm disease in a community is influenced more by the adequacy of the diet than the incidence of exposure.

The main health problems hookworms cause are bronchitis and pneumonia when in the lung, and nausea, abdominal discomfort, and sometimes diarrhea, but the principal effects are those of anemia. The effects of hookworm during pregnancy are especially severe when the demand for protein and iron by the developing fetus puts an extra drain upon the mother's nutritional state. Hookworm is implicated in a vast number of stillbirths and is considered a more severe complication of pregnancy than eclampsia.

Tapeworms (Various Species)

Tapeworms consist of extremely long chains of nearly independent, sexually capable segments. These chains may be anywhere from 6–60 ft (3–20 m) long The tapeworm attaches to the intestinal wall and absorbs food from the host. The life cycles vary with each species. The most common are spread by the host's eating uncooked or incompletely cooked pork, beef, or fish. They cause symptoms similar to other worm infections—abdominal pain, loss of weight, weakness, and particularly a severe anemia, especially the fish tapeworm, which uses up all the available vitamin B12, causing pernicious anemia.

TREATMENT

Drug therapy is recommended. It is rapid and fairly effective. Dietary therapies for these conditions are much slower. The role of diet and nutritional factors, however, should then be helpful in preventing reinfection. The exception to this is mild pinworm infestations, which are fairly easy to take care of with natural remedies. Some interesting references to botanicals sometimes used for other intestinal parasites are included for general interest.

Diet

Studies of those with high resistance to worm infestation show a diet high in unrefined carbohydrates, raw green vegetables, and adequate protein; with little meat, pork, or uncooked fish, and no sugar. It is clear that appropriate diet has a great deal to do with preventing worm infections by increasing host immunity and preventing obvious infection through proper preparation and cooking of food. Once infection has occurred, various regimens are useful to lower or completely remove the population.

A few useful diet regimens are as follows:

Day 1–3
Green cabbage (or carrots) plus pumpkin seeds eaten 3-4 times daily. Nothing else except garlic or garlic capsules three times daily. Take prescribed worm medication morning and evening. (Wormwood plus other prescriptions, depending on type of infection.)

Day 4
In morning take purging dose of Epsom salts, senna, or other cathartic. In the evening take an enema with bitterwood—1 fl oz (30 mL) to 1 pint (500 mL) of water. Same diet as above.

Day 5
Repeat Day 4.

Another version:
Day 1–3
As above

Day 4
Take ½ tsp Fletcher's castoria every ½ hour until half the bottle is used. next, take strong worm remedy specific to infection. when bowel movement occurs, finish castoria, plus half bottle more.

Another alternative is the all-garlic-and-onion diet instead of cabbage and pumpkin seeds. Follow the same directions as above for the worm medication and purge. Garlic water enemas may also be used.

Follow-up diet to include:
- No sweets or refined carbohydrates; increased raw greens, especially lettuce and cabbage.
- No milk; plenty of onions and garlic; 4 oz lb (120 g) pumpkin seeds daily; coconut meat and milk, if available; figs; raw pineapple; pomegranate: 1-3 daily when available.

It is important to change the intestinal environment by these measures. Worms love sugar, acid conditions, and constipation. High-fiber alkaline diets are the best prevention of infestation, and cure.

Physiotherapy

- Garlic clove inserted rectally at night.
- Garlic foot compresses at night.
- Abdominal exercise.
- Sit in bowl of warm milk after purge, for tapeworm

Therapeutic Agents

Garlic; papaya; onions; horseradish; pomegranate; fig; raw pancreas; lemons; pumpkin seeds; carrots; cabbage; pineapple; lettuce; bromelain.

Botanicals—Primary
Fresh papaya seeds: 1 tsp chewed on empty stomach.
Pumpkin seed tea: 1 fl oz (30 mL) to 1 pint (500 mL) water; 1-2 cups daily.
Wormwood: for pinworms, roundworms
1 teacup infusion morning and evening.
10-30 grains powder morning and evening
5-30 drops tincture morning and evening, then purge.
Santonica/wormseed: for pinworms, roundworms, tapeworms.
Pomegranate: for pinworms, roundworms, tapeworms. Decoction of root bark used.
Thymol: (tapeworm, roundworm).

Botanicals—Secondary

Wormseed: contains santonin. Useful with tapeworms. Use small doses frequently. $\frac{1}{2}$–$1\frac{1}{2}$ grains.

Male fern: $\frac{1}{2}$–1 tsp powder morning and evening, then purge (senna plus butternut purge) 30 drops oil morning and evening, then purge (for tapeworm). 1–$1\frac{1}{2}$ drams of tincture in morning, then purge.

American wormseed, Jerusalem oak: children: 20–30 grains powdered seeds or 3–10 drops oil; adults: 1–2 tsp powdered seeds or 10–20 drops oil (for roundworms, hookworms, tapeworms).

Tansy: $\frac{1}{2}$–1 cup infusion (especially seeds) morning and evening. Fluid extract: children: 1 tsp; adults: 3 tsp. Take cathartic 1 hour later

Prickly pear: for amebic dysentery. Use strong infusion of flowers. 1 cup morning and evening.

Kousso: for tapeworms.

Chips tea enema: for pinworms.

Bitterwood: enema or decoction. Use wood and bark: 1 tbsp to 1 cup water; boil 30 minutes. 1 tsp in 1 cup water 1–2 times daily.

Cascara (purge).

Senna (purge).

Epsom salts (purge).

Pinkroot with wormwood: for pinworms 15–30 drops twice daily.

Areca nut (betel nut) for tapeworms.

Aloe.

May-apple, or American mandrake (highly toxic; see p. 60).

Butternut: laxative.

Prescriptions:

Cina 6×; santoninum 3–6×; *Spigelia anthelmia* 1×; podophyllum: $\frac{1}{4}$ grain, twice daily with diet and purge; zymex 11 (Standard Process Labs); calomel: $\frac{1}{4}$ grain; senna: $\frac{1}{2}$ grain.

Santonin: $\frac{1}{4}$ grain; pomegranate; male fern; wormwood; sulfax (boericke and tafel).

WOUNDS, MINOR CUTS, BRUISES

All injuries that cause tissue damage should be placed in ice-cold water immediately. This will stop bleeding, reduce the chance of inflammation, and dramatically speed recovery. Cuts should be thoroughly cleaned while in the cold water, and freed of any dirt or foreign object. Apply tea tree oil to prevent infection, and reapply every 2–3 hours. Vitamin E may be used topically to accelerate healing and reduce scarring. Arnica tincture applied topically 3–4 times daily—is excellent for any bruise. Arnica in potency form should be taken internally at frequent intervals. Calendula cream can be applied to cuts once they are clean, as can fresh Aloe vera juice and/or a comfrey poultice, which will also accelerate healing of superficial wounds.

TREATMENT

Vitamins and Minerals— Primary

- Vitamin C: 5–10 g daily.
- Zinc: 25 mg 2–3 times daily.

Vitamins and Minerals— Secondary

- Vitamin A: 50,000–100,000 IU daily.
- Bioflavonoids: 300–1000 mg daily.
- Vitamin E: 400–800 IU daily.

YEAST INFECTION

DEFINITION

Local or systemic colonization of the skin or mucous membranes by the yeast *Candida albicans*, also referred to as *Monilia albicans*, or thrush.

SYMPTOMS

These depend on the severity of colonization, area affected, and tissue response. Common symptoms include the following: recurrent vaginal infections (see Vaginitis), fatigue, depression, inability to concentrate, constipation or diarrhea, gas, bloating, abdominal pain, muscle or joint pain, headaches, allergies, skin rashes (hives, eczema, psoriasis, rash under arms, in crotch, etc.), nail fungus, menstrual problems (premenstrual syndrome), prostatitis, hypoglygemia, hyperactivity, athlete's foot.

ETIOLOGIC CONSIDERATIONS

- Repeated antibiotic use
- Birth control pill use
- Consumption of refined carbohydrates or excess fruit or fruit juice
- Improper hygiene
- Nutritional deficiency due to improper diet or malabsorption
- IgA (gamma-A globulin) or other immune deficiencies
- Allergies
- Chemical exposure
- Pregnancy
- Menstrual cycle
- Constipation

DISCUSSION

Yeast infections have been recognized since the days of Hippocrates. Most women are aware of yeast problems since they are such a common cause of vaginitis. The yeast involved is *Candida albicans*, a common, usually non-pathogenic inhabitant of the skin and mucous membranes. Under normal circumstances, the body's defense barriers and immune system keep this fungus in check, allowing it only a limited existence. If, however, the body's defenses are weakened by improper diet, or if the general or local ecology of the body or tissues is severely altered, as it is by antibiotic use, Candida can begin to flourish throughout the body, causing the wide range of symptoms listed above.

The problem with Candida infections is diagnosis. Since Candida is a normal inhabitant of the vagina and gastrointestinal tract, a culture is of no use. The only diagnosis can be one suggested by the case history followed by a successful trial treatment of an antifungal system.

TREATMENT

Diet

Yeast seems to thrive on sugars and refined carbohydrates. This may be the reason that a history of hypoglycemia and sweets craving is so common in patients with Candida infections. By starving Candida of its favorite foods, a better internal ecology is favored. A diet composed mainly of vegetarian (fish is an exception) non-dairy protein (except for yoghurt), unrefined grains, and vegetables is best. Onions and garlic are particularly useful.

We prefer to avoid meat-based proteins, since these are associated with abnormal bowel flora development. Milk also can result in abnormal flora; however, fermented dairy products such as buttermilk, kefir, and yoghurt are beneficial. Yoghurt should be included in the diet once or twice daily, unless obvious dairy allergy exists. Although whole grains are suggested, yeasted grains should be avoided. Some question has arisen about yeast avoidance, since the type of yeast in bread and baked products is not the same as Candida. While this is true, it is a common clinical observation that these yeasts definitely do aggravate these conditions are best avoided. This also includes yeast-source multivitamins, or yeast-source B vitamins, and any foods commonly known to contain yeast. The following summary of acceptable foods may be of use:

Proteins
Yoghurt, kefir, buttermilk, seeds, nuts, eggs, tofu, beans, fish, chicken (less frequently), meat (less frequently).

Vegetables
Unrestricted, except for the following carbohydrate-containing vegetables, which should be eaten less frequently: potatoes, sweet potatoes, beans, squash, corn.

Fruit or fruit juice
Little or none, except for avocado and papaya.

Whole grains
All grains are allowed unless obvious allergy exists. The only restriction is the amount in the diet. Some patients respond best by reducing the proportion of grains dramatically, even excluding them altogether; others may handle unrestricted quantities and still re-establish good external ecology. While the whole grains are composed of significant carbohydrate, the fiber and protein components help re-establish proper bowel function, a major factor in the causation of altered bowel ecology in the first place.

Therapeutic Agents

Vitamins and Minerals
- Vitamin A: 25,000–50,000 IU 1–2 times daily.
- Yeast-free vitamin B complex: 25–50 mg 1–2 times daily.
- Vitamin B6: 100–250 mg 1–2 times daily, especially with premenstrual syndrome.
- Vitamin C: up to bowel tolerance.
- Vitamin E: 400–800 IU daily.
- Biotin.
- Caprilic acid.

Others
Garlic: We prefer pure clove garlic, however unsociable, in cases of yeast infections. One medium clove 2–3 times daily, although difficult to take, is the best preparation available. We question Kyolic in this instance and would prefer the products made by Arizona Natural Products if the clove garlic is not being used. Take garlic preparations at least 3 times per day.

Lactobacillus: Since this is one of the most important medications, it is essential that the preparation be *viable*. We use Super-dophilus or Megadophilus powder, 1 tsp 3–4 times daily. Other brands may be as, or more, useful, but the health food industry is not presently regulated to demand validated testing of product consistency and potency. This applies to all nutritional products in health food stores. How often is an unreliable product the cause of prescription failure? We presently cannot know.

Nystatin: Once Candida is entrenched, it can be very difficult to eradicate. Many cases will not be treatable with general internal ecology improvement, and will require nystatin or other anifungal medication. Since this is a prescription item, it must be prescribed by your doctor. Usual doses range from 50,000–100,000 units 3–4 times daily. Side-effects are minimal. Nystatin seems to be fairly non-toxic. Many of its side effects are in reality the result of massive Candida death, the body's sudden burden of breakdown products, and the body's imflammatory response to these materials.

Botanicals
Taheebo inner bark tea (antifungal): 1 cup infusion 4 times daily.

Tea tree oil (local use): useful in nail fungus. Add 1 tbs water-soluble tea tree (Melasol; Metabolic Products) to 1 cup hot water. Soak nail 20–30 minutes 1–2 times daily. Apply tea tree oil to nail and nail bed two to three times per day. Continue treatment for 30–60 days.

Aloe vera juice: 2 oz (60 g) 4 times daily.

See Vaginitis for local vaginal treatments.

NOTES

1 Drysdale, Ian, *Notes on Natural Therapeutics.*

2 Lindlahr, Henry, *Philosophy of Natural Therapeutics*, The Lindlahr Publishing Co., Chicago, Ill., 1919.

3 Ibid.

4 Ibid.

5 Lindlahr, Henry, op. cit.

6 Lindlahr, Henry, op. cit.

7 De Ropp, Robert, *Drugs and the Mind*, Grove Press, 1960, p. 72.

8 Williams, R. J., "The Concept of Genotrophic Disease", *Lancet*, 1:287, 1950.

9 Davis, Donald R., "Nutritional Needs and Biochemical Diversity", in Jeffrey Bland, *Medical Applications of Clinical Nutrition*, Keats Publishing Co., New Canaan, Conn., 1983, pp. 41–63.

10 Prasad, Ananda A., *Nutrition Reviews*, 41:197-208, 1983.

11 Beach, R., *Science*, 218:469-471, 1982.

12 Hahnemann, Samuel, *Organon of Medicine*, 6th ed., B. Jain Publishers, New Delhi, India, reprint 1982 (original 1921), p. 112.

13 Hahnemann, Samuel, op. cit., p. 97.

14 Kent, James Tyler, *Lectures on Homeopathic Philosophy*, B. Jain Publishers, New Delhi, India, 1979, p. 60.

15 Hahnemann, Samuel, op. cit., p. 112.

16 Stoddard, Alan, *Manual of Osteopathic Practice*, Hutchinson, London, 1969, p. 36.

17 Stoddard, Alan, op. cit., p. 38.

18 Bland, Jeffrey, *Medical Applications of Clinical Nutrition*, Keats Publishing Co., New Canaan, Conn., 1983, pp. 43-45.

19 Ibid.

20 Wright, Jonathon, *Dr Wright's Guide to Healing with Nutrition*, Rodale Press, Emmaus, Pa., 1984, p. 21.

21 Bland, Jeffrey, *Nutraerobics*, Harper & Row, San Francisco, 1983, p. 113.

22 Pfeiffer, Carl, *Mental and Elemental Nutrients*, Keats Publishing Co., New Canaan, Conn., 1975, pp. 380-383.

23 Airola, Paavo, *Hypoglycemia, a Better Approach*, Health Plus Publishing, Phoenix, Ariz., 1977, pp. 61-62.

24 *Annals of Allergy*, 51:296-299, 1983.

25 *Poisonous Prescriptions*, 1994, Podd Publishing, Western Australia.

26 Lindahl, O. et al. *Journal of Asthma*, 1985, 22, pp. 45-55)

27 Cayce, Edgar, *Physician's Reference Notebook,* A.R.E. Press, Virginia Beach, Virginia, 1968.

28 Allen, R.B., "Nutritional Aspects of Epilepsy", *International Clinical Nutrition Review*, 3(3):3-10, 1983.

29 Crowil, G.F., and Roach, E S., "Vitamin B, Dependent Seizures in Infants", *American Family Physician* 27 (3): pp. 183-187.

30 Pfeiffer, Carl, *Mental and Elemental Nutrients,* Keats Publishing,

31 Allen, R. B., op. cit., pp. 3-10.

32 Ibid.

33 *British Medical Journal*, 304; 6824, p.431.

34 See Trenev, N., *Probiotics, Nature's Internal Healers*, Avery Publishing, NY, 1998.

35 For proper testing of these muscles, the best book on this subject is *Muscles: Testing and Function* by Florence Peterson Kendall et al., Williams and Wilkins Publishers.

APPENDIX I

Remedies

DIETARY INSTRUCTION

MUCUS-CLEANSING DIET

This diet is extremely useful for all conditions of excess mucus such as asthma, bronchitis, catarrh, colds, pneumonia, salpingitis, ear infections, and many others.

Breakfast
Citrus fruit (especially grapefruit)

Midmorning
Fresh carrot juice

Lunch
A large plate of steamed onions with a little natural soy sauce for flavor. In some cases steamed carrots are also allowed (up to 25% of the meal), with the rest being onions.

Midafternoon
Potassium broth, or as midmorning

Supper
Same as lunch

Evening
As midafternoon

ALL-FRUIT DIET

Eat any unsprayed fruit or fruit juice other than banana. Banana is considered too starchy for an elimination regimen. Take only one type of fruit per meal. Alternate the juice and fruit every 1–2 hours.

HONEY/ONION SYRUP

Slice a large onion thinly, place in a bowl, and cover with 1–2 tbsp honey. Cover container tightly and allow to sit for 8 hours. Mash, strain, and take in 1 tsp doses 4–8 times daily. Excellent in mucous conditions.

POTASSIUM BROTH

Take ¼ inch (6 mm) of outer peelings of potatoes (including the skin), fresh parsley, unpeeled carrots, beet greens, onions, garlic, and any other organically grown green vegetables on hand. Prepare broth by washing and chopping the vegetables and then simmering in a large covered pot of water for 30–40 minutes. Strain and drink the essence, discarding the vegetables. Excess may be stored in glass containers in the refrigerator for up to 2 days.

AJ'S SALAD DRESSING

To make your own healthy *and* tasty formulation:
Put together equal amounts of balsamic (or apple cider) vinegar ($\frac{1}{4}$), flaxseed oil ($\frac{1}{4}$), (cold pressed, extra-virgin) olive oil ($\frac{1}{4}$), pure water ($\frac{1}{4}$), 1 tsp Celtic salt, then any/all the following as optional extras: 1 tsp whole-grain mustard seed, 1 clove finely chopped and crushed garlic, a little grated fresh ginger, 1 tsp of chilli sauce, a pinch of kelp. Shake together well before using each time.

PHYSIOTHERAPY INSTRUCTIONS

ENDONASAL TECHNIQUE

This is a method where obstructions from the upper parts of the respiratory system are removed by manipulating small bones in and surrounding the nasal area. The usual method is the introduction inside the nose of small balloons that are then suddenly inflated. Most naturopaths use this technique as well as many chiropractors and osteopaths.

COFFEE ENEMA

First thing in the morning prepare a pot of caffeinated coffee (not instant) using a glassware, enamelware, or stainless steel container. Use 2-4 tbsp of coffee grinds to 2 pints (1 liter) of water. Take a preliminary warm water enema to cleanse the lower bowel. When coffee has cooled to body temperature, place in enema container 18-20 inches (46-50 cm) higher than the body. Attach a 24-32 inch (60-80 cm) colon tube (obtainable from most drug stores) to the end of the enema tip. Lubricate tube with KY jelly and slowly insert 18-20 inches (46-50 cm) into the colon, slowly rotating the tube to prevent kinking. Lie on the left side as you allow the coffee to enter the colon. If fluid does not flow easily, the colon tube may be kinked. If so, slowly remove 4-8 inches (10-20 cm) of the tube until the flow of fluid is felt and slowly reinsert the entire 18-20 inches (46-50 cm). When all the coffee has entered the colon, remove the colon tube slowly and remain on the left side for 5 minutes. Roll onto the back for a further 5 minutes and finally on to the right side for 5 minutes. Finish by expelling the fluid into the toilet. The coffee enema removes toxins and opens the bile ducts.

GARLIC FOOT COMPRESS

This is an extremely valuable method to reduce excess mucus and combat systemic infections. It is especially useful with infants who cannot take garlic or onions by mouth. Care must be taken to follow these instructions explicitly to prevent severe blistering of the soles. It is entirely safe if applied correctly. Oil the soles of the feet with olive oil. Mash garlic and apply $\frac{1}{8}$-$\frac{1}{4}$ inch (3-6 mm) thick between gauze. Apply to soles with suitable non-stick tape and cover with a sock to secure. Leave poultice on all night.

"SALT GLOW"

Mix 1 lb (500 g) of fine salt in enough water to make a slurry. Begin with a warm shower and then with water off rub the salt all over the body firmly. Finish with an ice-cold shower. Your skin will "glow" for hours. A dry sand scrub is also wonderfully therapeutic, and beneficial for the blood, lymph, and the skin.

DRY BODY BRUSHING

Dry body brushing is done *before* a shower, while the body is still dry. There are many therapeutic benefits of dry body brushing. It exfoliates the outer layer of the skin and stimulates blood flow to the skin, enabling it better to breathe, and eliminate wastes carried in the bloodstream such as uric acid. The skin is the largest organ of the body, is a major eliminative organ (along with bowels, kidneys and lungs), and is often called the "third kidney" since sweat has almost the same constituents as urine.

Body brushing also stimulates blood flow to the epidermis cells, important especially to Langerhans cells which interact with helper T-cells in immune reactions, as well as epidermal growth factor (EGF) regulation (proper functioning of which prevents melanomas). Brushing also stimulates blood flow to the dermis (a deeper layer of skin), vital to the health of the skin. Skin aging can be defined in terms of dermis health.

Most importantly, body brushing helps decongest lymphatic capillaries which interface with blood capillaries in all connective tissue (including skin). Blockage in lymph flow can occur for many reasons, including sclerosing (thickening) of lymphatic tissue, mucus and fatty deposits, dehydration and electrolyte imbalance, blood thickening, and lymph node congestion. Dietary fats such as those in animal products, e.g. dairy, red meats, poultry, and trans fatty acids such as are in margarines, as well as poor protein digestion, are also implicated in a sluggish lymphatic system.

Buy a body brush made of natural plant fiber, or a coarse bath glove, or a loofah mitt. Pressure depends on skin sensitivity. Start gently and increase pressure until the body becomes more used to it. Brush vigorously making rotary motions, and massage every part of your body. Start with the feet and legs, then hands and arms, then back, abdomen, chest and neck. (Use a towel for the back if cannot reach with brush). Once finished, shower to clean off exfoliated skin cells. 5–10 minutes morning and evening is ideal.

There are many other benefits to dry body brushing as well. Dry brushing:

- Stimulates blood circulation in all underlying organs and tissues
- Stimulates hormone and oil-producing glands of the skin
- Has a powerful rejuvenating influence on the nervous system by stimulating nerve endings in the skin
- Contributes to a healthier muscle tone and better distribution of fats
- Rejuvenates the complexion, is anti-aging

EPSOM SALTS BATHS

Put 1–1½ lb (2–2.25 kg) of Epsom salts into a hot tub and soak for 15–20 minutes. Immediately go to bed under plenty of covers to sweat. Remain in bed 3 hours to all night. Rinse off with tepid water after the sweat and finish with a colder application, either a sponge bath or shower.

CASTOR OIL PACKS

Obtain undyed cotton or preferably wool flannel of sufficient size so that it will cover an area approximately 8 × 12 inches (20 × 30 cm) when folded to 2–4 thicknesses. Soak this flannel in a pan of unrefined cold-pressed castor oil. Wring out so that the cloth is just wet but not dripping, and apply to area of body to be treated. Cover this with plastic and apply a heating pad as warm as is comfortably bearable. Leave pack on for 1–1½ hours. After the pack is completed, wash the oil off with warm water and baking soda —1 tsp to 1 pint (500 mL) warm water. Store flannel in covered pan for future use. After 20 or 30 uses thoroughly cleanse the flannel and reuse. (Materials available from Cayce.)

BOWEL FIBER

Fiber comprises plant cell walls which are made up of cellulose and non-cellulose polysaccharides which include gums, mucilages, pectins and lignans, all of which were intended by Nature to benefit the consumer, by increasing fecal size, binding to bile acids, laxatives (ensuring proper transit time), heavy metal chelation, and the lignans act as antioxidants and have demonstrated anticarcinogenic effects.

Most importantly, intestinal flora ferment this fiber to produce acids such as acetic, butyric and propionic acids, important for a wide range of biochemical and physiological benefits, including the health and integrity of bowel wall cells, and provide an energy source for the health of the floral populations themselves, thus ensuring a healthy bowel.

As foods are becoming more and more refined, these valuable properties are being lost to us. In the past, naturopaths have generally recommended the addition of bran powder in many conditions requiring a bulking agent for the bowels. The medical profession and dietitians still routinely suggest it. The idea behind such a fiber is good and valid indeed, but there is something much better and less expensive.

Most proprietary brans contain wheat proteins. Wheat fiber irritates and scratches delicate bowel tissue, and for whatever the reasons might be, intolerance of wheat is implicit in the etiology of many disease states, not merely celiac disease.

So, we recommend the use of psyllium powder/husks/husks instead of wheat bran. Psyllium is a highly mucilaginous bulking agent, with soothing transitional effects, promotes peristalsis, and keeps the feces soft, bulky, and easy to pass.

Simply purchase from health food shops as powder. There are proprietary preparations of fiber that use psyllium, such as metamucil, but these are expensive and may not represent value for money.

Psyllium can be added to the diet in any liquid such as water, juice, soup/broth, smoothies, or sprinkled over food such as porridge, casserole, etc. If your bowels tend towards constipation, psyllium is best taken 3 times daily in water or juice. If the bowels are loose as in diarrhea, psyllium is best sprinkled over food with less water. We recommend a daily intake of 1–3 heaped tsp for good bowel maintenance. The bowel bacteria will thank you for such an excellent supply of food for them.

Oat bran is another bowel fiber with similar characteristics to psyllium, and is a good alternative if psyllium is unavailable.

Ensure your sources are organically grown.

APPENDIX II

Naturopathic Websites

www.standardprocess.com
Supplier of organically grown nutritional supplements including raw glandular "protomorphogen" supplements as recommended in this book.

www.are-cayce.com
The Association for Research and Enlightenment. Source of information about Edgar Cayce.

www.caycecures.com
Source of Edgar Cayce products.
E-mail at heritage@caycecures.com
Phone: 800-TO-CAYCE (800-862-2923)
The Heritage Store Inc.
PO Box 444 314 Laskin Road
Virginia Beach, VA 23458

www.cayce.com
Resource site for Edgar Cayce information and natural therapies.

www.natural-living.com
Go to heritage in catalogue. Supplier of Edgar Cayce products found in this book. Also a discount supplier of a huge selection of natural products from many other sources.

www.eclecticherb.com
Source of quality naturopathic products including pre-made depletion pack formulation

www.pandamedicine.com
Naturopathic medicine network. This web site is a superb source of resource information on naturopathic medicine and includes free access to medline search. They also can help you find a naturopathic physician in your area (US or Canada only at present).

www.naturalmed.net/
Excellent web site for those interested in naturopathy. You can obtain information on any condition or be put in contact with a naturopath near you or on the net. It has a detailed database for naturopathic research on individual disease conditions.

www.holisticmed.com
Useful links to diverse web sites on natural lifestyles and healing as well as schedules for holistic healing trade shows, festivals and expos. Includes an international directory of practitioners of holistic medicine.

www.altmedicine.com/
Alternative health news and information online.

www.healthy.net
Great web site for those interested in natural therapies and lifestyle. Links to a huge number of interesting sites on alternative healing.

www.americanyogaassociation.org
Information on yoga and source of books
and videos for home use.

**www.noah.cuny.edu/alternative/alter
native.html**
Excellent site with information on
alternative therapies.

www.acnt.edu
Australasian College of Natural Therapies
57 Foveaux Street
Surry Hills
Sydney, Australia
Ph: 02 9218 8850
Fax: 02 9291 4411

www.acnm.edu.au
Australian College of Natural Medicine
1 Nerang Street
Southport, Qld 4215
Ph: 07 5503 0977
This college also has branches in Brisbane,
and Melbourne.

www.safetherapies.com.au
Academy of SAFE Therapies
42 Junction Road
PO Box 2060
Burleigh Junction, Qld 4220
Ph: 07 5522 0404
Fax: 07 5522 0505

www.naturopath.org.nz
New Zealand Society of Naturopathy
Links to colleges, practitioners and
information including:
South Pacific College of Natural Thera-
peutics (NZ)
PO Box 11-311
Auckland, NZ
Ph: (09) 579 4997
Fax: (09) 579 4997
Naturopathic College of New Zealand
PO Box 5109
New Plymouth, NZ
Ph: (06) 759 0218
Fax: (06) 759 0281

www.naturopathycollege.com
Naturopathic College of New Zealand (and
Australia)
PO Box 5109
New Plymouth, NZ
Ph: (06) 759 0218
Fax: (06) 759 0281

www.naturopathy.org.uk
Information on naturopathy in the United
Kingdom. Contact site for the general
council and register of naturopaths in the
UK and a full listing of registered
naturopaths who have graduated from
four-year naturopathic medical schools.
This listing primarily lists naturopaths in
the UK but other countries are also listed.

www.bcno.org.uk
British College of Naturopathy and
Osteopathy
Offers 4-year full time course in
osteopathy and naturopathy.
6 Netherhall Gardens
London, England NW3

www.naturopathics.com
Worldwide directory of naturopathic
practitioners, colleges and organizations.

www.cnra.org/welcome.html
Council on Naturopathic Registration and
Accreditation
Suite 1600
3509 Connecticut Avenue, NW
Washington D.C. 20008-2402
Ph: (800) 200 9123

www.naturopathic.org
American Association of Naturopathic
Physicians.
General information on naturopathy,
colleges, state associations, books and
finding qualified naturopaths in the US and
other valuable links.

www.aanp.com
Alternate site for American Association of
Naturopathic Physicians with useful links.

www.anma.com
American Naturopathic Medical
Association
PO Box 96273
Las Vegas, Nevada 89193
Ph: (702) 897 7053
Fax: (702) 897 7140

www.tnaa.com/index.htm
The Naturopathic Association of America

www.canp.org
California Association of Naturopathic
Physicians
112 Douglas Blvd.
Roseville, CA 95678
Ph: (800) 521 1200

www.cnme.org
Council on Naturopathic Medical
Education
Programs leading to the Doctor of
Naturopathic Medicine (N.D.) degree for
the USA and Canada.

www.scnm.edu
Southwest College of Naturopathic
Medicine and Health Sciences.
2140 E. Broadway Road
Tempe, Arizona 85282
Ph: (480) 858 9100
Fax: (480) 858 0222

www.bastyr.edu
Bastyr University
Four-year fully accredited naturopathic
medical school.
14500 Juanita Drive NE
Kenmore, WA 98028-4966
USA

Ph: (425) 823 1300
Fax: (425) 823 6222

www.ncnm.edu
National College of Naturopathic Medicine
Four-year fully accredited naturopathic
medical school.
049 SW Porter Street
Portland, Oregon USA
Ph: (503) 499 4343
Fax: (503) 499 0022

www.bridgeport.edu
The University of Bridgeport
College of Naturopathic Medicine
221 University Avenue
Bridgeport, CT 06601
USA
Ph: (203) 576 4109

www.ccnm.edu
Canadian College of Naturopathic
Medicine
2300 Yonge Street
8th Floor
PO Box 2431
Toronto, Ontario
Canada MAP IE4
Ph: (416) 486 8584
Fax: (416) 484 6821

www.oand.com
Ontario Association of Naturopathic
Doctors
4174 Dundas Street West, Suite 304
Toronto, ON M8X 1X3
Ph: (416) 233 2001
Fax: (413) 233 2924

Botanical Names

Albizzia (*Albizzia lebbeck*)

Alfalfa (*Medicago sativa*)

Aloe (*Aloe vera*)

Amaranth (*Amaranthus hypochondriacus*)

American elder (*Sambucus canadensis*)

American saffron (*Carthamus tinctorius*)

Andrographis (*Andrographis panniculate*)

Angelica (*Angelica archangelica*)

Anise (*Pimpinella anisum*)

Aphanes (*Aphanes arvensis*)

Arrach (*Chenopodium olidum*)

Astragalus (*Astragalus membranaceus*)

Autumn crocus (*Colchicum autumnale*)

Avens (*Geum urbanum*)

Bacopa (*Bacopa monniera*)

Balm (*Melissa officinalis*)

Barberry (*Berberis vulgaris*)

Bayberry (*Myrica cerifera*)

Bearberry (*Arctostaphylos uva-ursi*)

Beech leaf (*Fagus* spp.)

Bergamot (*Citrus bergamia*)

Bethroot (*Trillium erectum*)

Betony (*Betonica officinalis*)

Bilberry (*Vaccinium myrtillus*)

Birch (*Betula* spp.)

Bistort (*Polygonum bistorta*)

Bitter orange (*Citrus aurantium*)

Bitterwood (*Picraena excelsa*)

Black bean (*Castanospermum* sp.)

Black cohosh (*Cimicifuga racemosa*)

Black currant (*Ribes nigrum*)

Black haw (*Viburnum prunifolium*)

Black root (*Leptandra virginica*)

Blackberry (*Rubus* spp.)

Bladderwrack (*Fucus vesiculosis*)

Blazing star (*Aletris farinosa*)

Blazing star root (*Chamaelirium luteum*)

Bloodroot (*Sanguinaria canadensis*)

Blue cohosh (*Caulophyllum thalictroides*)

Blue flag (*Iris versicolor*)

Blue vervain (*Verbena hastata*)

Boldo (*Peumus boldus*)

Boneset (*Eupatorium perfoliatum*)

Broom tops (*Cytisus scoparius*)

Buchu (*Barosma betulina*)

Bugle weed (*Lycopus virginica*)

Bupleurum (*Bupleurum falcatum*)

Burdock (*Arctium lappa*)

Butternut (*Juglans cinerea*)

Cactus (*Cactus grandiflorus*)

Cajuput (*Melaleuca cajuputi*)

Calendula (*Calendula officinalis*)

Caraway (*Carum carvi*)

Cardamom seeds (*Elettaria ardamomum*)

Cascara (*Cascara sagrada*)

Castor oil plant (*Ricinus communis*)

Catnip (*Nepeta cataria*)

Cat's claw (*Uncaria tomentosa*)

Cayenne (*Capsicum frutescens*)

Celandine (*Chelidonium majus*)

Celery (*Apium graveolens*)

Chamomile (*Anthemis nobilis*)

Chamomile (*Matricaria recutita*)

Chaparral (*Larrea tridentata*)

Chaste tree (*Vitex agnus castus*)

Chelendonium (*Chelendonium majus*)

Chia seed (*Salvia columbariae*)

Chickweed (*Stellaria media*)

Cinnamon (*Cinnamomum zeylanicum*)

Cleavers (*Calium aparine*)

Clivers (*Galium aparine*)

Cloves (*Eugenia carophyllus*)

Coleus (*Coleus forskolii*)

Coltsfoot (*Tussilago farfara*)

Columbo (*Frasera carolinensis*)

Comfrey (*Symphytum officinale*)

Common figwort (*Scrophularia*)

Coneflower (*Echinacea angustifolium*)
Coriander (*Coriandrum sativum*)
Cornsilk (*Zea mays*)
Corydalis (*Corydalis ambigua*)
Couch grass (*Agropyrum repens*)
Cramp bark or high-bush cranberry
   (*Viburnum opulus*)
Cranberry, High-bush (*Viburnum opulus*)
Cranesbill (*Geranium maculatum*)
Crataeva (*Crataeva nurvala*)
Crawley root (*Corallorhiza odontorhiza*)
Culver's root (*Leptandra virginica*)
Cumin (*Cuminum cyminum*)
Damiana (*Turnera diffusa*)
Dandelion (*Taraxacum officinale*)
Devil's claw (*Harpagophtum*
   procumbens)
Dill (*Anethum graveolens*)
Dogbane (*Apocynum androsaemifolium*)
Dong quai (*Angelica sinensis*)
Echinacea (*Echinacea angustifolia*)
Elder blossom (*Sambucus nigra*)
Elder leaf (*Sambucus* sp.)
Elderflower (*Sambucus* sp.)
Elecampane (*Inula helenium*)
Eucalyptus (*Eucalyptus globulus*)
European vervain (*Verbena officinalis*)
Eyebright (*Euphrasia officinalis*)
False unicorn root (*Helonia luteum*)
False unicorn root (*Helonias dioica*)
Fennel (*Foeniculum dulce*)
Fenugreek (*Trigoneela foenum-graecum*)
Feverfew (*Tanacetum parthenium*)
Figwort (*Scrophularia nodosa*)
Flaxseed (*Linum usitatissimum*)
Fotitieng (*Polygonum multifiorum*)
Foxglove (*Digitalis purpurea*)
Garlic (*Allium sativum*)
Gentian (*Gentiana lutea*)
Geranium (*Pelargonium* spp.)
Ginger (*Zingiber officinale*)
Ginger root (*Zingiber officinale*)
Ginkgo (*Ginkgo biloba*)
Ginseng (*Panax* spp.)
Ginseng Siberian (*Eleutherococcus*)
Globe artichoke (*Cynara scolymus*)
Goat's rue (*Galega officinalis*)
Goldenseal (*Hydrastis canadensis*)
Gotu kola (*Centella asiatica*)
Gravel root (*Eupatorium purpureum*)

Green hellebore (*Veratrum viride*)
Grindelia (*Grindelia camporium*)
Ground ivy (*Nepeta hederacea*)
Guaiacum (*Guaiacum officinale*)
Gum plant (*Grindelia squarrosa*)
Gymnema (*Gymnema sylvestre*)
Hops (*Humulus lupulus*)
Horehound (*Marrubium vulgare*)
Horse chestnut (*Aesculus*
   hippocastanum)
Horseradish (*Cochlearia armoracia*)
Horsetail (*Equisetum arvense*)
Hydrangea (*Hydrangea arborescens*)
Hyssop (*Hyssopus officinalis*)
Indian barberry (*Berberis aristata*)
Indian snakeroot (*Rauwolfia serpentina*)
Ipecacuanha (*Psychotria ipecacuanha*)
Irish moss (*Chrondrus crispus*)
Jaborandi (*Pilocarpus*)
Jalapa (*Ipomoea jalapa*)
Jamaica dogwood (*Piscidia erythrina*)
Jambul (*Syzygium jambdlanum*)
Jerusalem oak (*Chenopodium*
   anthelminticum)
Juniper (*Juniperus communis*)
Kava (*Piper methysticum*)
Kousso (*Brayera anthelmintica*)
Lady's slipper (*Cypripedium pubescens*)
Lavender (*Lavandula officinalis*)
Lemon balm (*Melissa officinalis*)
Licorice (*Glycyrrhiza glabra*)
Life root (*Senecio aureus*)
Lily-of-the-valley (*Convallaria majalis*)
Lime flowers (*Tilea* spp.)
Lobelia (*Lobelia inflata*)
Magnolia (*Magnolia officinalis*)
Male fern (*Dryopteris filixmas*)
Marigold (*Calendula officinalis*)
Marshmallow (*Althaea officinalis*)
May-apple or American mandrake
   (*Podophyllum peltatum*)
Melissa (*Melissa officinalis*)
Mistletoe (*Viscum album*)
Mother's wort (*Leonurus cardiaca*)
Mountain flax (*Linum cartharticum*)
Mugwort (*Artemisia vulgaris*)
Mullein (*Verbascum thapsus*)
Mustard seeds (*Brassica juncea*)
Myrrh (*Commiphora myrrha*)
Nasturtium (*Tropaeolum majus*)

Nettle (*Urtica dioica*)
Oak (*Quercus*)
Oats (*Avena sativa*)
Olive oil (*Olea europaea*)
Onion (*Allium cepa*)
Oregon grape root (*Berberis aquifolium*)
Paeonia (*Paeonia lactiflora*)
Papaya (*Carica papaya*)
Pareira root (*Chondrodendron tomentosum*)
Parsley (*Petroselinum sativum*)
Parsley piert (*Alchemilla arvensis*)
Passion flower (*Passiflora incarnata*)
Pau d'arco (*Tabebuia avellanedae*)
Pellitory-of-the-wall (*Parietaria officinalis*)
Pennyroyal (*Hedeoma pulegioides*)
Peony root (*Paeonia officinalis*)
Peppermint (*Mentha piperita*)
Peruvian bark (*Cinchona ledgeriana*)
Pheasant's eye (*Adonis vernalis*)
Phyllanthus (*Phyllanthus amarus*)
Picrorrhiza (*Picrorrhiza kurroa*)
Pine (*Pinus* spp.)
Pinkroot (*Spigelia marilandica*)
Pinus bark (*Tsuga canadensis*)
Pipsissewa (*Chimaphila umbellate*)
Plantain (*Plantago lanceolata*)
Pleurisy root (*Asclepias tuberosa*)
Poke root (*Phytolacca decandra*)
Pomegranate (*Puncia granatum*)
Poplar (*Populus tremuloides*)
Prickly ash (*Xanthoxylum americanum*)
Prickly pear (*Opuntia* spp.)
Psyllium (*Plantago ovata*)
Pulsatilla (*Anemone patens*)
Pulsatilla (*Anemone pulsatilla*)
Pumpkin (*Curcurbita pepo*)
Quebracho blanco (*Aspidosperma quebracho-blanco*)
Queen of the meadow (*Eupatorium purpureum*)
Queen's root (*Stillingia sylvatica*)
Raspberry leaves (*Rubus idaeus*)
Red clover (*Trifolium pratense*)
Red eyebright (*Euphrasia officinalis*)
Red raspberry (*Rubus strigosus* and *R. idaeus*)
Rehmannia (*Rehmannia glutinosa*)
Rhatany (*Krameria triandra*)
Rhubarb (*Rheum palmatum*)

Rosemary (*Rosmarinus officinalis*)
Rue (*Ruta graveolens*)
Sage (*Salvia miltiorrhiza*)
St John's wort (*Hypericum perforatum*)
St Mary's thistle (*Silybum marianum*)
Salicin willow (*Salix alba*)
Santonica (*Artemisia santonica*)
Sarsaparilla (*Smilax ornata*)
Sassafras (*Sassafras officinale*)
Saw palmetto (*Serenoa serrulata*)
Schisandra (*Schisandra chinensis*)
Scutellaria (*Scutellaria baicalensis*)
Senna (*Cassia acutifolia*)
Shepherd's purse (*Casella bursa-pastoris*)
Siberian ginseng (*Eleutherococcus*)
Skullcap (*Scutellaria lateriflora*)
Skunk cabbage (*Symplocarpus foetidus*)
Slippery elm (*Ulmus fulva*)
Snake root (*Aristolochia reticulata*)
Solomon's seal (*Polygonatum multiflorum*)
Southernwood (*Artemisia abrotanum*)
Spearmint (*Mentha viridis*)
Spotted cranesbill (*Geranium maculatum*)
Squaw vine (*Mitchella repens*)
Squill (*Urginea scilla*)
Stinging nettle (*Urtica urens*)
Stone root (*Collinsonia canadensis*)
Strawberry (*Fragaria vesca*)
Strophanthus (*Strophanthus hispidus*)
Sundew (*Drosera longifolia*)
Sweet clover (*Melilotus officinalis*)
Sweet flag (*Acorus calamus*)
Sweet sumach (*Rhus aromatica*)
Tansy (*Tanacetum vulgare*)
Thyme (*Thymus vulgaricus*)
Tormentil (*Potentilla tormentilla*)
Tree of life (*Thuja occidentalis*)
True unicorn root (*Aletris farinosa*)
Tylophera (*Tylophera asthmatica*)
Valerian (*Valeriana officinalis*)
Wahoo (*Euonymus atropurpureus*)
Watercress (*Nasturtium officinale*)
Watermelon seeds (*Citrullus vulgaris*)
White bryony (*Bryonia alba*)
White oak bark (*Quercus alba*)
White pine (*Pinus strobus*)
White pond lily (*Nymphaea odorata*)
White willow (*Salix alba*)

Wild black carrot (*Lomatia dissectum*)
Wild carrot (*Daucus carota*)
Wild cherry bark (*Prunus serotina*)
Wild cherry bark (*Prunus virginiana*)
Wild clover (*Trifolium pretense*)
Wild ginger (*Asarum canadensis*)
Wild indigo (*Baptisia tinctoria*)
Wild yam (*Dioscorea villosa*)
Willow bark (*Salix alba*)
Wintergreen (*Gaultheria procumbens*)
Witch hazel (*Hamamelis virginiana*)

Withania (*Withania somnifera*)
Worm grass (*Spigelia marilandica*)
Wormseed (*Chenopodium anthelminticum*)
Wormwood (*Artemisia absinthium*)
Yarrow (*Achillea millefolium*)
Yellow dock (*Rumex crispus*)
Yellow jasmine (*Gelsemium sempervirens*)
Zizyphus (*Zizyphus spinosa*)

GLOSSARY

Acid An organic or inorganic compound with a low pH. Generally sour to taste and corrosive. The balancing compound is called an alkali (or base).

Acidosis A condition in which the acidity of tissues and fluids becomes abnormally high. It creates excessive inflammation and mucous.

Achlorhydria A fairly common condition in which very little or no hydrochloric acid is produced by the parietal cells of the stomach.

Acute condition One which onsets rapidly, usually of short duration, but can cause severe symptoms, e.g. a fever.

Adaptogen A herb (usually) which helps to return a body to balance (homeo-stasis).

Adrenal glands A pair of important glands covering the superior face of the kidneys, and which secrete various hormones such as adrenaline (epinephrine) and noradrenaline, and corticosteroids.

Allergy A disorder in which the body becomes hypersensitive to a normally harmless substance (in this situation such a substance is called an allergen). An abnormal immune system response produces characteristic inflammation. Any body tissue can be affected.

Amino acid An organic compound containing an amino group. Amino acids are fundamental constituents of protein. The body can make some; others are essential (needed in the diet).

Anabolic (anabolism) The metabolic process of building complex structures from simple ones (for example, building fats from fatty acids). Opposite of catabolism.

Antacid An alkaline substance, which neutralizes gastric acid in the lower esophagus, stomach or duodenum.

Antibiotic Literally "against life". A substance that destroys bacteria and or fungi (not viruses).

Antibody An immune system protein molecule designed to attack an antigen and neutralize it.

Antigen Any substance the immune system regards as foreign or potentially dangerous.

Antioxidant Damage to tissue can be caused by "oxidative" reactions (can be caused by free radicals). Antioxidants help reduce such damage.

Arteriosclerosis When walls of arteries become thick and stiff causing poor blood circulation. Atherosclerosis is one form of arteriosclerosis, and is caused by damage (often free radical damage) to arterial walls, with consequent buildup of cholesterol plaque as the body attempts to heal itself.

Ascorbic acid/ascorbate Ascorbic acid is called vitamin C. In this form it can be quite harsh on the gastrointestinal tract. When combined with a mineral to form a salt (ascorbate — e.g. magnesium ascorbate), it is less acidic, and more bio-available (absorbable).

Autoimmune disease A condition in which the immune system becomes confused and becomes active against the body, creating antibodies that act against certain components or products of its own tissues.

Autonomic nervous system Part of the nervous system that governs those bodily functions not under the control of the conscious mind, such as the regular beating of the heart, intestinal movements and sweating. It is subdivided into the sympathetic and parasympathetic nervous systems.

Bacteria Usually single-celled organisms, which inhabit every surface and medium on the planet. Those on and in humans are generally beneficial, acting as they do elsewhere, as nature's ecologists, helping preserve the biosphere as a viable environment in which to live. If they cause problems, it is generally due to some man-made imbalance somewhere.

Basal metabolic rate (BMR) The minimum amount of energy required to be expended by the body to maintain vital processes such as respiration, circulation and digestion. Factors affecting the BMR include thyroid activity, age and sex.

Biochemical The chemistry of life forms. There are thousands of natural chemical reactions occurring in cells at any given moment.

Biofeedback Process helping one become more conscious of body processes so as to gain some measure of control over these (usually) involuntary activities (such as heart rate, body temperature, etc.).

Bioflavonoids Sometimes referred to as vitamin P, bioflavonoids are associated with vitamin C and are essential for the utilization of vitamin C in the body. Flavonoids are found in plants.

Biopsy A surgically acquired live tissue sample for laboratory examination.

Capillaries The tiniest of the fluid carrying vessels of the vascular and lymphatic systems. They allow exchange of fluids between these systems and body tissue.

Carcinogen A substance capable of causing cancer.

Carotene A yellowish plant pigment which can be converted in the body to vitamin A.

Chemotherapy Treatment of any disease (not just cancer) using synthetic chemicals (especially pharmaceutical drugs).

Chiropractic Use of physical manipulation of the bones to restore proper structure, hoping to restore proper nerve, muscle and vascular function.

Cholagogue A substance (usually a herb) which stimulates bile flow.

Cholesterol Substance produced by the liver, important to health. Acts as anti-oxidant; a constituent of cell membranes, and facilitates transport of the fatty acids.

Chronic illness (As distinct from acute) An illness which persists or recurs over a long time, sometimes for life. Often a sign of homeostatic imbalance.

Coenzyme A chemical molecule which works with an enzyme to facilitate a particular function.

Cold-pressed Food oils extracted from plant parts (often seeds) without the use of heat, to preserve nutrients and taste values.

Complex carbohydrate A type of carbohydrate, generally unrefined, which is not rapidly absorbed (unlike simple sugars), therefore releasing its sugar relatively slowly into the bloodstream.

Congenital Present from birth, but not necessarily inherited (genetic).

Debility A state of lowered vitality.

Demulcent A substance soothing especially to the mucous membranes.

Detoxification The process of reducing toxin buildup in body fluids, cells, tissues and organs.

Diuretic A substance that causes loss of body fluids.

DNA (deoxyribonucleic acid) The substance in cell nuclei that contains the genetic information of the particular species.

Edema Abnormal retention of body fluids causing (usually) visible swelling.

Electrolyte Mineral salts (ions) which dissolve in body fluids. Important for proper hydration, among other functions.

Embolus Something carried by the blood from one place to another; often a blood clot.

Endocrine gland A gland that manufactures one or more hormones which are secreted directly into the bloodstream. Includes the pituitary, adrenals, thyroid, ovaries and testes, placenta, and part of the pancreas.

Endorphin A brain-derived compound similar to encephalins which have pain-relieving properties similar to those of morphine or other opiates.

Enzyme A protein that speeds up biochemical reactions without itself being used up. Enzymes are relatively specific to the type of reaction they facilitate, so there are many different enzymes in the human body. Plant enzymes act in the human body, but are easily destroyed by heat (cooking; pasteurizing). Enzyme names usually end in "-ase".

Epstein-Barr virus (EBV) A common virus capable of causing debility especially within a weakened immune system. Often associated with glandular fever, and is implicated in chronic fatigue states.

Erythema Redness of the skin.

Essential Refers to substances required by the body which it cannot itself manufacture. Often refers to certain vitamins, minerals, amino acids and fatty acids.

Fatty acid The building blocks of fats, oils, cholesterols and hormones.

Fiber The indigestible parts of plants.

Flora Bacteria present within the length of the internal body tracts such as the gastrointestinal tract, urethral tract, vaginal tract, as well as the nasal, sinus and bronchial tracts, and the ears. Present on the skin surfaces as well. There are hundreds of different species, and trillions of members of the colonies; they act as Nature's ecologists, and do much for our health.

Free radical An atom or molecule which is unstable because it has at least one unpaired electron. Because they bind easily with other compounds, they can cause damage to body tissues (inflammation, even cancer). They often form when fats and oils are heated, or when exposed to environmental radiation and chemical pollution.

Gingivitis Inflammation of the gums (especially around the teeth margins).

Gland A tissue or organ which manufactures and secretes substances for use elsewhere in the body.

Globulin One of a group of simple proteins that act as antibodies and/or transporters of iron, copper or lipids around the body.

Glucose The form of sugar which the body uses to make energy. Is manufactured by the body from carbohydrates and can be stored as glycogen.

Gluten A protein found in grains.

Goiter A swelling on the neck due to thyroid gland enlargement. Is usually due to lack of iodine in the diet, and is common in areas where this mineral is absent from soil.

Hemo- Pertaining to the blood.

Hemoglobin The iron-containing red substance in the blood, responsible for the transport of oxygen from the lungs.

Hepatic Pertaining to the liver.

Hernia Protrusion of an organ or tissue out of its normal body cavity. The most common type is the hiatus hernia, where the stomach passes partly (or completely) into the chest cavity.

Histo- Prefix denoting tissue.

Histamine An immune system chemical causing inflammation of body tissue.

Hormone A substance produced by a gland which travels via the bloodstream for specific use elsewhere in the body.

Hydrochloric acid A strong acid designed to help in digestion, especially of proteins. Produced in stomach cells from hydrogen and chloride ions.

Hydrogenation A chemical process designed to turn liquid oils into solid form, as in the manufacture of margarine from vegetable oils.

Hydrotherapy Treatments using water,

externally and internally.

Hyper- Prefix denoting excessive.

Hypo- Prefix denoting deficiency, lack, or small size.

Iatrogenic A condition that has resulted from treatment (e.g. doctor-caused)

Idiopathic A disease of unknown cause(s).

Immunity Resistance or ability to overcome the threat of disease.

Infection An abnormal concentration of organisms that potentially can cause harm.

Inflammation Part of the immune response to injury which causes redness, pain, warmth and swelling. Can be acute or chronic.

Inguinal Pertaining to the groin area.

Insulin A hormone produced by the pancreas to help transport glucose from the bloodstream to sites of utilization.

Interferon An immune system protein produced in response to viral infection, able to prevent viral replication, thus limiting the viral spread to uninfected cells.

Intolerance The inability to digest a particular food. Sometimes referred to as a sensitivity. Can be mild to severe and life-threatening. See also Allergy.

Lactic acid Present in some foods (from lactose), and also a by-product of anaerobic muscle metabolism. Is usually recycled through the liver, but can persist in muscles causing inflammation and fatigue.

Lecithin One of a group of phospholipids, which are important parts of cell membranes, and help the liver in the metabolism of fats

Lipids Important natural substances with fat and oil-like qualities. Examples include choline, inositol, lecithin, and the omega-3 and omega-6 essential fatty acids.

Lipotropes Substances that prevent abnormal accumulation of fats in the liver, enhance fat metabolism, and assist in proper glucose metabolism.

They include methionine, choline and inositol.

Lymph Clear fluid derived from blood plasma, which bathes the interstitial areas (in between the cells of tissues). It is collected by the lymphatic system and returned to the blood stream via the subclavian veins. It collects wastes, and delivers nutrients to cells including cartilage.

Malignant Literally "evil". Often refers to cancer cells; opposite of benign.

Melanoma A tumor arising from the deeper pigment cells (melanocytes) of the skin. Often characterized as a coffee stain on the skin surface, and can become malignant.

Metabolism The various biological processes needed to sustain life, which include the production of energy, the synthesis of biological substances and the deployment of waste and pollutants.

Neuro- Pertaining to the nerves.

Organic (i) Pertaining to body organs and related systems; (ii) Pertaining to food produced (practically) without use of or contamination by pharmaceutical chemicals.

Oxidation A chemical reaction in which oxygen reacts with another substance occasioning deterioration of some type.

pH A scale used to measure the acidity or alkalinity of a substance. Acids have a low pH (from 1-7, where 1 is highly acidic), and alkalines have a high pH (from 7-14, where 14 is highly alkaline).

Parasite An organism which lives on or in another organism and feeds off it, often to the detriment of the host.

Phyto- Pertaining to plants.

Plaque An unwanted deposit of a substance on a particular tissue surface, usually with unhealthy results. Plaque can be different substances, such as that which might form on brain tissue (Alzheimer's disease), teeth and gums, or inside arteries leading to atherosclerosis.

Prostaglandins A group of hormone-like chemicals made from essential fatty acids that can positively and negatively affect health.

Proteolytic enzymes Digestive enzymes, which break down dietary proteins but do not attack structural proteins in body tissues.

Saturated fat A fat that is solid at room temperature. Usually of animal origin (exceptions include coconut and other palm oils). Generally not good for health. Chemically, these are fatty acid molecules that cannot take on any more hydrogen atoms.

Secondary An infection, a tumor or some other disease which develops after, and is made possible only by, the primary (first).

Serotonin A compound widely distributed in tissues, especially in blood platelets, intestinal wall, and central nervous system. Plays a role similar to histamine in inflammation; also acts as a neurotransmitter, essential for relaxation, sleep and mental concentration.

Steroid One of a group of fat-soluble organic compounds having a common structure. Naturally occurring steroids include androgens and estrogens, hormones of the adrenal cortex, bile salts and sterols including cholesterol.

Syndrome A combination of signs and/or symptoms that forms a distinct clinical picture characteristic of a particular disorder.

Synergy Literally "working together". A situation when two or more substances together have an action which is greater than the sum of their individual actions.

Systemic Pertaining to the whole system, the whole body.

Topical Pertaining to a surface of the body.

Toxin A compound which has a detrimental effect on living tissue; a poison.

Unsaturated fat A dietary fat that is liquid at room temperature. Generally from plant sources, and containing essential fatty acids.

Vascular Pertaining to the blood circulatory system.

Virus A minute particle capable of reproducing only within living cells. Each consists of a core of nucleic acid (DNA and/or RNA), surrounded by a protein shell, and some bear an outer lipid capsule. They are not considered to be living organisms because they cannot reproduce on their own. Antibiotics have no effect on them.

Vitamin A substance considered essential for life and health in small amounts. They cannot be synthesized by the body. There are water-soluble vitamins and fat-soluble vitamins. Lack of a vitamin can cause a specific "vitamin deficiency disease". Debate continues as to amounts required for optimal health.

INDEX

ABOUT THE AUTHORS

Dr Ross Trattler's premedical university degree was obtained at the University of Illinios and the University of New York. After four years of work and study at the Institute for Religious Development, a community in upstate New York that follows the esoteric methods of G.I. Gurdjieff, he attended the British College of Naturopathy and Osteopathy in London. Dr Trattler and his wife Nancy direct the Osteopathic Clinic of Mudgeeraba, located in the beautiful hinterland region of the Gold Coast, Queensland, Australia. He has been practicing as a naturopath and osteopath for over twenty years.

Dr Adrian Jones is a co-director of Total Health Centres Australia, a multi-disciplinary naturopathic health care clinic, and a Doctor of Naturopathy. As a child in the 1950s, his mother refused to allow any vaccines, pharmaceutical drugs or antibiotics into his system and raised him as a vegetarian on organic foods. Adrian says his immune system has never let him down. As well as running a busy naturopathic practice on Queensland's Gold Coast, Adrian is a noted speaker, writer, lecturer and public health educator. He holds degrees in theology and naturopathy, including nutrition, herbal and homoeopathic medicine, and enjoys practicing different massage modalities.